D1288625

Handbook of
Intellectual and
Developmental
Disabilities

Issues on Clinical Child Psychology

Series Editors: **Michael C. Roberts,** *University of Kansas—Lawrence, Kansas*
Lizette Peterson,[†] *University of Missouri—Columbia, Missouri*

A continuation Order Plan is available for this series. A continuation order will bring delivery of each new volume immediately upon publication. Volumes are billed only upon actual shipment. For further information please contact the publisher.

Handbook of
Intellectual and
Developmental
Disabilities

Edited by

John W. Jacobson

*NYS Office of Mental Retardation
and Developmental Disabilities
Albany, New York*

James A. Mulick

*The Ohio State University
Columbus, Ohio*

Johannes Rojahn

*George Mason University
Fairfax, Virginia*

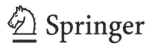 Springer

James A. Mulick
Department of Pediatrics and Psychology
The Ohio State University
Columbus, OH 43205
USA
mulick.1@osu.edu

Johannes Rojahn
Department of Psychology
George Mason University
Fairfax, VA 22030
USA
jrojahn@gmu.edu

Library of Congress Control Number: 2006923499

ISBN-10: 0-387-32930-7   e-ISBN-10: 0-387-32931-5
ISBN-13: 978-0-387-32930-7   e-ISBN-13: 978-0-387-32931-4

Printed on acid-free paper.

9 8 7 6 5 4 3 2 1

springer.com

Dedication

John W. Jacobson conceived of this book, recruited most of the contributors, and served as the Senior Editor until his untimely death from rapidly progressing lung cancer on May 8, 2004. The book was about two-thirds done at that point. He had recognized that this project, and a related work on controversial issues in developmental disabilities treatment that was actually nearly ready for submission when he died (Jacobson, Foxx, & Mulick, 2005), needed to be turned over to his coeditors for completion. The work of completing this book was daunting for a single editor and progress floundered, so Professor Johannes Rojahn of George Mason University was recruited to serve as coeditor. Professor Rojahn had collaborated with both Jacobson and Mulick on many projects in the past, shared many of the same philosophical and scientific values that guided the original selection of topics and contributors, and agreed that the work was both important and sorely needed for the field. The happy result of this collaboration is before you, and simply would not have been there without the dedicated work of Professor Rojahn and his students in moving the project forward to completion. But the book is fundamentally a result of Jacobson's vision, vast knowledge of the field, and many professional relationships with the best minds currently working in this area.

Jacobson was a civil servant, behavior analyst, scholar, editor, teacher, professional, futurist, and advocate for science and rational services for people with disabilities. His many contacts included leaders in government, professional psychology, and academe. He was generous with his time, frequently helping researchers to improve their research designs and parents to find and access high quality services for their children with developmental disabilities. He helped when he was asked, whether or not he knew previously the person requesting his assistance. He was genuinely friendly whenever friendship was offered to him. So many people sought his guidance in so many fields related to developmental disabilities, psychology, and applied research that his absence is sorely felt on at least three continents by scientists, professionals, and consumers of disability services alike. He was an internationalist and organizer, and consequently he earned recognition and leadership positions in learned societies, including the Association for Behavior Analysis International, the American

Psychological Association, the National Association for the Dually Diagnosed, the International Association for the Scientific Study of Intellectual Disabilities, and the American Association on Mental Retardation. There are many facets to his scientific and professional legacy, but perhaps none so fitting as a representative summary of his true avocation and life's work as this contribution to the next generation of scientists and professionals; hence, we, the editors and contributors will always think of this work in his memory as *Jacobson's Handbook of Intellectual and Developmental Disabilities*.

James A. Mulick
Johannes Rojahn

REFERENCE

Jacobson, J. W., Foxx, R. M., & Mulick, J. A. (Eds.). (2005). *Controversial therapies for developmental disabilities: Fad, fashion, and science in professional practice.* Mahwah, NJ: Author.

Contributors

James P. Acquilano, Comprehensive Geriatric Assessment Clinic, Finger Lakes Developmental Disabilities Service Office, 620 Westfall Road, Rochester, New York 14620.

Michael G. Aman, The Nisonger Center, Ohio State University, 1581 Dodd Drive, Columbus, Ohio 43210.

Jennifer Norins Bardon, Center for Social Development and Education, University of Massachusetts—Boston, 100 Morrissey Boulevard, Boston, Massachusetts 02125.

James W. Bodfish, Department of Psychiatry, University of North Carolina at Chapel Hill, J. Iverson Riddle Developmental Center, UNC Human Development Research Institute, 300 Enola Road, Morganton, North Carolina 28655.

John Borkowski, University of Notre Dame Department of Psychology, University of Notre Dame, Notre Dame, Indiana 46556.

Eric M. Butter, Department of Pediatrics, Columbus Children's Hospital and The Ohio State University, 700 Children's Drive, Columbus, Ohio 43205.

Shannon S. Carothers, University of Notre Dame Department of Psychology, University of Notre Dame, Notre Dame, Indiana 46556.

Janis G. Chadsey, Department of Special Education, University of Illinois at Urbana—Champaign, 1310 S. 6th Street, Champaign, Illinois 61820.

Mary Clair, Department of Psychology, Drexel University, 245 N 15th Street, MS 515, Philadelphia, Pennsylvania 19102-1192.

Robin S. Codding, May Institute, One Commerce Way, Norwood, Massachusetts 02062.

Philip W. Davidson, Pediatrics Department, Strong Center for Developmental Disabilities, Golisano Children's Hospital at Strong, Box 671, URMC, 601 Elmwood Avenue, Rochester, New York 14642.

Paula K. Davis, Rehabilitation Institute, Southern Illinois University, Carbondale, Illinois 62901-4609.

Shoumitro Deb, Neuropsychiatry & Intellectual Disability, Division of Neuroscience, Department of Psychiatry, University of Birmingham, Queen Elizabeth Psychiatric Hospital, Mindelsohn Way, Birmingham B15 2QZ United Kingdom.

Sharon Duffy, Graduate School of Education, UC Riverside, Riverside, California 92521.

Erin Dunn, May Institute, One Commerce Way, Norwood, Massachusetts 02062.

Maureen S. Durkin, Population Health Sciences, University of Wisconsin – Madison, 789 WARF, 610 Walnut Street, Madison, Wisconsin 53726.

Elisabeth M. Dykens, Vanderbilt Kennedy Center for Research on Human Development, Department of Psychology and Human Development, Vanderbilt University, Peabody Box 40, 230 Appleton Place, Nashville, Tennessee 37205.

Jaelyn R. Farris, University of Notre Dame Department of Psychology, University of Notre Dame, Notre Dame, Indiana 46556.

Bonnie Forman, Thursday's Child, Brooklyn, New York 11209

William I. Gardner, Rehabilitation Psychology Program, 432 N. Murray Street, University of Wisconsin – Madison, Madison, Wisconsin 53705.

Joanne Gerenser, The Eden II Programs, Staten Island, New York.

Christopher Gillberg, Department of Child and Adolescent Psychiatry, St. George's Hospital Medical School, University of London and Queen Silvia's Children's Hospital, University of Göteborg, Kungsgatan 12, SE 411 19 Gothenburg, Sweden.

Beth Glasberg, Douglass Developmental Disabilities Center, Rutgers, The State University of New Jersey, 151 Ryders Lane, New Brunswick, New Jersey 08901-8528.

Frances Page Glascoe, Pediatrics Department, Vanderbilt University, 25 Bragg Drive, East Berlin, Pennsylvania 17316.

Laraine Masters Glidden, Department of Psychology, St. Mary's College of Maryland, 18952 E. Fisher Road, St. Mary's City, Maryland 20686–3001.

Marc Goldman, Private Practice, 2310 Snowcrest Trail, Durham, North Carolina 27707.

Michael J. Guralnick, Center on Human Development and Disability, Psychology and Pediatrics Department, University of Washington, Box 357920, Seattle, Washington 98195-7920.

Sandra L. Harris, Douglass Developmental Disabilities Center, Rutgers, The State University of New Jersey, 151 Ryders Lane, New Brunswick, New Jersey 08901-8528.

Sigan L. Hartley, Dept. 3415, University of Wyoming, 1000 E. University Avenue, Laramie, Wyoming 82071.

Linda J. Hayes, Psychology Department, University of Nevada—Reno, Reno, Nevada 89557.

Robert M. Hodapp, Vanderbilt Kennedy Center Research Program on Families, Department of Special Education, Vanderbilt University, Peabody Box 328, 230 Appleton Place, Nashville, Tennessee 37205.

Sarah Christine Voss Horrell, Dept., 3415, University of Wyoming, 1000E. University Avenue, Laramie, Wyoming 82071.

Kimberly S. Howard, University of Notre Dame Department of Psychology, University of Notre Dame, Notre Dame, Indiana 46556.

Matthew P. Janicki, Technical Assistance Department, RRTC on Aging and Developmental Disabilities, University of Illinois at Chicago, 1640 West Roosevelt Road, Chicago, Illinois 60608.

James M. Kauffman, Department of Curriculum, Instruction, and Special Education, University of Virginia, 405 Emmet Street South, PO Box 400273, Charlottesville, Virginia 22904-4273.

Tamara L. Klein, Department of Psychology, Drexel University, 245 N 15th Street, MS 515 Philadelphia, Pennsylvania.

Richard J. Landau, Dykema Gossett PLLC, 2723 South State Street, Suite 400, Ann Arbor, Michigan 48104.

Timothy J. Landrum, Department of Curriculum, Instruction, and Special Education, University of Virginia, 617 West Main Street, Charlottesville, Virginia 22904.

Robin Gaines Lanzi, Georgetown University Center on Health and Education, 3700 Reservoir Rd., NW, St. Mary's Hall, Suite 134, Georgetown University, Washington, District of Columbia 20057.

Rinita B. Laud, Department of Psychology, Louisiana State University, Baton Rouge, Louisiana 70803.

James K. Luiselli, Applied Research, Clinical Training, and Peer Review, Internship Program in Clinical Psychology, The May Institute, Inc., Randolph, Massachusetts.

William E. Maclean Jr., Dept., 3415, University of Wyoming, 1000E. University Avenue, Laramie, Wyoming 82071.

Caroline I. Magyar, Pediatrics Department, Strong Center for Developmental Disabilities and STAART Center, University of Rochester School of Medicine and Dentistry, 601 Elmwood Ave., Box 671, Rochester, New York 14642.

Johnny L. Matson, Department of Psychology, Louisiana State University, Baton Rouge, Louisiana 70803.

Suzanne McDermott, Department of Family and Preventive Medicine, USC School of Medicine, Family Practice Center, 3209 Colonial Drive, Columbia, South Carolina 29208.

Amanda R. Mohler, Center for Social Development and Education, University of Massachusetts – Boston, 100 Morrissey Boulevard, Boston, Massachusetts 02125.

Arthur M. Nezu, Psychology, Medicine, & Public Health, Center for Behavioral Medicine & Mind/Body Studies, Drexel University, 245 N 15th Street, MS 515, Philadelphia, Pennsylvania 19102-1192.

Christine Maguth Nezu, Psychology, Medicine Departments, Center for Behavioral Medicine & Mind/Body Studies, Drexel University, Mail Stop 515, 245 N 15th Street; Philadelphia, Pennsylvania 19102-1192.

Gary Pace, May Institute, One Commerce Way, Norwood, Massachusetts 02062.

Vincent Pandolfi, School Psychology Program, College of Liberal Arts, Rochester Institute of Technology, 92 Lomb Memorial Drive, Rochester, New York 14623-5604.

Christine R. Peterson, Pediatrics Department, Strong Center for Developmental Disabilities, University of Rochester School of Medicine and Dentistry, 601 Elmwood Ave., Box 671, Rochester, New York 14642.

Yaser Ramadan, The Nisonger Center, The Ohio State University, 1581 Dodd Drive, Columbus, Ohio 43210.

Craig Thomas Ramey, Georgetown University Center on Health and Education, 3700 Reservoir Rd., NW, St. Mary's Hall, Suite 134, Georgetown University, Washington, District of Columbia 20057.

Sharon Landesman Ramey, Georgetown University Center on Health and Education, 3700 Reservoir Rd., NW, St. Mary's Hall, Suite 134, Georgetown University, Washington, District of Columbia 20057.

Ruth Anne Rehfeldt, Rehabilitation Institute, Southern Illinois University, Carbondale, Illinois 62901-4609.

Joseph N. Ricciardi, The National Autism Center, The May Institute, Inc., Randolph, Massachusetts.

Dennis C. Russo, May Institute, One Commerce Way, Norwood, Massachusetts 02062.

Richard R. Saunders, Schiefelbusch Institute for Life Span Studies, 1052 Robert Dole Human Development Center, 1000 Sunnyside Avenue, The University of Kansas, Lawrence, Kansas 66045.

Julie N. Schatz, University of Notre Dame Department of Psychology, University of Notre Dame, Notre Dame, Indiana 46556.

Sarah A. Schoolcraft, Department of Psychology, St. Mary's College of Maryland, 18952 E. Fisher Road, St. Mary's City, Maryland 20686–3001.

Nicole Schupf, Clinical Epidemiology, Sergievsky Center, Columbia University, 630 West 168th Street, New York 10032.

Gary N. Siperstein, Center for Social Development and Education, University of Massachusetts – Boston, 100 Morrissey Boulevard, Boston, Massachusetts 02125.

Robert L. Sprague, University of Illinois, 1306 Old Farm Road, Champaign, Illinois 61821-5940.

Zena A. Stein, Sergievsky Center, Columbia University, 630 West 168th Street, New York 10032.

Peter Sturmey, Department of Psychology, Queens College and The Graduate Center, City University of New York.

Denis G. Sukhodolsky, Child Study Center, Yale University School of Medicine, 230 South Frontage Road, New Haven, Connecticut 06520.

Jonathan Tarbox, Center for Autism and Related Disorders, 19019 Ventura Blvd., 3rd Floor, Tarzana, California 91356.

Sarah Winter, Columbus Children's Hospital, Ohio State University, 700 Children's Drive, Columbus, Ohio 43205.

Preface

This book is intended for use by graduate students, practitioners in clinical disciplines or management roles in developmental disabilities services and education, university faculty, and to a considerably lesser degree, advanced undergraduate and graduate students, parents, attorneys, and advocacy groups. Faculty will find this book useful as a primary course text at the graduate level. Practitioners and educators will make similar use of the book, in order to identify key research, but also as a resource they can point to when there is debate regarding desirable treatment or intervention practices for a particular individual they may serve. Researchers will find the coverage contained herein useful when they want a summary of contemporary thinking about a subarea of application or practice that is new to them or that intersects as a result of new findings with their own specialty in the wider field of developmental disabilities.

The purpose of this book is to provide readers with a complete and up-to-date overview of the state of knowledge in each topic area covered by the chapters. Authors were asked to emphasize conclusions and interpretations directly related to the status of the research in their assigned topic. In each case, they were urged to provide foundational conceptual information in their topic, to identify exceptionally valuable studies in the related literature, and to emphasize the latest research findings. Because research occurs in a social and political context, they were free to describe these other developments that might have affected research and practice during the past decade or so. Authors concluded their contributions with a brief summary of contemporary issues, concerns, or perspectives within the topic. As expected, the resulting contributions include not only a focus on intellectual disability (ID), but other developmental disabilities as well, and in some cases relevant research was drawn from other specialty areas (e.g., rehabilitation, child development, special education). Chapters were written for advanced readers, those having some knowledge of basic aspects of the topic assumed. The contributions to this book were original and provide readers with both a definitive synthesis and a guide to other important work on the various topics.

TERMINOLOGY

A word on terminology is required. The time this book spent in development spanned several years. In that time, changes in usage occurred with respect to the primary subject matter of this book; namely, the apparent delay in the normative acquisition of skills and knowledge by human beings. This condition, this *outcome* of human development, has been called *mental retardation* (MR) for the better part of the last century in North America. Scholars and researchers will need to use this terminology for the foreseeable future instead of ID as a search term in research and bibliographic search engines. The technical definition of this cognitive and developmental disability is still referenced against MR in the major diagnostic coding systems used worldwide, and the generally accepted defining characteristics of the condition remain significantly subaverage general intelligence and adaptive behavior as measured psychometrically, and that first occurs during the developmental period (see Jacobson & Mulick, 1996). Indeed, certain chapters in this book continue the MR terminology when the focus is on epidemiological issues or other topics referring to the specific aspects of disability that define MR and nothing more.

While terminology has not yet stabilized at this writing, and this state of affairs is reflected across the chapters in this book, the anticipated wide appeal of a reference text such as this one suggested to us that the term ID should be adopted as an editorial policy in as many places as possible because of its growing usage internationally in service organizations and agencies. These organizations and agencies are the very settings in which there is the greatest need for dissemination of the kind of research-based information and informed discussion contained herein. Advocacy groups and direct service providers in many parts of the world have increasingly expressed a desire to find an alternative to the term MR because of its derogatory connotations in common usage (Walsh, 2002), and it is true that the terminology has changed in both popular and scientific usage several times during the 19th and 20th centuries. We have, therefore, adopted the ID usage in the book in many places where the term MR would have been used in a similar reference work 10 or 15 years ago in order to extend the influence of this material as widely as possible. We hope this leads to no confusion on the part of readers, and that readers will understand that the value of consulting and studying research conducted using MR terminology far outweighs the value of political correctness for its own sake.

A SOUND BASIS FOR PROGRESS

This book is arranged in several sections corresponding to major domains of research and practice interest. Definition, classification, and etiology are discussed in Part I, with chapters on epidemiology, autism, cerebral palsy, genetic syndromes, epilepsy, brain injury, and the social aspects of developmental disabilities and associated disorders. The various organizing strategies typical of service delivery systems for people with developmental disabilities are considered in Part II. Chapters in Part II demonstrate that agency function, tradition, and outcome objectives, as well as the social and political landscape shape the culture and formats of service delivery. Before his untimely death in 2004, coeditor John Jacobson contributed a chapter on program evaluation in Part II, a subject in which he had been professionally engaged for over a quarter century. Part III is devoted to assessment. Psychologists in general have been the primary source of new knowledge and tools in individual assessment, and the section provides separate chapters on cognitive assessment and adaptive behavior assessment, the two critical aspects required for classification of MR when this is required for service eligibility in the United States. The section is rounded out with critical chapters on screening, educational assessment, family assessment, assessment of psychopathology, behavioral assessment, and forensic assessment. Part IV covers the many varieties of preventive and ameliorative interventions that are required to lessen the impact of ID on individuals, families, and society. The section begins with a review of the importance of evidence-based training for young professionals who wish to enter this exciting and complex field of professional practice. Finally, the last section, Part V, makes special note of the sensitivity required to be a helpful influence in this field. Ethical issues are considered in the last two chapters of this book by authors particularly noted for their wisdom and experience in identifying the things that matter to performing clinical services, research, and behavioral intervention with the vulnerable individuals with whom we work.

Not every issue relevant to this complex interdisciplinary field could be covered in a single volume. The topics that are included, like the thoughts and writings of the eminent contributors to this book, can be rightly considered essential reading as we move into a new century of discovery, effectiveness, and high quality care for people with intellectual and developmental disabilities.

James A. Mulick, Ph.D.
Columbus, OH
November 2005

REFERENCES

Jacobson, J. W., & Mulick, J. A. (Eds.). (1996). *Manual of diagnosis and professional practice in mental retardation.* Washington, DC: American Psychological Association.

Walsh, K. K. (2002). Thoughts on changing the term mental retardation. *Mental Retardation,* 40(1), 70–75.

Contents

PART III. ASSESSMENT AND DIAGNOSIS

PART IV. PREVENTION AND TREATMENT

PART V. ETHICAL ISSUES

I

Foundation

The focus of this section is on definition, epidemiology, and other causal influences that contribute to developmental disability.

1

Epidemiology and Etiology of Mental Retardation

SUZANNE McDERMOTT, MAUREEN S. DURKIN, NICOLE SCHUPF, and ZENA A. STEIN

Mental retardation (MR) is a manifestation of a heterogeneous set of impairments and conditions that result in cognitive limitation. It is a condition of medical, educational, and social importance. Physicians identify profound, severe, and moderate MR but rarely diagnose mild MR unless it is associated with a genetic or medical syndrome. From a medical perspective, the quest for etiology and the possibility of medical or surgical intervention to minimize deterioration are paramount. Educators, on the other hand are less concerned with causation than with academic achievement and school success. The majority of cases of mild MR is identified in school settings. Finally, the public uses the label to describe poor adaptive skills. Adults with MR who hold jobs, live independently, and participate in society are not always described as having MR. Thus some individuals characterized in childhood or adolescence as having mild MR become indistinguishable from the general population in adulthood.

There are numerous definitions of MR but the two most widely used in textbooks and research articles are the American Association on Mental Retardation [AAMR] (AAMR, 2002), recently revised and most often used in the United States, and the *International Classification of Diseases* (ICD-10) (World Health Organization [WHO], 1992) the most widely used classification in other countries of the world. The AAMR definition is a practical tool for the determination of service eligibility; the ICD-10 allows for levels of disability and is based on a medical model of classification.

SUZANNE McDERMOTT • Family Practice Center, Department of Family and Preventive Medicine, USC School of Medicine, Columbia, South Carolina 29208.   **MAUREEN S. DURKIN** • University of Wisconsin—Madison, Madison, Wisconsin 53726.   **NICOLE SCHUPF and ZENA A. STEIN** • Columbia University—New York, New York 10032.

Identification of the causes of MR has been a U.S. goal since the 1960s when the President's Committee on Mental Retardation was first formed by President John F. Kennedy. The search for etiology was fueled by the desire to prevent incident cases and this was coupled with the belief that scarce resources were needed for the lifelong care of individuals with MR. Research related to the search for causation requires a multidisciplinary approach, including the fields of neuroscience, genetics, epidemiology, and numerous medical specialties.

DEFINITIONS AND CLASSIFICATIONS

There are differences among the conceptual bases for defining MR and variations in the methods of ascertaining cases. The primary source of population-based data is household surveys. The United States conducts the *National Health Interview Survey* (NHIS) (National Center for Health Statistics, n.d.) which includes questions about impairments including MR. Administrative registries are often used to describe population rates of MR but these should be carefully interpreted because the criteria for participation in the program and its registry of needs vary. Some state and local programs are entitlements for eligible citizens, but not all citizens with the condition agree to be tested and deemed eligible. Other state programs are need-based with both economic and disability determinations. Thus, administrative registries are often not complete counts of individuals with MR but represent a combination of needy citizens and selective eligibility.

Age-specific rates of MR vary widely across different surveys. In order to appreciate the reasons for variability among age-specific rates of MR, definitions and classification systems must be considered. There are three main classification schemes used in the United States: the AAMR version is used by most adult service providers, the medical community uses the ICD-9 or ICD-10, the psychiatric practitioners use the *Diagnostic and Statistical Manual* (DSM) (American Psychiatric Association [APA], 1994), and state public education systems use variations of these. In addition, there has been a movement away from strict case-definitions that rely on standardized testing to a more functional and dynamic definition. Both the AAMR and the medical/rehabilitation international communities have moved from testing-based criteria to an assessment of needed supports.

CLASSIFICATION SCHEMES

Both national and international organizations have developed classifications for MR. These are summarized in Table 1.1.

In the United States the most widely accepted definition is taken from the 2002 version of the *Classification of Mental Retardation* published by the AAMR (AAMR, 2002): "MR is a disability characterized by significant limitations both in the intellectual functioning and in adaptive behavior as expressed in conceptual, social, and practical adaptive skills. This

Table 1.1. Principal Classification Systems for Mental Retardation in Common Use: 2005

Organization	Groups	Use
American Association on Mental Retardation (AAMR, 1992, 2002)	Mild, moderate, severe/profound intellectual deficit combined with intermittent, limited, extensive, and pervasive need for support	U.S. service agencies and institutions
World Health Organization (WHO, 1980a, 1980b, 1992), International Classification of Disease ICD-9 and ICD-10	Code groups: 317, 318, 319	Medical practice and research
World Health Organization (WHO, 1980a, 1980b, 2001), International Classification of Functioning (ICF) and ICIDH	Classification of functioning, disability, activity, and participation	International service agencies
American Psychiatric Association, Diagnostic and Statistical Manual (DSM-IV) (APA, 1994)	Multi-axial system of five domains—clinical mental disorders, general medical conditions, psychosocial and environmental problems, overall functioning	Psychiatry
Schools	Mild or educable, moderate or trainable, severe/profound	Public schools

disability originates before age 18." The AAMR classification recognizes that intellectual functioning is still best represented by IQ scores when obtained from appropriate assessment instruments. The criterion most widely used for labeling and diagnosis is two standard deviations below the mean score of a group of people thought to be representative of the entire population. Older definitions of MR have focused primarily on age at onset and intelligence. Adaptive behavior has become a second measurable component of the definition over the last 25 years and is viewed as a set of social and practical skills that have been learned by people to function independently. The classification of the AAMR commonly includes four categories of MR based on the statistical distribution of IQ scores. This categorization groups mild MR to an IQ range of 55–69, moderate MR to an IQ range of 40–54, severe MR to an IQ range of 25–39, and profound MR to an IQ below 25, although these subcategories have been omitted from the definition developed by AAMR (1992, 2002) and retained in a definition disseminated by the MR/DD division of the APA (Editorial Board, 1996).

The ICD, now in its 10th edition, was developed by the WHO to code health disorders, including impairments and disabilities (WHO, 1992). The ICD-10 is widely used by physicians and other health-care providers to code specific syndromes and impairments associated with MR, such as Down Syndrome (DS), Prader–Willi, Fragile X, and to code the level of intellectual disability (mild, moderate, and severe). The ICD codes are often combined with clinical procedure and therapeutic codes that are used for billing purposes. The DSM (APA, 1994) is used by U.S. psychiatrists to classify mental illnesses and is often considered analogous to the ICD for the field of psychiatry. The DSM includes MR (IQ and age of onset), the use of IQ ranges for levels of MR, and the assessment of adaptive skills as the defining criteria for diagnosis.

The WHO *International Classification of Functioning, Disability, and Health* (ICF) is the newest schema for classifying disability, including MR, and it was developed to describe a dynamic system in which impairment, function, and the environment interact (WHO, 2001). The ICF states that "an individual's disability may be characterized by marked and severe problems in the capacity to function ('impairments in body functions and structures'), the ability to function ('activity limitations'), and the opportunity to function ('participation restrictions')." The ICF codes have been used in some European countries since the early 1990s, and in selected sites in the United Sates.

The range of MR prevalence differs notably by etiology, degree of ability and disability, and behavioral characteristics. Individuals with mild MR predominate and constitute 75–90% of the group, and individuals with moderate to severe and profound MR make up 10–25%. The proportion in each category varies by the method of case acquisition, with school-based records favoring high proportions of mild cases and institutional registries reporting high proportions of severe and profound cases. Registries for adult services tend to report relatively more cases with moderate to severe MR than indicated by the proportions above. In addition, there are different proportions of severity by underlying impairment. For example, girls with Rett syndrome have a high proportion with severe and profound MR, while the range of intellectual disability is much wider for individuals with DS. There are also geographic and temporal variations that are a function of epidemics (e.g., rubella, influenza), poverty levels, environmental conditions (e.g., lead and mercury exposure), and access to prevention programs (e.g., early intervention for infants at risk, immunizations, dietary and therapeutic interventions).

It has been shown for the general population that IQ scores are relatively stable (Vernon, 1979; Zigler & Butterfield, 1966). Changes in scores greater than one standard deviation are usually attributed to removal of deprivation followed by intervention involving social and learning stimulation during early childhood (Clarke & Clarke, 1976; Dennis, 1973; Lazar & Darlington, 1982). In addition, the assumption of a normal distribution of IQ scores that underlie the assignment of an IQ of 70 as a cut point for MR is not based on epidemiological investigation. The empirical distribution obtained by researchers doing large-scale studies (e.g., Vernon, 1979; Zigler, 1967) has been bimodal with a second smaller peak in the lower tail of the curve. The explanation for this phenomenon is that there are two distributions of intelligence. One is for those whose intelligence is the result of an interaction of genetic and environmental influences and the other in which the brain has been damaged and the biological side of the interaction dominates (Lewis & Goldberg 1969; Zigler, 1967). The smaller mode in the left end of the distribution represents biologically induced MR. Many critics of intelligence testing and assignment of mental age argue that abstract intelligence cannot be forced into a linear model. The same argument has been applied to tests of adaptive functioning, which have been shown to have nonlinear progression (Jacobson & Mulick, 1996).

In general, in the field of MR there is a definite shift in the focus of classification schemes away from static definitions to dynamic models of functioning. These definitions, however, are not yet consistently used in the epidemiologic literature and there is little uniformity in their use in the service, medical, or educational arenas. Thus, it is important to recognize that although the AAMR definition of MR is widely known, many epidemiological studies of the prevalence of MR do not use measures of adaptive behavior and they most commonly report two categories of IQ. Epidemiologists use the term "mild" for an IQ between 50 and 70. They categorize all IQs below 50 as "severe" MR.

Epidemiologic research is based on the ability to count exposures and outcomes based on well-defined case definitions. When the outcome of interest is MR, the epidemiologist must specify the criteria used for designating cases and how the criteria were applied. Depending on whether the individuals were identified by a research testing protocol or ascertained from an administrative source such as a clinic, school, or service provider, the definition used was likely influenced by the year and the prevailing definition at that time.

INCIDENCE AND PREVALENCE

There have been extensive efforts to quantify the magnitude of the population with MR through the study of incidence and prevalence, a process that had used a number of approaches and yielded different results. The distinction between incidence and prevalence of MR is difficult to specify since MR identified at birth occurred during conception or gestation and many cases identified throughout childhood were probably also present at birth but not identified until delays in development were observed. There are a number of categories of causes that represent incident cases during childhood, such as postnatal encephalitis or trauma.

Prevalence is a function of incidence and duration and population dynamics such as immigration and emigration. Uneven prevalence rates throughout the lifespan are a result of delayed diagnosis for some mild cases, early death for some severe cases, and omission of mild cases from service registries during adulthood. These factors also make it impossible to determine incidence. The prevalence of MR in the United States during late childhood has been reported to be 1–2% of the population during the past decade, but there is substantial variation in the literature (Durkin & Stein, 1996). In the Netherlands, Sweden, and other countries, national registries track people throughout their lifetime in an effort to identify health, social problems, and service utilization and thus the disability associated with MR is captured more effectively (Kiely, 1987; Stein, Susser, & Saenger, 1976; Stein, Susser, Saenger, & Marolla, 1976). The United States has a birth defects surveillance system that captures only those cases identified in the first days of life, but the United States does not have a national disability registry; therefore prevalence rates for MR are usually calculated from cross-sectional data on children in public schools (Frankenberger & Harper, 1988; McDermott, 1994; McLaren & Bryson, 1987; Yeargin-Allsopp & Boyle, 2002).

Public school data on MR prevalence are not entirely reliable since intelligence tests are not administered universally and procedures for referral practices for testing and placement of children into special education vary among schools and by states, although they are all within guidelines from the U.S. Department of Education. Reports from the U.S. Department of Education include the number of children, aged 5–21, enrolled in special education programs and there are two and sometimes three programs for children with MR: Educable Mental Deficiency (EMD), Trainable Mental Deficiency (TMD), and Severe Mental Deficiency (SMD). In addition, some children with multiple disabling conditions are placed in other special education programs, i.e., multiply disabled, speech and language, orthopedic, or vision or hearing impairment, and are only counted in the one program with the highest level of reimbursement to the district, leading to an undercount of MR. Federal guidelines for placement of children with MR provide a definition of MR that includes significantly subaverage general intellectual functioning, with deficits in adaptive behavior. States provide guidance to local school districts in matters of referral, testing, and placement procedures. Research has shown that there are small-area (school district and county level) and large-area (national and state level) variations in MR prevalence rates (Baird & Sadovnick, 1987; Kiely, 1987; McDermott, 1994). The most widely used U.S. estimate of school-aged prevalence of MR is given in the *Healthy People 2010 Objectives for the Nation* (U.S. Department of Health and Human Services, 2000). The Metropolitan Atlanta Developmental Disabilities Surveillance System (MADDS) has set the benchmark for national prevalence of childhood MR at 131/10,000 8-year-old children, using an estimate from the 1991–1994 MADDS data (Yeargin-Allsopp & Boyle, 2002; Yeargin-Allsopp, Murphy, Cordero, Decoufle, & Hollowell, 1997).

Although MR is usually considered a lifelong disability, analysis of prevalence rates, especially for mild MR, indicates that the condition is less frequently identified in early life and it peaks during the school years, and that the label is not as often applied in later adulthood. Using the 1994/1995 *National Health Interview Survey Disability Supplements*, Larson et al. estimated the combined prevalence of MR or developmental disability to be 14.9 per 1000 in the noninstitutionalized population of the United States (Larson et al., 2001). Other estimates range from 1 to 10%, depending on the population surveyed and the methods used (Drillien, Pickering, & Drummond, 1988; Massey & McDermott, 1995; McLaren & Bryson, 1987; Simeonsson & Sharp, 1992; Stevenson, 1996).

ETIOLOGY

The AAMR 2002 states "etiology is a multifactorial construct composed of four categories of risk factors (biomedical, social, behavioral, and educational) that interact across time, including across the life of the individual and across generations from parent to child" (p. 123). Even gross genetic factors such as DS or mutation of a gene, can be viewed as highly associated with MR although not absolutely causal. In fact, with early intervention services some children with DS function in the low normal range on tests of IQ are not classified as having MR until they qualify for services later in childhood. Even more importantly, the cause of many genetic impairments remains unknown even when the underlying molecular pathways that cause neuronal processes involved in cognitive functions are understood.

In approximately half of the cases of MR the cause is unknown. Algorithms have been suggested for the evaluation of individuals that rely on family history, physical findings, and neurological functioning. The evaluation should include karyotyping and identification of anomalies. Then depending on the resources available to pursue the investigation there are a growing range of methods and technology available to make a diagnosis. Diagnostic techniques include chromosome microdissection, fluorescence in situ hybridization (FISH), interferometer spectral karyotyping (SKY), primed in situ labeling (PRINS), subtelomeric screening, magnetic resonance spectroscopy (MRS) of the brain, and other techniques in molecular genetics, neuroimaging and dysmorphology (Battaglia & Carey, 2003). The time when an insult occurs and leads to MR ranges from the time of conception through late childhood. A range of conditions associated with, and less often causally linked to MR, are described below in Table 1.2, in chronological order of occurrence.

SELECTED PERICONCEPTIONAL CAUSES

Telomeric Rearrangements

Chromosomal anomalies may be *numerical* or *structural*. Structural changes result from the breakage and rearrangement of chromosome parts, and animal experiments have shown that they can be induced by a variety of exposures, including ionizing radiation and certain viral infections and toxic substances. They occur as duplications, deletions, translocations, insertions, or inversions of chromosome parts or as rings on selected chromosomes. Numerical anomalies arise through nondisjunction during meiosis or mitosis, through lagging of chromosomes at anaphase of cell division, or through fertilization by two sperm (i.e., triploidy). Chromosomal anomalies as a whole contribute more to fetal loss than to live births and MR. Kline, Stein, and Susser (1989) estimated that from 8 weeks after the last menstrual period, the proportion of chromosomal aberrations lost by miscarriage exceeds 90% for all but trisomy 21 (DS), XXX, XXY (Klinefelter syndrome), and XYY. In survivors after birth in developed countries, chromosomal anomalies cause more than 30% of the cases of severe MR, with the majority of these having DS (Gustavson, Hagberg, Hagberg, & Sars, 1977a, 1977b).

Table 1.2. Categories of Causes of Mental Retardation, by Time of Insult (Adopted from Durkin et al., 2001)

Time	Category	Examples
Periconceptional	Genetic-chromosomal	Down syndrome, telometric rearrangements
	Sex linked-single gene	Fragile X syndrome, Rett syndrome
	Autosomal dominant	Phenylketonuria, neurofibromatosis, Tay Sacks
	Metabolic	Hypothyroidism
	Segmental autosomal syndromes	Prader–Willi syndrome, Angelman syndrome
	Genetic and nutritional	Neural tube defects
Intrauterine	Infection	Toxoplasmosis, rubella, cytomegalovirus, herpes, gonorrhea, group B streptococcus, Chlamydia, trichomonas vaginalis, bacterial vaginosis, herpes simplex virus, HIV
	Substances- prescribed and lifestyles	EtOH, antimicrobials (e.g., sulfonamides, isoniazid, ribavirin), anticonvulsants (e.g., phenytoin, carbamazepine), and other drugs- (e.g., warfarin, aminoptein, accutane)
	Metals and chemicals	Lead, mercury
	Nutritional	Iodine
Perinatal and postnatal	Birth complications and effects	Prematurity, low birth weight, asphyxia
Childhood	Infections	Encephalitis, meningitis, varicella
	Environmental exposures	Lead, mercury
	Injury	Traumatic brain injuries from vehicle crashes, child abuse and neglect
	Deprivation	Insufficient stimulation

In humans, *de novo* (presumed mutant) chromosomal rearrangements, whether balanced or unbalanced, occur in 2/1000 live births. This estimate is based on 63,000 fetal amniocenteses, which were diagnosed in the New York State Chromosome Registry (Hook & Cross, 1987). Of these, about 0.5 per 1000 are *de novo* markers; about 0.5 per 1000 other *de novo* unbalanced translocations and about 1.0 per 1000 *de novo* balanced rearrangements. The rate of inherited rearrangements was about 2.9 per 1000, including 0.3 per 1000 inherited markers, 0.2 per 1000 other inherited unbalanced rearrangements, and about 2.4 per 1000 inherited balanced abnormalities. Among fetuses studied because of maternal exposure to putative mutagens, there was an excess of mutants, 2.9–5.7 per 1000 versus 1.7–2.2 per 1000 (Hook & Cross, 1987). These findings suggest that workplace or environmental exposures may increase risk of structural cytogenetic abnormalities in the fetus that, in turn, may be associated with birth defects and neurodevelopmental delay in the infant.

Warburton (1984, 1987, 1991) reported the results of a 10-year collection of data from a series of over 377,000 amniocenteses in which the occurrence rate of *de novo* balanced reciprocal translocations, Robertsonian translocations, and inversions was estimated to be about 1 per 1000. The most common *de novo* balanced chromosomal anomalies were *de novo* reciprocal translocations (1 per 2000). The overall risk of a serious congenital anomaly, including but not limited to MR, for balanced reciprocal translocations and inversions was 6.7% (95% *CI* 3.1–10.3%). In this same study, *de novo* supernumerary markers were found in 1 in 2500 amniocenteses, and had a risk of approximately 15% of being associated with an abnormal fetal outcome. *De novo* unbalanced rearrangements, including supernumerary small markers, have been estimated to occur in about 1 in 1000 amniocenteses which were carried out for reasons other than suspected fetal anomalies (Hook & Cross, 1987). This rate increased to 1.8 per 1000 when amniocentesis was performed because of known or suspected fetal pathology.

However, these rates are based on cytogenetic methods that may miss small deletions or translocations and underestimate the impact of chromosomal anomalies on neurodevelopmental disorders. There is mounting evidence that chromosomal rearrangements involving the subtelomeric regions of chromosomes contribute to moderate to severe MR and are associated with dysmorphic phenotypic features (Flint et al., 1995; Knight et al., 1999). Flint and his colleagues (Knight et al., 1999) reported that subtelomeric abnormalities, requiring microassays or FISH to be detected, occurred in 7.4% (95% *CI* 4.4–10.4) of 284 children with previously unexplained moderate to severe MR. About half of the subtelomeric rearrangement cases were familial and the other half were isolated, apparently *de novo* cases. Approximately 10% of the de novo rearrangements had abnormal outcomes. In both the familial and *de novo* groups approximately 60% of the chromosomal anomalies were paternal and 40% were maternal in origin. If cases are selected to include dysmorphic features as well as developmental delay, chromosomal aberrations may be found in as many as 13.0% (Popp et al., 2002). On the other hand, van Karnebeek et al. (2002) screened 266 children in a consecutive cohort of cases with unexplained MR presenting to an academic tertiary center for diagnosis and found that the total frequency of cytogenetic anomalies was 10%, but the frequency of subtelomeric rearrangements was low (0.5%, van Karnebeek et al., 2002). Thus, screening for subtelomeric rearrangements is likely to be most effective when combined with targeted selection criteria, including unexplained MR, dysmorphic features, and a positive family history with two or more affected individuals (Popp et al., 2002).

DOWN SYNDROME

DS is the most common genetic cause of MR and the leading known cause of severe MR in developed countries (Nicholson & Alberman, 1992). All cases of DS result from partial or complete duplication of chromosome 21 in the genome (Epstein, 1986). The most common form (95% of cases at birth) is standard trisomy, involving duplication of chromosome 21. In over 90% of these cases, the extra chromosome is of maternal origin, due to nondisjunction during meiosis (Hassold, Chiu, & Yamane, 1984; Sherman et al., 1991; Stewart et al., 1988). Translocation of chromosome 21 material to another chromosome (usually 13 or 18) and mosaicism (transmission of a cryptic trisomy 21 cell line from an unaffected parent) are rare causes of DS (Hook, 1982; Staples, Sutherland, Haan, & Clisby, 1991).

The most striking epidemiological characteristic of DS is the marked increase in risk with increasing maternal age, from 1 per 1550 live births at ages 20–24 years to 1 per 700 live births at ages 30–34 years to 1 per 50 live births at ages 41–45 years (Cuckle, Wald, & Thompson, 1987). Despite this strong association with maternal age, most DS births are to women aged less than 35 years because younger women contribute the great majority of births. Thus, the crude birth rate of DS in a population will depend on the maternal age distribution and the availability and use of prenatal diagnosis followed by selective abortion.

Except for advanced maternal age, factors that increase risk for having a child with DS are not well established. Recently, variants in two folate metabolizing enzymes, the 677C → T polymorphism in the gene for methylenetetrahydrofolatereductase (MTHFR) and the 66A → G polymorphism in the gene for methionine reductase (MTRR), have been found to be more prevalent among mothers of children with DS than among control mothers (Hobbs et al., 2000; James et al., 1999; O'Leary et al., 2002). The combined presence of both the MTHFR and MTRR polymorphisms increased risk of having child with DS to a greater extent than either polymorphism alone (Hobbs et al., 2000; O'Leary et al., 2002). The MTHFR 677C → T mutation affects both folate metabolism and cellular methylation reactions. James and colleagues hypothesized that gene–nutrient interactions associated with abnormal folate metabolism and reduced DNA methylation might increase risk of nondisjunction DS (Hobbs et al., 2000; James et al., 1999). As Hobbs has noted, the reduction in enzyme activity in carriers of the 677C → T mutation may raise dietary requirements for folic acid. This is the first risk factor to be identified for DS in young women and raises the possibility of intervention and prevention for DS (Hassold et al., 2001).

Virtually all persons with DS have a cognitive impairment, with the majority functioning in the moderate to profound range of MR. Observations of children living at home with their families or enrolled in infant stimulation programs suggest that the cognitive intellectual potential of children with DS may have been underestimated (Bennett, Sells, & Brand, 1979; Centerwall & Centerwall, 1960; Clements, Bates, & Hafer, 1976; Connolly, Morgan, & Russell, 1984; Melyn & White, 1973; Rynders, Spiker, & Horrobin, 1978; Sharav & Shlomo, 1986). However, early intervention has not been effective in altering the trajectory of development for all children who receive it, and some children with severe MR do not benefit substantially from it.

Adults with DS show a variety of age-related changes in physical and functional capacities suggestive of premature or accelerated aging (Martin, 1978), including changes in skin tone, hypogonadism, increased frequency of cataracts, increased frequency of hearing loss, hypothyroidism, seizures, degenerative vascular disease, and Alzheimer's disease (AD) (Oliver & Holland, 1986; Sare, Ruvalcaba, & Kelly, 1978; Schupf & Sergievsky, 2002; Wisniewski, Wisniewski, & Wen, 1985; Zigman, Schupf, Sersen, & Silverman, 1996). The most extensively studied aspect of aging in DS is their high risk for the development of AD. Virtually all individuals with DS have key neuropathological changes consistent with a diagnosis of AD by the time they reach 40 years of age, including deposition of beta amyloid (Aβ) in diffuse and neuritic plaques (Wisniewski, Wegiel, & Popovitch, 1994), and most will develop dementia by the end of their seventh decade of life (Lai et al., 1999). The neuropathological manifestations of AD in DS have been attributed to triplication and overexpression of the gene for amyloid precursor protein (APP) located on chromosome 21 (Rumble et al., 1989). The increased risk of dementia in DS may be mediated by an increased substrate for cellular production of Aβ. Neuropathological studies have shown that diffuse plaques, the most prevalent "Alzheimer-type" lesion seen in individuals with DS before age 50, are not associated with dementia. In contrast, increase in the numbers of neuritic plaques, containing substantial amounts of fibrillized Aβ peptides, is observed in adults with DS predominantly after 50 years of age (Wisniewski et al., 1994) and all incidence studies agree that risk of AD increases primarily after 50 years of age (Holland, Hon, Huppert, & Watson, 1998; Lai et al., 1999; Visser et al., 1997). In addition, not all adults with DS will develop dementia even if they reach ages when the presence of high densities of neuritic plaques and neurofibrillary tangles can be presumed. Thus, factors, which modify the rate and degree of Aβ deposition, rather than overexpression of APP, may be the important determinants of risk for dementia in DS (Schupf & Sergievsky, 2002).

SEX-LINKED SINGLE GENE

Mutations in 14 X-linked genes have been identified in both syndrome and nonsyndrome conditions. These are AGTR2, ARHGEF6, ATRX, FACL4, FMR2, GD11, ILRIRAPL, MECP2, OPHNI, PAK3, RSK2, TM4SF2, and VCX-A. Other X-linked genes and those that map to X will likely be identified in the future (Chechlacz & Gleeson, 2003). The fragile X syndrome, a non-syndrome MR with a transcription factor (FMR2), primarily affects males. This syndrome, which results from mutations in the MECP2 gene located at Xq28, is both syndromic and nonsyndromic and the prevalence is estimated to be at least as high as 1 in 10,000 females (Hagberg & Hagberg, 1997; Kerr & Ravine, 2003).

Fragile X Syndrome

The fragile X syndrome is the most common form of inherited MR. In addition to cognitive disability, the fra(X) phenotype includes macroorchidism, a long face, prominent jaw, large ears, thickening of the nasal bridge, and joint hypermobility. Behavioral abnormalities may include autistic-like features, repetitive speech patterns, social anxiety, perseveration, and gaze aversion (Brown, Jenkins, & Friedman, 1982; Hagerman & Silverman, 1991; Opitz & Sutherland, 1984; Reiss & Freund, 1990). Neuroimaging has demonstrated a small posterior cerebellar vermis, and enlarged hippocampus, caudate nucleus, thalamus, and lateral ventricles and Reiss and colleagues have shown correlations between these structural abnormalities and IQ (Reiss, Abrams, Greenlaw, Freund, & Denckla, 1995; Reiss, Aylward, Freund, Joshi, & Bryan, 1991; Reiss, Lee, & Freund, 1994). A fragile site on the X chromosome, fra(X), was first identified in males from families with X-linked MR (Lubs, 1969; Sutherland, 1977). The proportion of cells showing the fragile X site in cytogenetic studies is quite variable and may be characteristic of each individual. About 80% of male carriers of the mutation and about 30% of female carriers show some degree of MR (Chudley et al., 1983; Sherman, Morton, Jacobs, & Turner, 1984).

An unusual pattern of inheritance emerged from segregation analysis of families affected with fra(X), which followed the intergenerational passage of the gene (Sherman, Jacobs, et al., 1985; Sherman, Morton, et al., 1984). About 20% of males who carry the genotype are clinically unaffected and do not express the fra(X) site on cytogenetic testing. Mothers of these nonpenetrant males are rarely affected. These nonpenetrant normal transmitting males transmit the mutation to daughters who, although unaffected themselves, will have affected children. Thus, grandsons of nonpenetrant normal transmitting males have MR and granddaughters may show some cognitive impairment (Sherman, Jacobs, et al., 1985; Sherman, Morton, et al., 1984). Brothers of nonpenetrant normal transmitting males are at low risk (approximately 9%) while grandsons and great grandsons are at high risk (approximately 40–50%).

The molecular basis of Fragile X syndrome was elucidated with the isolation of the fra(X) gene, FMR1, in 1991 (Bell et al., 1991; Fu et al., 1991; Kremer et al., 1991; Oberle et al., 1991; Verkerk et al., 1991; Vincent et al., 1991). At the molecular level the FRAXA site contains an exon of the FMR1 gene responsible for the fragile X, a repetitive CGG sequence, which demonstrates length variation in normal and in fra(X) individuals, and a cytidine phosphate guanosine (CpG) island that shows preferential methylation in fra(X) cases (Bell et al., 1991; Vincent et al., 1991). The length of the CGG repeat in genomic DNA is correlated with risk for the fragile X syndrome (Kremer et al., 1991). Normal individuals have CGG repeat lengths of 6–50 repeats and affected individuals show dramatic amplification of the CGG repeat (from 200 to 1000) and hypermethylation of the repeat and adjacent CpG region, resulting in a shutdown of transcription of FMR1 and absence of the FMR1 protein (Bell et al., 1991; Oberle et al., 1991; Pieretti et al., 1991; Sutcliffe et al., 1992; Verheij et al., 1993). The full mutation, when fully methylated, results in cognitive disability in all males and in 50–70% of affected females (de Vries et al., 1997; Hagerman et al., 1992; Rousseau et al., 1994).

Expansion of the premutation to the full mutation occurs only in female meiotic transmission (Oberle et al., 1991; Smits et al., 1992; Yu et al.,

1991) and risk for expansion to the full mutation increases with the number of repeats (Fu et al., 1991). As amplification of the gene increases, it becomes more unstable, leading to mitotic instability as well as meiotic instability (Fu et al., 1991; Oberle et al., 1991; Pieretti et al., 1991). The mitotic instability of the full repeat causes longer and shorter expansions, resulting in mosaicism with respect to size (premutation together with a full mutation) or with respect to degree of methylation (from 10 to 100% of leukocytes with an unmethylated full mutation). Several cases of intellectually normal males with a high proportion of unmethylated leukocytes have been reported, suggesting that methylation is critical for lack of transcription of FMR1 gene and expression of the phenotype (de Vries et al., 1996; Hagerman, Hull et al., 1994; Nolin, Glicksman, Houck, Brown, & Dobkin, 1994; Rousseau et al., 1994). In addition, several cases have been found with atypical mutations at the FRAXA site, two involving a deletion and one a point mutation in the FRM1 gene (Gedeon et al., 1992; Wohrle et al., 1992). Other fragile sites (FRAXE, FRAXD, FRAXF) are found close to the FRAXA site. FRAXE is associated with learning disabilities, but is caused by a different expanding trinucleotide repeat (Feldman, 1996).

Prevalence of the Fragile X Syndrome

Prevalence studies in defined populations have employed cytogenetic or DNA testing for fra(X) among individuals with MR. Prevalence estimates from these studies have ranged from 0.5 to 4.2% of patients with MR (de Vries et al., 1997; Hagerman, Wilson, et al., 1994; Jacobs et al., 1993; Meadows et al., 1996; Murray et al., 1996; Turner, Webb, Wake, & Robinson, 1996; van den Ouweland et al., 1994). The wide range of these estimates is likely to be due to differences in the distribution of MR causes in the samples studied, as well as variability in the DNA analysis. Within the general population, the prevalence of fra(X) has been estimated to range from 1/4000 to 1/6045 males (de Vries et al., 1997; Morton et al., 1997; Turner et al., 1996). Estimates of the prevalence of the FRAXA premutation carrier frequency among females in the general population have also ranged widely, from 1/248 women to 1/1000 women (Holden, Percy, et al., 1999; Reiss et al., 1994; Rousseau, Rouillard, Morel, Khandjian, & Morgan, 1995; Spence et al., 1996).

SEGMENTAL AUTOSOMY SYNDROMES

Segmental autosomy syndromes result from abnormalities in gene dosage caused by structural defects (deletion, duplication) or functional imbalance (imprinting defects, uniparental disomy) of critical genes (Budarf & Emanuel, 1997). Recent molecular studies have shown that three syndromes involving early onset cognitive disability are within this class of disorders: Williams, Prader–Willi, and Angelman syndromes.

Williams Syndrome

Williams syndrome (WS) is a multisystem disorder characterized by developmental and language delays, pixie-like facial features, cardiovascular abnormalities, elevated calcium levels, problems in gross motor skills, and a distinctive cognitive profile that includes mild MR with relatively good language and face-processing skills. The frequency of WS has been estimated to be about 1/10,000 live births (Beuren, Apitz, & Harmajanz, 1962; Williams, Barratt-Boyes, & Lowe, 1961). Individuals with WS have an approximately 2 Mb deletion of chromosomal region 7q11.23 (Ewart et al., 1993; Perez-Jurado, Peoples, Kaplan, Hamel, & Francke, 1996). Variability in deletion size may be related to variable phenotypic presentation. The majority of patients with WS is hemizygous for 7q11.23 and in more than 90% of cases, the deletion includes the locus for the elastin gene (*ELN*), a protein kinase LIM-kinase1 (*LIMK1*), and a replication factor C subunit (*RFC2*) (Frangiskakis et al., 1996; Osborne et al., 1996; Peoples, Perez-Jurado, Wang, Kaplan, & Francke, 1996). Families with "partial WS," involving smaller deletions that include only *ELN* and *LIMK1*, show the cognitive and cardiovascular profiles but lack other features of WS, suggesting that the loss of at least three genes is required for the full WS phenotype (Budarf & Emanuel, 1997; Frangiskakis et al., 1996). There is no evidence of imprinting in WS, but if the gene deletion is of maternal origin, patients have more severe growth retardation and microcephaly (Perez-Jurado et al., 1996).

Prader–Willi/Angelman Syndrome

Prader–Willi syndrome (PWS) and Angelman syndrome (AS) are characteristics of disorders resulting from genomic imprinting in which the phenotypic expression of the disorder depends on the parent from whom the genetic abnormality is inherited. Both syndromes involve structural or functional loss of expression of genes in the chromosome 15q11-q13 region, including deletions, uniparental disomy, and mutations in an imprinting center. Paternally inherited abnormalities result in PWS while maternally inherited abnormalities result in AS (Knoll et al., 1989; Ledbetter et al., 1981). PWS is characterized by developmental delay, hypotonia, and feeding problems in infancy followed by excessive and rapid weight gain resulting in severe obesity, cryptoorchidism, short stature, and mild MR. Behavioral characteristics include temper tantrums and ritualistic or obsessive-compulsive behavior (Clarke, Boer, Cheung, Sturney, & Webb, 1996; Dykens, Leckman, & Cassify, 1996; Webb et al., 2002). The frequency of PWS is approximately 1/15,000 live births. In contrast, AS is characterized by severe MR, microcephaly, hypermotoric behavior with hand-flapping, and jerky movements in association with outbursts of laughter, short attention span, hypopigmented skin and eyes, and seizures with onset under 3 years of age.

It appears that different genes are responsible for the two syndromes, all of them imprinted in the germ line. The 15q11-q13 region contains four paternally expressed genes whose loss of expression causes PWS;

small nuclear ribonucleoprotein-associated polypeptide N (Ozcelik et al., 1992), zinc finger protein (Mowery-Rushton, Driscoll, Nicholls, Locker, & Surti, 1996), a gene designated as imprinted in Prader–Willi (Wevrick, Kerns, & Francke, 1994) and two less well-characterized transcripts, PAR1 and PAR5 (Sutcliffe et al., 1994). The 15q11-q13 region also contains the gene for E6-AP ubiquitin-protein ligase 3A (*UBE3A*) which is biallelically expressed in somatic tissue but is imprinted with preferential maternal expression in the brain (Albrecht et al., 1997; Jiang, Tsai, Bressler, & Beaudet, 1998; Matsuura et al., 1997); mutations in UBE3A are found in a small subset of patients with AS.

The effects of imprinting are also seen in cases of uniparental disomy (UPD) where maternal UPD represents loss of paternally expressed genes and is associated with PWS, while paternal UPD represents loss of maternally expressed genes and is associated with AS. Seventy percent of cases in PWS are associated with a 4 Mb deletion in 15Q11-q13, an additional 27% display maternal uniparental disomy and 1–2% of cases are associated with mutations and deletions in the imprinting center (Sutcliffe et al., 1994). As in PSW, 70% of AS cases have maternal deletions in the 15q11-q13 region, 3–5% have paternal uniparental disomy, 7–9% have imprinting mutations, 2–4% have mutations in UBE3A, while in 10–20% of cases, the molecular defect is still unknown (Nicholls, 1993; Wagstaff et al., 1992).

COMBINATIONS OF GENETIC AND NUTRITIONAL FACTORS

Neural tube defects (NTD), including spina bifida, anencephaly, and meningomyelocele, result from failure of neural tube closure during the third to eighth week of gestation. The cause of a majority of cases of NTD is related to a nutritional deficit of folate and a small proportion of cases is related to a genetic problem (Czeizel, 1995; MRC Vitamin Study Group, 1991; Wild et al., 1986). The incidence of all levels of NTDs in the United States is 1–3 per 1000 births and 2–5% in children with a previous affected sibling (Cohen, 2000). NTDs are associated with a wide range of intellectual function and only a small proportion of MR is attributable to NTDs. Hydrocephalus occurs in 95% of high lumbar and thoracic lesions and 60–85% of low lumbar and sacral defects. Since shunting of cerebral spinal fluid is now a well-established surgical intervention, only a small proportion of these children has MR. The use of preconception and early conceptual folate supplementation through diet or vitamin pills can prevent a substantial proportion of occurrence and reoccurrence of NTDs.

Phenyketonuria (PKU) deficiency is a rare defect of amino acid metabolism with a frequency of about 1 per 15,000 in White populations. Because it is a single gene defect and PKU deficiency is identified during newborn screening in all states in the United States, the sequella of MR can be prevented with adherence to a strict diet during infancy and early childhood. The realization that the sequella of PKU can be prevented by strict diet during childhood unfortunately overlooked the fact that the female survivors who then became pregnant needed to go onto the diet perinatally, so the intrauterine environment of the fetus is not toxic with phenyke-tones (Baumeister & Woodley-Zanthos, 1996; Hanley et al., 1999; Lenke & Levy, 1980; Levy & Ghavami, 1996; Levy & Waisbren, 1983; Rouse et al., 1997; Waisbren, Chang, et al., 1988; Waisbren, Doherty, Bailey, Rohr, & Levy, 1998). Severe MR and microcephaly are observed in 75–90% of children of mothers with classic PKU (defined as blood phenylalanine level >1200 mol/l). Less severe cognitive deficit may affect children of moth-ers with atypical PKU (elevations of blood phenylalanine levels to between 594 and 1194 mol/l, Levy & Ghavami, 1996). Dietary restrictions dur-ing pregnancy to reduce maternal blood phenylalanine levels and prevent phenylalanine metabolite accumulation can improve the outcome in off-spring if the diet is started prior to conception and maintained throughout pregnancy.

A third nutritionally related cause of MR is hypothyroidism during pregnancy. A genetic form of hypothyroidism (which, when untreated is referred to as cretinism), unrelated to iodine deficiency, can result in pro-gressive neurological deficits after 3 months of age. In the United States, screening of all newborns is mandatory in all states and thus the occur-rence of cretinism is rare. Cretinism can also result when there is maternal, fetal, or neonatal nutritional thyroid hormone deficiency; the supplementa-tion of iodine in the mother needs to occur prior to conception. Cretinism can result in neurodevelopmental deficits in the newborn, including MR and a number of other sensory and motor impairments. When both fetal and maternal hypothyroxinemia are present, such as in iodine-deficient regions of China, it has been shown that iodine replacement in the first trimester of pregnancy was necessary to prevent neurological deficits (Cao et al., 1994; Liu, Momotani, & Yoshimura, 1994; O'Donnell et al., 2002; Wasserstrum & Anania, 1995). Iodine deficiency can range from mild to se-vere, and the associated outcomes range from mild cognitive impairments and cerebral palsy to death. Worldwide iodine deficiency is estimated to affect over 20 million people and it has been reported as a leading cause of MR (Hetzel, 1989).

Children with PKU and hypothyroidism can be identified at birth, so their parents can receive instruction about the appropriate diet or med-ication needed to prevent the onset of MR. The effectiveness of newborn screening strategies to identify and treat infants with PKU and hypothy-roidism has resulted in a significant decline in children with MR from these causes in the United States during the past 25 years.

INFECTIONS

Infections during pregnancy have long been recognized as contributors to maternal and infant mortality and morbidity, including long-term neuro-logical impairments. The significant role of infection in early child survival and wellness has led to the development of a number of vaccines. During the later part of the 1990s and in the decade of 2000–2010 the infective process during gestation has received a significant amount of attention.

The route of infection of the fetus following maternal infection is through transplacental transmission or from the genital tract by the cervical amniotic route. The effect of a maternal infection on the fetus may be due to direct actions of toxins or organisms or it can be an indirect consequence of interference with placental or uterine function (Leviton & Gilles, 1996; Leviton & Paneth, 1990). The effect of a specific infection on fetal development is likely to depend on maternal and fetal factors including genetics, nutrition, stage of development, anatomical site of the infection, and the integrity of the placenta. After implantation interaction between the mother and fetus is mediated through the trophoblast, which has distinct immunological characteristics. In addition, the endometrium of pregnancy is unique and the general maternal response to major histocompatability complex (MHC) antigens in the conceptus is downregulated by maternal antifetal HLA (human leukocyte antigen) antibody production (Johnson, 1995). Other factors that influence the outcome include the characteristics of the organism, portal of entry, time of exposure, and dose of the infectious organism. One group of intrauterine infections, which has contributed to MR and other adverse consequences, is collectively known by the acronym TORCH: toxoplasmosis, other, rubella, cytomegalovirus (CMV), and herpes. The impact of these infections is dependent on the time of exposure during gestation.

CMV is one of the most ubiquitous viral infections in humans in the world, with prevalence rates reported from 20 to 95%. In some countries of Southeast Asia, Africa, and the South Pacific islands prevalence rates are reported above 90%, while in the United States and parts of Europe the prevalence is reported to be around 50%. Transmission occurs through shedding of the virus from nasopharyngeal secretions, urine, saliva, tears, genital secretions, breast milk, and blood. Maternal infections usually occur because of sexual transmission, and high number of sexual partners and early age of intercourse are predictors of occurrence of CMV. Perinatal transmission occurs through exposure of the fetus, in utero, to virus from reactivated or acute maternal disease. The virus can remain dormant in the host and cause latent infection and its sequella are exacerbated if the host has immune compromise. Exposure of the fetus to a primary CMV infection poses a risk of adverse outcome at any stage of pregnancy (Peckham, 1991). Approximately 10% of infants with asymptomatic infections at birth develop serious sequella, such as optic atrophy, learning disabilities, and MR (Faro & Soper, 2001). Congenital CMV is reported in 0.2–2.2% of all live births (Baumeister & Woodley-Zanthos, 1996). The mortality rate among symptomatic newborns is about 30%, and more than 90% of survivors have neurological impairments including microcephaly, seizures, MR, and hearing and vision problems. The pathway of transmission of congenital CMV is probably through the placenta and the critical period of exposure appears to be in the first trimester.

Toxoplasmosis is a disease caused by a protozoan, often transmitted through maternal handling of cat feces when changing a litter box or through the ingestion of raw or undercooked meat that contains the protozoa. It can be acquired either pre- or postnatally although the prenatal infection appears to have the most critical impact during the first trimester. Transmission of toxoplasma to the fetus occurs only when the mother has been infected for the first time during gestation, except if the mother has severe immune compromise. The outcomes associated with untreated prenatal exposure to the fetus include microcephaly, hydrocephalus, cerebral palsy, epilepsy, and MR (Baumeister & Kupstas, 1991; Remington, McLeod, & Desmonts, 1995; Roizen, Swisher, & Stein, 1995). Infant sequella of a maternal infection can be prevented if it is detected and treated with spiramycin early in gestation or with pyrimethamine and sulfadiazine later in gestation. Although prevalence of congenitally infected infants in the United States is not available it has been estimated that 1–10 per 10,000 infants born annually have toxoplasmosis, and the majority is asymptomatic at birth and does not develop the sequella until later in life (Dunn et al., 1999; Guerina et al., 1994; Lebech et al., 1999).

The viral disease rubella has severe consequences when the infection occurs early in pregnancy. When a mother is infected in the first 12 weeks of pregnancy the fetus has an 80% chance of getting the infection, and the rate declines progressively to 25% during the 26th week. In infected fetuses, rubella-associated defects occur in all cases during the first 11 weeks and 35% of cases infected during weeks 13–16; risk to the fetus is negligible after the 16th week (Martin & Schoub, 2000; Morgan-Capner, 1999). The last major epidemic of rubella in the United States occurred in 1964–1965 and resulted in approximately 31,000 cases of rubella and congenital rubella infections. It is reported that 11,000 of these cases resulted in fetal death or therapeutic abortion and 20,000 infants were born with congenital rubella syndrome (CRS). Since 1969 the incidence of rubella declined by more than 99% (Centers for Disease Control and Prevention [CDC], 1997a).

Varicella and herpes zoster are different manifestations of the same virus. The primary infection produces chickenpox during childhood in the United States, although varicella is a disease of the reproductive years in subtropical and tropical climate countries. Chickenpox is a highly contagious disease and humans are the only reservoir. It is transmitted by droplets from vesicular fluid or secretions from the upper respiratory tract. There are approximately 1–7 cases per 10,000 pregnancies (Freij & Sever, 1997; Gilstrap, 1997; Paryani & Arvin, 1986; Preblud, Cochi, & Orenstein, 1986). The manifestations of congenital varicella include cortical atrophy and other neurological findings. *Varivax*, the live attenuated varicella vaccine, was approved in the United States in 1995 (Gibbs & Sweet, 1999).

Another important maternal infection that has consequences for the developing fetus is urinary tract infection. Urinary tract infections represent the most common medical complication of pregnancy, occurring in approximately 4–7% of all pregnancies. When all potentially offending genitourinary pathogens are included, and when the spectrum of asymptomatic bacteriuria is considered, these factors may increase the frequency of maternal bacteriuria to 25%. Recent research using an inception cohort design with Medicaid maternal and infant-linked records and Vital Records for 41,090 pregnancies during 1995–1998 found the relative risk

(RR) for MR or developmental delay among children of mothers with urinary tract infection without an antibiotic (i.e., based on Medicaid pharmacy reimbursement claims) was significantly elevated compared to the group without an urinary tract infection and compared to children of mothers with urinary tract infection and an antibiotic claim. Similar analyses of the National Collaborative Perinatal Project provide comparable results (McDermott, Callaghan, Szwejbka, Mann, & Daguise, 2000; McDermott, Daguise, Mann, Szwejbka, & Callaghan, 2001).

There is an increasing body of evidence suggesting that prematurity is a consequence of maternal infections including those that are sexually transmitted: gonorrhea, Group B streptococcus, Chlamydia trachomatis, trichomonas vaginalis, bacterial vaginosis, and herpes simplex virus. Premature rupture of the membranes (PROM), a precursor of early delivery, is often accompanied by the presence of one of these organisms, which could cause the fetal membranes in utero to weaken and rupture. Thus it is often suggested that PROM is a symptom of an existing infection, which was not treated (Creasy & Iams, 1999; Iams, Talbert, Barrows, & Sachs, 1985). Bacteria in amniotic fluid are found in approximately 10% of women with PROM and PROM occurs in approximately 5% of all pregnancies (Aries, Rodriquez, Rayne, & Kraus, 1993; Romero, Yoon, et al., 1993).

Worldwide another serious and widespread threat to cognitive development results from the transmission of human immunodeficiency virus (HIV) infection from the mother to the developing fetus. Perinatally acquired HIV infection and pediatric autoimmune deficiency syndrome (AIDS) emerged as a cause of MR in the late 1980s (Boylan & Stein, 1991). AIDS has become a major public health problem in many countries of Africa, where high HIV prevalence among childbearing women is combined with lack of access to antenatal antiretroviral therapy and cesarean delivery, causing vertical transmission of HIV (*intrauterine, intrapartum,* or neonatal) (European Mode of Delivery Collaboration, 1999). The neurodevelopmental effects of pediatric AIDS include microcephaly and significant delays in cognitive and motor development (Belman, 1992; Macmillan et al., 2001). These effects have been reported to be greater when transmission of the virus from mother to child occurs in utero versus during parturition (Smith et al., 2000). In developed countries, improvements in postnatal treatment and survival of children with HIV may be associated with a reduction in adverse neurodevelopmental outcomes. One U.S. study of HIV infected children aged 3–5 years found no detriment in verbal or performance IQ when compared to controls matched on ethnicity and prenatal drug exposure (Fishkin et al., 2000). Another study, without controls, of children with AIDS surviving to school age in Philadelphia, found no more than 12% to have developmental scores in the range for MR (Mialky, Vagnoni, & Rutstein, 2001). Estimates are not available of the prevalence of pediatric HIV-associated neurodevelopmental disorders from low-income countries, where the vast majority of HIV-infected children reside but where few have access to antiretroviral therapy. In addition to direct effects of AIDS on the developing nervous system, the AIDS epidemic may be a causal factor in mild MR to the extent that it increases children's exposure to social, emotional, and economic deprivation during critical periods of development. Cost-effective and accessible methods of prevention and treatment of HIV in developing countries are needed to control this emerging cause of MR. Although administration of antiretroviral therapy and other medications to the pregnant woman can dramatically reduce HIV transmission, this form of treatment and preventive intervention is not widely practiced in the continents of Asia and Africa, due to poverty and political will (Amar, Ho, & Mohan, 1999; Boylan & Stein, 1991). In low-income countries which include the majority of HIV-infected women worldwide and in which prenatal screening, counseling, and treatment options are limited, the probability of vertical transmission from mother to infant is 30–40%.

In addition to infections known to directly damage the developing nervous system, other prenatal and perinatal infections associated with perinatal complications may contribute to developmental disabilities either directly or indirectly. Perinatal complications that occur more frequently in the presence of maternal and fetal infections include premature birth, low birth weight, intrauterine growth restriction, and asphyxia (Donders, Desmyter, De Wet, & Ban Assche, 1993). Infants born with perinatal complications, in turn, are at increased risk for developmental disabilities (Broman, Nichols, Shaughnessy, & Kennedy, 1987). The role of maternal and intrauterine infections in the etiology of perinatal brain disorders is an area of active investigation (O'Shea & Dammann, 2000).

PREMATURITY AND LOW BIRTH WEIGHT

Some of the risk factors associated with MR are a mixture of causes that are highly correlated. These include poverty, prematurity, low birth weight, and intrauterine infection. Since the 1970s the proportion of infants born in the United States weighing less than 2500 g has remained around 7% of all births. Premature and low birth weight infants have three times the risk for neurodevelopmental impairments compared to babies weighing more than 2500 g at birth (Teplin, Burchinal, Johnson-Martin, Humphry, & Kraybill, 1991; Whitaker et al., 1996). It is not clear, in most cases, if intrauterine problems precipitated the premature birth or the early delivery was responsible for the development of subsequent problems. However, it is clear that the relationship between birth weight and risk for developmental delay is inverse, so the greatest risk is at the lowest weight. Risk factors associated with prematurity include young maternal age, minority racial or ethnic status, poverty, and unmarried status, several of which are likely to be concurrent factors. As noted previously, the role of bacteria in premature labor has been an important area of research in the last decade. Bacteria are found in the amniotic cavity in over 10% of patients with PROM, which occurs in approximately 5% of all pregnancies and accounts for 30–40% of all premature deliveries (Baumeister & Woodley-Zanthos, 1996; Cohen, 2000). However when Romero and colleagues compared randomized antibiotic treatment to placebo, in a multicenter trial, there was no difference between the two groups in postponing birth (Romero, Sibai, et al., 1993).

FETAL STOKE

Fetal stroke has emerged as another identifiable pregnancy event that can result in MR. Fetal stroke is defined as an ischemic, thrombotic, or hemorrhagic event occurring between 14 weeks of gestation and the onset of labor. A recent literature review suggests that in 50% of the identified cases, the cause of the stroke is unknown. For the cases where risk factors were identified the most common maternal condition was ischemic injury, hemorrhagic disturbances of coagulation, and fetal disorders such as pyruvate carboxylase deficiency (Ozduman et al., 2004).

BIRTH TRAUMA AND ASPHYXIA

Birth injuries occur at the rate of approximately 2–7 per 1000 live births. The risk factors include macrosomy, prematurity, amniocentesis, cordocentesis, fetal surgical manipulations, dystocia, cephalopelvic disproportion, and the prolonged labor (Fanaroff & Hack, 1999). The most common consequences of birth injuries include blood clots, paralysis, and fracture. Neurological consequences are considered rare and are usually attributed to asphyxia.

Asphyxia is a combination of acidemia, hypoxia, and metabolic acidosis. An infant who exhibits acute neurological injury proximate to asphyxia usually has had profound metabolic or mixed academia (pH < 7) on an umbilical cord arterial blood sample, an Apgar score of 0–3 for longer than 5 min, neonatal neurological manifestations of seizures, coma, or hypotonia, and dysfunction on a multisystem level. The neurological outcome of asphyxiated infants is difficult to determine in the immediate postnatal period since the sequella are related to the period during development when the event occurred. Fetal asphyxia is associated with cerebral palsy although experts estimate that no more than 15% of cases of CP are explained by this mechanism (Goldenberg & Nelson, 1999).

HARMFUL CHEMICAL AND COMPOUNDS

A number of common chemicals and compounds, e.g., alcohol (EtOH) and lead, are known to be teratogenic and neurotoxic to human embryo and fetal development. Many other chemicals, such as mercury and polychlorinated biphenyls (PCBs), are known to have neurodevelopmental effects that cannot be detected until later in life; therefore they are not classified as teratogens (substances that produce harmful effects detected at birth).

Alcohol

Alcohol has been shown to be associated with a wide array of birth defects ranging from dysmorphia, growth deficiency, and behavioral and cognitive deficits. Heavy alcohol exposure or binge drinking has been associated with fetal alcohol syndrome (FAS) and lower doses of alcohol exposure have been associated with the milder version of symptoms characteristic of fetal alcohol effects (FAE) and alcohol-related neurodevelopmental disorder (ARND). Establishing the rates of these effects is dependent on the admission of alcohol use during pregnancy and the identification of the syndrome by an examining physician. The CDC has estimated FAS affected 6.7 per 10,000 live births in the United States in 1993 (CDC, 1995a). Research indicates that the outcome of intrauterine exposure is associated with the time of exposure and the sensitivity of the mother and fetus to EtOH (Sampson, Streissguth, Bookstein, & Barr, 2000).

THERAPEUTIC AND DIAGNOSTIC AGENTS

The Food and Drug Administration (FDA) has established five categories of drugs based on their potential for causing birth defects in infants born to women who use the drugs during pregnancy. Birth defects are structural defects that can be recognized at birth, and thus exclude cognitive deficits, which cannot be detected until later infancy and early childhood. Five categories (A, B, C, D, X) range from the safest, (A) controlled studies in women fail to demonstrate a risk to the fetus in the first trimester, and fetal harm appears remote, to (X) studies or experience have shown fetal risk that clearly outweighs any possible benefits. For each presenting problem there are medications that are preferred by most prescribing physicians, based on the FDA categories. Few of the drugs considered unsafe for use during pregnancy that have possible links to MR, include antimicrobials (e.g., sulfonamides, isoniazid, ribavirin), anticonvulsants (e.g., phenytoin, carbamazepine), and warfarin, aminoptein, and accutane. Unfortunately, the inability to detect subtle cognitive limitations in infants results in inconclusive recommendations for many drugs (Jones, 1999; McGuigan & Bailey, 2001) and, more generally, knowledge of potential fetal risk presented by a wide range of medications is incomplete.

ENVIRONMENTAL CHEMICALS

The fetus and the developing child need special consideration in the assessment of safety of environmental chemicals since the mitotic activity of cerebral neuronal development occurs prenatally and in the first 2 years of postnatal life. Dose and timing of the chemical exposure are critical variables in predicting neurotoxic outcomes and in many cases human data are insufficient to make accurate assessments of metals and chemicals (Sullivan & Krieger, 2001). Toluene, nitrous oxide, carbon monoxide, organochlorines, organophosphates, methanol, xylene, trichloroethylene, perchloroethylene, carbon disulfide, lead, mercury, arsenic, manganese, thallium, aluminum, carbon tetrachloride, methylene chloride, n-Hexane, and ethylene glycol have all been associated with some neurobehavioral dysfunctions (Filley & Kelly, 2001). In addition, others report that only 7% of high-volume chemicals have actually been tested for potential neurodevelopmental toxicity (Goldman & Koduru, 2000). In humans, the environmental metals and chemicals for which there are the most data are lead, methyl mercury (MeHg), and PCBs.

Lead has been one of the most widely studied neurotoxic substances with respect to neurodevelopmental disorders and recommendations for lead screening, abatement of environmental exposures, and activities for the prevention of lead poisoning in children are numerous. Lead can cross the placenta beginning at 12 weeks of gestation and it accumulates in fetal tissues. Reports of neurobehavioral problems have been associated with blood lead levels higher than 10 mg/dl (Baghurst et al., 1992; CDC, 1997b; Keogh & Boyer, 2001; Tong, 1998). In the last 30 years lead levels in children have decreased in the United States due to the abandonment of leaded gasoline use; however, children living in older homes with leaded paint and other exposures continue to be exposed. Attention deficits and hyperactivity, IQ decreases, and memory deficits are among the neurologic manifestations of lead exposure (Agency for Toxic Substances and Disease Registry [ATSDR], 2000; Wasserman, Graziano, et al., 1994; Wasserman, Liu, et al., 1997). The ATSDR also indicates that pregnant women and children can absorb far more ingested lead than the general adult population: up to 70% of lead is absorbed by the former group compared to 20% by the latter group.

Mercury is found in three states—elemental mercury, inorganic mercury salts, and organic mercury. Small amounts of elemental mercury are found in dental amalgams, thermometers, sphygmomanometers, and batteries. In addition, there are natural sources of elemental mercury such as the degassing of the earth's crust, forest fires, the evaporation of seawater, and volcanoes. Mercury also gets into the environment as a result of the combustion of fossil fuels that contain mercury. Inorganic mercury salts are present in some pesticides and disinfectants and in some medications as a preservative. Mercury is constantly cycling through the environment, evaporating into the atmosphere, and returning to the ground and water sources as the result of gravity or precipitation. Both elemental and inorganic mercury can be transformed by microorganisms in water and soil into organic mercury; and the most common organic mercury in the environment is MeHg. Bioaccumulation in the food chain results from MeHg taken up by bacteria and plankton eaten by small fish, subsequently eaten by larger fish, which are caught and eaten by humans and animals. All forms of mercury cross the placenta into the fetal circulation. Maternal exposure usually occurs from the consumption of fish containing MeHg and through inhalation and skin absorption of elemental and inorganic mercury. All forms of mercury can be toxic to the developing brain and the spectrum of effects range from deficits in learning and memory to a cerebral palsy-like syndrome, MR, and microcephaly (McGuigan & Bailey, 2001). The effects on infants born to mothers with high exposure to MeHg are mainly neurological, including developmental delay and altered muscle tone and tendon reflexes. At low doses, expected in human consumption of fish, there is no population-based evidence of risk (Davidson et al., 1998). There is human evidence of neural degeneration and glial proliferation occurring throughout the cerebral and cerebellar cortices at high exposure levels, and the clinical manifestations are related to the age of fetal exposure with the effects most pronounced in the second and third trimesters.

PCBs are a group of more than 100 chemicals, which are fat soluble and bioaccumulate in the food chain. The consumption of fish and shellfish is thought to be a major route of human exposure (Landrigan, 2001). Some of the earliest evidence of neurodevelopmental deficits produced by PCBs is from an incident in Taiwan where prenatal exposure to PCB-contaminated cooking oil resulted in lower IQs, spatial reasoning deficits, and developmental delays (Longnecker, Rogan, & Lucier, 1997). However at least one published study (Schell, Budinsky, & Wernke, 2001) refutes the association between PCBs and neurodevelopmental effects in humans. Long-term environmental exposures have been studied in pregnant women eating contaminated fish from Lake Michigan and the results suggest a long-term impact on intellectual function (Buck, 1996; Jacobson & Jacobson, 1996; Jacobson, Jacobson, & Humphrey, 1990). Children with PCB exposures were at greater risk of fetal and postnatal growth deficit and had lower full-scale and verbal IQs in infancy and at age 11 when compared to non-exposed children (Ribas-Fito, Sala, Kogevinas, & Sunyer, 2001). The latest study (Walkowiak et al., 2001; Winneke, Walkowiak, & Lilienthal, 2002) estimated the prenatal and perinatal PCB exposures of newborns in cord blood and maternal milk and followed the infants until 42 months of age, when PCB concentrations were measured in serum. This study found lower cognitive function in the children with higher levels of PCBs, after controlling for the home environment.

POSTNATAL INFECTIONS

Postnatal meningitis and encephalitis are associated with a variety of infectious agents and leave a proportion of children with permanent cognitive disability, particularly in less developed countries where access to vaccination and treatment is limited or delayed. In the U.S. immunization of infants against tetanus, pertussis, diphtheria, and influenza have reduced the occurrence of these vaccine-preventable diseases.

Hemophilus influenzae type b (HiB), an invasive bacterium that can cause meningitis, was one of the most significant infectious causes of MR, deafness, and death in the United States from 1980 to the mid-1990s. The peak incidence, 150/100,000 per year, was in 1986 among children 6–7 months of age. Since 1991 the conjugate vaccine has been available for infants at 2 months of age and the incidence has dramatically declined (CDC, 1995b; Wenger et al., 1990).

ENVIRONMENTAL EXPOSURES IN INFANCY AND EARLY CHILDHOOD

Lead exposure in early childhood, through ingestion of paint chips, inhalation of lead in dust, and ingestion of ground dirt contaminated with lead from automobile and industrial emissions, is associated with learning and behavior problems. Lead is ubiquitous in the environment and in many parts of the world a significant level of lead has been detected in breast milk (Rabinowitz, Leviton, & Needleman, 1985). Several studies have found higher blood lead levels in formula-fed infants than in breast-fed infants probably because of contaminated formula cans or tap water with high lead levels. Lead is known to affect the central nervous system and leads to reduction in cognitive functioning. The impact of lead exposure is reported to impact the cognitive functioning of 1.7 million children, 1–5 years of age, in the United States.

INJURIES

Severe, traumatic brain injury (i.e., with loss of consciousness for longer than 24 h) during childhood can result in long-term cognitive deficits and thus is a preventable cause of MR. In the United States, the leading causes of traumatic brain injury include falls, motor vehicle collisions, sport-related injuries, and assaults (including shaken-baby syndrome and gunshot wounds, Ewing-Cobbs, Prasad, Kramer, & Landry, 1999; Kraus, Fife, Cox, Ramstein, & Conroy, 1986; Thurman, Alverson, Dunn, Guerrero, & Sniezek, 1999). Despite the relatively high incidence of traumatic brain injuries to children in the population (2–3/1000 per year), evidence from epidemiologic studies indicates that trauma is an infrequent cause of MR (Annegers, Grabow, Kurland, & Laws, 1980; Blomquist, Gustavson, & Holmgren, 1981; Bower, Leonard, & Petterson, 2000; Durkin, Olsen, Barlow, Virella, & Connolly, 1998; Durkin, Schupf, Stein, & Susser, 1998; Gustavson et al., 1977a, 1977b; Kraus et al., 1986; Thurman & Guerrero, 1999). One possible explanation for the relatively minor role of trauma in the etiology of MR is that the majority of head injuries severe enough to result in MR is fatal. Another is that nonfatal brain injuries during childhood are followed by considerable recovery of function (Tomlin, Clarke, Robinson, & Roach, 2002). From a review of the literature, it appears that: (a) long-term sequella of traumatic brain injuries to children commonly include problems with memory, behavior, mood, and sleep, but rarely include significant deficits in general cognition (i.e., intelligence per se) and adaptive behavior (Emanuelson, von Wendt, Lundalv, & Larsson, 1996; Luis & Mittenberg, 2002); and (b) most studies of the relationship between trauma and MR focus on MR as a risk factor for trauma rather than trauma as a risk factor for MR (Konarski, Sutton, & Huffman, 1997; Sherrard, Tonge, & Ozanne-Smith., 2002). The fact that cognitive disability is a risk factor for injury makes it difficult from follow-up studies of brain-injured children to distinguish cognitive sequella from preexisting cognitive deficits.

DEPRIVATION

Deprivation in childhood includes children living in extreme poverty, those who experience disordered parenting because of mental illness or MR of a parent, and children faced with family stress, crisis, or neglect for any reason. The actual parent–child problems can include inadequate stimulation, deficient interpersonal nurturance, physical abuse, or malnutrition. In addition, there can be a confounding effect when children with disabilities and low cognitive function live in family chaos or in families with insufficient support systems. Societal advances that decrease the percentage of children living in poverty or increase the proportion of children attending stimulating child care can reduce deprivation and the exacerbating effect it has on children with established developmental deficits. Efficacious programs targeted at families without adequate resources to provide early stimulation can improve outcomes in these children. However, research has shown variability in the effectiveness of in home and out of home programs, and the effects do not extend far beyond the length of attendance (Garber, 1988; Gorman & Pollitt, 1996; Ramey & Ramey, 1998).

Effective prevention of MR must be accomplished by a multifaceted approach of both health-care delivery and educational interventions involving parents and young children. For example, an existing program, WIC—*The Special Supplemental Food Program for Women, Infants, and Children*, is a potentially effective, existing mechanism to define and reach the population at high risk. Expanding WIC services, already in place and staffed, to provide parent education or referral to high quality child stimulation programs would represent an adjustment of that program rather than the creation of a new bureaucratic service and delivery system. An MR-prevention intervention associated with WIC could reach children early in life, motivate both parent and child involvement, and combine health and education service components.

CONCLUSION

It is essential to take into account the synergistic effect of environmental and biologic factors which determine MR. The interplay among child and parental medical and social characteristics, poverty, and deprivation must be addressed both in program planning and in research. At the present time, there are established strategies to prevent some environmental and heritable causes of MR, although for religious, social, and ethical reasons they are not always carried out. Identification of causation is fundamental to developing prevention strategies. Prevention of MR challenges the established domains of education, medicine, basic science, and social service to work across discipline and organizational lines.

REFERENCES

Agency for Toxic Substances and Disease Registry. (2000). *Case studies in environmental medicine: Lead toxicity*. Atlanta, GA: Author.

Albrecht, U., Sutcliffe, J. S., Cattanach, B. M., Beechey, C.V., Armstrong, D., Eichele, G., et al. (1997). Imprinted expression of the murine Angelman syndrome gene, *UBE3A*, in hippocampal and Purkinje neurons. *Nature Genetics, 17*(1), 75–78.

Amar, H. S., Ho, J. J., & Mohan, A. J. (1999). Human immunodeficiency virus prevalence in women at delivery using unlinked anonymous testing of newborns in the Malaysian setting. *Journal of Paediatrics and Child Health, 35*(1), 63–66.

American Association on Mental Retardation. (1992). *Mental retardation: Definition, classification, and systems of supports* (9th ed.). Washington, DC: Author.

American Association on Mental Retardation. (2002). *Mental retardation: Definition, classification, and systems of supports* (10th ed.). Washington, DC: Author.

American Psychiatric Association. (1994). *Diagnostic and statistical manual of mental disorders* (4th ed.). Washington, DC: Author.

Annegers, J. F., Grabow, J. D., Kurland, L. T., & Laws, E. R. (1980). The incidence, causes, and secular trends of head trauma in Olmsted County, Minnesota, 1935–1974. *Neurology, 30*(9), 912–919.

Aries, F., Rodriquez, I., Rayne, S. C., & Krausu, F. T. (1993). Maternal placental vasculopathy and injection: Two distinct subgroups among patients with preterm labor and preterm ruptured membranes. *American Journal of Obstetrics and Gynecology, 168*(2), 585–591.

Baghurst, P. A., McMichael, A. J., Wigg, N. R., Vimpani, G. V., Robertson, E. F., Roberts, R. J., et al. (1992). Environmental exposure to lead and children's intelligence at the age of seven years. *New England Journal of Medicine, 327*(18), 1279–1284.

Baird, P. A., & Sadovnick, A. D. (1987). Life expectancy in Down's syndrome. *Journal of Pediatrics, 110*(6), 849–854.

Battaglia, A., & Carey, J. C. (2003). Diagnostic evaluation of developmental delay/mental retardation: An overview. *American Journal of Medical Genetics, 117C*, 3–14.

Baumeister, A. A., & Kupstas, F. D. (1991). The new morbidity: Implications for prevention and amelioration. In A. D. B. Clarke & P. Evan (Eds.), *Combating mental handicap: A multidisciplinary approach* (pp. 46–72). London: A.B. Academic .

Baumeister, A. A., & Woodley-Zanthos, P. (1996). Prevention: Biological factors. In J. W. Jacobson & J. A. Mulick (Eds.), *Manual of diagnosis and professional practice in mental retardation*. Washington, DC: American Psychological Association.

Bell, M. V., Hirst, M. C., Nakahori, Y., MacKinnon, R. N., Roche, A., Flint, T. J., et al. (1991). Physical mapping across the fragile X: Hypermethylation and clinical expression of the fragile X syndrome. *Cell, 64*, 861–866.

Belman, A. L. (1992). Acquired immunodeficiency syndrome in the child's central nervous system. *Pediatric Clinics of North America, 39*(4), 691–714.

Bennett, F. C., Sells, C. J., & Brand, C. (1979). Influences on measured intelligence in Down's syndrome. *American Journal of Diseases in Children, 133*(7), 700–703.

Beuren, A. J., Apitz, J., & Harmajanz, D. (1962). Supravalvular aortic stenosis in association with mental retardation and a certain facial appearance. *Circulation, 26*, 1235–1240.

Blomquist, H. K., Gustavson, K. H., & Holmgren, G. (1981). Mild mental retardation in children in a northern Swedish county. *Journal of Mental Deficiency Research, 25*(Pt. 3), 169–186.

Bower, L., Leonard, H., & Petterson, B. (2000). Intellectual disability in Western Australia. *Journal of Paediatrics and Child Health, 36*(3), 213–215.

Boylan, L., & Stein, Z. (1991). The epidemiology of HIV infection in children and their mothers—vertical transmission. *Epidemiologic Reviews, 13,* 143–177.

Broman, S., Nichols, P. L., Shaughnessy, P., & Kennedy, W. (1987). *Retardation in young children: A developmental study of cognitive deficit.* Hillsdale, NJ: Erlbaum.

Brown, W. T., Jenkins, E. C., & Friedman, E. (1982). Autism is associated with the fragile-X syndrome. *Journal of Autism and Developmental Disorders, 12*(3), 303–308.

Buck, G. M. (1996). Epidemiologic perspective of the developmental neurotoxicity of PCBs in humans. *Neurotoxicology and Teratology, 18*(3), 239–241; discussion 271–276.

Budarf, M. L., & Emanuel, B. S. (1997). Progress in the autosomal segmental aneusomy syndromes (SASs): Single or multi-locus disorders? *Human Molecular Genetics, 6*(10), 1657–1665.

Cao, X. Y., Jiang, X. M., Dou, Z. H., Rakeman, M. A., Zhang, M. L., O'Donnell, K., et al. (1994). Timing of vulnerability of the brain to iodine deficiency in endemic cretinism. *New England Journal of Medicine, 331*(26), 1739–1744.

Centers for Disease Control and Prevention. (1995a). Update: Trends in fetal alcohol syndrome—United States, 1979–1993. *JAMA, 273*(18), 1406.

Centers for Disease Control and Prevention. (1995b). Progress toward elimination of *Haemophilus influenzae* type b disease among infants and children—United States, 1993–1994. *Morbidity and Mortality Weekly Report, 44*(29), 545–550.

Centers for Disease Control and Prevention. (1997a). Rubella and congenital rubella syndrome—United States, 1994–1998. *Morbidity and Mortality Weekly Report, 46*(16), 350–354.

Centers for Disease Control and Prevention. (1997b). Update: Blood lead levels—United States, 1991–1994. *JAMA, 277*(13), 1031–1032.

Centerwall, S. A., & Centerwall, W. R. (1960). A study of children with Mongolism reared in the home compared to those reared away from the home. *Pediatrics, 25,* 678–685.

Chechlacz, M., & Gleeson, J. G. (2003). Is mental retardation a defect of synapse structure and function? *Pediatric Neurology, 29,* 11–17.

Chudley, A. E., Knoll, J., Gerrard, J. W., Shepel, L., McGahey, E., & Anderson, J. (1983). Fragile (X) X-linked mental retardation. I. Retardation between age and intelligence and the frequency of expression of fragile (X) (q28). *American Journal of Medicine Genetics, 14*(4), 699–712.

Clarke, A. M., & Clarke, A. D. B. (1976). *Early experience: Myth and evidence.* New York: Free.

Clarke, D., Boer, H., Cheung, M., Sturney, P., & Webb, T. (1996). Maladaptive behavior in Prader–Willi syndrome in adults life. *Journal of Intellectual Disability Research, 40*(Pt. 2), 159–165.

Clements, P. R., Bates, M. V., & Hafer, M. (1976). Variability within Down's syndrome (trisomy-21): Empirically observed sex differences in IQs. *Mental Retardation, 14*(1), 30–31.

Cohen, W. (Ed.). (2000). *Cherry and Merkatz's complications of pregnancy* (5th ed.). Philadelphia, PA: Lippincott.

Connolly, B. H., Morgan, S. B., & Russell, F. F. (1984). Evaluation of children with Down syndrome who participated in an early intervention program. *Physical Therapy, 64*(10), 150–151.

Creasy, R. K., & Iams, J. D. (1999). Preterm labor and delivery. In R. K. Creasy & R. Rasnik (Eds.), *Maternal-fetal medicine* (4th ed., pp. 498–531). Philadelphia, PA: Saunders.

Cuckle, H. S., Wald, N. J., & Thompson, S. G. (1987). Estimating a woman's risk of having a pregnancy associated with Down's syndrome using her age and serum alpha-fetoprotein level. *British Journal of Obstetrics and Gynaecology, 94*(5), 387–402.

Czeizel, A. E. (1995). Folic acid in the prevention of neural tube defects. *Journal of Pediatric Gastroenterology and Nutrition, 20*(1), 4–16.

Davidson, P. W., Myers, G. J., Cox, C., Axtell, C., Shamlaye, C., Sloane-Reeves, J., et al. (1998). Effects of prenatal and postnatal methylmercury exposure from fish consumption on neurodevelopment: Outcomes at 66 months of age in the Seychelles Child Development Study. *JAMA, 280*(8), 701–707.

Dennis, W. (1973). *Children of the crèche.* New York: Appleton-Century-Croft.

de Vries, B. B., Jansen, C. C., Duits, A. A., Verheij, C., Willemsen, R., van Hemel, J. O., et al. (1996). Variable *FMR1* gene methylation of large expansion leads to variable phenotype in three males from one fragile X family. *Journal of Medical Genetics, 33*(12), 1007–1010.

de Vries, B. B., van den Ouweland, A. M., Mohkamsing, S., Duivenvoorden, H. J., Mol, E., Gelsema, K., et al. (1997). Screening and diagnosis for the fragile X syndrome among the mentally retarded: An epidemiological and psychological survey. Collaborative Fragile X Study Group. *American Journal of Human Genetics, 61*(3), 660–667.

Donders, G. G., Desmyter, J., De Wet, D. H., & Ban Assche, F. A. (1993). The association of gonorrhoea and syphilis with premature birth and low birthweight. *Genitourinary Medicine, 69*(2), 98–101.

Drillien, C. M., Pickering, R. M., & Drummond, M. B. (1988). Predictive value of screening for difficult areas of development. *Developmental Medicine and Child Neurology, 30*, 294–305.

Dunn, D., Wallon, M., Peyron, F., Peterson, E., Peckham, C., & Gilbert, R. (1999). Mother-to-child transmission of toxoplasmosis: Risk estimates for clinical counseling. *Lancet, 353*(9167), 1829–1833.

Durkin, M., Schupf, N., Susser, M., & Stein, Z. (2001). Epidemiology of mental retardation. In M. Levene, R. Lilford, M. J. Bennet & J. Punt. (Eds.), *Fetal neurology and neurosurgery* (3rd ed., pp. 719–818). London: Churchill Livingstone.

Durkin, M. S., Olsen, S., Barlow, B., Virella, A., & Connolly, E. S. (1998). The epidemiology of urban, pediatric, neurological trauma: Evaluation of, and implications for, injury prevention programs. *Neurosurgery, 42*(2), 300–310.

Durkin, M. S., Schupf, N., Stein, Z. A., & Susser, M. W. (1998). Mental retardation. In R. B. Wallace (Ed.), *Public health and preventive medicine* (pp. 1049–1058). Stamford, CT: Appleton & Lange.

Durkin, M. S., & Stein, Z. A. (1996). Classification of mental retardation. In J. W. Jacobson & J. A. Mulick (Eds.), *Manual of diagnosis and professional practice in mental retardation.* Washington, DC: American Psychological Association.

Dykens, E. M., Leckman, J. F., & Cassify, S. B. (1996). Obsession and compulsions in Prader–Willi syndrome. *Journal of Child Psychiatry, 37*(8), 995–1002.

Editorial Board. (1996). Definition of mental retardation. In J. W. Jacobson & J. A. Mulick (Eds.), *Manual of diagnosis and professional practice in mental retardation* (pp. 13–38). Washington, DC: American Psychological Association.

Emanuelson, I., von Wendt, L., Lundalv, E., & Larsson, J. (1996). Rehabilitation and follow-up of children with severe traumatic brain injury. *Childs Nervous System, 12*(8), 460–465.

Epstein, C. M. (1986). *The consequences of chromosome imbalance.* Cambridge, UK: Cambridge University Press.

European Mode of Delivery Collaboration. (1999). Elective caesarean-section versus vaginal delivery in prevention of vertical HIV-1 transmission: A randomized clinical trial. *Lancet, 353*(9158), 1030–1031.

Ewart, A. K., Morris, C. A., Atkinson, D., Jin, W., Sternes, K., Spallone, P., et al. (1993). Hemizygosity at the elastin locus in a developmental disorder, Williams syndrome. *Nature Genetics, 5*(1), 11–16.

Ewing-Cobbs, L., Prasad, M., Kramer, L., & Landry, S. (1999). Inflicted traumatic brain injury: Relationship of developmental outcome to severity of injury. *Pediatric Neurosurgery, 31*(5), 251–258.

Fanaroff, A. A., & Hack, M. (1999) Periventricular leukomalacia—prospects for prevention. *New England Journal of Medicine, 341*(16), 1229–1231.

Faro, S., & Soper, D. E. (2001). Infectious diseases in women (1st ed.). Philadelphia, PA: WB Saunders.

Feldman, E. J. (1996). The recognition and investigation of X-linked learning disability syndromes. *Journal of Intellectual Disability Research, 40*(Pt. 5), 400–411.

Filley, C. K., & Kelly, J. P. (2001). Clinical neurotoxicology and neurobehavioral toxicology. In J. B. Sullivan & G. R. Krieger (Eds.), *Clinical environmental health and toxic exposures.* Denver, CO: Lippincott, Williams & Wilkins.

Fishkin, P. E., Armstrong, F. D., Routh, D. K., Harris, L., Thompson, W., Miloslavich, K., et al. (2000). Brief report: Relationship between HIV infection and WPPSI-R performance in preschool-age children. *Journal of Pediatric Psychology, 25*(5), 347–351.

Flint, J., Wilkie, A. O., Buckle, V. J., Winter, R. M., Holland, A. J., & McDermid, H. E. (1995). The detection of subtelomeric chromosomal rearrangements in idiopathic mental retardation. *Nature Genetics, 9*(2), 132–140.

Frangiskakis, J. M., Ewart, A. K., Morris, C. A., Mervis, C. B., Bertrand, J., Robinson, B. F., et al. (1996). LIM-kinase1 hemizygosity implicated in impaired visuospatial constructive cognition. *Cell, 86*(1), 59–69.

Frankenberger, W., & Harper, J. (1988). States' definitions and procedures for identifying children with mental retardation: Comparison of 1981–1982 and 1985–1986 guidelines. *Mental Retardation, 26*(3), 133–136.

Freij, B. J., & Sever, J. L. (1997). Varicella. In J. T. Queenan & J. C. Hobbins (Eds.), *Protocols for high risk pregnancies* (3rd ed., pp. 387–397). Cambridge, MA: Blackwell Science.

Fu, Y. H., Kuhl, D. P., Pizzuti, A., Pieretti, M., Sutcliffe, J. S., Richards, S., et al. (1991). Variation of the CGG repeat at the fragile X site results in genetic stability: Resolution of the Sherman paradox. *Cell, 67*(6), 1047–1058.

Garber, H. (1988). *The Milwaukee project: Preventing mental retardation in children at risk.* Washington, DC: American Association on Mental Retardation.

Gedeon, A. K., Baker, E., Robinson, H., Partington, M. W., Gross, B., Manca, A., et al. (1992). Fragile X syndrome without CGG amplification has an *FMR1* deletion. *Nature Genetics, 1*(5), 341–344.

Gibbs, R. S., & Sweet, R. L. (1999). Maternal and fetal infectious disorders. In R K Creasy & R. Rasnik (Eds.), *Maternal-fetal medicine* (4th ed., pp. 685–689). Philadelphia, PA: Saunders

Gilstrap, L. C. (1997). *Infections in pregnancy* (2nd ed.). New York: Wiley.

Goldenberg, R. L., & Nelson, K. G. (1999). In R. K. Creasy & R. Rasnik (Eds.), *Maternal-fetal medicine* (4th ed., pp. 1194–1214). Philadelphia, PA: Saunders.

Goldman, L. R., & Koduru, S. (2000). Chemicals in the environment and developmental toxicity to children: A public health and policy perspective. *Environmental Health Perspectives, 108*(Suppl. 3), 443–448.

Gorman, K. S., & Pollitt, E. (1996). Does schooling buffer the effects of early risk? *Child Development, 67*(2), 314–326.

Guerina, N. G., Hsu, H. W., Meissner, H. C., Maguire, J. H., Lynfield, R., Stechenburg, B., et al. (1994). Neonatal serological screening and early treatment for congenital Toxoplasma gondii infection. *New England Journal of Medicine, 330*(26), 1858–1863.

Gustavson, K. H., Hagberg, B., Hagberg, G., & Sars, K. (1977a). Severe mental retardation in a Swedish county. I. Epidemiology, gestational age, birth weight and associated CNS handicaps in children born 1959–1970. *Acta Paediatrica Scandinavica, 66,* 373–379.

Gustavson, K. H., Hagberg, B., Hagberg, G., & Sars, K. (1977b). Severe mental retardation in a Swedish county: Etiological and pathogenic aspects of children born 1959–1970. *Neuropadiatrie, 8*(3), 293–304.

Hagberg, B., & Hagberg, G. (1997). Rett syndrome: Epidemiology and geographical variability. *European Child and Adolescent Psychiatry, 6*(Suppl. 1), 5–7.

Hagerman, R. J., Hull, C. E., Safanda, J. F., Carpenter, I., Staley, L. W., O'Connor, R. A., et al. (1994). High functioning fragile X males: Demonstration of an unmethylated fully expanded FMR-1 mutation associated with protein expression. *American Journal of Medical Genetics, 51*(4), 298–308.

Hagerman, R. J., Jackson, C., Amiri, K., Silverman, A. C., O'Conner, R., & Sobesky, W. (1992). Girls with fragile X syndrome physical and neurocognitive status and outcome. *Pediatrics, 89*(3), 395–400.

Hagerman, R. J., & Silverman, A. C. (Eds.). (1991). Fragile X syndrome, diagnosis, treatment and research. Baltimore: Johns Hopkins University Press.

Hagerman, R. J., Wilson, P., Staley, L. W., Lang, K. A., Fan, T., Uhlhorn, C., et al. (1994). Evaluation of school children at high risk for fragile X syndrome utilizing bucal cell FMR-1 testing. *American Journal of Medical Genetics, 51*(4), 474–481.

Hanley, W. B., Platt, L. D., Bachman, R. P., Buist, N., Geraghty, M. T., Isaacs, J., et al. (1999). Undiagnosed maternal phenylketonuria: The need for prenatal selective screening or case finding. *American Journal of Obstetrics and Gynecology, 180*(4), 986–994.

Hassold, T. J., Burrage, L. C., Chan, E. R., Judis, L. M., Schwartz, S., James, J., et al. (2001). Maternal folate polymorphisms and the etiology of human nondisjunction. *American Journal of Human Genetics, 69*(2), 434–439.

Hassold, T., Chiu, D., & Yamane, J. A. (1984). Parental origin of autosomal trisomies. *Annals of Human Genetics, 48*(Pt. 2), 129–144.

Hetzel, B. S. (1989). *The story of iodine deficiency: An international challenge in nutrition.* Oxford: Oxford University Press.

Hobbs, C. A., Sherman, S. L., Yi, P., Hopkins, S. E., Torfs, C. P., Hine, R. J., et al. (2000). Polymorphisms in genes involved in folate metabolism as maternal risk factors for Down syndrome. *American Journal of Human Genetics, 67*(3), 623–630.

Holden, J. J., Percy, M., Allingham-Hawkins, D., Brown, W. T., Chiurazzi, P., Fisch, G., et al. (1999). Conference Report: Eighth International Workshop on the fragile X syndrome and X-linked mental retardation, August 16–22, 1997. *American Journal of Medical Genetics, 83*(4), 221–236.

Holland, A. J., Hon, J., Huppert, F. A., & Watson, P. (1998). Population-based study of the prevalence and presentation of dementia in adults with Down syndrome. *British Journal of Psychiatry, 172,* 493–498.

Hook, E. B. (1982). Epidemiology of Down syndrome. In S. M. Pueschel & J. E. Rynders (Eds.), *Down syndrome: Advances in biomedicine and the behavioral sciences* (pp. 11–18). Cambridge, MA: Ware .

Hook, E. B., & Cross, P. K. (1987). Rates of mutant and inherited structural cytogenetic abnormalities detected at amniocentesis: Results of about 63,000 fetuses. *Annals of Human Genetics, 51,* 27–55.

Iams, J. D., Talbert, M. L., Barrows, H., & Sachs, L. (1985). Management of preterm rupture of the membranes: A prospective randomized comparison of observation versus use of steroids and timed delivery. *American Journal of Obstetrics and Gynecology, 151*(1), 32–38.

Jacobs, P. A., Bullman, H., Macpherson, J., Youings, S., Rooney, V., Watson, A., et al. (1993). Population studies of fragile X: A molecular approach. *Journal of Medical Genetics, 30*(6), 454–459.

Jacobson, J., & Jacobson, S. (1996). Intellectual impairment in children exposed to polychlorinated biphenyls in utero. *New England Journal of Medicine, 335*(11), 783–789.

Jacobson, J., Jacobson, S., & Humphrey, H. (1990). Effects of in utero exposure to polychlorinated biphenyls and related contaminants on cognitive functioning in young children. *Journal of Pediatrics, 116*(1), 38–45.

Jacobson, J. W., & Mulick, J. A. (1996). *Manual of diagnosis and professional practice in mental retardation.* Washington, DC: American Psychological Association.

James, S. J., Pogribna, M., Pogribny, I. P., Melnyk, S., Hine, R. J., Gibson, J. B., et al. (1999). Abnormal folate metabolism and mutation in the methylenetetrahydrofolate reductase gene may be maternal risk factors for Down syndrome. *American Journal of Clinical Nutrition, 70*(4), 495–501.

Jiang, Y.-H., Tsai ,T.-F., Bressler, J., & Beaudet, A. L. (1998). Imprinting in Angelman and Prader–Willi syndromes. *Current Opinion in Genetics and Development, 8*(3), 334–342.

Johnson, P. M. (1995). Immunology of pregnancy. In G. Chamberlain (Ed.), *Turnbull's obstetrics* (2nd ed., pp. 143–159). Edinburgh, UK: Churchill Livingstone.

Jones, K. L. (1999). Effects of therapeutic, diagnostic and environmental agents. In R. K. Creasy & R. Rasnik (Eds.), *Maternal-fetal medicine* (4th ed., pp. 132–144). Philadelphia, PA: Saunders.

Keogh, J. P., & Boyer, L. V. (2001). Lead. In J. B. Sullivan & G. R. Krieger. (Eds.), *Clinical environmental health and toxic exposures* (pp. 879–889). Baltimore: Lippincott Williams & Wilkins.

Kerr, A. M., & Ravine, D. (2003). Review article: Breaking new ground with Rett syndrome. *Journal of Intellectual Disability Research, 47*(8), 580–587.

Kiely, M. (1987). The prevalence of mental retardation. *Epidemiologic Reviews, 9,* 194–218.

Kline, J., Stein, Z., & Susser, M. (1989). *Conception to birth: Epidemiology of prenatal development.* New York: Oxford University Press.

Knight, S. J., Regan, R., Nicod, A., Horsely, S. W., Kearney, L., Homfray, T., et al. (1999). Subtle chromosomal rearrangements in children with unexplained mental retardation. *Lancet, 354*(9191), 1676–1681.

Knoll, J. H., Nicholls, R. D., Magenis, R. E., Graham, J. M., Jr., Lalande, M., & Latt, S. A. (1989). Angelman and Prader–Willi syndromes share a common chromosome 15 deletion but differ in parental origin of the deletion. *American Journal of Medical Genetics, 32*(2), 285–290.

Konarski, E. A., Sutton, K., & Huffman, A. (1997). Personal characteristics associated with episodes of injury in a residential facility. *American Journal of Mental Retardation, 102*(1), 37–44.

Kraus, J. F., Fife, D., Cox, P., Ramstein, K., & Conroy, C. (1986). Incidence, severity, and external causes of pediatric brain injury. *American Journal of Diseases of Children, 140*(7), 687–693.

Kremer, E. J., Pritchard, M., Lynch, M., Yu, S., Holman, K., Baker, E., et al. (1991). Mapping of DNA instability at the fragile X to a trinucleotide repeat sequence p(CCG)n. *Science, 252*(5013), 1711–1714.

Lai, F., Kammann, E., Rebeck, G. W., Anderson, A., Chen, Y., & Nixon, R. A. (1999). APOE genotype and gender effects on Alzheimer disease in 100 adults with Down syndrome. *Neurology, 53*(2), 331–336.

Landrigan, P. J. (2001). Pesticides and polychlorinated biphenyls (PCBs): An analysis of the evidence that they impair children's neurobehavioral development. *Molecular Genetics and Metabolism, 73*(1), 11–17.

Larson, S. A., Lakin, K. C., Anderson, L., Kwak, N., Lee, M., & Anderson, D. (2001). Prevalence of mental retardation and developmental disabilities: Estimates from the 1994/1995 National Health Interview Survey Disability Supplements. *American Journal of Mental Retardation, 106*(3), 231–252.

Lazar, I., & Darlington, R. (1982). Lasting effects of early education: A report from the consortium for longitudinal studies. *Monographs of the Society for Research in Child Development, 47*(2–3), 1–151.

Lebech, M., Andersen, O., Christensen, N. C., Hertel, J., Nielsen, H. E., Peitersen, B., et al. (1999). Feasibility of neonatal screening for toxoplasma infection in the absence of prenatal treatment. Danish Congenital Toxoplasmosis Study Group. *Lancet, 353*(9167), 1834–1837.

Ledbetter, D., Riccardi, V., Airhart, S., Strobel, R., Keenean, B., & Crawford, J. (1981). Deletions of chromosome 15 as a cause of the Prader–Willi syndrome. *New England Journal of Medicine, 304*(6), 325–329.

Lenke, R. R., & Levy, H. L. (1980). Maternal phenylketonuria and hyperphenylalaninemia: An international survey of the outcome of untreated and treated pregnancies. *New England Journal of Medicine, 303*(21), 1202–1208.

Leviton, A., & Gilles, F. (1996). Ventriculomegaly, delayed myelination, white matter hypoplasia, and "periventricular" leukomalacia: how are they related? *Pediatric Neurology, 15*(2), 127–136.

Leviton, A., & Paneth, N. (1990). White matter damage in preterm newborns—an epidemiologic perspective. *Early Human Development, 24*(1), 1–22.

Levy, H. L., & Ghavami, M. (1996). Maternal phenylketonuria: A metabolic teratogen. *Teratology, 53*(3), 176–184.

Levy, H. L., & Waisbren, S. E. (1983). Effects of untreated maternal phenylketonuria and hyperphenylalaninemia on the fetus. *New England Journal of Medicine, 309*(21), 1269–1274.

Lewis, M., & Goldberg, S. (1969). Perceptual-cognitive development in infancy: A generalized expectancy model as a function of mother–infant interaction. *Merrill-Palmer Quarterly, 15*, 81–100.

Liu, H., Momotani, N., & Yoshimura, J. (1994). Maternal hypothyroidism during early pregnancy and intellectual development of the progeny. *Archives of Internal Medicine, 154*(7), 785–787.

Longnecker, M. P., Rogan, W. J., & Lucier, G. (1997). The human effects of DDT and PCBs and an overview of organochlorines in public health. *Annual Review of Public Health, 18*, 211–244.

Lubs, H. A. (1969). A marker-X chromosome. *American Journal of Human Genetics, 21*(3), 231–244.

Luis, C. A., & Mittenberg, W. (2002). Mood and anxiety disorders following pediatric traumatic brain injury: A prospective study. *Journal of Clinical and Experimental Neuropsychology*, 24(3), 270–279.

Macmillan, C., Magder, L. S., Brouwers, P., Chase, C., Hittelman, J., Lasky, T., et al. (2001). Head growth and neurodevelopment of infants born to HIV-1 infected drug-using women. *Neurology*, 57(8), 1402–1411.

Martin, D., & Schoub, B. (2000). Rubella infection in pregnancy. In M. L. Newell & J. McIntyre. (Eds.), *Congenital and perinatal infections: Prevention, diagnosis and treatment*. Cambridge, UK: Cambridge University Press.

Martin, G. M. (1978). Genetic syndromes in man with potential relevance to pathobiology of aging. *Birth Defects Original Articles Series*, 14(1), 5–39.

Massey, P. S., & McDermott, S. (1995). State-specific rates of mental retardation—United States, 1993. *Morbidity and Mortality Weekly Report*, 45, 61–65.

Matsuura, T., Sutcliffe, J. S., Fang, P., Galjaard, R. J., Jiang, Y. H., Benton, C. S., et al. (1997). De novo truncating mutations in E6-AP ubiquitin-protein ligase gene (*UBE3A*) in Angelman syndrome. *Nature Genetics*, 15(1), 74–77.

McDermott, S. (1994). Explanatory model to describe school district prevalence rates for mental retardation and learning disabilities. *American Journal of Mental Retardation*, 99(2), 175–185.

McDermott, S., Callaghan, W., Szwejbka, L., Mann, H., & Daguise, V. (2000). Urinary tract infections during pregnancy and mental retardation and developmental delay. *Obstetrics and Gynecology*, 96(1), 113–119.

McDermott, S., Daguise, V., Mann, H., Szwejbka, L., & Callaghan, W. (2001). Perinatal risk for mortality and mental retardation associated with maternal urinary-tract infections. *Journal of Family Practice*, 50(5), 433–437.

McGuigan, M. A., & Bailey, B. (2001). In J. B. Sullivan & G. R. Krieger (Eds.), Clinical environmental health and toxic exposures (pp. 289–299). Baltimore: Lippincott Williams & Wilkins.

McLaren, J., & Bryson, S. E. (1987). Review of recent epidemiological studies of mental retardation: Prevalence, associated disorders, and etiology. *American Journal of Mental Retardation*, 92(3), 243–254.

Meadows, K. L., Pettay, D., Newman, J., Hersey, J., Ashley, A. E., & Sherman, S. L. (1996). Survey of the fragile X syndrome and the fragile X E syndrome in a special education needs population. *American Journal of Medical Genetics*, 64(2), 428–433.

Melyn, M. A., & White, D. T. (1973). Mental and developmental milestones of noninstitutionalized Down's syndrome children. *Pediatrics*, 52(4), 542–545.

Mialky, E., Vagnoni, J., & Rutstein, R. (2001). School-age children with perinatally acquired HIV infection: Medical and psychosocial issues in a Philadelphia cohort. *AIDS Patient Care and STDS*, 15(11), 575–579.

Morgan-Capner, P. (1999). Rubella. In D. J. Jeffries & C. N. Hudson (Eds.), *Viral Infections in obstetrics and gynaecology*. London: Arnold.

Morton, J. E., Bundey, S., Webb, T. P., Macdonald, F., Rindl, P. M., & Bullock, S. (1997). Fragile X syndrome is less common than previously estimated. *Journal of Medical Genetics*, 34(1), 1–5.

Mowery-Rushton, P. A., Driscoll, D. J., Nicholls, R. D., Locker, J., & Surti, U. (1996). DNA methylation patterns in human tissues of uniparental origin using a zinc-finger gene (*ZNF127*) from the Angelman/Prader–Willi region. *Human Molecular Genetics*, 61(2), 140–146.

MRC Vitamin Study Group. (1991). Prevention of neural tube defects: Results of the Medical Research Council vitamin study. *Lancet*, 338(8760), 131–137.

Murray, A., Youings, S., Dennis, N., Latsky, L., Linehan, P., McKechnie, N., et al. (1996). Population screening at the FRAXA and FRAXE loci: Molecular analyses of boys with learning difficulties and their mothers. *American Journal of Medical Genetics*, 5(6), 727–735.

National Center for Health Statistics. (2000). National Health Interview Survey. Retrieved December 3, 2002, from National Center for Health Statistics, National Health Interview Survey (NHIS) Web site: http://www.cdc.gov/nchs/nhis.htm

Nicholls, R. D. (1993). Genomic imprinting and candidate genes in the Prader–Willi and Angelman syndromes. *Current Genetic Developments, 3*(3), 445–456.

Nicholson, A., & Alberman, E. (1992). Prediction of the number of Down's syndrome infants to be born in England and Wales up to the year 2000 and their likely survival rates. *Journal of Intellectual Disability Research, 36*(Pt. 6), 505–517.

Nolin, S. L., Glicksman, A., Houck, G., Brown, W. T., & Dobkin, C. S. (1994). Mosaicism in fragile X affected males. *American Journal of Medical Genetics, 51*(4), 509–512.

Oberle, I., Rousseau, F., Heitz, D., Kretz, C., Devys, D., Hanauer, A., et al. (1991). Instability of a 550-base pair DNA segment and abnormal methylation in fragile X syndrome. *Science, 252*(5010), 1097–1102.

O'Donnell, K. J., Rakeman, M. A., Zhi-Hong, D., Xue-Yi, C., Mei, Z. Y., DeLong, N., et al. (2002). Effects of iodine supplementation during pregnancy on child growth and development at school age. *Developmental Medicine and Child Neurology, 44*(2), 76–81.

O'Leary, V. B., Parle-McDermott, A., Molloy, A. M., Kirke, P. N., Johnson, Z., Conley, M., et al. (2002). MTRR and MTHFR polymorphism: Link to Down syndrome? *American Journal of Medical Genetics, 107*(2), 151–155.

Oliver, C., & Holland, A. J. (1986). Down syndrome and Alzheimer's disease: A review. *Psychological Medicine, 16*(2), 307–322.

Opitz, J. M., & Sutherland, G. R. (1984). Conference report: International Workshop on the fragile X and X-linked mental retardation. *American Journal of Medical Genetics, 17*(1), 5–94.

Osborne, L. R., Martindale, D., Scherer, S. W., Shi, X. M., Huizenga, J., Heng, H. H., et al. (1996). Identification of genes from a 500-kb region at 7q11.23 that is commonly deleted in Williams-syndrome patients. *Genomics, 36*, 328–336.

O'Shea, T. M., & Dammann, O. (2000). Antecedents of cerebral palsy in very low birth weight infants. *Clinics in Perinatology, 27*(2), 285–302.

Ozcelik, T., Leff, S., Robinson, W., Donlon, T., Lalande, M., Sanjines, E., et al. (1992). Small nuclear ribonucleoprotein polypeptide N (SNRPN), an expressed gene in the Prader–Willi syndrome critical region. *Nature Genetics, 9*, 395–400.

Ozduman, K., Pober, B. R., Barnes, P., Copel, J. A., Ogle, E. A., Duncan, C. C., et al. (2004). Fetal stroke. *Pediatric Neurology, 30*, 151–162.

Paryani, S. G., & Arvin, A. M. (1986). Intrauterine infection with varicella-zoster virus after maternal varicella. *New England Journal of Medicine, 314*(24), 1542–1546.

Peckham, C. (1991). Cytomegalovirus infection, congenital and neonatal disease. *Scandinavian Journal of Infectious Diseases, 80*(Suppl.), 82–87.

Peoples, R., Perez-Jurado, L., Wang, Y.-K., Kaplan, P., & Francke, U. (1996). The gene for replication factor C subunit (RFC2) is within the 7q11.23 Williams syndrome deletion. *American Journal of Human Genetics, 58*(6), 1370–1373.

Perez-Jurado, L. A., Peoples, R., Kaplan, P., Hamel, B. C. J., & Francke, U. (1996). Molecular definition of the chromosome 7 deletion in Williams syndrome and parent-of-origin effects on growth. *American Journal of Human Genetics, 59*(4), 781–792.

Pieretti, M., Zhang, F. P., Fu, Y. H., Warren, S. T., Oostra, B. A., Caskey, C. T., et al. (1991). Absence of expression of the *FMR-1* gene in fragile X syndrome. *Cell, 66*, 817–822.

Popp, S., Schulze, B., Granzow, M., Keller, M., Holtgreve-Grez, H., Schoell, B., et al. (2002). Study of 30 patients with unexplained developmental delay and dysmorphic features or congenital abnormalities using conventional cytogenetics and multiplex FISH telomere (MTEL) integrity assay. *Human Genetics, 111*(1), 31–39.

Preblud, S., Cochi, S., & Orenstein, W. (1986). Varicella-zoster infection in pregnancy. *New England Journal of Medicine, 315*(22), 1415–1417.

Rabinowitz, M., Leviton, A., & Needleman, H. (1985). Lead in Milk and Infant Blood: A dose-response model. *Archives of Environmental Health, 40*(5), 283–286.

Ramey, C. T., & Ramey, S. L. (1998). Prevention of intellectual disabilities: Early interventions to improve cognitive development. *Preventive Medicine, 27*(2), 224–232.

Reiss, A. L., Abrams, M. T., Greenlaw, R., Freund, L., & Denckla, M. B. (1995). Neurodevelopmental effects of the FMR-1 full mutation in humans. *Nature Medicine, 1*(2), 159–167.

Reiss, A. L., Aylward, E., Freund, L. S., Joshi, P. K., & Bryan, R. N. (1991). Neuroanatomy of fragile X syndrome: The posterior fossa. *Annals of Neurology, 29*, 26–32.

Reiss, A. L., & Freund, L. (1990). Fragile X syndrome, DSM-III-R and autism. *Journal of the American Academy of Child and Adolescent Psychiatry, 29*(6), 885–891.

Reiss, A. L., Lee, J., & Freund, L. (1994). Neuroanatomy of fragile X syndrome: The temporal lobe. *Neurology, 44*(7), 1317–1324.

Remington, J. S., McLeod, R., & Desmonts, G. (1995). Toxoplasmosis. In J. S. Remington & J. O. Klein (Eds.), *Infectious diseases of the fetus and newborn infant* (4th ed., pp. 140–267). Philadelphia: WB Saunders.

Ribas-Fito, N., Sala, M., Kogevinas, M., & Sunyer, J. (2001). Polychlorinated biphenyls (PCBs) and neurological development in children: A systematic review. *Journal of Epidemiology and Community Health, 55*(8), 537–546.

Roizen, N., Swisher, C. N., & Stein, M. A. (1995). Neurologic and developmental outcome in treated congenital toxoplasmosis. *Pediatrics, 95*, 11–20.

Romero, R., Sibai, B., Caritis, S., Paul, R., Depp, R., Rosen, M., et al. (1993). Antibiotic treatment of preterm labor with intact membranes: A multicenter, randomized, double-blinded, placebo-controlled trial. *American Journal of Obstetrics and Gynecology, 169*(4), 764–774.

Romero, R., Yoon, B. H., Mazor, M., Gomez, R., Diamond, M. P., Kenney, J. S., et al. (1993). The diagnostic and prognostic value of amniotic fluid white blood cell count, glucose, interleukin-6, and Gram-stain in patients with preterm labor and intact membranes. *American Journal of Obstetrics and Gynecology, 169*(4), 805–816.

Rouse, B., Azen, C., Koch, R., Matalon, R., Hanley, W., de la Cruz, F., et al. (1997). Maternal Phenylketonuria Collaborative Study (MPKUCS) offspring: Facial anomalies, malformations, and early neurological sequelae. *American Journal of Medical Genetics, 69*(1), 89–95.

Rousseau, F., Heitz, D., Tarleton, J., MacPherson, J., Malmgren, H., Dahl, N., et al. (1994). A multicenter study on genotype–phenotype correlation in the fragile X syndrome, using direct diagnosis with probe StB12.3: The first 2253 cases. *American Journal of Human Genetics, 55*(2), 225–237.

Rousseau, F., Rouillard, P., Morel, M. L., Khandjian, E. W., & Morgan, K. (1995). Prevalence of carriers of premutation-size alleles of the *FMR1* gene and implications for the population genetics of the fragile X syndrome. *American Journal of Human Genetics, 57*(5), 1006–1018.

Rumble, B., Retallack, R., Hilbich, C., Simms, G., Multhaup, G., Martins, R., et al. (1989). Amyloid A4 protein and its precursor in Down's syndrome and Alzheimer's disease. *New England Journal of Medicine, 320*(22), 1446–1452.

Rynders, J. E., Spiker, D., & Horrobin, J. M. (1978). Underestimating the educability of Down's syndrome children: Examination of methodological problems in recent literature. *American Journal of Mental Deficiency, 82*(5), 440–448.

Sampson, P. D., Streissguth, A. P., Bookstein, F. L., & Barr, H. M. (2000). On categorization in analyses of alcohol teratogenisis. *Environmental Health Perspectives, 108*(Suppl. 3), 421–428.

Sare, Z., Ruvalcaba, R. H., & Kelly, V. C. (1978). Prevalence of thyroid disorder in Down syndrome. *Clinical Genetics, 14*(3), 154–158.

Schell, J. D., Jr., Budinsky, R. A., & Wernke, M. J. (2001). PCBs and neurodevelopmental effects in Michigan children: An evaluation of exposure and dose characterization. *Regulatory Toxicology and Pharmacology, 33*, 300–312.

Schupf, N., & Sergievsky, G. H. (2002). Genetic and host factors for dementia in Down syndrome. *British Journal of Psychiatry, 180*, 405–410.

Sharav, T., & Shlomo, L. (1986). Stimulation of infants with Down syndrome: Long-term effects. *Mental Retardation, 24*(2), 81–86.

Sherman, S. L., Jacobs, P. A., Morton, N. E., Froster-Iskenius, U., Howard-Peebles, P. N., Nielsen, K. B., et al. (1985). Further segregation analysis of the fragile X syndrome with special reference to transmitting males. *Human Genetics, 69*(4), 289–299.

Sherman, S. L., Morton, N. E., Jacobs, P. A., & Turner, G. (1984). The marker X syndrome: A cytogenetic and genetic analysis. *Annals of Human Genetics, 48*(Pt. 1), 21–37.

Sherman, S. L., Takaesu, N., Freeman, S. B., Grantham, M., Phillips, C., Blackston, R. D., et al. (1991). Trisomy 21: Association between reduced recombination and nondisjunction. *American Journal of Human Genetics, 49*(3), 608–620.

Sherrard, J., Tonge, B. J., & Ozanne-Smith, J. (2002). Injury risk in young people with intellectual disability. *Journal of Intellectual Disability Research, 46*(Pt. 1), 6–16.

Simeonsson, R. J., & Sharp, M. C. (1992). Developmental delays. In R. A. Hockelman, S. B. Friedman, N. M. Nelson & H. M. Seidel (Eds.),*Primary pediatric care* (2nd ed., pp. 867–870). St. Louis, MO: Mosby-Year Book.

Smith, R., Malee, K., Charurat, M., Magder, L., Mellins, C., Macmillan, C., et al. (2000). Timing of perinatal human immunodeficiency virus type 1 infection and rate of neurodevelopment. The Women and Infant Transmission Study Group. *Pediatric Infectious Disease Journal, 19*(9), 862–871.

Smits, A., Smeets, D., Dreesen, J., Hamel, B., de Haan, A., & van Oost, B. (1992). Parental origin of the Fra(X) gene is a major determinant of the cytogenetic expression and the CGG repeat length in female carriers. *American Journal of Medical Genetics, 43*(1–2), 261–267.

Spence, W. C., Black, S. H., Fallon, L., Maddalena, A., Cummings, E., Menapace-Drew, G., et al. (1996). Molecular fragile X screening in normal populations. *American Journal of Medical Genetics, 64*(1), 181–183.

Staples, A. J., Sutherland, G., Haan, E. A., & Clisby, S. (1991). Epidemiology of Down syndrome in South Australia, 1960–1989. *American Journal of Human Genetics, 49*(5), 1014–1024.

Stein, Z. A., Susser, M. W., & Saenger, G. (1976). Mental retardation in a national population of young men in The Netherlands: 2. Prevalence of mild mental retardation. *American Journal of Epidemiology, 104*(2), 159–169.

Stein, Z. A., Susser, M. W., Saenger, G., & Marolla, F. (1976). Mental retardation in a national population of young men in The Netherlands: 1. Prevalence of severe mental retardation. *American Journal of Epidemiology, 103*(5), 477–489.

Stevenson, R. (1996). Mental retardation: Overview and historical perspective. *Proceedings of the Greenwood Genetic Center, 15*, 9–18.

Stewart, G. D., Hassold, T. J., Berg, A., Watkins, P., Tanzi, R., & Kurnit, D. M. (1988). Trisomy 21 (Down syndrome): Studying nondisjunction and meiotic recombination by using cytogenetic and molecular polymorphisms that span chromosome 21. *American Journal of Human Genetics, 42*(2), 227–236.

Sutcliffe, J. S., Nakao, M., Christian, S., Orstavik, K. H., Tommerup, N., Ledbetter, D. H., et al. (1994). Deletions of a differentially methylated CpG island at the SNRPN gene define a putative imprinting control region. *Nature Genetics, 8*(1), 52–58.

Sullivan, J. B., & Krieger, G. R. (2001). *Clinical environmental health exposures* (2nd ed.). Philadelphia: Lippincott Williams & Wilkins.

Sutcliffe, J. S., Nelson, D. L., Zhang, F., Pieretti, M., Caskey, C. T., Saxe, D., et al. (1992). DNA methylation represses FMR-1 transcription in fragile X syndrome. *Human Molecular Genetics, 1*(6), 397–400.

Sutherland, G. R. (1977). Fragile sites on human chromosomes. Demonstration of their dependence on the type of tissue culture medium. *Science, 197*(4300), 265–266.

Teplin, S. W., Burchinal, M., Johnson-Martin, N., Humphry, R. A., & Kraybill, E. N. (1991). Neurodevelopmental, health, and growth status at age 6 years of children with birth weights less than 1001 grams. *Journal of Pediatrics, 118*(5), 768–777.

Thurman, D., Alverson, C., Dunn, K., Guerrero, J., & Sniezek, J. (1999).Traumatic brain injury in the United States: A public health perspective. *Journal of Head Trauma and Rehabilitation, 14*(6), 602–615.

Thurman, D., & Guerrero, J. (1999). Trends in hospitalization associated with traumatic brain injury. *JAMA, 282*(10), 954–957.

Tomlin, P., Clarke, M., Robinson, G., & Roach, J. (2002). Rehabilitation in severe head injury in children: Outcome and provision of care. *Developmental Medicine and Child Neurology, 44*(12), 828–837.

Tong, S. (1998). Lead exposure and cognitive development: Persistence and a dynamic pattern. *Journal of Paediatrics and Child Health, 34*(2), 114–118.

Turner, G., Webb, T., Wake, S., & Robinson, H. (1996). Prevalence of fragile X syndrome. *American Journal of Medical Genetics, 64*(1), 196–197.

U.S. Department of Health and Human Services. (2000). *Healthy People 2010: Understanding and improving health and objectives for improving health* (2nd ed., 2 Vols). Washington, DC: U.S. Government Printing Office.

van den Ouweland, A. M., de Vries, B. B., Bakker, P. L., Deelen, W. H., de Graaff, E., van Hemel, J. O., et al. (1994). DNA diagnosis of the fragile X syndrome in a series of 236 mentally retarded subjects and evidence for a reversal of mutation in the *FMR-1* gene. *American Journal of Medical Genetics, 51*(4), 482–485.

van Karnebeek, C. D., Koevoets, C., Sluijter, S., Bijlsma, E. K., Smeets, D. F., Redeker, E. J., et al. (2002). Prospective screening for subtelomeric rearrangements in children with mental retardation of unknown aetiology: The Amsterdam experience. *Journal of Medical Genetics, 39*(8), 546–553.

Verheij, C., Bakker, C. E., de Graaff, E., Keulemans, J., Willemsen, R., Verkerk, A. J., et al. (1993). Characterization and localization of the *FMR-1* gene product associated with fragile X syndrome. *Nature, 363*(6431), 722–724.

Verkerk, A. J., Pieretti, M., Sutcliffe, J. S., Fu, Y. H., Kuhl, D. P., Pizzuti, A., et al. (1991). Identification of a gene (*FMR-1*) containing a CGG repeat coincident with a breakpoint cluster region exhibiting length variation in Fragile X syndrome. *Cell, 65*(5), 905–914.

Vernon, M. (1979). Variability in reading retardation. *British Journal of Psychology, 70*(1), 7–16.

Vincent, A., Heitz, D., Petit, C., Krietz, C., Oberle, I., & Mandel, J. L. (1991). Abnormal pattern detected in fragile X patients by pulsed field gel electrophoreses. *Nature, 349*(6310), 624–626.

Visser, F. E., Aldenkamp, A. P., van Huffelen, A. C., Kuilman, M., Overweg, J., & van Wijk, J. (1997). Prospective study of the prevalence of Alzheimer-type dementia in institutionalized individuals with Down syndrome. *American Journal of Mental Retardation, 101*(4), 400–412.

Wagstaff, J., Knoll, J. H., Glatt, K. H., Shugart, Y. Y., Somer, A., & Lalande, M. (1992). Maternal but not paternal transmission of 15q11-q13 linked nondeletion Angelman syndrome leads to phenotypic expression. *Nature Genetics, 1*(4), 291–294.

Waisbren, S. E., Chang, P., Levy, H. L., Shifrin, H., Allred, E., Azen, C., et al. (1998). Neonatal neurological assessment of offspring in maternal phenylketonuria. *Journal of Inherited Metabolic Diseases, 21*(1), 39–48.

Waisbren, S. E., Doherty, L. B., Bailey, I. V., Rohr, F. J., & Levy, H. L. (1988). The New England Maternal PKU Project: Identification of at-risk women. *American Journal of Public Health, 78*(7), 789–792.

Walkowiak, J., Wiener, J. A., Fastabend, A., Heinzow, B., Kramer, U., Schmidt, E., et al. (2001). Environmental exposure to polychlorinated biphenyls and quality of the home environment: Effects on psychodevelopment in early childhood. *Lancet, 358*(9293), 1602–1607.

Warburton, D. (1984). Outcome of case of de novo structural rearrangements diagnosed at amniocentesis. *Prenatal Diagnosis, 4*, 69–80.

Warburton, D. (1987). De novo structural rearrangements at amniocentesis: Outcome and nonrandom position of breakpoints. *American Journal of Human Genetics, 41*(Suppl.), A145.

Warburton, D. (1991). De novo balanced rearrangements and extra marker chromosomes identified at prenatal diagnosis: Clinical significance and distribution of breakpoints. *American Journal of Human Genetics, 49*(5), 995–1013.

Wasserman, G. A., Graziano, J. H., Factor-Litvak, P., Popovac, D., Morina, N., Musabegovic, A., et al. (1994). Consequences of lead exposure and iron supplementation on childhood development at age 4 years. *Neurotoxicology and Teratology, 16*(3), 233–240.

Wasserman, G. A., Liu, X., Lolacono, N. J., Factor-Litvak, P., Kline, J. K., Popovac, D., et al. (1997). Lead exposure and intelligence in 7-year-old children: The Yugoslavia prospective study. *Environmental Health Perspectives, 105*(9), 956–962.

Wasserstrum, N., & Anania, C. A. (1995). Perinatal consequences of maternal hypothyroidism in early pregnancy and inadequate replacement. *Clinical Endocrinology, 42*(4), 353–358.

Webb, T., Whittington, J., Clarke, D., Boer, H., Butler, J., & Holland, A. (2002). A study of the influence of different genotypes on the physical and behavioral phenotypes of children and adults ascertained clinically as having PWS. *Clinical Genetics, 62*(4), 273–281.

Wenger, J. D., Hightower, A. W., Facklam, R. R., Gaventa, S., Broome, C. V., & the Bacterial Meningitis Study Group (1990). Bacterial meningitis in the United States, 1986: Report of a multistate surveillance study. *Journal of Infectious Diseases, 162*(6), 1316–1323.

Wevrick, R., Kerns, J. A., & Francke, U. (1994). Identification of a novel paternally expressed gene in the Prader–Willi syndrome region. *Nature Genetics, 3*(10), 1877–1882.

Whitaker, A. H., Feldman, J. F., VanRossem, R., Schonfeld, I. S., Pinto-Martin, J. A., Torre, C., et al. (1996). Neonatal cranial ultrasound abnormalities in low birth weight infants: Relation to cognitive outcomes at six years of age. *Pediatrics, 98*(4 Pt. 1), 719–729.

Wild, J., Read, A. P., Sheppard, S., Seller, M. J., Smithells, R. W., Nevin, N. C., et al. (1986). Recurrent neural tube defects, risk factors and vitamins. *Archives of Disease in Childhood, 61*(5), 440–444.

Williams, J. C., Barratt-Boyes, B. G., & Lowe, J. B. (1961). Supravalvular aortic stenosis. *Circulation, 24,* 1311–1318.

Winneke, G., Walkowiak, J., & Lilienthal, H. (2002). PCB-induced neurodevelopmental toxicity in human infants and its potential mediation by endocrine dysfunction. *Toxicology, 181-182,* 161–165.

Wisniewski, H. M., Wegiel, J., & Popovitch, E. (1994). Age-associated development of diffuse and thioflavin-S-positive plaques in Down syndrome. *Developmental Brain Dysfunction, 7,* 330–339.

Wisniewski, K. E., Wisniewski, H. M., & Wen, G. Y. (1985). Occurrence of neuropathological changes and dementia of Alzheimer's disease in Down's syndrome. *Annals of Neurology, 17*(3), 278–282.

Wohrle, D., Kotzot, D., Hirst, M. C., Manca, A., Korn, B., Schmidt, A., et al. (1992). A microdeletion of less than 250 kb, including the proximal part of the *FMR-1* gene and the fragile site, in a male with the clinical phenotype of fragile X syndrome. *American Journal of Human Genetics, 51*(2), 299–306.

World Health Organization. (1980a). *International classification of impairments, disabilities and handicaps.* Geneva, Switzerland: Author.

World Health Organization. (1980b). *International statistical classification of diseases* (9th ed.). Geneva, Switzerland: Author.

World Health Organization. (1992). *International statistical classification of diseases* (10th ed.). Geneva, Switzerland: Author.

World Health Organization. (2001). *International classification of functioning, disability and health (ICF).* Geneva, Switzerland: Author.

Yeargin-Allsopp, M., & Boyle, C. (2002). Overview: The epidemiology of neurodevelopmental disorders. *Mental Retardation and Developmental Disabilities Research Reviews, 8*(3), 113–116.

Yeargin-Allsopp, M., Murphy, C. C., Cordero, J. F., Decoufle, P., & Hollowell, J. G. (1997). Reported biomedical causes and associated medical conditions for mental retardation among 10-year-old children, metropolitan Atlanta, 1985 to 1987. *Developmental Medicine and Child Neurology, 39*(3), 142–149.

Yu, S., Pritchard, M., Kremer, E., Lynch, M., Nancarrow, J., Baker, E., et al. (1991). Fragile X genotype characterized by an unstable region of DNA. *Science, 252*(5010), 1179–1181.

Zigler, E. (1967). Mental retardation. *Science, 157*(788), 578–579.

Zigler, E., & Butterfield, E. C. (1966). Rigidity in the retarded: A further test of the Lewin–Kounin formulation. *Journal of Abnormal Psychology, 71*(3), 224–231.

Zigman, W. B., Schupf, N., Sersen, E., & Silverman, W. (1996). Prevalence of dementia in adults with and without Down syndrome. *American Journal on Mental Retardation, 100*(4), 403–412.

2

The Autism Spectrum

CHRISTOPHER GILLBERG

Autism was first delineated as a syndrome of childhood onset by Leo Kanner in the United States in the 1940s (Kanner, 1943). Long before that—at the turn of the 18th century—classic autism cases had been described by John Haslam in the United Kingdom and Jean Itard in France. The word autism (from the Greek autos for self) was introduced by Eugen Bleuler to depict the self-cantered thinking believed to be typical of schizophrenia. Believed by Kanner to be a discrete disease entity, early infantile autism was conceptualized as an extremely rare disorder, and one that would be easy to identify and diagnose. It was only in the early 1980s that the concept of an autism spectrum was introduced by Wing (Waterhouse, Wing, & Fein, 1989; Wing, 1981, 1988) and Gillberg (Gillberg & Steffenburg, 1987). Wing put forward the notion of a fairly specific triad of impairments of social, communicative, and imaginative functioning as being at the basis of all autism spectrum disorders. She also coined the term Asperger's syndrome for the kind of "high-functioning" autism spectrum disorder originally described by Hans Asperger (1944) (who used the term *autistic psychopathy*) at about the same time that Kanner described his more "low-functioning" variant of autism.

CLASSIFICATION

Terminology in the field of autism spectrum disorders is problematic. Diagnostic manuals do not use the term autism spectrum, but instead refer to pervasive developmental disorders (PDD). PDD is a misnomer in that not all autism spectrum disorders are pervasive. Furthermore, profound learning disability (a.k.a. mental retardation in the United States), the most

---

CHRISTOPHER GILLBERG • St. George's Hospital Medical School, University of London, London, United Kingdom and Queen Silvia's Children's Hospital, University of Göteborg, Gothenburg, Sweden.

pervasive of all developmental disorders, is not considered a PDD. In clinical practice, autism spectrum disorders remain the preferred term. However, some authorities in the field speak of autism *and* autism spectrum disorders, whereas others include the core syndrome of autism (childhood autism or autistic disorder) as a subgroup *within* the autism spectrum disorders. The latter definition is used here. Under this model, autism spectrum disorders and PDD can be seen as synonymous concepts. Both the ICD-10 (World Health Organization [WHO], 1992) and DSM-IV (American Psychiatric Association [APA], 1994) list five different subtypes of PDD: the core syndrome of *autism, Asperger syndrome, childhood disintegrative disorder, atypical autism or PDD Not Otherwise Specified (PDD-NOS)*, and *Rett syndrome*. The inclusion of Rett syndrome as one specific variant of autism spectrum disorder makes little sense as Rett syndrome is one of the many medical disorders that are often associated with autistic symptomatology. It belongs instead on the medical disorder axis of the multiaxial classification system.

ICD-10 and DSM-IV Criteria

The ICD-10 category for the core syndrome of autism is *childhood autism*. The DSM-IV *autistic disorder* is virtually identically defined. The definition is based upon the simultaneous presence of all three of the *triad of severe impairment of reciprocal social interaction, severe impairment of reciprocal communication (including but not exclusive to problems with language use), and severe restriction of imagination and behavioral repertoire*. The problems need to be at a level that is out of keeping with the child's overall chronological and developmental age. Problems must have been present before age 3 years. In ICD-10 there is also an exclusion criterion that leads to diagnostic confusion if strictly adhered to and prevents clinicians from making appropriate diagnoses and interventions for comorbid problems (such as Attention Deficit and Hyperactivity Disorder [ADHD]). This criterion is less stringent in the DSM-IV. The exclusion criterion should be disregarded in clinical practice.

The ICD-10 and DSM-IV category of *Asperger syndrome* or *Asperger's disorder* is a theoretical construct not consistent with clinical realities. For instance, Asperger's own cases do not meet criteria for this category. The criteria for social and behavioral impairments are the same as for childhood autism. Nothing is said about the communication impairment (so striking in the typical case of Asperger syndrome). The major problem with this set of criteria resides in the requirement for normal development in the first 3 years of life, something almost unheard of in autism spectrum disorders. In clinical practice, the criteria by Gillberg and Gillberg (1989) are the ones most commonly used. Many individuals meet criteria both for autism and Asperger syndrome. It is often best in such cases to make the diagnosis of autism but equally to provide the information that it is the variant referred to as Asperger syndrome.

Childhood disintegrative disorder is an autism spectrum disorder with the typical clinical presentation emerging only after a period of a few or several years of normal or near-normal development.

Atypical autism is an autism spectrum disorder that cannot be classified as childhood autism, Asperger syndrome, or Childhood disintegrative disorder. The corresponding terminology of the DSM-IV is *PDD-NOS*.

Comments

"High-functioning autism" is a term often applied to cases meeting ICD-10 or DSM-IV criteria for autism and who test at near-normal, normal, or superior levels of IQ. Most clinicians would argue that such cases fit Asperger's description, particularly if the level of spoken language is superior. The term "high functioning" is inappropriate because it suggests that the affected individual is "well functioning," which is almost never the case in an individual with a clinically diagnosed autism spectrum disorder. The individual with this "diagnosis" is usually *relatively* high functioning as regards overall IQ, but in respect of the autism symptomatology, functional disability is often major.

In clinical practice it would seem reasonable to diagnose children and adolescents as having an *autism spectrum disorder* if and only if there are severe problems in at least two of the three triad domains or if there are mild to moderate problems in two domains and severe problems in a third domain. Subgrouping according to ICD-10 or DSM-IV could then be achieved for autism, childhood disintegrative disorder, and atypical autism or PDD NOS. If the clinical gestalt of Asperger syndrome is invoked, then thorough review of the Gillberg criteria might be helpful before concluding that this category is applicable. The word autism (such as in autism spectrum disorder) should always be mentioned in the diagnostic formulation. Many countries require this diagnostic specification for the provision of adequate services.

EPIDEMIOLOGY

Autistic disorder and the other conditions referred to the autism spectrum disorder or PDD category are much more common than was suspected until the 1990s. The prevalence for all autism spectrum disorders is in the range of 0.5–1.0% of the general school age population (Wing & Potter, 2002). Core autism cases account for about one-third of this proportion and Asperger syndrome or atypical autism for the vast majority of the remainder. Childhood disintegrative disorder is extremely rare. Most of the available evidence suggests that the relatively high rates now reported for autism spectrum disorders are due to increased awareness, new autism concepts and diagnostic criteria, and "diagnostic overshadowing" (i.e., if there is already a diagnosis of, e.g., epilepsy, learning disability, or tuberous sclerosis, an additional diagnosis of autism is less likely to be made) rather than to any real increase in the population.

Sex Ratios

Clinical studies show a very high boy:girl ratio for autism. This drops to considerably lower levels (around 1.5–3:1) in the general population. Girls with autism spectrum disorders are probably underdiagnosed and may receive other diagnoses such as depression, personality disorder, or eating disorder. Girls may also be less likely than boys to be referred for help at an early age. Girls in the general population show less of hyperactive and violent behaviors (commonly encountered in autism spectrum disorders and often part of the reason for referral) and talk more and at an earlier age. Therefore, it would require a more severe variant of an autism spectrum disorder to produce the "full-blown" clinical picture manifested by boys at an early age. Girls who receive an early diagnosis of autism are often among those most severely affected, with major signs of brain dysfunction including epilepsy. More moderate and mild variants are the ones most likely to be missed or misdiagnosed.

CLINICAL PICTURE

The triad of impairments typical of all autism spectrum disorders affect social, communicative (including language), and behavioral or imaginative functioning (Gillberg & Gillberg, 1989; Wing, 1996). There are usually additional symptoms, including a range of perceptual abnormalities, but these are not currently considered necessary features for the diagnosis.

The Severe Impairment of Reciprocal Social Interaction

The severe impairment of reciprocal social interaction may be observed in the staring, fixed or "wide-open" gaze—often directed at the lower portion of the face rather than the eyes—which is not used to regulate social interaction, the reduced ability to take the cognitive and emotional perspective of another person, disregard for needs of age-peers and adults alike, a complete lack of turn-taking in social interactions or games, and failure to understand the need for social overtures. Many are perceived as lacking in empathy, even though this does not necessarily imply "coldness." Many have strong affects, but with their problems understanding the perspective of the other person, they misinterpret social signals, as, in turn, others misunderstand their affects. Some are "sweet," "naive," and "easy to love" so long as demands are kept to a minimum or within an accepted routine. Social "style" may vary from complete "aloofness" and autistic aloneness, through a "friendly and passive" interactive style to an impulsive, intruding "active but odd" pattern of interaction. The group showing the active but odd style (and sometimes those who are aloof) may be severely hyperactive from a very early age. They may receive a diagnosis of ADHD or hyperkinetic disorder, and it is only when this has come under control with treatment or at a later age that the underlying severe social interaction impairment of autism comes to attention.

The child with an autism spectrum disorder usually has no "real" friend, even though some may be passive members of a group where very little interaction is demanded. The lack of concern about the absence of friends is sometimes the most striking feature, even though, in other cases or at a later age, the person with an autism spectrum disorder may have come to realize that it is "normal" for young people to have friends and therefore may worry about "not being normal" because there are no friends. Some may insist that their parents call up a "friend and bring him over" and will go on and on about the time the friend will arrive, only to ignore the "friend" completely once he or she has arrived in the house.

The Severe Impairment in Reciprocal Communication

The severe impairment in reciprocal communication can present as complete muteness or the reduction of spoken language down to a few words or sentences, but it may equally show as extremely repetitive complex language. About one-third of those with the core syndrome of autism never speak in communicative phrases. Some acquire single word skills at the expected time but then do not progress beyond this stage for many months or years. This is often perceived as a "set-back" even in cases where there have been some documented abnormalities in the social domain at an earlier age. Even those with the clinical presentation of Asperger syndrome (who often progress to a stage of elaborate, even "perfect" language) often go through such a stage of a language development plateau and may be perceived as very late speakers (particularly perhaps as compared with brothers or sisters), only to "explode" in their acquisition of spoken language skills around age 3–5 years, when, within a period of only some months they go from "almost mute" to "adult type" expressive language. The vast majority—even those with the clinical presentation of Asperger syndrome—have great difficulty understanding the meaning of what other people tell them or ask them in conversation, even when they themselves are able to speak in grammatically perfect sentences. Again, their reduced capacity for taking the other person's cognitive and emotional perspective is severely limiting for their ability to grasp the meaning of communication.

The Severe Restriction in the Behavioral Repertoire

The severe restriction in the behavioral repertoire is seen by many to reflect the *lack of flexible imaginative skills*. In children with marked degrees of learning disability, repetitive motor behaviors (e.g., stereotypies such as hand flapping, finger flickering, body rocking, and head banging) are the rule. Such behaviors may occur in those with higher IQ as well, but usually to a less conspicuous degree. Fixation on routines, rituals, pedantry, and a variety of symptoms that might equally be described as obsessive-compulsive are almost universal, but may be obscured or lacking in those with severe comorbid inattention and hyperactivity. Some throw extreme tantrums when routines are broken or demands of any kind are made. In older individuals, these are often referred to as "violent outbursts" (or even "aggressiveness," a term that should usually not be employed, because it is very difficult to determine whether the violence is intentional or not). Play is usually rigid, stilted, or lacking altogether. Hard objects are often much preferred over soft and cuddly things. Because, at least when very young, they do not seem to appreciate the existence of other people's minds, they do not go to them for comfort or for sharing positive or negative experiences.

Many have elaborate routines involving feeding behaviors (e.g., will only eat one particular type of food and only if seated on a particular stool with one elbow resting on the table) and bathroom activities (e.g., can only brush teeth in front of mirror at home, cannot manage in front of other mirrors in other bathrooms). Those with IQs in the normal or superior range very often develop narrow interests (e.g., in meteorology, dinosaurs, opera singers, Chinese pottery, Rommel's desert wars, the Paris Metro system, train time tables, telephone directories, or computers) that come to occupy so much of their time that there is little left over for any other kind of meaningful activity. They tend to talk endlessly about these special interests and appear to be unaware that others may not share them. Many are extremely interested in details and are very astute in memorizing matters concerned with the observable world. They may remember in the most astounding detail what people were wearing 10 years ago or the particulars of a building not visited for more than a few minutes many years previously. Those with the highest levels of IQ are often expert at picking up other people's "weak spots." They may also have "emotional radar" and observe minute change in social atmosphere even while not being able to make the slightest sense of what is going on. Such skills may lead the clinician to exclude erroneously even considering a diagnosis in the autism spectrum.

Not part of the triad but extremely common in autism are perceptual distortions or abnormalities of various kinds. One or more of oversensitivity to touch, certain sounds, smells, tastes, or visual stimuli is an almost universal phenomenon. Abnormal reactions to auditory stimuli (e.g., strong reactions to barely audible sounds and little or no reaction to loud noise) are often among the presenting symptoms of autism in the first year of life. Decreased pain sensitivity is another common symptom, which may or may not be accompanied by a variety of self-injurious behaviors. These behaviors can be the most debilitating problem in the set of symptoms shown by a child with autism. As already mentioned, hyperactivity, often amounting to full symptomatic diagnostic criteria for ADHD or Hyperkinetic Disorder, is a very common handicapping symptom, especially in the preschool child. In other cases hypoactivity can be the major problem with lack of initiative, lack of interest in new things (which may be shown, for example, in relation to gifts that may trigger extreme temper tantrums), and "resistance to change and learning." Sleep problems are also very common, and constitute a handicapping problem in about one in three of all preschool children with one or other of the autism spectrum disorders.

Subjectively, children with autism spectrum disorders may be extremely psychologically frustrated by overstimulating environments, perceptual overreactions, verbal interactions, common demands for social interaction, and, in some cases, demands of any kind. In a structured, calm environment with predictable routines, they are usually "happy," although they tend not to share this experience with others in a spontaneous fashion. Some of those with very high IQ seem to have little memory of around— perhaps—age 7, 8, or 9 years. Others appear to have the opposite problem of not being able to forget anything they ever experienced.

The early course and clinical presentation of autism spectrum disorders differ quite considerably from one case to another. About two in three of all cases have shown some social, communicative, or typical behavioral change before their first birthday. Others appear to develop normally up until 12–24 months of age and then suffer real or seeming regression, sometimes, but not always in temporal association with onset of seizures. Until recently, it was considered very rare for autism not to present with the full-blown clinical picture before age 5 years, but new studies of adults and follow-up studies of children with atypical autistic features and language disorders in early childhood indicate that not infrequently autism emerges more clearly only after the first years. Children with very early onset extreme hyperactivity and motor control problems constitute other risk groups in whom the clinician must be prepared to assess features of autism at later follow-up.

DIFFERENTIAL DIAGNOSIS AND COMORBIDITY

Many problems of differential diagnosis in the field of autism include those pertaining to differentiating between the various forms of conditions within the spectrum. The most common comorbid or overlapping *syndromes* are ADHD, Developmental Coordination Disorder (DCD), tic disorders, depression, bipolar disorder, anxiety disorders, and eating disorders (Gillberg & Billstedt, 2000). Common associated *symptoms* are perceptual abnormality, violent outbursts, self-injury, and sleep problems, which have been briefly dealt with already. Medical disorders are very commonly associated with autism spectrum disorders and should be coded on a separate diagnostic axis.

Attention Deficit and Hyperactivity Disorder

Hyperactivity, inattention, and handicapping impulsiveness are almost universally occurring problems in all autism spectrum disorders. When, from the point of view of symptom threshold, they amount to combined ADHD (and especially when symptom criteria for Hyperkinetic Disorder are met), a separate diagnosis for this category should be considered. Many children with autism spectrum disorders, perhaps particularly those with IQs above 50, may benefit from the same type of intervention approaches that are advantageous for other children with ADHD. Children with the combination of ADHD and DCD have a relatively high risk of also meeting criteria for an autism spectrum disorder. It is not always appropriate to give the autism spectrum disorder diagnosis priority over ADHD. The syndrome that, from the point of view of treatment need, is the most handicapping should be named as the primary diagnosis. Thus, one child might correctly receive the diagnosis of ADHD at age 3 years, of ADHD with atypical autism at age 4 years, and Autistic disorder with ADHD at age 9 years.

Developmental Coordination Disorder

In the past children with autism were believed to be exceptionally talented in the field of motor performance. This is now known to be a mistaken notion. To the contrary, the vast majorities have mild, moderate, or severe motor control problems, and many meet criteria for DCD. Mild DCD problems are part of the Asperger syndrome diagnosis, but when the motor control problems are moderately or severely debilitating, they may require specific intervention and a separate diagnosis of DCD should be made.

Tic Disorders

Tics are very common in children in the general population, but are definitely much overrepresented among those with autism spectrum disorders. They may be motor tics (in which case they can be very difficult to separate from motor stereotypies), vocal tics, simple or complex (in which case they can be indistinguishable from complex stereotypies or stereotyped utterances), transient or chronic. When motor and vocal tics occur together and are handicapping in their own right (as separate from autism), a diagnosis of Tourette syndrome might be warranted. Having said this, it also needs to be added that tics are only rarely severely handicapping.

Depression

Depression is common in teenagers with autism spectrum disorders. A change in behavior (such as hyperactivity turning to hypoactivity), loss of appetite, or severely disrupted sleep patterns may all indicate depression in autism. Interpersonal loss and bullying are common precipitants of depression in autism spectrum disorders. For instance, the death of a parent might not seem to affect the child with autism at all early on. However, as weeks pass and the child gradually realizes that the routine of having someone catering to his or her particular and peculiar needs has disappeared, depressive symptoms set in. As in the case of the child being victimized by bullies, he or she is unlikely to communicate anything about his feelings to other people, and the depressed mood may therefore go unnoticed or undiagnosed for longer periods.

Bipolar Disorder

It seems likely that bipolar disorder is overrepresented in families who have children with autism and clinical experience suggests that bipolar disorder is a common comorbidity in both autism and Asperger syndrome. Mood swings, periods of extreme hyperactivity, "intermittent explosive behaviors," and abrupt sleep disturbance are all possible indicators of bipolar disorder, especially in the presence of a positive family history for such a disorder.

Anxiety Disorders

Children with autism spectrum disorders are often anxious, particularly in situations when they do not know what is expected of them. "Panic attacks" amounting to confused states are often seen in settings of perceptual overload such as in the middle of a busy street or in crowds of people making all sorts of verbal demands. The individual with autism might then cover his ears and start screaming, hitting himself, or running out in front of oncoming vehicles. DSM-IV Panic Disorder or Generalized Anxiety does occur occasionally and is most commonly diagnosed in those with higher IQ, but it is unclear whether the rate of such problems is increased over and above that of the general population. *Selective mutism*—often categorized as an anxiety disorder—is strongly associated with autistic features.

Eating Disorders

Food fads, food refusal, and overeating are all common, perhaps almost universal phenomena in autism spectrum disorders. *Anorexia nervosa* has been shown to be associated with autism spectrum disorders. Ten to twenty percent of a general population group of adolescent girls with anorexia nervosa meet full criteria for an autism spectrum disorder. Such cases are usually missed cases of early onset autism or Asperger syndrome who develop extreme routines and rituals around food in teenage (as part of a life-long proclivity for rituals and routines), and who do meet diagnostic criteria for anorexia nervosa, but will not benefit from interventions unless the underlying autistic problems are acknowledged.

Other Developmental, Psychiatric, and Personality Disorder Diagnoses

During the young adult years, many individuals with autism spectrum disorders apply for help within adult psychiatric services. It is then very common for them to receive diagnoses of "schizophreniform disorder" or of "personality disorder." The underlying autism diagnosis may be disregarded or may have been missed altogether.

Semantic Pragmatic Disorder

Semantic pragmatic disorder is a diagnostic term used mostly by speech-language therapists (Rapin & Allen, 1983). Many individuals in the autism spectrum suffer from semantic pragmatic disorder or, at least, pragmatic disorder. It is unclear what proportions of those with so-called semantic pragmatic disorder meet some or all criteria for an autism spectrum disorder.

Nonverbal Learning Disability

Nonverbal learning disability is a neuropsychological concept used in cases with much poorer results on performance than on verbal portions of IQ-tests (e.g., who score 20 points or more lower on the performance than the verbal part of the WISC—Rourke, 1988). This test profile is quite common in Asperger syndrome. It is believed often to reflect right hemisphere dysfunction.

Medical Disorders

In classic autism in the general population, as many as one in four individuals may have a medical disorder which, in one way or another is strongly associated with the autistic symptomatology (Gillberg & Coleman, 1996). In specialized autism clinics, to which those with an already "overshadowing" medical disorder diagnosis (such as tuberous sclerosis or fragile X syndrome) are less likely to be referred, the rate may be lower, but it is certainly not negligible there either (Rutter, Bailey, Bolton, & Le Couteur, 1994). This means that all individuals with a diagnosis of an autism spectrum disorder will need a medical assessment by a clinician well trained in the field, who knows which disorders to look out.

Epilepsy is very common in childhood autism and in atypical autism cases with mental retardation, occurring in 25–40% of all cases depending on the duration of follow-up. Slightly under half of this proportion is contributed by cases with seizure onset in the first 5 years of life. The epilepsy in such cases is often severe and presents with a combination of several different types of seizures. The majority of the remainder has adolescent onset of seizures, which are usually of a more benign type. A small number of additional cases of epilepsy emerge in early adult life. Epilepsy is much rarer in Asperger syndrome, but it does occur at rates considerably higher than in the general population.

Moderate hearing deficits occur in about 10% of all individuals with childhood autism and complete deafness is present in a few percent (which is much higher than in the general population). Extreme acoustic hypersensitivity is very common and occurs in 30–50% of all cases. Visual deficits are also much overrepresented. Certain kinds of congenital blindness with brain damage (e.g., retinopathy of prematurity) are strongly associated with autism spectrum disorders.

Tuberous sclerosis, the fragile X syndrome, and the partial tetrasomy 15 syndrome are probably the most commonly encountered specific brain disorders in autism cases with an IQ of about 50 and below. Together they account for 10–15% of all such cases. Other relatively common medical conditions in autism spectrum disorders, across the board of intellectual functioning, are Moebius syndrome, 22q11 deletion syndrome, and sex chromosome aneuploidies.

DIAGNOSTIC INSTRUMENTS

Rating scales for autism can be subdivided into those that have been developed for screening typical cases, and those that are geared rather toward finding cases of "high-functioning" autism, Asperger syndrome, and atypical autism. The most widely used rating scales for people in the autism spectrum with IQ under 70 is the Autistic Behavior Checklist (ABC—Krug, Arick, & Almond, 1980) which provides a good measure of the level of symptoms and severity. There is also a brief Autism Screen based on the ADI-R (see Berument, Rutter, Lord, Pickles, & Bailey, 1999). A mixture of observation and interview is usually required for the completion of the Childhood Autism Rating Scale-Revised (CARS-R—Schopler, Reichler, & Renner, 1988). This scale, which takes about 45 min to complete, is the most widely empirically studied instrument in the autism field. It provides a summary score in the range of 15–60, with cutoff for a preliminary diagnosis of autism at 30 and for severe variants of autism at 36. For individuals in the autism spectrum with an IQ of about 60 and above, the best validated screening instrument in school age children is the Autism Spectrum Screening Questionnaire (ASSQ) for completion by parents or teachers in less than 10 min (Ehlers & Gillberg, 1993). Finally, there is the Asperger Syndrome Diagnostic Interview (ASDI—Gillberg, Rastam, & Wentz, 2001) that takes about 40 min to complete and provides a good indication whether or not diagnostic criteria for Asperger syndrome (or another "high-IQ autism spectrum disorder") are met.

Detailed clinical interview with a close carer (usually one of the parents) is the most important single measure of any in the diagnostic process. This is often best accomplished by using a structured or semistructured psychometrically tested diagnostic interview. One of the best clinical interviews of this kind is the Diagnosis of Social and Communication Disorders-10th Revision (DISCO-10—Wing, Leekam, Libby, Gould, & Larcombe, 2002) which covers not only autism spectrum disorders but many of the overlapping or comorbid conditions as well, as providing a detailed picture of the individual's early development. The Autism Diagnostic Interview- Revised (ADI-R—Lord, Rutter, & Le Couteur., 1994) is an excellent interview for tapping into classic autism cases, but has been developed specifically for research, not clinical, purposes, and does not cover all of the spectrum disorders or comorbidities. Use of the DISCO-10 and ADI-R require diploma training.

Observation of the child's behavior is the most important component of the diagnostic process. The Autism Diagnostic Observation Schedule (ADOS) and the Pre-Linguistic ADOS (PL-ADOS—DiLavore, Lord, & Rutter, 1995) are excellent research instruments for structured rating of social interaction and communication behaviors in the child, but again have been developed for research, rather than clinical purposes. Observation of the child in a naturalistic setting (such as in preschool or school, at home or in the playground) may sometimes be the best, and only way of definitely determining whether he or she actually meets criteria for autism or not.

Psychological tests are not required for the diagnosis of autism as such, but they are necessary components of the diagnostic evaluation. One of the Wechsler scales for estimation of IQ (or the Leiter scale in nonverbal children) should be tried in all cases. Occasionally in children with severe mental retardation, one has to settle for an estimate of overall functioning based on Vineland Adaptive Behavior Scale interview (Sparrow, Balla, & Cicchetti, 1984).

ASSESSMENT

The multifactorial nature of autism makes it mandatory to perform an expert medical evaluation by a doctor (e.g., child neuropsychiatrist, child neurologist, or developmental pediatrician) with state-of-the-art skills in syndromology, learning disability, autism, and the comorbidities so often associated with it.

Psychometric evaluation, including a measure of the child's overall intellectual level of functioning, must be done in all cases. The clinical medical-neurological examination (which must always include head circumference, height, weight, and evaluation of minor physical anomalies, skin abnormalities, and hearing and visual problems) is crucial for deciding on what further laboratory investigations need to be performed (e.g., karyotyping, DNA tests, MRI scanning, and EEG being the tests most commonly indicated). The clinical examination must also include a systematic psychiatric screen for ADHD, tics, motor control problems, sleep disorders, self-injurious behaviors, and the other common comorbidities listed in the foregoing. The results of the medical and psychiatric examination and the tests performed should be conveyed to all concerned both orally and in writing.

CAUSES AND RISK FACTORS

There are multiple causes of autism spectrum disorders (Gillberg & Coleman, 2000). Genetic factors are very important (Turner, Barnby, & Bailey, 2000). The sibling rate for the core syndrome given a child with core syndrome autism is about 5%, but the rate for an autism spectrum disorder in such cases is probably of the order of 15–25%. Twin studies have shown concordance rates of 60–89% in monozygotic twins and under 5% in dizygotic twins (similar to nontwin siblings), suggesting a heritability of close to 100% in cases that are not associated with specific medical disorders. It is not clear exactly what it is that is inherited, but it now seems likely that aberrant or variant genes (such as neuroligin and glutamate genes) may act in concert that more than 30 different genes are likely to be involved, and that the individual genes may increase liability for a particular autism *feature* rather than for the full syndrome of autism.

The frontotemporal portions of the brain are often dysfunctional in autism (bilaterally or, typically in more "high-functioning" cases, in the right hemisphere). The brainstem and cerebellum have also been shown to be abnormal in relatively large subgroups of individuals with autism. Dysfunction of the fusiform gyrus might be specifically related to the unusual processing of faces and facial features so often encountered in autism. Autopsy studies have revealed abnormalities in the amygdala and cerebellum, in particular. Megalencephalus is much overrepresented in autism spectrum disorders, apparently more so among those with IQs above 70. Hyperserotonemia in the blood, dopamine and endorphin dysfunction, and excess of glial fibrillary acidic protein in the cerebrospinal fluid have all been shown to be associated with autism in group studies, but it is not clear what relevance, if any, these "markers" may have for the understanding of autism etiology (Gillberg & Coleman, 2000).

It has been demonstrated convincingly in many case studies that certain acquired brain lesions, such as in connection with herpes encephalitis, can cause autism without there being any known genetic susceptibility. However, many of the associated medical disorders that are currently believed to be etiologically related to autism (such as tuberous sclerosis) are themselves genetic. In addition, some studies suggest that even when there is an associated medical disorder that is believed to be important in the pathogenetic chain of events, interaction with autism susceptibility genes may occur. It has been suggested that in certain cases there might have been genetic predisposition for a "mild autistic-like condition" but that additional (prenatal or possibly perinatal) brain damage has led to the full-blown syndrome of autism. It is unlikely that psychosocial factors themselves cause autism, but conditions with some similar symptoms have been reported in children exposed to severe emotional and psychosocial deprivation in the first years of life. If such factors play a role in some autism cases, they would do so by impinging (perhaps irreversibly) on brain systems that are crucial for social and communicative functioning. It is likely that autism spectrum disorders will be shown to be the "final common behavioral presentation" of a multitude of different etiologies, and that only after more sophisticated subgrouping than can currently be achieved, will it be possible to find *the* cause in an individual case.

COGNITIVE NEUROPSYCHOLOGY

Neuropsychologically, children in the autism spectrum usually have *executive function deficits* showing clinically as poor planning ability, low motivational level, and difficulty with time concepts. Sustaining attention may be very difficult, and there appear to be general problems with shifting of attention from one object of focus to another. *Mentalizing ("theory of mind")deficits* occur almost universally, particularly in preschool children. These deficits are connected to lack of empathy and inability to take the cognitive and emotional (though not necessarily perceptual) perspective of other people. There is also usually a *decreased drive for central coherence*, meaning that individuals with autism may have no difficulty remembering details or amassing concrete factual knowledge about the observable world (at which they actually be better than individuals without autism at similar IQ levels), but may have major problems fitting the details into a coherent "whole" or to make sense of all the facts (Frith & Happe, 1994). On cognitive tests (Ehlers et al., 1997; Gillberg, 1999), those with a diagnosis of childhood autism (and of atypical autism) usually fall below an IQ of about 80, whereas the majority of those with Asperger syndrome test at or above IQ 70. The former group frequently does better on performance than verbal parts of tests, whereas the opposite pattern is more likely to be encountered in those with Asperger syndrome. On the Wechsler scale, core autism cases often have relatively better results on the subtest of Block Design, while showing a trough on the Comprehension subtest. Those with a diagnosis of Asperger syndrome often show a similar pattern when young (although, unlike those with classic autism, the better result on Block Design may well be coupled with a poor result on Object Assembly), but as they grow older, they tend to do progressively better on the Comprehension subtest. Slow processing appears to be typical of Asperger syndrome. Many individuals with this diagnosis would pass on most tasks if they were not timed.

INTERVENTIONS

The evidence base for interventions in autism spectrum disorders is limited (Howlin, 1998). No one treatment will lead to a cure and it is unlikely that a single mode of intervention will ever dominate the arena, given the multifactorial contribution to autism pathogenesis. A child with a diagnosis within the autism spectrum and his or her family will need the continued support of an expert team consisting of a medical doctor, psychologist, and a special education expert (at the very least) for many years, usually throughout childhood and into adult life. It is usually to be preferred that this service is offered within a slightly broader child neuropsychiatric or developmental pediatric clinic rather than in a highly specialized autism center, in which the experts may not have enough skills in the neighboring fields of comorbidity.

Education

Those with childhood autism and an IQ of 70 or under almost always need to attend specialist autism classrooms, whereas those with Asperger syndrome may well benefit from attending a mainstream classroom. Nevertheless, in this intellectually better functioning group it is important to be able to offer a choice, and some, for instance, many of those who are victims of bullying, will do much better and have a better quality of life in a classroom for intellectually normal, able, or gifted children with autism spectrum disorders. Others may do better in mixed special education classrooms. The most important considerations pertain to the knowledge of autism on the part of the teachers. All children in the autism spectrum will need a considerably greater amount of structure, concreteness, and systematic, well-planned skills training (both as regards school day structure and overview and in all individual subjects) than is usually considered to be required (or even helpful) for other children.

Specific education programs, such as that developed under the acronym of TEACCH (Treatment and Education of Autistic and Communication handicapped Children—Schopler, 1990), are available and provide a very good basis for training teachers and parents to become proponents for and providers of an "autism-friendly" environment (rich in structure, concreteness, and, usually, though not always, including much more visual material than ordinarily provided in education). Continuity as regards time, place, and people is the most important aspect of autism education, and one, which is strongly emphasized in the TEACCH philosophy.

Psychological Interventions

Psychoeducation is perhaps the most important part of any intervention scheme for autism spectrum disorder. Parents, siblings, and, depending on the intellectual capacity, the affected individual, all need detailed up-to-date information about autism, its causes, prognosis, and possible intervention strategies. They need to be well informed about relevant support groups, books, pamphlets, conferences, Internet addresses, and other ways to access information. *Applied behavior analysis* (ABA) has been shown to reduce effectively some problem behaviors in autism and to improve social and communication skills (Department of Health, 1999; National Research Council, 2001; Smith, Groen, & Wynn, 2000). Some parents want to have their children in a stringent ABA-protocol for 40 hr a week or more, and seem to find this very helpful. Others would not be happy with such a demanding and time-consuming intervention, and would rather have their child involved for 10–15 hr a week, or in a behaviorally orientated education program of the TEACCH variant. *Individual talks* with teenagers with autism spectrum disorders of the Asperger variant can be beneficial so long as the psychologist or doctor is well acquainted with the basic problems typical of autism. Psychoanalytically orientated psychotherapies have little place in the overall intervention program for people in the autism spectrum.

Neuropsychopharmacology

No currently known drugs are likely to affect the ultimate outcome of autism spectrum disorders. However, many pharmacological interventions are available for symptoms associated with autism spectrum disorders (van Buitelaar & Willemsen-Swinkels, 2000).

Severe ADHD will sometimes respond favorably to typical stimulant treatment in autism spectrum disorder cases with IQs above 50. In those with severe and profound learning disability, a positive response is not excluded, but the odds are not very favorable. Severe hyperactivity when combined with violent behaviors and self-injury is more likely to respond to an atypical neuroleptic, such as risperidone (often in doses of 0.5–3.0

mg/day in one dose for children under 12 years, increasing to about 1.0–4.5 mg/day for older individuals).

In depression and social withdrawal, particularly in autism spectrum disorder with normal IQ, and especially when there is also a high degree of obsessionality or ritualism, a trial of a serotonin reuptake inhibitor such as fluoxetine (10–40 mg/day in one dose for those under 12 years, 20–80 mg/day for those of about 13 and above) may be valuable. Associated bipolar disorder, not exceedingly rare in autism, is often best treated with risperidone in doses as suggested, followed by the addition of a mood stabilizer such as valproic acid, or, in some cases, lithium. Tics only rarely require separate pharmacologic intervention in autism, but if they are extreme, risperidone, again, is quite likely to be effective. Sleep disorders are difficult to treat. Melatonin (3 mg half an hr before projected sleep onset) can be very effective in inducing sleep, but if used on a regular basis, tends to lose its effect. After a "drug holiday" of a few months, parents report that the drug can be used again with good effect for a similar amount of time.

Those with epilepsy should be treated for their seizure disorder in close collaboration with a child neurologist. Lamotrigine and valproic acid sometimes appear to have beneficial effects not only on the seizure disorder, but also on mood swings and violent behavior. Carbamazepine is probably the antiepileptic drug most widely used in the treatment of epilepsy in autism (Gillberg, 1991). It is often effective, but there is a tendency for perseverative symptoms to become more pronounced in some individuals.

Information to Parents and Patients

As has already been outlined information to all those concerned is extremely important. Very often the easiest way of accessing good information about autism is through a support group such as the National Autism Society (NSA) in the United Kingdom or the Autism Society of America (ASA), or Families for Early Autism Treatment (FEAT) in the United States. Having said that, it is also important to be aware that some information about autism is unscientific and, occasionally, outright unhelpful, spreading myths about the causes and cures. Rather than trying to persuade parents to avoid such information, one should inform them of their existence, so that, when they come across it, they may be better prepared to form their own opinion, distance themselves from it, or come back asking about it.

OUTCOME

Diagnoses of conditions within the autism spectrum are stable over the shorter term. In the very long-term perspective they are also stable, even though conditions diagnosed as atypical or as falling just outside the spectrum are more likely to be considered typical at later evaluation. Of those with classic autism, it is likely that, in adult life, the majority will continue to be dependent on other adults for work, activities, and dwelling (Billstedt,

Gillberg, & Gillberg, submitted). Even the most recent follow-up studies, in which, at least partly adequate interventions have been provided from early childhood, suggest that only a few percent of all affected individuals will be completely independent at age 20–40 years. However, these studies also suggest that with good early programs, the number needing medication or long-term stay in psychiatric hospitals may be greatly reduced. Quality of life in an autism-friendly environment can be good even when independence has not been achieved. Mortality is increased in the classic group. Mortality can usually be attributed to epilepsy, a severe associated medical disorder, or accidents (including drowning). Nevertheless, the vast majority of all with autism will live to old age.

Outcome in Asperger syndrome is much less well understood (Szatmari et al., 2000). However, it varies enormously, with some people doing very well indeed in adult life, who have made excellent careers for themselves, living with a partner, and even having children. Unfortunately, some of these children themselves have autism spectrum disorders. A large subgroup of those with Asperger syndrome has major psychiatric and academic problems in adult life.

Many people (as many as one in three) with autism spectrum disorders show severe symptom aggravation around the time of adolescence. About half of this proportion actually deteriorates, and may never again attain the level of functioning they had reached before puberty.

Prognostic Factors

It has long been recognized that IQ above 70 and some communicative speech at early school age are the strongest predictors of a relatively better outcome in autism (Howlin, 1997). An associated severe medical disorder and the presence of epilepsy, particularly if of early childhood onset, tend to predict a worse outcome. It is likely that an early diagnosis will help increase the odds for a positive outcome.

REFERENCES

American Psychiatric Association. (1994). *Diagnostic and statistical manual of mental disorders: DSM-IV.* Washington, DC: Author.

Asperger, H. (1944). Die autistischen Psychopathen im Kindesalter. *Archiv für Psychiatrie und Nervenkrankheiten, 117,* 76–136.

Berument, S. K., Rutter, M., Lord, C., Pickles, A., & Bailey, A. (1999). Autism screening questionnaire: Diagnostic validity. *British Journal of Psychiatry, 175,* 444–451.

Billstedt, E., Gillberg, I. C., & Gillberg, C. (submitted). Autism after adolescence population-based 13–22-year follow-up study of 118 individuals with autism diagnosed in childhood.

Department of Health. (1999). *Clinical practice guideline: The guideline technical report. Autism/pervasive developmental disorders, Assessment and intervention for young children (age 0–3 years).* Publication No. 4217. Albany, NY: Early Intervention Program. Retrieved from http://www.health.state.ny.us/nysdoh/eip/menu.htm

DiLavore, P. C., Lord, C., & Rutter, M. (1995). The pre-linguistic autism diagnostic observation schedule. *Journal of Autism and Developmental Disorders, 25,* 355–379.

Ehlers, S., & Gillberg, C. (1993). The epidemiology of Asperger syndrome. A total population study. *Journal of Child Psychology and Psychiatry, 34,* 1327–1350.

Ehlers, S., Nyden, A., Gillberg, C., Dahlgren-Sandberg, A., Dahlgren, S.-O., Hjelmquist, E., et al. (1997). Asperger syndrome, autism and attention disorders: A comparative study of the cognitive profiles of 120 children. *Journal of Child Psychology and Psychiatry, 38*, 207–217.

Frith, U., & Happe, F. (1994). Autism: Beyond "theory of mind." *Cognition, 50*, 115–132.

Gillberg, C. (1991). The treatment of epilepsy in autism. *Journal of Autism and Developmental Disorders, 21*, 61–77.

Gillberg, C. (1999). Neurodevelopmental processes and psychological functioning in autism. *Developmental Psychopathology, 11*, 567–587.

Gillberg, C., & Billstedt, E. (2000). Autism and Asperger syndrome: Coexistence with other clinical disorders. *Acta Psychiatrica Scandinavia, 102*, 321–330.

Gillberg, C., & Coleman, M. (1996). Autism and medical disorders: A review of the literature. *Developmental Medicine and Child Neurology, 38*, 191–202.

Gillberg, C., & Coleman, M. (2000). *The biology of the autistic syndromes* (3rd. ed.). London, UK: Mac Keith.

Gillberg, C., Rastam, M., & Wentz, E. (2001). The Asperger Syndrome (and high-functioning autism) Diagnostic Interview (ASDI): A preliminary study of a new structured clinical interview. *Autism, 5*, 57–66.

Gillberg, C., & Steffenburg, S. (1987). Outcome and prognostic factors in infantile autism and similar conditions: A population-based study of 46 cases followed through puberty. *Journal of Autism and Developmental Disorders, 17*, 273–287.

Gillberg, I. C., & Gillberg, C. (1989). Asperger syndrome—some epidemiological considerations: A research note. *Journal of Child Psychology and Psychiatry, 30*, 631–638.

Howlin, P. (1997). Prognosis in autism: Do specialist treatments affect long-term outcome? *European Child and Adolescent Psychiatry, 6*, 55–72.

Howlin, P. (1998). Practitioner review: Psychological and educational treatments for autism. *Journal of Child Psychology and Psychiatry, 39*, 307–322.

Kanner, L. (1943). Autistic disturbances of affective contact. *Nervous Child, 2*, 217–250.

Krug, D. A., Arick, J., & Almond, P. (1980). Behavior checklist for identifying severely handicapped individuals with high levels of autistic behavior. *Journal of Child Psychology and Psychiatry, 21*, 221–229.

Lord, C., Rutter, M., & Le Couteur, A. (1994). Autism Diagnostic Interview-Revised: A revised version of a diagnostic interview for caregivers of individuals with possible pervasive developmental disorders. *Journal of Autism and Developmental Disorders, 24*, 659–685.

National Research Council. (2001). *Educating children with autism.*Committee on Educational Interventions for Children with Autism, Division of Behavioral and Social Sciences and Education. Washington, DC: National Academy Press. Retrieved from www.nap.eduhttp://www.health.state.ny.us/nysdoh/eip/menu.htm

Rapin, I., & Allen, D. (1983). Developmental language disorders: Nosologic considerations. In U. Kirk (Ed.), *Neuropsychology of language reading and spelling* (pp. 155–180). New York: Academic.

Rourke, B. P. (1988). The syndrome of non-verbal learning disabled children: Developmental manifestations of neurological disease. *Clinical Neuropsychology, 2*, 293–330.

Rutter, M., Bailey, A., Bolton, P., & Le Couteur, A. (1994). Autism and known medical conditions: Myth and substance. *Journal of Child Psychology and Psychiatry, 35*, 311–322.

Schopler, E. (1990). *Individualized assessment and treatment for autistic and developmentally disabled children.* Austin, TX: Pro-ed.

Schopler, E., Reichler, R. J., & Renner, B. R. (1988). *The Childhood Autism Rating Scale* (CARS—Rev. ed.). Los Angeles: Western Psychological Services.

Smith, T., Groen, A. D., & Wynn, J. W. (2000). Randomized trial of intensive early intervention for children with pervasive developmental disorder. *American Journal on Mental Retardation, 105*, 269–285.

Sparrow, S. S., Balla, D. A., & Cicchetti, D. V. (1984). *The Vineland Adaptive Behavior Scales.* Circle Pines, MN: American Guidance Service.

Szatmari, P., Bryson, S. E., Streiner, D. L., Wilson, F., Archer, L., & Ryerse, C. (2000). Two-year outcome of preschool children with autism or Asperger's syndrome. *American Journal of Psychiatry, 157*, 1980–1987.

Turner, M., Barnby, G., & Bailey, A. (2000). Genetic clues to the biological basis of autism. *Molecular Medicine Today, 6*, 238–244.

van Buitelaar, J. K., & Willemsen-Swinkels, S. H. (2000). Medication treatment in subjects with autistic spectrum disorders. *European Child and Adolescent Psychiatry, 9*(Suppl. 1), 185–197.

Waterhouse, L., Wing, L., & Fein, D. (1989). Re-evaluating the syndrome of autism in the light of empirical research. In G. Dawson (Ed.), *Autism: Nature, diagnosis, and treatment* (pp. 263–281). New York: Guilford.

Wing, L. (1981). Language, social, and cognitive impairments in autism and severe mental retardation. *Journal of Autism and Developmental Disorders, 11*, 31–44.

Wing, L. (1988). The continuum of autistic characteristics. In E. Schopler & G. B. Mesibov (Eds.), *Diagnosis and assessment in autism. Current issues in autism* (pp. 91–110). New York: Plenum.

Wing, L. (1996). *The autistic spectrum: A guide for parents and professionals.* London, UK: Constable.

Wing, L., Leekam, S. R., Libby, S. J., Gould, J., & Larcombe, M. (2002). The Diagnostic Interview for Social and Communication Disorders: Background, inter-rater reliability and clinical use. *Journal of Child Psychology and Psychiatry, 43*, 307–325.

Wing, L., & Potter, D. (2002). The epidemiology of autistic spectrum disorders: Is the prevalence rising? *Mental Retardation and Developmental Disabilities Reviews, 8*, 151–161.

World Health Organization. (1992). *International statistical classification of diseases and related health problems: ICD-10.* Geneva, Switzerland: Author.

3

Cerebral Palsy

SARAH WINTER, MD

Cerebral palsy (CP) is a handicapping condition that can present with such vastly different expressions that it is easy to question the appropriateness of the term. Despite these misgivings, CP does exist. There are common understandings of its definition, a generally accepted classification system, increasing knowledge about its etiology, a body of knowledge about its epidemiology, and increasing numbers of treatment options.

CP is often described as a group of nonprogressive, but often changing, motor impairment syndromes secondary to lesions or anomalies of the brain arising at any time during early brain development (Mutch, Alberman, Hagberg, Kodama, & Perat, 1992). The tone abnormalities of CP can range from spasticity to hypotonicity, can be mixed, and can vary in one child throughout the day. An important component of the definition of CP is that it is nonprogressive. In fact, many children improve functionally over time consistent with the nature of pediatric neurologic maturation. Central to the definition of CP is the concept that it is a disorder of the brain and not of the musculoskeletal system. Understanding that CP is a neurodevelopmental disability with its primary impact on the motor system will assist families in understanding the impact of CP on a child's or adult's functional skills.

CP was first described in the medical literature in the late 19th century by Dr William Little. Little's description of the condition in his article, "On the Influence of Abnormal Parturition, Difficult Labours, Premature Birth . . ." set the stage for our understanding of CP as a condition that results from anoxia during labor and delivery (Little, 1862, article reprinted in (not alive in 1958) 1958). Unfortunately, a half century of epidemiologic research refuting that conclusion has not changed the lay perception that CP is caused by a bad labor and delivery experience with anoxic damage

SARAH WINTER • Section of Developmental and Behavioral Pediatrics, Columbus Children's Hospital, The Ohio State University, Columbus, Ohio 43210

to the brain. While hypoxic ischemic encephalopathy occurs, it is only an infrequent cause of CP (Nelson & Grether, 1999).

Currently, as in the case for most developmental disabilities, a cure for CP is not available. The neurologic damage cannot be undone nor can a surgeon create new neuronal tissue. Nevertheless, medical professionals do provide assistance to the child and family through diagnosis, case management, and interventions that minimize impairment and disability and prevent secondary disabilities, as do related healthcare and rehabilitation or habilitation professionals. The majority of CP research and clinical activities support the use of interventions to maximize each individual's physical well-being and functional skills, and thereby their potential to live life to its fullest.

EPIDEMIOLOGY AND PREVENTION EFFORTS

Much of the information regarding the prevalence and trends in CP comes from population databases in Sweden, Western Australia, and England. Over a period of 40 years, these databases show the prevalence rate of CP to be between 1.5 and 2.5 per 1000 live births (Hagberg, Hagberg, Beckung, & Uvebrant, 2001; Pharoah, Cooke, Cooke, & Rosenbloom, 1990; Stanley, Blair, & Alberman, 2000). Data from the United States are consistent with these studies showing the prevalence of CP at 2.4 per 1000 live births (Boyle et al., 1991). Trend analysis over a 16-year period shows no significant change in the overall prevalence of CP per 1000 live births and 1-year survivors between 1975 and 1991 (Winter, Autry, Yeargin-Allsopp, & Boyle, 2002). This remains consistent despite the fact that neonatal intensive care lowers the risk of mortality among low birth weight infants. A recent report of infants born at 500–1500 g showed that despite a declining mortality rate in this group of low birth weight infants born from 1979 through 1994, the rate of CP did not increase (O'Shea, Preisser, Klinepeter, & Dillard, 1998).

Preventing CP is a large and complex task because there are multiple etiologies. Much attention has been paid to the prevention of premature birth as more than half of children with CP are born at low birth weight or less than 2500 g. Recent information regarding the successful use of progesterone injections to prevent premature labor in women who had already had one premature delivery is promising (Meis et al., 2003). Theories regarding uterine irritability leading to premature delivery with the presence of subclinical or overt infection have led to many trials using antibiotics in pregnant women. These studies have shown benefit to the mother and infant in preventing postnatal morbidity but have not yet been shown to decrease the prevalence of CP. Specific interventions for the premature infant that may reduce CP, such as the use of surfactant that has increased survival and has prevented chronic lung disease, have yet to demonstrate an effect on the overall or birth weight specific prevalence of CP (Soll & Morely, 2001).

CLASSIFICATION OF CEREBRAL PALSY

The classification system for CP serves to highlight consistent differences in the types of CP, the associated conditions, and similarities in etiology. CP is most often congenital, meaning that the cause is presumed to be prenatal or perinatal (with perinatal defined as the time period beginning at the initiation of labor and ending at 30 days postdelivery). CP is less often acquired. Examples of acquired CP include a postnatal infection, trauma, and shaken baby syndrome. CP is classified in two ways. Attempts have been made to classify CP in degrees of severity such as mild, moderate, and severe. The use of this terminology is subjective and is not universally accepted. Most often, CP is described by the terms extrapyramidal and spastic types. Within the spastic types, CP is described by location of the affected area. About 75% of children with CP have spasticity with spastic hemiplegia, diplegia, and quadriplegia being evenly distributed amongst all children with spastic CP.

Extrapyramidal versus Spastic CP. The descriptions extrapyramidal versus spastic refer to the location of the abnormality or damage to the brain. Movement is initiated and regulated by the motor control system of the brain. The pyramidal tracts carry the signal for muscle contraction. The extrapyramidal system, including the basal ganglia, provides regulatory influences on that contraction.

Extrapyramidal CP is a term used to describe the abnormal movement patterns that are caused by damage to areas of the brain outside of the pyramidal tracts. Extrapyramidal CP is often further subdivided into dyskinetic and ataxic types. Dyskinetic movement disorders within CP classification systems include dystonia, athetosis, chorea, rigidity, and hypotonia. Often, more than one of these movement patterns are present.

Choreoathetoid CP, an example of extrapyramidal CP, occurs when the damage to the brain is located in the basal ganglia, classically kernicterus (Sugama, 2001) (Centers for Disease Control and Prevention, 2001). The brief, jerking, purposeless movements of chorea and the long axial writhing movements of athetosis characterize choreoathetoid movements.

Dystonic CP is characterized by the simultaneous involuntary contraction of agonist and antagonist muscle group. This pattern is often fluctuating.

Hypotonic CP is a term that creates confusion. Hypotonia is described as low resting muscle tone. When hypotonia is generalized throughout the body, the term CP is often applied. In these cases, it impairs function, is nonprogressive, is a result of damage to the developing brain, and is not due to a known other cause. When this low muscle tone accompanies a condition like Down Syndrome or Prader–Willi Syndrome, the term hypotonic CP is not added to the diagnosis but hypotonia is understood to be an aspect of the underlying primary, genetic condition.

Ataxic CP, a subtype of extrapyramidal CP, results when damage occurs in the cerebellum. Ataxia is characterized by difficulties performing finely controlled movements and results in overshooting when reaching for objects and a wide-based, unsteady gait.

Spastic CP is a movement disorder characterized by velocity-dependent increase in resistance. Approximately 75% of cases are primarily *Spastic CP*, which is a movement disorder characterized by velocity-dependent increase in resistance. Spasticity results when damage occurs along the pyramidal tract. Attempts to localize the spasticity and describe spastic CP in terms of where on the body it is expressed aid understanding; in general, of the etiology, functional impairment, associated conditions, and potential treatments for children with spastic CP.

Diplegic CP describes spasticity that occurs in the lower extremities. An individual with diplegic CP, however, will often experience coordination difficulties of the upper extremities or even spasticity of the upper extremities. But, the predominant impairment is in the lower extremities.

Hemiplegic CP is when the spasticity is on one side of the body. Typically, the arm is more affected than the leg and may assume a triple flexion posture. The term triple flexion posture describes the classic position of the involved upper extremity with flexion of the wrist and elbow, and adduction of the shoulder.

Quadriplegic CP involves all four extremities. Generally, the legs are more involved than the arms. Individuals with quadriplegic CP frequently present with truncal hypotonia and extremity hypertonicity.

Monoplegic CP is a term used to describe spasticity found in only one extremity. Practically, this situation is likely the result of a hemiplegia in which the impairment of the leg is imperceptible.

As with any classification system, the present nomenclature does not completely describe what is seen in practice. Many individuals with CP have a combination of the previously described movement abnormalities. This is referred to *as mixed pattern CP* and is present in many individuals with CP. Because epidemiologic studies often use a primary diagnosis for classification, mixed pattern CP is likely to be underreported. Additionally, as children grow and develop, the pattern of CP, and specific diagnosis, may change.

DIAGNOSING CEREBRAL PALSY

Many types of physicians are called upon to make this diagnosis including primary pediatricians, family practitioners, developmental pediatricians, pediatric neurologists, rehabilitation specialists, pediatric orthopedists, and geneticists. Diagnosing and imparting the diagnosis requires an understanding of the risk factors for CP, experience with the neurologic examination that is unique to the developing child, use of imaging studies, and the ability to give the diagnosis to the family and child in a compassionate, realistic, but hopeful manner.

In reviewing the patient history, it is helpful to gather information about factors that are related to CP as an outcome. Oftentimes, it is easiest to consider these risk factors in three broad categories as, prenatal, perinatal, and postnatal risk factors. Infants born with intrauterine growth retardation are at risk for a variety of developmental disabilities including CP. Growth retardation may be a result of an injury or developmental abnormality of the brain or a genetic defect. Recently more genetic disorders have been identified as causes for CP. Congenital malformations of the brain are most often idiopathic, but a few of these disorders have been found to have specific chromosomal abnormalities, such as the deletion in the short arm of chromosome 17 in the Miller–Dieker form of lissencephaly (Dobyns et al., 1996). Stroke or hemorrhage occurs in the prenatal period. Occasionally the cause of such an event is known, such as maternal anticoagulation therapy resulting in fetal CNS hemorrhage or Factor V Leiden mutation, which causes resistance to activated protein C, causing fetal stroke (Thorarensen, Ryan, Hunter, & Younkin, 1997). Often, evidence for the stroke is found on head imaging studies without a specific reason being evident. The presence of calcifications on a head computer tomography (CT) may suggest an intrauterine infection such as cytomegalovirus or toxoplasmosis.

Thorough investigation into the circumstances of the child's birth is important. The neonatal discharge summary should be scanned for information on birth weight and gestational age, Apgar scores, head ultrasound results, and presence of neonatal seizures. It is known that the risk of CP increases with decreasing birth weight. Nevertheless, even in the majority of children born at extremely low birth (<1000 g) only 17%, showed signs of CP at age 18 months in one recent study (Vohr et al., 2000). In premature infants, the presence of an intraventricular hemorrhage and parenchyma involvement on head ultrasound studies is predictive of CP (Msall et al., 1994; Pinto-Martin et al., 1995; Vohr et al., 1999).

Although the prevalence of neonatal asphyxia is low, it is devastating. The cause of the asphyxia may be known, such as prolonged hypoxia (in the event of a placenta abruption). In other cases, its onset is less defined but the neonate was clearly affected as evidenced by severely depressed Apgar scores and or neonatal seizures within the first 24 hr of life. Postnatal causes for CP tend to be more obvious and dramatic such as a shaking injury, accidental trauma, and bacterial meningitis.

Diagnosis of CP

The diagnosis of CP consists of specific neurologic exam findings present in the developing child and a history that confirms the motor delay or deviance is not deteriorating. The neurologic findings include the following: (1) abnormality of muscular tone, (2) abnormalities of posture/movement, and (3) persistence of primitive reflexes. Findings consistent with central nervous system injury or congenital brain anomaly on head imaging studies are supportive but not diagnostic of CP.

Motor delay in a child is most notable when a child fails to accomplish known gross motor milestones. Fine motor milestones receive less attention by both parents and medical professionals but can signal the presence of CP. Normal gross and fine motor milestones are listed in Table 3.1.

Table 3.1. Motor Milestones in Normal Child Development

Gross motor milestone	Age	Fine motor milestone	Age
Head off table	1 month	Retain rattle	1 month
Chest up	2 months	Hands unfisted	3–4 months
Roll	3–5 months	Transfers objects	5 months
Sitting without support	7 months	Immature pincer grasp	7–8 months
Cruising	9–10 months		
Walking alone	12 months	Release	12 months
Jump in place	24 months	Hand preference	18 months
Pedal tricycle	30 months		

Walking is the most recognized developmental milestone and occurs in most children at 12 months with the upper limit of the normal range being at 16 months. The presence of persistent head lag, poor sitting balance, inability to bear weight on the legs, and the inability to walk by the appropriate time are other common triggers for an evaluation. Hand preference should not occur prior to 18 months. Hand preference at 6–12 months is often misinterpreted by parents as early hand preference rather than an abnormality of neurologic function in the nondominant hand. This is a frequent presentation of hemiplegic CP and should prompt a neurologic evaluation.

Assessing muscular tone in a child is a skill that requires experience and exposure to children and adults with abnormal tone. Spasticity is the clasp knife response or velocity-dependent increased resistance to passive stretch. When severe, it is an obvious finding. It is often accompanied by increased deep tendon reflexes. Spasticity is more pronounced when a child is anxious or ill. Hypotonia, or low resting muscle tone, can also be present to a greater or lesser degree. It can often be elicited in the smaller child by noticing slip through when holding a child under the arms in vertical suspension. Deep tendon reflexes are either decreased or increased with hypotonia. Rigidity is classically described as lead pipe hypertonia, a persistence of increased tone throughout the range of motion about the joint. Children with rigidity tend to have more fluctuation in tone and have persistent primitive reflexes. Muscular tone can change as a child develops. This is commonly seen in infants with hypotonia who evolve to have spasticity by 12–18 months of age. This change is not due to a progression in the neuronal injury or abnormality but rather reflects maturation of the central nervous system.

The diagnosis of CP requires the examiner to observe movements and postural control that are not typically noted in a neurologic exam. A neurodevelopmental exam of the gross and fine motor systems must be added. Abnormal movements should be noted. Unless specific attention is paid to how a child moves, abnormal movements and postures will be missed on the typical neurologic exam such as combat crawling, dragging one side, or standing on toes. Abnormal postural control is often present in children with CP. The infant exam should assess the quality of head control, rolling, sitting balance, crawling, cruising, and walking. This exam will pick up abnormalities even if the motor developmental milestones are intact. Attention to the fine motor exam will permit the examiner to detect the persistence of fisting or the presence of ataxic hand movements long before delays in walking are noticed.

Knowledge of primitive reflex patterns is essential. The newborn child has primitive reflexes that are normal and diminish over a period of approximately 6 months. These reflexes must disappear to allow a child to attain normal postural and righting responses acquired from approximately 3–9 months. With CP, this normal evolution is disrupted. The persistence of a startle response or Moro reflex prohibits good sitting balance. The presence of a plantar grasp impedes an infant's ability to cruise. These abnormal patterns will be noticed when specific attention is paid to the neurodevelopmental exam.

Brain Imaging

As previously mentioned, imaging studies can be supportive to but are not diagnostic of CP. Significant changes are occurring in the ability to image the central nervous system. Magnetic resonance imaging (MRI) is the single most useful tool to enhance the history and physical exam in the diagnosis of CP. In children with a major motor delay, the majority will have abnormalities on MRI (Candy, Hoon, Capute, & Bryan, 1993). Head ultrasound is limited to the neonate and young infant while the fontanels remain open. Since MRI is superior to CT in differentiating soft tissue differences such as gray and white matter, the MRI is the recommended study beyond infancy. Positron emission tomographic (PET) scans, functional MRI, and diffusion-weighted imaging may add to our understanding in the future. Currently they are not used as a clinical tool (Chugani, 1993; Hoon & Melhem, 2000; Inder et al., 1999). Magnetic resonance spectroscopy, the observation of intracellular cerebral metabolites, is being used as an adjunct to the information provided by the MRI.

Giving the Diagnosis

For most parents, the moment they hear the diagnosis of CP applied to their child, is a profound event. The diagnosis should be given in terms that can be understood by the parents. Information should be given in written form to provide support to what was discussed in the clinical setting. References for parent/caregiver focused information are included in Appendix A. A follow-up visit to review this information is recommended.

There are certain factors that must be appreciated surrounding the diagnosis of CP. Sometimes, the diagnosis of CP is the least of a parent's concern. Describing CP and its functional implications, its causes, and its treatment may be secondary in the minds of parents who are facing a diagnosis of mental retardation or autism in addition to CP. Hearing that a child has CP and may limp when it walks may be good news to a family faced with the possible death of their child from extreme prematurity. The clinician must try to understand how the diagnosis fits in the context of what the parent has experienced up to the moment of diagnosis, which will help when trying to gauge the language and terminology that will be most helpful to a parent's understanding.

INTERVENTIONS: A MULTIDISCIPLINARY PROCESS

Facilitating the growth, development, and ongoing progress into adulthood of people with CP requires an integration of family, medical, educational, therapeutic, and technologic support systems. Most major urban areas have a multispecialty clinic that serves many of the needs of individuals with CP and has information and connections to other CP-specific services. Usually these clinics have nursing, orthopedics, developmental pediatrics, psychiatry, physical therapy consultation, and orthotic vendors. Many clinics also have psychology, neurology, occupational therapy, social work, and nutrition as well as close working relationships with many other subspecialists.

While every person presents with a unique set of circumstances, there are common conditions that occur within each type of CP. Broad generalizations about associated conditions can be made to help organize proactive planning for assessment of needs and services for individuals with CP. Table 3.2 shows frequently associated conditions occurring with the common subtypes of spastic CP. As a group, these conditions are associated with these types of CP. In any individual person, all or none of these conditions may exist.

Cognitive Impairment and Learning Disability

Overall, approximately 50% of individuals with CP have some degree of cognitive impairment (Murphy, Yeargin-Alsopp, Decoufle, & Drews, 1993).

Table 3.2. Conditions that are Associated with Specific Types

Hemiplegic cerebral palsy	Spastic diplegia	Spastic quadriplegia
General health good	General health good	Multiple medical conditions:
Unilateral spasticity	Spasticity of the lower extremities	Constipation
Unilateral muscle contractures		Oromotor dysfunction
	Muscle contractures lower extremities	Aspiration and/or pneumonia
Unilateral growth disturbances		
	Learning disabilities	Failure to thrive
Epilepsy	Strabismus	Epilepsy
Visual disturbance:		Orthopedic problems:
Hemianopsia		Muscle contractures
Learning disability		Hip dislocation
		Spine curvature
		Cognitive impairment of CP

Often, CP is erroneously linked with intellectual disability as if the two conditions always occur together. In addition to intellectual disability, another 25–30% has specific learning disabilities. Evaluation of these concerns is conducted by standardized intelligence and achievement testing usually performed by psychologists. Specialized testing materials, procedures, and interpretation may be required for individuals with significant motor impairment and oromotor dysfunction. Physicians, psychologists, and educators should be vigilant for these learning problems and proactively initiate testing early in the child's educational course so that the findings can be translated to the best individualized education program for the child and individualized services for adults.

Role of Schools

Many advances in the education of children with CP have occurred in the last 30 years. Most of them are the direct result of Individuals with Disabilities Education Act (IDEA) of 1975 also known as Public Law-142. Under this legislation and its amendments, standards are set and some financial support is provided to direct states to provide free and appropriate education to all children with disabilities. The fundamental features of these laws include inclusive education, early intervention, assistive technology, and transition planning. Children with CP qualify for early intervention services based on developmental delay judged by defined criteria. Usually children with CP qualify based on motor delay but may also qualify in other domains. Services to the infant and toddler can be provided in a home-based model or a center-based model. A transition plan is then provided through the individualized family service plan (IFSP) for a preschool program. Some children with CP have no educational needs at this stage but need related services, usually physical therapy. This can be arranged. However, many children will need educational services that will be provided based on the individualized education program (IEP). The IEP will be reviewed and updated periodically throughout the child's educational years. Children with CP often need services such as, physical, occupational, and speech and language therapy. All children with CP will need adaptive physical education, even the child with the minimal functional limitations. In 1991, as a part of PL-102-199, children with CP and other disabilities were made eligible for technology-based assistive devices for educational purposes. Devices commonly used by children with CP include augmentative communication devices, powered mobility, ambulation devices, computers, prescription lenses, and environmental controls. School systems can vary greatly with respect to the extent to which they acquire and utilize assistive technology. Part of transition planning services and providing inclusive education is the ability of the child with CP to move about in the educational environment. Accessible classrooms, bathrooms, and playgrounds are essential to the education of children with these physical disabilities. It is the responsibility of the clinical team assisting the family to advise them about needed services, environmental modifications, and assistive devices, and to advocate with the family as necessary.

Another feature of transition planning is the transition out of the secondary education into higher education, vocational training, and supported employment and other adult services. This planning should and typically does begin years before the end of high school. For the student who is college bound, accessibility should be addressed prior to enrollment. States provide through lead state agencies for vocational rehabilitation services, programs to support vocational training to persons with disabilities. These programs are made available by federal funds dispersed to states meeting the standards set by law. These programs are unlike IDEA, in that this legislation is not enforceable by rights and procedures, as entitlements. However, many private foundations, commercial businesses, and community agencies provide opportunities for persons with CP to find supported employment and alternative day involvements and services.

Social Adjustment

Children with CP may go through a pattern of adjustment to their disability that is fairly predictable depending on their cognitive abilities. Typically, the toddler or preschooler does not notice the difference between them and other children. When the child approaches the later years of preschool and certainly by elementary school, the child with CP realizes these differences and may experience frustration, sadness, and anger at their limitations. Fortunately, other children who are able-bodied are very accepting of differences at this stage. As the child approaches middle school, prejudices against persons with disabilities may develop. Cognitive immaturity or a disruption of what is expected in a peer may account for the negative attitudes about persons with disabilities (Harper, 1999). Hopefully, the child with CP has strong family support to validate their worth as a person and value to their family. Family, educators, and medical professionals can limit the lack of knowledge that can stimulate cruel comments or treatment of the child with CP. This can be done by honest and appropriate sharing of information about CP and education in the schools and in the community.

Adolescence is a turbulent time for all teens, including those with CP. Extended periods of normalizing activities, like clubs, church, music and sports lessons, and opportunities for independence help children with CP accept their differences. Counseling may be necessary at any of these stages of adjustment, and may include a focus on alleviation of distress or teaching of coping and social skills.

MEDICAL MANAGEMENT

Every individual with CP should have a primary physician and medical home. The complexity of medical care is more easily addressed with the assistance of someone who is charged with overseeing the medical care. While this person need not be an expert in CP, an interest in the individual, a willingness to learn, and expertise in general medical healthcare are necessary to provide an optimal medical home.

Growth

Unlike other children in the United States, those with CP often struggle to maintain or gain weight and are rarely overweight. Many factors contribute to the common problem of failure to thrive that is usually described as weight for height that is less than the 5 percentile on the growth chart (Hamill et al., 1979). There are limitations to the growth chart. Experts in the field of CP and growth recommend the use of skin fold thickness as a measure of nutritional status, because it is a more sensitive measure of failure to thrive (Samson-Fang & Stevenson, 2000).

Most often the cause of failure to thrive in children with CP is organic. Weight gain is based on consuming a larger number of calories than are expended. Children with CP have problems with both energy intake and energy expenditure. A child may be in constant motion or use a large amount of energy to move expending a large number of kilocalories daily. In addition, problems with oromotor function may cause gagging, choking, and/or aspiration of food into the lungs. These factors inhibit ingestion of adequate calories. Oftentimes, a combination of multiple factors such as oromotor dysfunction, muscle spasms with pain, poor sleep, constipation, and behavioral refusal conspire to prevent adequate nutrition and subsequent growth. Addressing all of the factors contributing to poor growth in the individual case will be more effective than concentrating on one single factor. Ultimately, a gastrostomy tube may be a necessary intervention on either a temporary or permanent basis. Parents will often express a sense of relief once a gastrostomy tube is placed.

Oromotor Dysfunction

Oromotor dysfunction is often present in individuals with spastic quadriplegia and children with extrapyramidal CP. Language delay may indicate cognitive delays or may instead be a sign of oromotor dysfunction. Expressive language delay with relatively higher receptive language skills may indicate significant oromotor dysfunction. Children with oromotor dysfunction often benefit from assistive communication devices but need professional expertise to teach a child how to use the device (Downey & Hurtig, 2003).

Drooling is another manifestation of poor oromotor control. Drooling may be worsened by poor head and neck control and decreased sensitivity to saliva in the mouth. The presence of drooling can be very socially limiting for the individual with CP. Multiple interventions are possible for this problem including therapy, medications, and surgery (Blasco & Allaire, 1992).

Oromotor dysfunction may result in aspiration of food or saliva into the lungs. The symptoms of aspiration may be obvious such as choking and/or cyanosis with eating. Aspiration may also occur silently, causing no discomfort to the individual at all. In this case, a child may experience failure to thrive, frequent pneumonia, or recurrent wheezing. Chronic aspiration should be considered when CP, oromotor dysfunction, and recurrent wheezing are present.

Gastrointestinal Dysmotility

Problems with delayed gastric emptying, gastroesophageal reflux, and constipation are frequent in individuals with spastic quadriplegic CP. These disorders are interrelated and compound one another. The child who has delayed gastric emptying is likely to reflux from the stomach causing pain and discomfort. Thus, eating becomes more difficult resulting in decreased intake of food and fluids causing constipation that, in turn, causes bloating, distension of the abdomen, and poor gastric emptying. This is a problem most often seen in children who have poor mobility and poor nutritional status. Improving nutritional status and hydration through dietary supplements, feeding therapy, and or a gastrostomy tube can break this cycle. Increasing movement and exercise can also improve gastrointestinal dysmotility.

Spasticity Management

Treatment to minimize spasticity does not address the primary pathology of CP that resides in the brain, but it may decrease the sequelae of the increased tone. Problems such as musculoskeletal deformity, limitations of movement, and pain may be minimized by the use of interventions to reduce tone. Historically, diazepam and related medications were the only options for management of spasticity. Within the past two decades, selective medications and surgical interventions have become available. Treatment options for spasticity currently include oral medications, injection of medication into the affected muscle, intrathecal medication, and neurosurgical intervention.

Oral Medications

Common oral medications used to decrease spasticity include diazepam, baclofen, and dantrolene. Diazepam (Valium™) is readily available, inexpensive, and has a long history of use. Unfortunately, diazepam acts centrally and sedating side effects usually make this drug an undesirable choice for managing the problems of spasticity (Young, Robert, & Delwaide, 1981).

Baclofen (Lioresal™) acts at the spinal cord stimulating gamma aminobutyric acid (GABA) inhibitory pathways to reduce spasticity. In large doses it may cause central nervous system sedation. Acute withdrawal from the drug may cause serious central nervous system effects such as hallucinations and seizures or acute increase in spasticity. No intravenous preparation of baclofen is available. Therefore, it is recommended to taper use of this drug prior to surgery or procedure that results in an ileus

(Krach, 2001). Dantrolene sodium (Dantrium™) produces muscle relaxation by interfering with the release of calcium from the sarcoplasmic reticulum of the skeletal muscle. Dantrolene does not directly affect the central nervous system but has central side effects. Dantrolene has the potential for fatal and nonfatal liver toxicity and may cause excessive weakness (Gormley, 2001).

Intrathecal Baclofen

Severe spasticity can be controlled by placing baclofen in a hockey puck-sized device in the abdominal cavity, a treatment called continuous intrathecal baclofen. The baclofen is delivered from the reservoir through a catheter into the spinal canal. The tip of the catheter is usually positioned on the low thoracic area. This externally programmable device pumps very small amounts of baclofen on a continuous basis and can be varied throughout the day by the programmable pump. Complications may include mechanical failure, CNS side effects of lethargy and sedation, and operative complications including infection, disconnected tubing, catheter breakage, cerebrospinal fluid (CSF) leak (Albright, 1996). Despite these limitations, many centers report improvements in muscle tone, range of motion, and functional activities in patients receiving the intrathecal baclofen (Butler & Campbell, 2000).

Nerve blocks

Nerve blocks can be used to affect muscle tone in a localized way. Two examples of chemical neurolysis are phenol blocks and botulism toxin A injections. Phenol, alcohol, and localized anesthetics have long been used to provide a local motor point block. Phenol denatures protein in the myelin sheath of the nerve, destroying the axon. Because nerves are capable of regeneration within 3–6 months, this effect is temporary. Botulism toxin acts to irreversibly block the cholinergic receptors of the neuromuscular junction thus inhibiting the release of acetylcholine, which is required for muscle contraction. This too is temporary, in effect, lasting approximately 2–3 months. Botulism toxin can be rapidly administered without the need for electrical stimulation, and requires a much smaller volume and smaller needle for infusion, thereby causing less pain than the process of injecting phenol. The cost of botulism toxin is quite high compared to other neurolytic agents. The efficacy of single or repeated botulism toxin injections on functional abilities in the long run is unknown. However, use of botulism toxin injections has demonstrated short-term improvement in range of motion, muscle tone, and functional abilities (Koman et al., 2001).

Selective Dorsal Rhizotomy

Finally, spasticity may be permanently addressed with the selective dorsal rhizotomy. This procedure involves the selective cutting of sensory nerves returning from the lower extremities to the lumbosacral spine. Following the surgery, an intensive rehabilitative program is undertaken by the child to "relearn how to walk." Outcome studies of the selective dorsal rhizotomy show that it helps reduce spasticity and has a positive effect of gross motor function (McLaughlin et al., 2002).

ORTHOPEDIC MANAGEMENT

Orthopedic intervention involves managing the sequelae of increased muscular tone that includes treating and preventing skeletal deformity and addressing muscle, ligament, tendon, and surrounding soft tissue contracture. Orthopedic treatment and spasticity management are not mutually exclusive but rather complimentary components of an appropriate medical intervention plan. Surgical intervention to correct deformity or contracture does not equate to normalization of gait pattern or cure of CP. Correction of a deformity of the musculoskeletal system does not eliminate the cause of the deformity. Orthopedic management of children with CP involves complex decisions integrating surgical skills, knowledge about the patterns of CP pathology, natural progression of the different subtypes of CP, and an understanding of child development. This type of surgery is best done by the surgeon who has pediatric expertise and experience in CP. Finally, orthopedic management of CP takes time and consistent follow-up.

Hip

Children with spastic quadriplegia will frequently have problems with growth about the hip due to increased and abnormal balance of tone around the hip joint. Since bones grow according to the forces placed on them, the femoral head and acetabulum may gradually become dysplastic under the influence of spasticity. These forces may cause the hip to dislocate posteriorly and superiorly out of the joint. This is most likely to occur in nonambulatory children with spastic quadriplegia. If the hip is identified as at risk, hip positioning, soft tissue surgery, and osteotomies are considerations.

Foot

The goal of orthopedic intervention on the foot is to preserve a plantigrade (flat on the ground) foot position. This provides the best biomechanical and proprioceptive position for both ambulation and positioning in a wheelchair or stander. Spasticity works against that ideal often pushing the foot into an equinovarus (plantarflexed and medially deviated) position. Bracing with ankle foot orthoses, serial casting, and botulism toxin injections have been effective in treating the plantar flexion contracture. Orthopedic intervention is often necessary and effective when the contracture has become fixed. Gait analysis laboratories can be used to assist in the decision making process (Schwartz, 2004).

Spine

Treatment of spine curvature in individuals with CP is increasingly limited to pediatric orthopedists with a special interest in spinal surgery. Observation, orthoses, and surgical intervention are treatment options. In general terms, bracing is considered at curves measuring approximately 20–25° but less than 40° (Lonstein, Winter, Bradford, & Ogilvie, 1995). Spine braces should be used to hold a curve rather than providing correction. Progression of the curve is likely in children with neuromuscular curves. A decision to operate, which includes fusion of vertebral bodies to prevent progression and sometimes correction of the curve, is complex.

THERAPEUTIC INTERVENTION

The goal of therapy is to allow a child to participate as fully and developmentally appropriate as possible in their lives. This is done in many ways but traditionally this involves initiating physical therapy, occupational therapy, and speech language therapy. Therapy is provided in a variety of models. It can be provided in the context of a home-based model, a center-based program, a hospital outpatient model, and a multidisciplinary educational model. Therapy can be provided in group sessions or as individual therapy. Finally, therapy can be provided as a direct service or in an indirect consultative fashion.

Specific principles of therapy related to CP are beginning to emerge with new research on the efficacy and outcomes of therapeutic intervention. The goal with all children with CP is to establish normal motor development and function and to prevent contractures and deformity. Therapeutic goals include teaching a developmental sequence of acquiring skills and preparing the child with tone abnormalities to perform specific functional tasks in real life settings. Specific techniques are being studied in children with CP. Forced used or constraint-induced therapy is when the affected side is forced to be used by restraining, by tying back, or casting the typical side of the body. This is a therapeutic approach being tried in adults with hemiplegia resulting from a stroke (van der Lee, 1999). It is also being evaluated for efficacy in children with hemiplegic CP (Willis, 2002). Strength training for a person with spasticity is being promoted now rather than discouraged as had been in the past. Evidence exists that spastic muscles that are weak can improve in strength without increasing the spasticity (Dodd, Taylor, & Damiano, 2002). Therapists may guide the family into thinking about occasional episodes of therapy rather than years of commitment to a therapy program as an expected course of treatment.

INTERVENTION AND SUPPORT FOR ADULTS WITH CP

High functioning adults with CP have a life expectancy close to that of the general population. However, life expectancy can be reduced by factors that impair an individual's functional level such as low cognitive level, involvement of all four extremities, poor mobility, and dependent feeding (Strauss & Shavelle, 2001). As most individuals with CP live a long life, planning for adulthood is important.

Medical Care

Caring for the medical issues of adults is often overlooked. Adults with CP are often concerned about pain, decline in mobility, fatigue, and loss of independence. In one survey of adults with CP, 35% reported decreased walking ability and 9% reported having stopped walking (Andersson & Mattsson, 2001). Eighteen percent of these respondents reported pain everyday. Pain in individuals with CP is likely to come from the hip and in nonambulatory individuals pain is very common. One survey of nonambulatory adults, with a mean age of 27 years, reported that hip pain was present in 47% of respondents. Of that group only 13.6% of those with pain had received medical treatment for the pain (Hodgkinson et al., 2001).

Osteoporosis is a concern for all adults, but especially for those with CP. In fact, osteopenia was found in 77% of a population-based cohort of children and adolescents with CP and 97% of the subgroup of children who were older than 9 years and could not stand (Henderson et al., 2002). Given this knowledge and the known patterns of bone density loss in the general adult population, concern for increased bone fractures, subsequent pain, and functional limitation, more research into treatment is needed.

The medical care and treatment of patients with CP has usually been provided by pediatricians and pediatric subspecialists. The medical needs of the adults with CP may be left untreated, as few medical professionals caring for adults are familiar with CP and its related conditions. Oftentimes, unrelated acute and chronic conditions go untreated as adults with CP find it difficult to find routine medical care and dental care. Routine care also may be limited by financial disincentives to care for individuals with disabilities and physical barriers present in clinic settings.

Vocational Services

Employment for adults with CP and other disabilities, including intellectual disabilities and epilepsy has improved through vocational services. An increasing number of individuals with CP are gaining competitive employment (Gilmore, 2000). Successful employment is partly related to type and severity of disability, intelligence level, functional independence, and whether or not assistive technology is needed (O'Grady, 1995). Community integrated employment must include an appropriate and reliable means of transportation. Driver assessments through the Bureau of Motor Vehicles and handicapped-accessible public transportation are means to overcome obstacles to competitive employment. Unfortunately, despite the increased prevalence of competitive employment, there was a decrease in real earnings when earnings were adjusted for inflation (Gilmore, 2000). Private groups such as United Cerebral Palsy, professional groups such as the Academy of Cerebral Palsy and Developmental Medicine, and federal agencies such as the Administration of Developmental Disabilities and the Centers for Disease Control and Prevention are trying to address the concerns of these adults. Other advocacy groups also exist to help adults with CP.

SUMMARY

CP, present in approximately 2 per 1000 live births, is a group of motor impairment syndromes caused by an injury or abnormality of the brain that is nonprogressive. CP is classified by two main categories; spastic and extrapyramidal. The diagnosis is made by physical exam and a thorough history. Taken together, the presence of abnormal tone, abnormal movements and postures, and persistence of primitive reflexes in an infant with motor delays, which are nonprogressive, constitutes the diagnosis of CP. MRI is a helpful adjunct but is not diagnostic of CP. Educational services and related services such as physical therapy and assistive technology are available in school systems as a result of the IDEA legislation. Adjusting to having CP is difficult. A strong family that is able to validate the child's worth and contribution to the family will make this process easier.

Most children access the services of a multidisciplinary CP clinic to address the many associated conditions and needs related to CP. These issues include but are not limited to initial diagnosis, musculoskeletal problems, spasticity management, feeding difficulties, weight problems, respiratory infections and aspiration, epilepsy, and impaired communication, learning, and mobility. Relatively new treatments for spasticity include selective dorsal rhizotomy, intrathecal baclofen pump placement, and botulism toxin injection. Research has demonstrated that spastic muscles do benefit by strengthening despite earlier concerns that strengthening would only result in increasing spasticity.

Adults with CP are concerned about persisting or chronic pain, osteoporosis, and inadequate primary medical care due to misunderstandings about CP, paucity of providers available to care for their specialized needs, and financial barriers to providing care.

APPENDIX A

References for Parents of Children With Cerebral Palsy

1. Batshaw, M. (1998). *Your child has a disability: A complete sourcebook of daily and medical care*. Baltimore, MD: Paul H. Brookes.
2. Geralis, E. (Ed.). (1998). *Children with cerebral palsy—A parent's guide*. Bethesda, MD: Woodbine House.
3. Internet Resources
   CP: Resource Center: Retrieved from www.twinenterprises.com/cp5/30/06

Cerebral Palsy: Retrieved from www.comeunity.com/disability/
cerebral_palsy/index.html5/30/06

4. Magazine: *Exceptional parent magazine* by Psy-Ed Corp. Retrieved
from http://www.eparent.com5/30/06

REFERENCES

Albright, A. L. (1996). Baclofen in the treatment of cerebral palsy. *Journal of Child Neurology,
11*(2), 77–83.

Andersson, C., & Mattsson, E. (2001). Adults with cerebral palsy: A survey describing
problems, needs, and resources, with special emphasis on locomotion. *Developmental
Medicine and Child Neurology, 43*(2), 76–82.

Blasco, P. A., & Allaire, J. H. (1992). Drooling in the developmentally disabled; management
practices and recommendations. Consortium on Drooling. *Developmental Medicine and
Child Neurology, 34*(10), 849–862.

Boyle, C. A., Yeargin-Allsopp, M., Doernberg, N. S., Holmgreen, P., Murphy, C. C., Schendel,
D. E., et al. (1996). Prevalence of selected developmental disabilities in children 3–10
years of age: The Metropolitan Atlanta Developmental Disabilities Surveillance Program,
1991. *Mortal Weekly Report CDC Surveillance Summary, 45*, 1–14.

Butler, C., & Campbell, S. (2000). Evidence of the effects of intrathecal baclofen for spastic and dystonic cerebral palsy. *Developmental Medicine and Child Neurology, 42*, 634–
645.

Candy, E. J., Hoon, A. H., Capute, A. J., & Bryan, R.N. (1993). MRI in motor delay: Important
adjunct to classification of cerebral palsy. *Pediatric Neurology, 9*(6), 421–429.

Centers for Disease Control and Prevention (2001). Kernicterus in full-term infants—United
States, 1994–1998 (June 15, 2001). *Morbidity and Mortality Weekly Report, 50*(23), 491–
494.

Chugani, H. (1993). Position emission tomography scanning: Applications in newborns. *Clinics in Perinatology, 20*(2), 395–409.

Dobyns, W. B., Andermann, E., Andermann, F., Czapansky-Beilman, D., Dubeau, F., Dulac,
O., et al. (1996). X-linked malformations of neuronal migration. *Neurology, 47*(2), 331–
339.

Dodd, K. J., Taylor, N. F., & Damiano, D. L. (2002). A systematic review of the effectiveness
of strength-training program for people with cerebral palsy. *Archives of Physical Medicine
and Rehabilitation, 83*(8), 1157–1164.

Downey, D., & Hurtig, R. (2003). Alternative Communication. *Pediatric Annals, 32*(7), 467–
474.

Gilmore, D. S. (2000). An analysis of trends for people with MR, CP, and epilepsy. *Rehabilitation Counseling Bulletin, 44*(1), 30–38.

Gormley, M. E. (2001). Treatment of neuromuscular and musculoskeletal problems in cerebral palsy. *Pediatric Rehabilitation, 4*(1), 5–16.

Hagberg, B., Hagberg, G., Beckung, E., & Uvebrant, P. (2001). Changing panorama of cerebral
palsy in Sweden. VIII. Prevalence and origin in the birth year 1991/94. *Acta Paediatrics,
90*, 271–277.

Hamill, P., Drizd, T., Johnson, C., Reed, R., Roche, A., Moore, W., et al. (1979). Physical growth:
National Center for Health Statistics percentiles. *American Journal of Clinical Nutrition,
32*, 607–629.

Harper, D. (1999). Social Psychology of difference: Stigma, spread, and stereotypes in childhood. *Rehabilitation Psychology, 44*(2), 131–144.

Henderson, R. C., Lark, R. K., Gurka, M. J., Worley, G., Fung, E. B., Conaway, M., et al.
(2002). Bone density and metabolism in children and adolescents with moderate to severe
cerebral palsy. *Pediatrics, 1109*, 5.

Hodgkinson, I., Jindrich, M. I., Duhaut, P., Vadot, J. P., Metton, G., Berard, C., et al.
(2001). Hip pain in 234 non-ambulatory adolescents and young adults with cerebral: A

cross-sectional multicentre study. *Developmental Medicine and Child Neurology, 43*(12), 806–808.

Hoon, A. H., & Melhem, E. R. (2000). Neuroimaging: Application in disorders of early brain development. *Journal of Developmental and Behavioral Pediatrics, 21*(4), 291–302.

Inder, T., Huppi, P., Zientara, G., Maier, S., Jolesz, F., & Disalvo, D. (1999). Early detection of periventricular leucomalacia by diffusion-weighted magnetic resonance imaging techniques. *Journal of Pediatrics, 134,* 631–634.

Koman, L. A., Brashear, A., Rosenfeld, S., Chambers, H., Russman, B., Rang, M., et al. (2001). Botulism toxin type A neuromuscular blockade in the treatment of equines foot deformity in cerebral palsy: A multicenter, open-label clinical trial. *Pediatrics, 108*(5), 1062–1071.

Krach, L. (2001). Pharmacotherapy of spasticity. *Journal of Child Neurology, 1*(16), 31–36.

Little, W. J. (1862). On the influence of abnormal parturition, difficult labor, premature birth and asphyxia neonatorum on mental and physical conditions of the child, especially in relation to deformities. *Transactions of the Obstetrical Society of London, 3,* 293–344 (reprinted in *Cerebral Palsy Bulletin,* 1958, *1,* 5–34).

Lonstein, J. E., Winter, R. B., Bradford, D. S., & Ogilvie, J. (1995). *Moe's textbook of scoliosis and their spinal deformities.* Philadelphia: W.B. Saunders.

McLaughlin, J., Bjornson, K., Temken, N., Steinbok, P., Wright, V., Reiner, A., et al. (2002). Elective dorsal rhizotomy: Meta-analysis of three randomized controlled trials. *Developmental Medicine and Child Neurology, 44,* 17–25.

Meis, P. J., Klebanoff, M., Thom, E., Dombrowski, M. P., Sibai, B., Moawad, A. H., et al. (2003). Prevention of recurrent preterm delivery by 17 alpha-hydroxyprogesterone caproate. *New England Journal of Medicine, 348*(24), 2453–2455.

Msall, M. E., Buck, G. M., Rogers, B. T., Merke, D. P., Wan, C. C., Catanzara, N. L., et al. (1994). Multivariate risks among extremely premature infants. *Journal of Perinatology, 14*(1), 41–47.

Murphy, C. C., Yeargin-Allsopp, M., Decoufle, P., & Drews, D. C. (1993). Prevalence of cerebral palsy among ten-year-old children in metropolitan Atlanta, 1985 through 1987. *Journal of Pediatrics, 123*(5), S13–S20.

Mutch, L., Alberman, E., Hagberg, B., Kodama, K., & Perat, M. V. (1992). Cerebral palsy epidemiology: Where are we now and where are we going? *Developmental Medicine and Child Neurology, 34,* 547–551.

Nelson, K. B., & Grether, J. K. (1999). Causes of cerebral palsy. *Current Opinion in Pediatrics, 11,* 487–491.

O'Grady, R. S. (1995). The prediction of long-term functional outcomes of children with cerebral palsy. *Developmental Medicine and Child Neurology, 37,* 997–1005.

O'Shea, T. M., Preisser, J. S., Klinepeter, K. L., & Dillard, R. G. (1998). Trends in mortality and cerebral palsy in a geographically based cohort of very low birth weight neonates born between 1982 to 1994. *Pediatrics, 101,* 642–647.

Pharoah, P. O. D., Cooke, T., Cooke, R. W. I., & Rosenbloom, L. (1990) Birthweight specific trends in cerebral palsy. *Archives of Disease in Childhood, 65,* 602–606.

Pinto-Martin, J. A., Riolo S., Cnaan A., Holzman, C., Susser, M. W., & Paneth, N. (1995). Cranial ultrasound prediction of disabling and nondisabling cerebral palsy at age two in a low birth weight population. *Pediatrics, 108*(2), 238.

Samson-Fang, L., & Stevenson, R. (2000). Identification of malnutrition in children with cerebral palsy: Poor performance of weight-for height centiles. *Developmental Medicine and Child Neurology, 42,* 162–168.

Schwartz, M. H. (2004). Comprehensive treatment of ambulatory children with cerebral palsy: An outcome assessment. *Journal of Pediatric Orthopaedics, Jan–Feb 24*(1), 45–53.

Soll, R. F., & Morley, C. J. (2001). Prophylactic versus selective use of surfactant in preventing morbidity and mortality in preterm infants. *Cochrane Database System Review,* (2): CD00510.

Stanley, F., Blair, E., & Alberman, E. (2000). *Cerebral palsies: Epidemiology and causal pathways* (1st ed.). London: Mac Keith.

Strauss, D., & Shavelle, R. (2001). Life expectancy in cerebral palsy. *Archives of Disease in Childhood, 85*(5), 76–82.

Sugama, S. (2001). MRI in three children with kernicterus. *Pediatric Neurology, 25*(4), 358–331.

Thorarensen, O., Ryan, S., Hunter, J., & Younkin, D. P. (1997). Factor V Leiden mutation: An unrecognized cause of hemiplegic cerebral palsy, neonatal stroke, and placental thrombosis. *Annals of Neurology, 42*(3), 372–375.

van der Lee, J. H., (1999). Forced use of the upper extremity in chronic stroke patients: Results from a single-blind randomized clinical trial. *Stroke, 31*(4), 69–75.

Vohr, B., Allan, W. C., Scott, D. T., Katz, K. H., Schneider, K. C., Makuch, R. W., et al. (1999). Early-onset intraventricular hemorrhage in preterm neonates: Incidence of neurodevelopmental handicap. *Seminars in Perinatology, 23*(3), 212–217.

Vohr, B., Wright, L., Dusick, A., Mele, L., Verter, J., Steichen, J., et al. (2000). Neurodevelopmental and functional outcomes of extremely low birth weight infants in the National Institute of Child Health and Human Development neonatal research network. *Pediatrics, 105*, 1216–1226.

Willis, J. K., (2002). Forced use treatment of childhood hemiparesis. *Pediatrics, 110*(1), 94–96.

Winter, S., Autry, A., Yeargin-Allsopp, M., & Boyle, C. (2002). Prevalence of cerebral palsy in a population based study. *Pediatrics, 110*(6), 1220–1225.

Young, Robert, R., & Delwaide, P. J. (1981). Drug therapy spasticity. *New England Journal of Medicine, 304*(2), 96–99.

4

Epilepsy in People With Mental Retardation

SHOUMITRO DEB

PREVALENCE OF EPILEPSY IN PEOPLE WHO HAVE MENTAL RETARDATION

Epilepsy is a tendency of occurrence of transient recurrent abnormal electrical discharges in the brain affecting one or more of the following brain functions: motor, sensory, cognitive, speech, behavioral, emotional, and psychological. The lifetime prevalence of epilepsy in the general population is between 2 and 3%. The prevalence of epilepsy among people who have mental retardation is much higher. Although it is difficult to determine the exact figure, the reported prevalence of lifetime epilepsy among people with mental retardation (IQ< 70) varies between 13 and 24% (Deb, 1997a; Forsgren, Edvinsson, Blomquist, Heijbel, & Sidenvall, 1990; Goulden, Shinnar, Koller, Katz, & Richardson, 1991; McGrother, Hauck, Bhaumik, Thorp, & Taub, 1996; Rutter, Tizard, Yule, Graham, & Whitmore, 1976).

However, the prevalence varies depending on the age of the person, severity and cause of mental retardation, and the presence and absence of associated neurological conditions. For example, Goulden et al. (1991) found cumulative incidence of epilepsy was 9%, 11%, 13%, and 15% among people with mental retardation at age 5, 10, 15, and 22 years, respectively. Among studies of adults who have mental retardation, Lund (1985) found 18.2% of a Danish population, McGrother et al. (1996) among 24% of an English population, and Deb (1997a) among 14–19% of a Welsh population in the United Kingdom with a lifetime history of epilepsy.

The prevalence of epilepsy among people with mental retardation increases with the severity of mental retardation. Steffenburg, Hagberg, and

SHOUMITRO DEB • Division of Neuroscience, Department of Psychiatry, University of Birmingham, Birmingham, United Kingdom

Kyllerman (1996) found, among 378 children with mental retardation between age 6 and 13, that 15% of those with mild mental retardation as opposed to 45% of those with severe mental retardation had epilepsy. Similarly, Shepherd and Hosking (1989) found 7% of children with mild to moderate mental retardation, and 67% of those with severe mental retardation had epilepsy. The reported rate of epilepsy among people with profound mental retardation (IQ<20) varies between 50 (Michelucci et al., 1989) and 82% (Suzuki, Aihara, & Sugai, 1991).

The prevalence of epilepsy rises if mental retardation is associated with other neurological disorders. In Benedetti, Dov, Hauser, Shinnar, and Cohen's (1986) study in New York about 10% of those who had mild (IQ 50–70) to moderate (IQ<50) mental retardation but without motor handicap had epilepsy. Similarly, Goulden et al. (1991) found the cumulative incidence of epilepsy in people with mental retardation but without associated neurological disability was 2.6%, 3.2%, 3.9%, and 5.2% at 5, 10, 15, and 22 years, respectively, whereas among children with mental retardation and cerebral palsy the cumulative risk was 28%, 31%, and 38% at age 5, 10, and 22 years, respectively.

The prevalence of epilepsy also varies depending on the cause of mental retardation. In Down syndrome, which is the most common chromosomal cause of mental retardation, epilepsy is reported among 5–10% of individuals (see Stafstorm, 1999). Infantile spasm is the most common seizure type among children who have Down syndrome. The rate of epilepsy increases, as people with Down syndrome grow older. It is reported that as many as 75% of older individuals with Down syndrome may develop epilepsy, and this is not always believed to be associated with the increased rate of Alzheimer's disease that is known to affect these people after age 35 years. Generalized tonic clonic seizure is the most common seizure type in late onset epilepsy in people with Down syndrome, but an increased incidence of myoclonic seizures is also observed. Interestingly, the genes for both Unverricht–Lundborg disease that causes a form of myoclonic seizure and the glutamate subunit GluR5 that may play a role in neuronal excitability are localized at the distal long arm of chromosome 21, within the critical Down syndrome region (Eubanks et al., 1993; Lehesjoki et al., 1991—cited in Stafstorm, 1999).

Different seizure types, especially generalized tonic clonic seizure, have been reported in about 25% of people with fragile X syndrome, which is a common inherited cause for mental retardation. Seizures usually start after infancy and before midadolescence, the frequency of which tends to decrease with age. In people with fragile X syndrome, no direct relationship between seizure occurrence and the severity of mental retardation or the presence of autistic feature is reported (Wisniewski et al., 1985). Electroencephalograph (EEG) examination in children with fragile X syndrome shows either a normal pattern or some nonspecific abnormalities such as diffuse slowing. However, a characteristic EEG similar to those seen in benign rolandic epilepsy is reported in a significant proportion of people who have fragile X syndrome (Stafstorm, 1999). There are also many rare conditions associated with mental retardation in which a higher rate of epilepsy is reported. For example, epilepsy is reported in around 75% of people with Rett syndrome, 86% with Angelman syndrome, in a high proportion of people with Aicardi syndrome, about 50% of people with Lesch–Nyhan syndrome, about 30% cases of Lowe syndrome, over 80% cases of Tuberous Sclerosis and Sturge–Weber syndrome, and about 25% cases of Rubenstein–Taybi syndrome (Deb & Ahmed, 2000).

ETIOLOGIES OF EPILEPSIES AND MENTAL RETARDATION

Diagnosis of epilepsy syndrome depends on the combination of seizure types, age of onset, association with other clinical features, course of epilepsy, and characteristic EEG abnormalities. Certain epilepsy syndromes such as West syndrome and Lennox–Gastaut syndrome are commonly associated with mental retardation. Lennox–Gastaut syndrome usually starts between 3 and 5 years of age, involves multiple seizure types such as atypical absences, myoclonic, myoclonic-atonic (sudden falls), and axial tonic, and shows characteristic EEG abnormalities in the form of diffuse spike-waves (2–3 Hz) while awake and bursts of 10 Hz rhythm during sleep. It is important to distinguish this syndrome from other childhood myoclonic seizures. This syndrome carries a poor prognosis in that complete recovery is unusual; mental retardation is the rule, and a proportion (5%) die within 10 years. Seizure types may change in adulthood and include generalized tonic clonic, tonic, myoclonic, absence, and partial seizures. This syndrome constitutes 5% of childhood epilepsies (Sillanpää, 1973), and Trevathan, Murphy, and Yeargin-Allsopp (1997) reported Lennox–Gastaut syndrome among 17% of patients with profound mental retardation (cited in Sillanpää, 1999).

Malformation of cerebral cortical development (also known as neuronal migration disorders or NMDs) such as hemimegalencephaly, lissencephaly, pachygyria, polymicrogyria, and heterotopia are important causes of mental retardation and epilepsy. More than 25 syndromes associated with cerebral dysgenesis have been identified; most have a genetic basis (Dobyns & Truwit, 1995). Cerebral dysgenesis can also be seen as an isolated finding rather than as part of a genetic syndrome. Lesions may be focal or generalized and may affect one or both cerebral hemispheres. Li et al. (1995) found evidence of cerebral dysgenesis in magnetic resonance imaging (MRI) in 12% of adults with partial or secondary generalized epilepsy who attended a specialist epilepsy unit. Cerebral dysplasias also include neuroectodermal dysplasias such as Tuberous Sclerosis and Sturge–Weber disease. These are rare conditions but are usually associated with epilepsy. In the past when evidence of cerebral dysgenesis primarily came from autopsy studies, it was thought that these conditions were only compatible with resistant epilepsy and severe mental retardation. However, with the advancement of neuroimaging techniques, it has become apparent that even some people who do not have epilepsy or mental retardation may show evidence of NMDs in MRI scans (see review by Deb, 1997b). Although cerebral dysgenesis is often associated with resistant and partial seizures, neurosurgical

interventions such as focal resection, hemispherectomy, and corpus callosotomy may prove beneficial for some of these patients (Cataltepe &
Comair, 1999; Holthausen et al., 1999; Roberts, 1999).

DIAGNOSIS OF EPILEPSY

The diagnosis of epilepsy depends on an eyewitness account of the
seizures, examination of the person who has epilepsy, and investigations.
Of these, a detailed eyewitness account is perhaps the most crucial component. Diagnosis of epilepsy, particularly the seizure type, can be difficult
in people with mental retardation, and therefore it is possible for clinicians
to make both a false positive and a false negative diagnosis in a number
of cases. Nonepileptic seizure disorders (pseudoseizures) are known to be
present in a proportion of patients in the general population who have a
diagnosis of epilepsy (Betts, 1990). Similarly, behavioral disorder could be
misdiagnosed as an epileptic seizure in some people with mental retardation (Coulter, 1993). On the other hand, partial and absence seizures
could remain underdiagnosed in people with mental retardation. It is imperative to gather a thorough description of the seizure activities from an
eyewitness including activities before and after the seizure.

A thorough examination of the person who has mental retardation
using standardized methods is necessary (see practice guideline by Deb,
Matthews, Holt, & Bouras, 2001). Physical examination may detect organic
factors that may cause or precipitate seizure disorders. A thorough assessment of the person's adaptive and maladaptive behavior, mental and physical health, and social circumstances is necessary to estimate the effect of
epilepsy on their quality of life (Kerr, Scheepers, Bowely, & Working Group,
2001). Sabaz, Cairns, Lawson, Bleasley, and Bye (2001) found that both
children with and without mental retardation who had epilepsy were more
likely to have psychosocial problems compared with their respective reference populations. They also found that children with mental retardation
had reduced health-related quality of life (HRQOL) compared with intellectually normal children, a finding independent of epilepsy. The HRQOL
of children with refractory epilepsy is greatly affected, and the presence
of mental retardation in children with epilepsy independently depressed
HRQOL outcomes. Espie et al. (2001) developed a measure for use with
adults with epilepsy and mental retardation capable of assessing both
clinical and care concerns and of quantifying treatment outcomes. The
35-item Glasgow Epilepsy Outcome Scale (GEOS-35) comprises four subscales: concerns about seizures, treatment, caring, and social impact each
explaining about 70% of variance. Espie et al. (2001) established the validity and reliability of the GEOS-35 for use with clinical populations of
people with epilepsy and mental retardation.

INVESTIGATIONS

EEG is the main investigational method in relation to the diagnosis of
epilepsy. Other possible investigational methods include neuroimaging and

specific investigations necessary to determine the cause of mental retardation. It is also necessary to investigate any underlying physical condition that may be contributing to the epilepsy. Interictal (in the interval between seizure episodes) EEGs do not show any abnormality in a proportion of patients who have epilepsy. In many people with mental retardation, it is difficult to perform an EEG. As well, in a high proportion of cases, abnormal EEGs in people with mental retardation constitute nonspecific abnormalities such as an excess of the background slow activities, which could be a possible manifestation of an underlying brain damage rather than specific epileptic changes (Deb, 1995; Deb & Joyce, 1999a). A proportion of people with mental retardation who manifest generalized seizures show focal epileptic changes in their EEG, indicating the possibility of secondary generalization of focal seizures in many people with mental retardation. Video telemetry and 24-hr EEG recordings are also helpful in confirming a seizure diagnosis.

Structural neuroimaging such as computed tomography (CT) and MRI are not necessary in most cases. The recent advances in MRI technology have made it possible to detect subtle focal brain malformation that was not possible before. This has led to successful neurosurgery for many patients who have epilepsy. The sensitivity of functional neuroimaging such as single photon emission computerized tomography or positron emission tomography (SPECT/PET) in detecting epileptic abnormality in the interictal phase is low. The sensitivity increases if an ictal EEG can be performed. A combination of ictal and interictal EEG is likely to detect abnormality in a high proportion of patients with epilepsy. The usefulness of neuroimaging investigations in people with mental retardation has not been explored. Magneto-encephalograph (MEG), which could be useful in the investigation of epilepsy, is not available in most centers.

MANAGEMENT OF EPILEPSY

Treatment of epilepsy with antiepileptic drugs constitutes only part of the management regime for epilepsy in people with mental retardation. The primary emphasis of management should be to provide a better quality of life for the person who has epilepsy and their carers. Some special considerations for the use of antiepileptic drugs in people with mental retardation are mentioned in Table 4.1 (see Alvarez, Besag, & Livanianen 1998). A high proportion of people with mental retardation receive antiepileptic drugs because of the high rate of epilepsy among this population. The use of polypharmacy of antiepileptic medication is also common in these patients (Deb & Hunter, 1992). A recent study found 42% of 143 adults with mental retardation and epilepsy received polypharmacy; 28% received two, 12.6% received three, and 1.4% received four antiepileptic drugs concurrently (Deb & Joyce, 1999b). Polypharmacy was significantly associated with multiple seizure type, longer duration of epilepsy, active epilepsy (seizure within the past 12 months), and female gender. Prospective studies have shown that through an active effort it is possible to achieve a reduction of polypharmacy and introduction of modern generation of less toxic

Table 4.1. Special Considerations for the Use of Antiepileptic Drugs in People with Mental Retardation

1. Difficulty of diagnosis of epilepsy (both false positive and false negative diagnoses are possible).
2. Difficulty of diagnosing the seizure-type (because of difficulty of performing EEG in some people with mental retardation).
3. Common occurrence of multiple seizure-type.
4. Long duration of seizures.
5. A high proportion of treatment-resistant epilepsy (possibly because of underlying brain damage).
6. A higher sensitivity to cognitive and behavioral adverse effects of antiepileptic drugs (many people with mental retardation have concurrent mental health problems).
7. Likelihood of drug interactions (many people with mental retardation receive antipsychotic and antidepressant drugs that are potentially epileptogenic).
8. Difficulty in detecting adverse effects of drugs (because of communication problems).
9. Possibility of central nervous system adverse effects of drugs being more pronounced in this population (because of preexisting brain damage).

antiepileptic drugs (Collacott, Dignon, Hauck, & Ward, 1989). The reduction of polyphramacy not only achieves a reduction in seizure frequency but also is also associated with an improvement in patients' behavior (Pellock & Hunt, 1996).

USE OF SPECIFIC ANTIEPILEPTIC MEDICATIONS IN PEOPLE WHO HAVE MENTAL RETARDATION

Barbiturates

The two main barbiturates used in the treatment of epilepsy are primidone and phenobarbitone. There is a widespread anxiety about using these drugs because of well-publicized cognitive and behavioral adverse effects of these medications (Alvarez, 1998). Clinicians treating epilepsy in people with mental retardation have reported a higher frequency of behavioral adverse effects from the use of phenobarbitone in this population. It is thus suggested that where possible barbiturates should not be used to treat epilepsy in people with mental retardation, particularly if an alternative is available (Alvarez, 1998).

Phenytoin

Because of its well-known severe adverse effects on the central nervous system, it has been suggested that phenytoin should not be recommended as a first line treatment of epilepsy in people with mental retardation, many of whom have underlying brain damage (Livanianen, 1998). Phenytoin is effective in both focal and generalized seizures. Important adverse effects include encephalopathy, megaloblastic and aplastic anemia, acne, hirsutism, agranulocytosis, gingival hyperplasia, and liver dysfunction. Regular monitoring of phenytoin serum level is advisable because of its "zero-order kinetics" and the wide variability of metabolic rates among different individuals.

Sodium Valproate

Valproate is a broad-spectrum antiepileptic drug. This drug is particularly relevant in the treatment of people with mental retardation because of its effect on the Lennox–Gastaut syndrome. This drug is also shown to be effective in the treatment of West syndrome. Important adverse effects are weight gain, thrombocytopenia, hyperammonemia, liver dysfunction, tremor, hair loss, and possible amenorrhoea. In rare cases, hepatotoxicity could cause a major problem; however, its teratogenic adverse effect is of less concern for people with mental retardation. Valproate is also shown to be effective as an add-on therapy for the treatment of so-called therapy resistant epilepsy. On the basis of the evidence available so far, sodium valproate can be recommended as a first line of choice of antiepileptic drug for those people with mental retardation who suffer from generalized tonic clonic seizures, typical and atypical absences, Lennox–Gastaut syndrome, juvenile myoclonic epilepsy, tonic, atonic seizures (drop attacks), and infantile spasms (Friis, 1998). Along with carbamazepine and oxcarbazepine, valproate could also be used as a first line antiepileptic drug for the treatment of partial seizures with or without secondary generalization.

Carbamazepine

Carbamazepine is a potent antiepileptic drug although is not as broad spectrum as sodium valproate. Carbamazepine is also indicated in the treatment of trigeminal and occipital neuralgia, and in the prophylaxis of bipolar affective disorder. Because of its better cognitive adverse effect profile and possible positive effect on behavior and mood, this drug is popular among physicians treating epilepsy in people with mental retardation. Psychiatric illness and behavior disorders are common in people with mental retardation (Deb, 1997c). However, because of its lack of effect on Lennox–Gastaut syndrome and multiple types of seizures, it is not indicated for many people with mental retardation and epilepsy (Weisburg & Alvarez, 1998). Carbamazepine may make some seizure types such as absence, myoclonic, and atonic seizures worse. Important adverse effects are drowsiness, skin rash, dizziness, ataxia, aplastic anemia, thrombocytopenia, hyponatremia, and agranulocytosis. Skin rash usually disappears on a rechallenge with a lower dose of carbamazepine. However, carbamazepine can cause a paradoxical increase in behavioral problems in some people with mental retardation and epilepsy.

Oxcarbazepine

Oxcarbazepine has a similar mode of action to, and clinical indications like those for, carbamazepine with fewer adverse effects and drug interactions. It thus appears to be a better alternative to carbamazepine particularly in people with mental retardation (Gaily, Granstrom, & Lliukkonen, 1998). However, so far experience with use of this drug in people with mental retardation is limited.

Lamotrigine

Lamotrigine, a relatively new antiepileptic drug that was initially introduced as an add-on therapy for partial seizures, is now indicated as a monotherapy and also for the treatment of generalized seizures. In a recent review on the topic, Besag (1998) proposed that lamotrigine should be a favored drug of choice in the treatment of epilepsy in people with mental retardation for several reasons. Lamotrigine is a broad-spectrum antiepileptic drug and is effective in treating many different types of seizures including generalized tonic clonic seizures, partial seizures with or without generalization, typical and atypical absences, atonic seizures (drop-attacks), and myoclonic jerks, particularly if associated with Lennox–Gastaut syndrome. In some cases, however, lamotrigine may worsen myoclonic seizures (Genton, Dravet, Bureau, Formosa, & Mesdjian, 1997). It has a favorable adverse effect profile, particularly having minimum effect on intellectual functioning and sedation. Important adverse effects are skin rash, dizziness, tremor, and ataxia. It is advisable to start lamotrigine at a low dose and very gradually titrate the dose to its optimum effective level to avoid adverse effects like the skin rash. Although in general lamotrigine's adverse effect profile on behavioral disorder is favorable, some clinicians have reported a paradoxical increase in behavioral problems in some people with mental retardation who were treated with lamotrigine.

Vigabatrin

Vigabatrin is indicated as an add-on therapy for the treatment of partial seizures. One study has reported the use of vigabatrin in people with mental retardation (Ylinen, 1998). This drug is also effective in the treatment of infantile spasms. Its overall profile on cognition and behavior seems favorable, although psychosis and paradoxical increase in behavioral disorders have been reported anecdotally (Ramsay & Slater, 1993). A recent observational study has found no difference in the rate of behavioral disorders in three groups of people with mental retardation and epilepsy treated respectively with vigabatrin, lamotrigine, and gabapentine (Bhaumik, Branford, Duggirala, & Ismail, 1997). Despite its favorable drug interaction profile, there is major anxiety about the reported visual field defect (bilateral visual field constriction) associated with the use of this drug. Visual field defect may occur in as many as 30% patients treated with vigabatrin and may remain initially asymptomatic. The fact that visual field examination could be particularly difficult to perform in people with mental retardation is likely to limit severely the use of this drug in people with mental retardation.

Gabapentin

Gabapentin is indicated as an add-on therapy for drug-resistant partial seizures. A recent study has reported the use of gabapentin in children with and without mental retardation (Mikati et al., 1998). This study found that the clinical effect of gabapentin was similar in both groups of children. Its lack of interaction with other antiepileptic drugs makes it an attractive choice for use in people with mental retardation; however, this drug has no particular effect on Lennox–Gastaut syndrome and generalized seizures. Its effect on cognition is minimal and common adverse effects include somnolence, dizziness, ataxia, fatigue, and nystagmus. Some have reported an increase in behavioral problems in the form of hyperactivity, moodiness, unprovoked outbursts of anger, and uncooperative behavior among children with and without mental retardation who were treated with gabapentin.

Topiramate

This antiepileptic drug was initially shown to be effective as an add-on therapy for partial seizures. However, subsequent studies have shown its efficacy in the treatment of generalized seizures and also as a monotherapy. Its particular effectiveness in Lennox–Gastaut syndrome will make it popular for use among people with mental retardation and epilepsy. However, in a small proportion of cases nephrolithiasis may cause particular problem in people with mental retardation. A recent study has shown efficacy of topiramate in the treatment of drop attacks in people with mental retardation (Kerr, 1998). Important adverse central nervous system related effects include somnolence, dizziness, ataxia, psychomotor slowing, speech disorder, nervousness, nystagmus, and paresthesia but also non-CNS effects such as weight loss are reported. However, its reported adverse effect on cognition, particularly difficulty in word finding, may prove to be a restrictive factor for its use in people who have mental retardation.

Zonisamide

Zonisamide is a new broad-spectrum antiepileptic drug that is effective in both partial as well as generalized seizures, primarily used in Japan and South Korea, and recently in the United States with some encouraging results. A recent study has shown somewhat lesser efficacy of this drug in the treatment of both partial and generalized seizures among children with mental retardation when compared with efficacy in children without mental retardation (Linuma, Minami, Cho, Kajii, & Tachi, 1998). Common adverse effects include drowsiness, ataxia, anorexia, gastrointestinal symptoms, loss or decrease in spontaneity, and slowing of mental activity. However, adverse effects such as nephrolithiasis and leukopenia may restrict its use in Caucasians. This drug may be particularly effective in myoclonic seizures.

Tiagabine

Tiagabine is shown to be effective as an add-on therapy in patients suffering from partial seizures. It is unlikely to be useful in treatment of absence or myoclonic seizure. Tiagabine may cause dizziness and other central nervous system related adverse effects. Although its efficacy in people with mental retardation and epilepsy has not been studied, considering its minimum adverse effect on cognition this could become a drug of choice for use in this population (Kälväiinen, 1998). Limiting factors for its use in people with mental retardation are the fact that this drug is less broad spectrum and there is currently not enough evidence for its efficacy on infantile spasms and Lennox–Gastaut syndrome.

Felbamate

This drug is effective in the treatment of complex partial seizures and also in Lennox–Gastaut syndrome (Leppik & Wolff, 1995). Common adverse effects include nausea, vomiting, headache, insomnia, and anorexia. Recent reports of fatal aplastic anemia and hepatotoxicity have halted wider use of this drug (Ben-Menachem, Henriksen, & Johannessen, 1999). Although no specific trial of this drug in people with mental retardation exists, because of its potent effect on Lennox–Gastaut syndrome, this drug could be used as a last resort in this population under strict monitoring of adverse effects.

Levetiracetam

This derivative of piracetam is a relatively new antiepileptic drug, which is licensed for use as an add-on therapy for resistant partial seizures. Several double-blind placebo-controlled clinical trials showed 30–40% response rate in patients with intractable partial seizures with favorable adverse effect profile (see review by Ben-Menachem, 2000). However, there are relatively less data available for its efficacy for people who have mental retardation. However, on the basis of current evidence this drug looks promising for use among people with mental retardation. There is also anecdotal evidence of increased behavior disorders in the form of aggression associated with the use of levetirecetam in adults with mental retardation.

Benzodiazepines

Within the benzodiazepine group, drugs such as diazepam, clonazepam, and lorazepam are commonly used in the management of acute seizures and status epilepticus (Isojärvi & Tokola, 1998). The role of midazolam in this respect is also being increasingly recognized. Rectal diazepam is widely used in the treatment of prolonged seizures and status epilepticus in people with mental retardation as a prehospital treatment option. As an alternative to rectal diazepam, intranasal or buccal midazolam has been proposed recently (Scheepers, Scheepers, & Clough, 1998). Drugs such as clobazam, nitrazepam, and clonazepam are also used in epilepsy as a prophylaxis (Isojärvi & Tokola, 1998). Clonazepam and nitrazepam are used mostly among children and clobazam is used as an add-on therapy, particularly where anxiety and stress seem to play an important role in epileptic seizures. Clobazam has also been used periodically during menstrual cycles in women who tend to have an increased seizure frequency during their menstrual periods. As the overall adverse effect of benzodiazepines apart from sedation is minimal, these drugs could be favored for the treatment of people with mental retardation. However, benzodiazepines could not be recommended for long-term use because patients develop tolerance, and there are problems associated with the withdrawal of these drugs.

Polypharmacy

As far as possible people with mental retardation and epilepsy should be treated with a single antiepileptic drug. If combination of antiepileptic drugs is necessary, a possible combination with sodium channel blocker and GABA-ergic drugs (affecting available concentrations of gamma aminobutyric acid) or drugs with mixed mode of action is preferable. As such, a combination of lamotrigine with either valproate or topiramate or gabapentine is recommended as well as a combination of carbamazepine with valproate or topiramate or gabapentine.

Vagus Nerve Stimulation (VNS)

This device, developed by Cyberonics Incorporation, has been shown to be effective in a proportion of individuals (approximately 30%) with intractable epilepsy. In almost all cases antiepileptic drugs had to be continued even after the insertion of VNS. There are no data available on people with mental retardation (see review by Schachter & Wheless, 2002).

Neurosurgical Treatment

Henriksen, Bjørnaes, and Røste's (1999) recent review of studies of epilepsy surgery on patients with mental retardation clearly demonstrates that a substantial proportion of people with mental retardation improve following epilepsy neurosurgery and some become totally seizure free. Benefits on both epilepsy control and cognitive development are most apparent when surgery is instigated early in life, particularly in childhood. On average, the overall success rate of epilepsy surgery is higher in the general population compared with the patients with mental retardation. However, good results can be achieved in selected patients with a clearly unifocal disease even if they have mental retardation. Therefore, mental retardation per se is no longer considered a contraindication to epileptic surgery. The risk–benefit of each case must be individually ascertained. Extensive investigations including neurophysiological, neuroimaging, and neuropsychological tests, necessary before epilepsy surgery, will require patient cooperation that may not be easily available from some patients who have mental retardation. As in the general population, the success of epilepsy surgery will depend on many factors such as associated neurological disorders, etiology of epilepsy and mental retardation, and social support services available for these patients.

CONCLUSIONS

The true prevalence of epilepsy in people who have mental retardation remains difficult to determine. Further careful studies are needed in this area. More important is the identification of predisposing, precipitating, and perpetuating risk factors for which interventions could be developed or implemented. Clinicians should remain vigilant to the possibility of a false positive diagnosis of epilepsy that could lead to unnecessary lifelong medication as well as a false negative diagnosis that leads to a missed opportunity for proper treatment in some patients with mental retardation. Despite the evidence that with an active effort, polypharmacy of antiepileptic drugs could be reduced, which subsequently improves seizure frequency and behavioral problems, this practice still seems common. Although some have highlighted the possibility of using rational polypharmacy of antiepileptic drugs (Brodie, Yuen, and the 105 Study Group, 1997), the evidence base for conjoint use of two or more antiepileptic medications is not comprehensive.

While treating patients with mental retardation, certain considerations that specifically affect the antiepileptic treatment in this population should be borne in mind. The National Institute for Clinical Excellence in the United Kingdom has recently produced guideline for epilepsy treatment (nice.org.uk), an adapted version of which is shown in Table 4.2 for

Table 4.2. A Proposed Guideline for the Use of Antiepileptic Drugs in the Treatment of Different Seizure Types in People Who Have Mental Retardation (Adapted from the NICE Guideline on Epilepsy; www.nice.org.uk)

Seizure type	1st line therapy	2nd line/add-on therapy
GTCS (generalized tonic clonic seizure)	Valproate Carbamazepine Lamotrigine Topiramate	Levetiracetam Oxcarbazepine Phenytoin Clobazam
Partial (simple and complex with and without generalization)	Oxcarbazepine Carbamazepine Valproate Lamotrigine Topiramate	Gabapentin Tiagabine Levetiracetam Clobazam Phenytoin
Absence (typical and atypical)	Valproate Ethosuximide Lamotrigine	Topiramate Clobazam Clonazepam
Myoclonic	Valproate	Topiramate Lamotrigine Levetiracetam Clobazam Conazepam
Atonic (drop-attacks) + tonic	Valproate Lamotrigine	Topiramate Levetiracetam Clobazam Conazepam

Note. Vigabatrin and felbamate have not been included in the table because of their severe adverse effects.

use among people with mental retardation. Because of the introduction of newer antiepileptic treatments in future, availability of effective neurosurgical treatments, and new treatments such as vagus nerve stimulation, this guideline will need to be revised at regular intervals. Deb and Fraser (1994) proposed a common sense, rational approach to the psychopharmacology for people with mental retardation. It is also worth emphasizing that seizure control constitutes only one part of the treatment strategy, the ultimate aim of the treatment should be to provide a better quality of life for these patients.

REFERENCES

Alvarez, N. (1998). Barbiturates in the treatment of epilepsy in people with intellectual disability. *Journal of Intellectual Disability Research, 42*(S1), 16–23.

Alvarez, N., Besag, F., & Livanianen, M. (1998). Use of antiepileptic drugs in the treatment of epilepsy in people with intellectual disability. *Journal of Intellectual Disability Research, 42*(S1), 1–15.

Benedetti, B. D., Dov, I., Hauser, W. A., Shinnar, S., & Cohen, H. J. (1986). Frequency of seizures among children with cerebral palsy and mental retardation. *Developmental Medical Child Neurology, 28*(Suppl. 53), 36.

Ben-Menachem, E. (2000). New antiepileptic drugs and non-pharmacological treatments. *Current Opinion in Neurology, 13*, 165–170.

Ben-Menachem, E., Henriksen, O., & Johannessen, S. I. (1999). Diagnosis and treatment of partial seizures. *CNS Drugs, 11*(1), 23–39.

Besag, F. M. C. (1998). Lamotrigine in the treatment of epilepsy in people with intellectual disability. *Journal of Intellectual Disability Research, 42*(S1), 50–56.

Betts, T. (1990). Pseudoseizures: Seizures that are not epilepsy. *Lancet, 336*, 163–164.

Bhaumik, S., Branford, D., Duggirala, C., & Ismail, I. A. (1997). A naturalistic study of the use of vigabatrin, lamotrigine and gabapentin in adults with learning disabilities. *Seizure, 6*, 127–133.

Brodie, M. J., Yuen, A. W. C., & the 105 Study Group. (1997). Lamotrigine substitution study: Evidence for synergism with sodium valproate? *Epilepsy Research, 26*, 423–432.

Cataltepe, O., & Comair, Y. G. (1999). Focal resection in the treatment of neuronal migrational disorders. In P. Kotagal & H. O. Lüders (Eds.), *The epilepsies: Etiology and prevention* (pp. 87–92). San Diego, CA: Academic.

Collacott, R. A., Dignon, A., Hauck, A., & Ward, J. W. (1989). Clinical and therapeutic monitoring of epilepsy in a mental handicap unit. *British Journal of Psychiatry, 155*, 522–525.

Coulter, D. L. (1993). Epilepsy and mental retardation: An overview. *American Journal of Mental Retardation, 98*, 1–11.

Deb, S. (1995). Electrophysiological correlates of psychopathology in individuals with mental retardation and epilepsy. *Journal of Intellectual Disability Research, 39*, 129–135.

Deb, S. (1997a). Epilepsy and mental retardation. *Epilepsie Bulletin, 25*, 91–94.

Deb, S. (1997b). Structural neuroimaging in mental retardation. *British Journal of Psychiatry, 171*, 417–419.

Deb, S. (1997c). Mental disorder in adults with mental retardation and epilepsy. *Comprehensive Psychiatry, 38*, 179–184.

Deb, S., & Ahmed, Z. (2000). Special conditions leading to mental retardation. In M. G. Gelder, N. Andreasen, & J. J. Lopez-Ibor (Eds.), *New Oxford textbook of psychiatry* (pp. 1953–1963). Oxford, UK: Oxford Press.

Deb, S., & Fraser, W. I. (1994). The use of psychotropic medication in people with learning disability: Towards rational prescribing. *Human Psychopharmacology, 9*, 259–272.

Deb, S., & Hunter, D. (1992). The effect of anticonvulsant medication on the psychopathology of adults with a mental handicap and epilepsy. *Human Psychopharmacology, 7*, 129–134.

Deb, S., & Joyce, J. (1999a). Characteristics of epilepsy in a population bases cohort of adults with learning disability. *Irish Journal of Psychological Medicine, 16*(1), 5–9.

Deb, S., & Joyce, J. (1999b). The use of anti-epileptic medication in a population based cohort of adults with learning disability and epilepsy. *International Journal of Psychiatry in Clinical Practice, 3*, 129–133.

Deb, S., Matthews, T., Holt, G., & Bouras, N. (Eds.). (2001). *Practice guidelines for the assessment and diagnosis of mental health problems in adults with intellectual disability.* London, UK: Pavilion.

Dobyns, W. B., & Truwit, C. L. (1995). Lissencephaly and other malformations of cortical development: 1995 update. *Neuropediatrics, 26*, 132–147.

Espie, C. A., Watkins, J., Duncan, R., Espie, A., Sterrick, M., Brodie, M. J., et al. (2001). Development and validation of the Glasgow Epilepsy Outcome Scale (GEOS): A new instrument for measuring concerns about epilepsy in people with mental retardation. *Epilepsia, 42*(8), 1043–1051.

Eubanks, J. H., Puranam, R. S., Kleckner, N., Bettler, B., Heinemenn, B., & McNamara, J. O. (1993). The gene encoding the glutamate receptor subunit GluR5 is located on human chromosome 21q21.1-22.1 in the vicinity of the gene for familial amyotrophic lateral sclerosis. *Proceedings of National Academy of Science (USA), 90*, 178–182.

Forsgren, L., Edvinsson, S. O., Blomquist, H. K., Heijbel, J., & Sidenvall, R. (1990). Epilepsy in a population of mentally retarded children and adults. *Epilepsy Research, 6*(3), 234–248.

Friis, M. L. (1998). Valproate in the treatment of epilepsy in people with intellectual disability. *Journal of Intellectual Disability Research, 42*(S1), 32–35.

Gaily, E., Granstrom, M.-L., & Lliukkonen, E. (1998). Oxcarbazepine in the treatment of epilepsy in children and adolescents with intellectual disability. *Journal of Intellectual Disability Research, 42*(S1), 41–45.

Genton, P., Dravet, C., Bureau, N., Formosa, F., & Mesdjian, E. (1997). Aggravation of severe myoclonic epilepsy of infancy by lamotrigine. *Epilepsia, 38*(Suppl. 3), 32.

Goulden, K. J., Shinnar, S., Koller, H., Katz, M., & Richardson, S. A. (1991). Epilepsy in children with mental retardation: A cohort study. *Epilepsia, 32*, 690–697.

Henriksen, O., Bjørnaes, H., & Røste, G. K. (1999). Epilepsy surgery in mental retardation: The role of surgery. In M. Sillanpää, L. Gram, S. I. Johannessen, & T. Tomson (Eds.), *Epilepsy and mental retardation* (pp. 105–113). Philadelphia, PA: Wrightson Biomedical.

Holthausen, H., Tuxhorn, I., Pieper, T., Pannek, H., Lahl, R., & Oppel, F. (1999). Hemispherectomy in the treatment of neuronal migrational disorders. In P. Kotagal & H. O. Lüders (Eds.), *The epilepsies: Etiology and prevention* (pp. 93–102). San Diego, CA: Academic.

Isojärvi, J. I. T., & Tokola, R. A. (1998). Benzodiazepine in the treatment of epilepsy. *Journal of Intellectual Disability Research, 42*(S1), 80–92.

Kälväiinen, R. (1998). Tiagabine: A new therapeutic option for people with intellectual disability and partial epilepsy. *Journal of Intellectual Disability Research, 42*(S1), 63–67.

Kerr, M., Scheepers, M., Bowely, C., & Working Group of the International Association of the Scientific Study of Intellectual Disability. (2001). Clinical guidelines for the management of epilepsy in adults with an intellectual disability. *Seizure, 10*, 401–409.

Kerr, M. P. (1998). Topiramate: Uses in people with an intellectual disability who have epilepsy. *Journal of Intellectual Disability Research, 42*(S1), 74–79.

Lehesjoki, A.-E., Koskiniemi, M., Sistonen, P., Miao, J., Hästbacka, J., Norio, R., et al. (1991). Localisation of a gene for progressive myoclonus epilepsy to chromosome 21q22. *Proceedings of National Academy of Science (USA), 88*, 3696–3699.

Leppik, J. E., & Wolff, D. L. (1995). The place of felbamate in the treatment of epilepsy. *CNS Drugs, 4*, 294–301.

Li, L. M., Fish, D. R., Sisodiya, S. M., Shorvon, S. D., Alsanjari, N., & Stevens, J. M. (1995). High resolution magnetic resonance imaging in adults with partial or secondary generalised epilepsy attending a tertiary referral unit. *Journal of Neurology, Neurosurgery, and Psychiatry, 59*, 384–387.

Linuma, K., Minami, T., Cho, K., Kajii, N., & Tachi, N. (1998). Long term effects of Zonisamide in the treatment of epilepsy in children with intellectual disability. *Journal of Intellectual Disability Research, 42*(S1), 68–73.

Livanianen, M. (1998). Phenytoin: Effective but insidious therapy for epilepsy in people with intellectual disability. *Journal of Intellectual Disability Research, 42*(S1), 24–31.

Lund, J. (1985). Epilepsy and psychiatric disorder in the mentally retarded adults. *Acta Psychiatrica Scandinavica, 72*, 557–562.

McGrother, C. W., Hauck, A., Bhaumik, S., Thorp, C., & Taub, N. (1996). Community care for adults with learning disability and their carers: Needs and outcome from the Leicestershire register. *Journal of Intellectual Disability Research, 40*, 183–190.

Michelucci, R., Forti, A., Rubboli, G., Plasmati, R., Volpi, L., & Tassinari, C.-A. (1989). Mental retardation and behavioural disturbances related to epilepsy: A review. *Brain Dysfunction, 2*(1), 3–9.

Mikati, M. A., Choueri, R., Khurana, D. S., Riviello, J., Helmers, S., & Holmes, G. (1998). Gabapentin in the treatment of refractory partial epilepsy in children with intellectual disability. *Journal of Intellectual Disability Research, 42*(S1), 57–62.

Pellock, J. M., & Hunt, P. A. (1996). A decade of modern epilepsy therapy in institutionalised mentally retarded patients. *Epilepsy Research, 25*, 263–268.

Ramsay, R. E., & Slater, J. D. (1993). Antiepileptic drugs in clinical development [In J. A. French, M. A. Dichter, & I. E. Leppik (Eds.), New anti-epileptic drug development, preclinical and clinical aspects]. *Epilepsy Research,* (Suppl. 10), 45–67.

Roberts, D. W. (1999). Corpus callosotomy in the treatment of neuronal migrational disorders. In P. Kotagal & H. O. Lüders (Eds.), *The epilepsies: Etiology and prevention* (pp. 103–112). San Diego, CA: Academic.

Rutter, M., Tizard, J., Yule, W., Graham, P., & Whitmore, K. (1976). Research report: Isle of Wight studies 1964–1974. *Psychological Medicine, 76*, 313–332.

Sabaz, M., Cairns, D. R., Lawson, J. A., Bleaseley, A. F., & Bye, A. M. E. (2001). The health-related quality of life of children with refractory epilepsy: A comparison of those with and without intellectual disability. *Epilepsia, 42*(5), 621–628.

Schachter, S. C., & Wheless, J. W. (2002). Vagus nerve stimulation therapy 5 year after approval: A comprehensive update. *Neurology, 59*(6, Suppl. 4), S1–S61.

Scheepers, M., Scheepers, B., & Clough, P. (1998). Midazolam via the intranasal route: An effective rescue medication for severe epilepsy in adults with learning disability. *Seizure, 7*, 509–512.

Shepherd, C., & Hosking, G. (1989). Epilepsy in school children with intellectual impairment in Sheffield: The size and nature of the problem and its implications in service provision. *Journal of Mental Deficiency Research, 33*, 511–514.

Sillanpää, M. (1973). Medico-social prognosis of children with epilepsy. Epidemiological study and analysis of 245 cases. *Acta Paediatrica Scandinavica,* (Suppl. 237), 1–104.

Sillanpää, M. (1999). Definitions and epidemiology. In M. Sillanpää, L. Gram, S. I. Johannessen, & T. Tomson (Eds.), *Epilepsy and mental retardation* (pp. 1–6). Philadelphia, PA: Wrightson Biomedical.

Stafstorm, C. E. (1999). Mechanisms of epilepsy in mental retardation: Insight from Angelman syndrome, Down syndrome and fragile X syndrome. In M. Sillanpää, L. Gram, S. I. Johannessen, & T. Tomson (Eds.), *Epilepsy and mental retardation* (pp. 7–40). Philadelphia, PA: Wrightson Biomedical.

Steffenburg, U., Hagberg, G., & Kyllerman, M. (1996). Characteristics of seizures in a population-based series of mentally retarded children with active epilepsy. *Epilepsia, 37*, 850–856.

Suzuki, H., Aihara, M., & Sugai, K. (1991). Severely retarded children in a defined area of Japan: Prevalence rate, associated disabilities and causes. *Brain and Development, 23*, 4–8.

Trevathan, E., Murphy, C. C., & Yeargin-Allsopp, M. (1997). Prevalence and descriptive epidemiology of Lennox–Gastaut syndrome among Atlanta children. *Epilepsia, 38*, 1283–1288.

Weisburg, H., & Alvarez, N. (1998). Carbamazepine in the treatment of epilepsy in people with intellectual disability. *Journal of Intellectual Disability Research, 42*(S1), 36–40.

Wisniewski, K. E., French, J. H., Fernando, S., Brown, W. T., Jenkins, E. C., Friedman, E., et al. (1985). Fragile X syndrome: Associated neurological abnormalities. *Annals of Neurology, 18*, 665–669.

Ylinen, A. (1998). Antiepleptic efficacy of Vigabatrin in people with severe epilepsy and intellectual disability. *Journal of Intellectual Disability Research, 42*(S1), 46–49.

5

Pediatric Brain Injury

DENNIS C. RUSSO, ERIN DUNN, GARY PACE, and ROBIN S. CODDING

Brain injury is a health problem of major proportion. Affecting physical, cognitive, and behavioral function, brain injuries can occur as a result of a number of circumstances. For example, it is estimated that each year 1.5 million Americans sustain a traumatic brain injury (TBI) resulting from such causes as injury, accident, toxic exposure, or assault. According to the Brain Injury Association of America (2002), more people experience TBI each year than breast cancer, HIV/AIDS, multiple sclerosis, and spinal cord injuries combined.

The impact of TBI can be measured by both its effect on society, and its effect on the individual with brain injury. Traumatic brain injuries result in an annual cost of $9–10 billion dollars (National Institute of Child Health and Human Development [NICHD] Consensus Report, 1999). They also result in a significant decrease in quality of life for many TBI survivors and their families. Although the effects of brain injuries can be temporary, in some individuals the physical, cognitive, and behavioral changes associated with brain injury can be persistent or permanent. Accordingly, it is estimated that as many as 6.5 million people currently have a TBI (NICHD Consensus Report, 1999). The purpose of this chapter is to describe the epidemiology, potential long-term effects, and treatment strategies for children and adolescents with brain injury.

CLASSIFICATION AND INCIDENCE

Definition

Historically there has not been a universally accepted definition of brain injury. Academy for the Certification of Brain Injury Specialists

DENNIS C. RUSSO, ERIN DUNN, GARY PACE, and ROBIN S. CODDING • The May Institute, Norwood, Massachusetts 02062.

(2004) has suggested the following definitions and these will be the definitions used in this chapter. The term *acquired brain injury* (ABI) is a general term for an injury to the brain that has occurred after birth, and results in total or partial functional disability and/or psychosocial impairment that adversely affects an individual's performance. A *TBI* is defined as an ABI caused by an external force such as motor vehicular accidents, falls, physical assaults, or sports accidents. A *non-TBI* is defined as an ABI resulting from nontraumatic factors such as malignancy, infections, degenerative processes, or stoke.

There are two types of TBI. In an *open* TBI, brain tissue is penetrated from outside the skull, resulting in a localized injury and a somewhat predictable outcome. An example of an open TBI is a gunshot injury. Since the path of bullet into the brain is clear, the parts of the brain that are damaged are identifiable and the outcome is relatively predictable.

On the other hand, in a *closed* TBI the damage to the brain tends to be diffuse, and the outcome is less predictable. Closed TBIs often result from impact accidents. For example, a rapidly moving automobile suddenly stops, resulting in a person's head forcefully coming in contact with a stationary object such as the automobile's windshield or dashboard. In this example, damage to the brain occurs not only at the point of contact of the head and the stationary object, but also from the movement of the brain within the skull. Since the skull consists of many bony protrusions, in these types of impact accidents the brain can "bounce" back and forth (termed coup/contracoup injury) resulting in focal impact damage at the point of impact and on the opposite side of the brain. Additional damage can result from upward forces and the "twist" of the brain itself side to side within the skull. These actions can produce diffuse tearing and shearing of the brain leading to coma and to damage of multiple brain areas influencing cognitive and behavioral functions.

Clinically, nontraumatic brain injuries may show similar "focal" and diffuse effects. Certain medical conditions (e.g., stroke, and tumor), which are diagnosable via imaging, may leave specific or focal injury at the site of the event, while other secondary causation (anoxia, edema, high fever) may result in more diffuse damage with concomitant pervasive dysfunction. Because each brain injury is a unique event, careful studies of the injury itself and the behavioral manifestations in the patient are necessary to ascertain the proper course of treatment, including behavioral approaches. All references to brain injury in this chapter will refer to both types of ABI unless specifically referred to as traumatic and nontraumatic.

Incidence of Brain Injuries in Children

According to the National Center for Injury Prevention and Control, TBI is the leading cause of injury-related death and disability in children and adolescents (Bergman, 2003). It is estimated that 165,000 children a year are hospitalized with traumatic brain injuries. Each year 5000–10,000 of these children die, while 20,000–30,000 are left with lifelong deficits as a result of their TBI. Overall TBI is consistently found to be more

Table 5.1. Student Demographics at The May Center

	No. of students (%)
Infant/toddler	36
Age at the time of injury (years)	
2–6	24
7–10	17
11–14	6
15–18	17
Type of injury	
-Traumatic	47
-Nontraumatic	53
Source of injury	
Traumatic brain injury	
-Motor vehicle accident	57
-Falls	20
-Abuse	8
-Assaults	8
-Sports injuries	7
Non-TBI	
-Acquired neurological disorder	62
-Neurotoxic poisoning	15
-Anoxia	12
-Infectious disease	7
-Diabetic coma	2
-Vascular injury	2

common in males than females (National Institutes of Child Health and Human Development [NICHD] Consensus Report, 1999). The incidence of TBI is highest in individuals 15–24 years of age, with peaks in children under 5 (Kraus, Rock, & Hemyari, 1990). Although these statistics begin to illustrate the significance of the problem of ABI, they likely represent underestimates of the incidence of ABI. Surveillance systems are just beginning to be established to accurately document the incidence of TBI, and therefore many individuals with TBI are still being excluded from these national statistics (NIH Consensus Report, 1999). Additionally these national incidence data typically only include traumatic brain injuries; they do not include nontraumatic brain injuries.

Epidemiological data from our own program both support and complement these national incidence data. Approximately 10 years ago, the May Institute established a school and community residential program for children and adolescents with ABI. Since the school opened we have served approximately 130 students from 5 to 21 years of age with an average at admission of 16 years. Consistent with national statistics, the majority of the students we have served have been male (78%). Table 5.1 also shows that the majority of our students had acquired their injuries by the age of 6 years.

Table 5.1 also presents additional demographic information concerning the students we have served. We have experienced admissions of children with relatively equal numbers of traumatic and nontraumatic brain injuries over our 10 years of operation. The nontraumatic injuries are the result of a wide variety of illnesses such as diabetic coma, encephalitis, or meningitis; medical complications including anoxia; and secondary effects of treatment such as functional loss postcranial radiation for cancer treatment. If these incidence data are at all reflective of national occurrence, it would suggest that a much larger group of children who present with problems secondary to undiagnosed ABI exists and requires identification and treatment.

CHILDREN AND BRAIN INJURIES

Contrary to common perceptions, children's recovery from brain injury may be slower and less complete than that of adults (The University of the State of New York, 1995). Brain injury often affects new learning more than information that has been learned prior to the injury. It is hypothesized that recovery is enhanced in older patients who utilize previously learned information to assist in compensating for the challenge of acquiring new information. Since the child's brain is developing at the time of injury, children have less learned information to build upon, and therefore recovery may be slow. It also may be the case that structural damage to parts of the brain responsible for the processing, understanding, or management of information may be damaged, making new learning difficult or impossible. Additionally, accurate assessment of the long-term effects of brain injury is more complicated in children because the full residual effects of the injury may not be apparent for many years. For example, a child who sustains a brain injury at 5 years of age may not demonstrate deficits in problem solving until age 12 or 13 when she, and her noninjured peers, are typically expected to perform the skills at a higher cognitive level.

Causes of Traumatic Brain Injury in Children

Motor vehicle accidents account for the majority of TBI (Centers for Disease Control, 1997). However, a clearer developmental understanding of the causes of TBI in children and adolescents emerges when one compares the most common causes of injury across various age ranges. The most common cause of TBI for infants is physical abuse or neglect. In the preschool years physical abuse and falls represent the most common causes. Once children move into the early elementary school years, pedestrian motor vehicle accidents emerge as most common, while in late elementary school, bicycle and sports accidents are added to pedestrian motor vehicle accidents as the primary causes of TBI. In high school, motor vehicle accidents are the primary cause of TBI.

Our data support these national data indicating that motor vehicle accidents are responsible for a majority of our students' traumatic brain injuries. Table 5.1 presents the source of injury for all of our students, across traumatic and nontraumatic acquired brain injuries. Across the 10 years of program operation, we have seen relatively equal numbers of traumatic and nontraumatic brain injuries. While many different types of injury are responsible for TBIs, an even greater number of diseases produce specific neurological deficits and many treatment courses may lead to iatrogenic consequences in the form of specific learning and behavioral deficits. Despite these factors, our data document that 80% of our students are able to return to less restrictive placements after an average of 2.67 years.

In all cases we have found that careful history taking is crucial to correct diagnosis. The event or illness that leads to deficits is often removed in time from its outcomes. In this way medical and family focus on initial somatic damage and physical healing may hide or obscure the relationships between injury and neurocognitive deficit (Lash et al., 1996). Over time, these sequelae may be rediagnosed as psychiatric or behavioral problems often after repeated failures have taken a progressive toll on both child and family (Savage, Russo, & Gardner, 1997).

CONSEQUENCES OF BRAIN INJURY

The long-term deficits associated with brain injury generally cluster around three domains: physical, cognitive, and behavioral (Luiselli et al., 1998). It is the complex interrelations among the deficits associated with each of these domains that result in each child or adolescent having a unique and clinically significant pattern of strengths and needs. Table 5.2 presents typical physical, cognitive, and behavioral sequelae of ABI.

Although no child experiences all of these deficits, many of the symptoms of ABI, such as short-term memory loss, attention deficits, poor organization, impulsivity, difficulties in judgement and decision-making, reduced strength and endurance, and disruptive outbursts are present in the majority of the students we see at our school. Clearly, many of these deficits can also be displayed by students with diagnoses other than brain injury, but it is the concurrent presence of several deficits in many cases that renders learning and intervention difficult or complex.

Students with brain injuries do tend to differ from students with other disabilities in several ways that have important implications for treatment. While topographically behaviors may be similar to those seen in nonbrain injured children, their function or causation may differ, therefore requiring different methods of treatment for successful outcome. It must be recognized that a common problem secondary to the physical damage sustained in ABI is behavioral dysfunction and explicit assessment and treatment is required to allow children to return successfully to community living after their injuries (Russo & Navalta, 1995; Savage & Wolcott, 1988).

Given the complexity of the combined cognitive, physical, and behavioral deficits displayed by individuals with brain injury, it is prudent to assume that children and adolescents with brain injury differ significantly from those with other disabilities and, therefore, that assessment and treatment of these individuals should be different (Russo, 1990). In our experience, this assumption is true. For example, unlike individuals with developmental disabilities (DD), those with brain injury tend to show wide

Table 5.2. Long-term Residual Deficits Following ABI

Cognitive deficits
Difficulty in attention and concentration
Slowed information processing
Difficulty in thinking and reasoning
Difficulty with communication, language, and speech
Impaired memory, particularly for new information
Difficulty in judgement and decision making
Impaired planning and organization
Difficulty adjusting to change
Impaired perception
Unawareness of cognitive strengths and weaknesses

Physical deficits
Changes in vision and hearing
Difficulties in spatial coordination
Reduced speed and coordination
Impaired balance and equilibrium
Reduced strength and endurance
Changes in speech
Difficulties in eye–hand coordination
Changes in muscle tone

Common behavioral changes
Disruptive outbursts
Physical aggression
Noncompliance
Lethargy
Blunting of social skills
Loss of activities of daily living

scatter or splinter skills. That is, while an individual with a DD might be expected to have pervasive and diffuse delays across skills, individuals with brain injury may demonstrate ability in one area (e.g., academic skills) while displaying significant deficits in another area (e.g., social skills). Similarly, an individual with brain injury may appear to have a particular skill in certain situations, but under other specific conditions may not be able to display the skill effectively.

In addition to the scatter that can be anticipated within individuals with brain injury, the population as a whole is characterized by heterogeneity. The deficits associated with ABI depend on a number of factors including type, cause, severity, and location of the injury as well as age, gender, and premorbid characteristics of the individual (Ylvisaker, Szekeres, & Hartwick, 1994). For children and adolescents with brain injury, whose development is in progress, deficits are even more difficult to anticipate.

Further complicating the predictability of deficits with individuals with brain injury is the variability in the course of recovery (The State University of New York, 1995). That is, when working with children and adolescents with brain injury during the acute phases of recovery, it is possible that skills will be regained, whereas when working with their peers with developmental delays de novo acquisition, rather than recovery, skills will be the focus. In addition, it may be the case that the recovery, like deficits, occurs in some skills but not in others. For each child, which skills return and which exhibit continued deficit will be a function of initial injury, preinjury skills or deficits, effective intervention by professionals, and patient motivation for recovery. For example, a student may regain the ability to walk, but may continue to struggle with social or behavioral deficits. Similarly, the individual's memory of their life prior to injury can compound difficulties (The State University of New York, 1995). As a result, in some cases interventions meant to improve student's skills may be aversive as children and adolescents resist the stigma of using techniques entailing adaptive equipment or increased staff supervision.

TREATMENT STRATEGIES

Behavioral Assessment and ABI

As a result of the complexity of deficits, scatter within individuals, and the heterogeneity of the population, it is imperative that the assessment and treatment of individuals with brain injury be individualized. This need for an individualized approach lends itself to the use of the principles of Applied Behavior Analysis (ABA) (Pace & Nau, 1993). While the population of individuals with brain injury is distinct from other populations, the assumption that the tools of ABA assessment and treatment for ABI individuals will work less effectively is mistaken.

Because of the complexity of the deficits displayed by individuals with brain injury, the development of sound interventions with this population may require (1) a more thorough examination of a wider range of causes or conditions under which deficits emerge, and (2) integration of these causes into the treatment formulation (Ylvisaker et al., 1994). Selective damage to perceptual, memory, motivational, and executive functions of the brain may as well influence the selection of treatments and suggest a need for consideration of heightened antecedent as well as consequence-based intervention (Carnevale, Amselmi, Busichio, & Millis, 2002; Savage et al., 1997; Schlund & Pace, 1999).

Caveats in the Use of ABA Assessment

Since the clinical assessment of these individuals is more elaborate, it may require consideration of variables not typically explored when using ABA with other disorders (Russo & Navalta, 1995). For example, a child who fails to comply with requests may appear noncompliant suggesting treatment procedures, based upon a consequence analysis, such as timeout, might be effective. However, careful antecedent assessment, particularly neuropsychological testing, may indicate such behavior to be potentially the result of deficits in short-term memory, organization, or the ability to understand and operate on verbal information, all frequent outcomes of ABI. The use of consequence-based ABA is not only likely to be ineffective in such cases, but actually may worsen the behavior. In addition, because of this broader functional causation, treatment procedures may be more idiosyncratic than those attempted with other populations requiring, for example, the inclusion of visual stimuli, compensatory skills training, or prompting to help the child.

Identifying Targets and Taking Baselines

Regardless of the locus, causation, or extent of the brain injury, the initial steps of a behavioral assessment of ABI require the precise identification of the target behavior(s) as well as the establishment of a data collection system. Because of the difficulty in anticipating the deficits associated with brain injury in children and adolescents, a baseline period, usually after the acute phase of recovery, during which the student is observed in a variety of settings and under specific conditions will be helpful. In our program, for example, each student admitted participates in a 3-week baseline period during which skills, deficits, and problem behaviors are recorded by estimating the frequency and severity of their impact on the student's functioning in the school and community (see Figure 5.1). During this time, intervention procedures are minimized in order to better estimate the student's functioning in a typical environment. In addition, narrative data are collected regarding academic and social skills as well as activities of daily living. Based on the results of this baseline period, a data sheet is developed that is specific to the individual student.

Functional Assessment

Following this baseline period, the focus of assessment becomes determining the function of the identified problem behaviors and skill deficits. Informal and formal, descriptive and experimental methods for assessing the function of the target behavior(s) have been established (Iwata, Dorsey, Slifer, Bauman, & Richman, 1982; O'Neill et al., 1997). Much initial effort of these techniques has focused primarily on assessing how consequences may be maintaining the target behavior. That is, behavioral researchers and therapists, often initially trained in areas other than brain injury, are typically interested in establishing whether the function of the behavior is controlled by its consequences—whether attention, escape, access to tangibles, or automatic reinforcement seems to be responsible for the problem.

While any assessment of the function of a behavior requires thorough examination of consequences, a more refined assessment of individuals with brain injury is necessary, including a thorough examination of antecedents in a variety of domains including behavioral, social, and neurological. As with consequences, the assessment of antecedents can be conducted informally or formally, through descriptive or experimental analysis (Luiselli, Pace, & Dunn, 2003; Pace, Ivancic, & Jefferson, 1994). Particularly in applied settings where resources may be limited, descriptive analyses or a combination of experimental and descriptive analyses can be beneficial (Savage et al., 1997).

☐ Home   ☐ School

Baseline Data Sheet

Student's Name: _____   Date: _____   Staff Initials: _____

Behavior	Frequency Check the box corresponding to the approximate number of times the behavior was observed		Severity Check the box corresponding to the level of severity of the behavior observed				
	Tally Record each observed instance of behavior between 1 and 11	Summarize Note the number of occurrences of the behavior for the day/shift.	1 Not Severe at all	2	3	4	5 Very Severe
Self-Injurious Behavior: Any instance of a student injuring or attempting to injure him or herself.		☐ 0 ☐ 1–5 ☐ 6–10 ☐ 11+					
Aggressive Episode: Any instance of a student attempting to hit, kick, bite, scratch, spit at, or throw objects at others.		☐ 0 ☐ 1–5 ☐ 6–10 ☐ 11+					
Destructive Episode: Any instance of a student attempting to cause damage to objects in their environment.		☐ 0 ☐ 1–5 ☐ 6–10 ☐ 11+					
Inappropriate Social: Any verbalization out of context, making noises out of context, mimicking peers, staring at others, making faces at others, or laughing out loud out of context.		☐ 0 ☐ 1–5 ☐ 6–10 ☐ 11+					
Inappropriate Speech: Swearing, yelling, name calling, back talk, demanding speech, condescending remarks, raising their voice above conversational level in anger, or use of argumentative statements.		☐ 0 ☐ 1–5 ☐ 6–10 ☐ 11+					
Other:		☐ 0 ☐ 1–5 ☐ 6–10 ☐ 11+					
Other:		☐ 0 ☐ 1–5 ☐ 6–10 ☐ 11+					

The student follows directions approximately _____% of the time: 0–25%   26–50%   51–75%   76–100%

Protective Holds (Record time of incident and duration)

Figure 5.1. An example of a baseline data sheet that measures problem behaviors.

One example of a descriptive data sheet used to collect information regarding antecedents and consequences that most practitioners are familiar with is an Antecedents, Behavior Consequences (ABC) data sheet. However, this type of data collection does not lend itself to easy analysis. In addition, the quality, timeliness, and specificity of the information provided may be suspect. Therefore, for a more structured, direct, descriptive assessment of antecedents and consequences, a checklist method for conducting ABC data, such as that presented in Miltenberger (1997) and shown in Figure 5.2, may provide more information, while minimizing the demand on resources such as time and personnel.

Figure 5.3 presents the data collected using the checklist ABC data sheet presented in Figure 5.2. The information collected suggests that differentiation among antecedent events can be achieved using a checklist method for collecting ABC data. In this particular example, it is apparent

☐ Home   ☐ School

Student: Nathan   *Date: _____*   *Day: M T W Th F*

Antecedents: Record by placing a ✔ in the box any antecedent that occurred within 30 seconds of the target behavior.

1. Peer engaged in problem behavior
2. Group Instruction
3. Independent Seatwork
4. Seatwork with a 1:1

5. Verbal Demand from staff
6. Transition: in between activities or from one activity to another
7. Free Time / Free choice
8. Verbal prompt to be appropriate

Target Behaviors: Verbal Outburst (Mimicking, Inappropriate Speech, Screeching, and/or Inappropriate Social), Aggression, and/or Bolting

Record episodes that occur more than one minute apart as separate episodes. Record by placing a ✔ in the box any of the target behaviors that occur within the episode.

1. INAPPROPRIATE SOCIAL: Verbalization out of context, or laughing out loud out of context
2. INAPPROPRIATE SPEECH: Swearing, yelling, name calling, back talk, demanding speech, condescending remarks, raising voice above conversation level in anger, or use of argumentative statements.
3. MIMICKING: Repetition of a word or phrase or a physical gesture within 2 minutes of a peer or staff
4. SCREECHING: High pitched vocalization
5. AGGRESSION: Swatting or pulling hair that is directed at peers or staff.
6. BOLTING: Leaving morning group or the classroom without permission.

Episode	Time	Antecedents	Target Behaviors	Staff Initials
1	____ ☐ AM ☐ PM	☐1 ☐2 ☐3 ☐4 ☐5 ☐6 ☐7 ☐8	☐1 ☐2 ☐3 ☐4 ☐5 ☐6 ☐7 ☐8	
2	____ ☐ AM ☐ PM	☐1 ☐2 ☐3 ☐4 ☐5 ☐6 ☐7 ☐8	☐1 ☐2 ☐3 ☐4 ☐5 ☐6 ☐7 ☐8	
3	____ ☐ AM ☐ PM	☐1 ☐2 ☐3 ☐4 ☐5 ☐6 ☐7 ☐8	☐1 ☐2 ☐3 ☐4 ☐5 ☐6 ☐7 ☐8	
4	____ ☐ AM ☐ PM	☐1 ☐2 ☐3 ☐4 ☐5 ☐6 ☐7 ☐8	☐1 ☐2 ☐3 ☐4 ☐5 ☐6 ☐7 ☐8	
5	____ ☐ AM ☐ PM	☐1 ☐2 ☐3 ☐4 ☐5 ☐6 ☐7 ☐8	☐1 ☐2 ☐3 ☐4 ☐5 ☐6 ☐7 ☐8	
6	____ ☐ AM ☐ PM	☐1 ☐2 ☐3 ☐4 ☐5 ☐6 ☐7 ☐8	☐1 ☐2 ☐3 ☐4 ☐5 ☐6 ☐7 ☐8	
7	____ ☐ AM ☐ PM	☐1 ☐2 ☐3 ☐4 ☐5 ☐6 ☐7 ☐8	☐1 ☐2 ☐3 ☐4 ☐5 ☐6 ☐7 ☐8	
8	____ ☐ AM ☐ PM	☐1 ☐2 ☐3 ☐4 ☐5 ☐6 ☐7 ☐8	☐1 ☐2 ☐3 ☐4 ☐5 ☐6 ☐7 ☐8	
9	____ ☐ AM ☐ PM	☐1 ☐2 ☐3 ☐4 ☐5 ☐6 ☐7 ☐8	☐1 ☐2 ☐3 ☐4 ☐5 ☐6 ☐7 ☐8	
10	____ ☐ AM ☐ PM	☐1 ☐2 ☐3 ☐4 ☐5 ☐6 ☐7 ☐8	☐1 ☐2 ☐3 ☐4 ☐5 ☐6 ☐7 ☐8	
11	____ ☐ AM ☐ PM	☐1 ☐2 ☐3 ☐4 ☐5 ☐6 ☐7 ☐8	☐1 ☐2 ☐3 ☐4 ☐5 ☐6 ☐7 ☐8	
12	____ ☐ AM ☐ PM	☐1 ☐2 ☐3 ☐4 ☐5 ☐6 ☐7 ☐8	☐1 ☐2 ☐3 ☐4 ☐5 ☐6 ☐7 ☐8	
13	____ ☐ AM ☐ PM	☐1 ☐2 ☐3 ☐4 ☐5 ☐6 ☐7 ☐8	☐1 ☐2 ☐3 ☐4 ☐5 ☐6 ☐7 ☐8	
14	____ ☐ AM ☐ PM	☐1 ☐2 ☐3 ☐4 ☐5 ☐6 ☐7 ☐8	☐1 ☐2 ☐3 ☐4 ☐5 ☐6 ☐7 ☐8	
15	____ ☐ AM ☐ PM	☐1 ☐2 ☐3 ☐4 ☐5 ☐6 ☐7 ☐8	☐1 ☐2 ☐3 ☐4 ☐5 ☐6 ☐7 ☐8	
16	____ ☐ AM ☐ PM	☐1 ☐2 ☐3 ☐4 ☐5 ☐6 ☐7 ☐8	☐1 ☐2 ☐3 ☐4 ☐5 ☐6 ☐7 ☐8	
17	____ ☐ AM ☐ PM	☐1 ☐2 ☐3 ☐4 ☐5 ☐6 ☐7 ☐8	☐1 ☐2 ☐3 ☐4 ☐5 ☐6 ☐7 ☐8	
18	____ ☐ AM ☐ PM	☐1 ☐2 ☐3 ☐4 ☐5 ☐6 ☐7 ☐8	☐1 ☐2 ☐3 ☐4 ☐5 ☐6 ☐7 ☐8	
19	____ ☐ AM ☐ PM	☐1 ☐2 ☐3 ☐4 ☐5 ☐6 ☐7 ☐8	☐1 ☐2 ☐3 ☐4 ☐5 ☐6 ☐7 ☐8	
20	____ ☐ AM ☐ PM	☐1 ☐2 ☐3 ☐4 ☐5 ☐6 ☐7 ☐8	☐1 ☐2 ☐3 ☐4 ☐5 ☐6 ☐7 ☐8	
21	____ ☐ AM ☐ PM	☐1 ☐2 ☐3 ☐4 ☐5 ☐6 ☐7 ☐8	☐1 ☐2 ☐3 ☐4 ☐5 ☐6 ☐7 ☐8	
22	____ ☐ AM ☐ PM	☐1 ☐2 ☐3 ☐4 ☐5 ☐6 ☐7 ☐8	☐1 ☐2 ☐3 ☐4 ☐5 ☐6 ☐7 ☐8	
23	____ ☐ AM ☐ PM	☐1 ☐2 ☐3 ☐4 ☐5 ☐6 ☐7 ☐8	☐1 ☐2 ☐3 ☐4 ☐5 ☐6 ☐7 ☐8	

Figure 5.2. An example of an ABC checklist to identify antecedent and consequences of various target behaviors.

that antecedents associated with decreased attention (i.e., peer engaged in problem behavior, group instruction, independent seatwork) preceded inappropriate behavior more than antecedents associated with demands (i.e., verbal prompt, transition, verbal demand, seatwork with 1:1 instruction) or preferred activities (i.e., freetime).

Similarly, Figure 5.4 presents data collected during a formal functional analysis conducted with the same student. It is apparent that the data collected using the checklist ABC form corresponds directly to the function of the behavior as determined by the formal functional analysis.

However, in addition to information regarding the function of the student's behavior, the checklist ABC was able to provide information relative to the specific conditions (antecedents) under which the student was more likely to exhibit problem behavior. With children and adolescents with brain

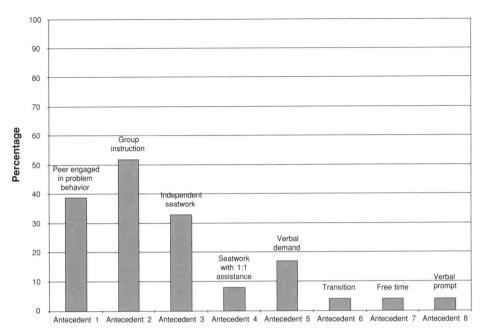

Figure 5.3. Percentage of antecedent events that preceded Nathan's target behaviors.

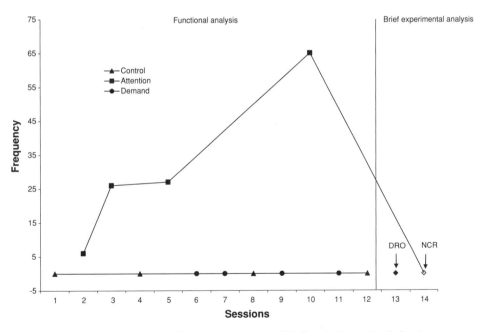

Figure 5.4. Results of a functional analysis of Nathan's disruptive behavior.

injury this antecedent information is imperative in developing comprehensive behavior support plans.

Antecedents and Consequences

As we have stated earlier, it is misleading to suggest that consequences are not an integral part of behavior support plans developed for use with students with brain injury. In many cases, however, we have observed that the combined use of antecedents and consequences or the use of antecedents alone to be most effective (Smith & Iwata, 1997). For example, Figure 5.5 presents data suggesting the use of combined consequence and antecedent-based procedures may be helpful in decreasing rates of noncompliance. Noelle, for whom data are presented in Figure 5.5, is a 15-year-old female student diagnosed with atypical Landau–Kleffner Syndrome. This neurological syndrome is associated with language deficits accompanied by seizures.

In addition, this student had undergone surgery to remove a tumor in Broca's area and bilaterally in the temporal lobes. Through an informal functional assessment it was determined that her noncompliance (i.e., failure to initiate a directive within 15 s) was maintained by escape. In order to decrease noncompliance a procedure was developed in which consequences (extinction) were combined with antecedents. The antecedent procedures included the use of transition warnings, a predictable schedule of activities, modifications to the language in which demands were presented, and clarifications of expectations of task engagement. In addition,

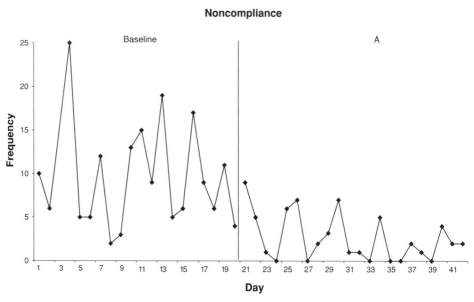

Figure 5.5. An example of the combined use of antecedent and consequent procedures on noncompliance.

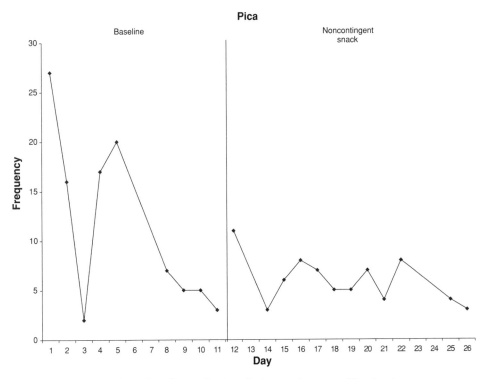

Figure 5.6. The effects of antecedent procedures on Albert's pica.

a break program was implemented so that the student could appropriately delay activities. The results of this intervention suggest that the combined use of consequences and antecedents can be effective at reducing noncompliance.

Similarly, Figure 5.6 presents data supporting the use of an antecedent procedure to target pica. Albert, for whom data are presented here, is a 6-year-old male student previously diagnosed with a pervasive developmental disorder who subsequently suffered from pneumococal meningitis, which resulted in substantial cognitive, communication, and behavioral deficits. Upon admission it was noted that Albert frequently engaged in attempts to eat nonedible items such as toys, buttons, and crayons. He had a history of a limited diet and behavior problems during meals. In addition, based on an informal functional assessment it was determined that his caloric intake was poor, suggesting the pica may have been associated with hunger.

Therefore, in order to target the pica, an antecedent-based procedure was implemented in which Albert was allowed noncontingent access to preferred food items. Food items were presented at scheduled times during the day and evening. In addition, at any time he could request food items by a verbal approximation "Foo." The results of this intervention suggest that the use of a noncontingent access to food was successful at decreasing rates of pica.

Input From Multiple Sources

Just as antecedents are an important, yet not always fully appreciated, element of ABA, so is the involvement of an interdisciplinary team. Like antecedent interventions, the use of an interdisciplinary team becomes imperative when working with individuals with brain injury. In ruling out trauma damage or exploring medical disorders that may be affecting a student's behavior, input from occupational therapy (OT), physical therapy (PT), and speech and language therapy (SLP), as well as the neuropsychological assessment of cognitive and academic deficits is integral to effective brain injury treatment. In attempting to change behavior it may be necessary to determine through further assessment whether the individual has the physical, cognitive, or academic prerequisite skills to perform the activity, the cognitive capability to understand the context and meaning of the task, and the ability to respond correctly. Other factors, including evaluating the influences of medications on behavior and utilizing the child's intact skills and functions to compensate for deficits, are also facilitated by this collaboration between members of the clinical team.

Direct assessment of these prerequisite skills, such as those provided by medical and allied health departments or through the use of Curriculum-Based Measurement (Shinn, 1989) when assessing academic prerequisites can provide the information necessary for determining effective interventions. With behaviors that are maintained by automatic reinforcement, OT, PT, and SLP services can be resources for determining the sensory input provided by the behavior and generating more socially acceptable alternatives. Similarly, with students whose behaviors are maintained by access to social reinforcement or tangibles, OT, PT, and SLP services may be beneficial, particularly in cases where verbal and nonverbal communication are a concern. For example, in the case of Albert presented earlier, the use of noncontingent access to food was effective at reducing pica. However, when this intervention was combined with a total communication approach developed in consultation with the SLP a further reduction in pica was noted (see Figure 5.7). Similarly, the use of an interdisciplinary team can help to determine what interventions are less likely to be of value.

Given the complexity of the individuals' needs that are served in a brain injury program as well as the finite amount of time available to provide services, comprehensive assessment is essential to evaluate how resources should best be allocated. It also sets the occasion to push the behavioral technology down to other treatment personnel and families, thus providing a more consistent and pervasive treatment environment. The assessment methodology of ABA is, in this regard, particularly important in evaluating what works and what does not. Figure 5.8 presents a sample of a case in which the Certified Occupational Therapy Assistant implemented a noncontingent schedule of brushing and joint compressions; a procedure designed to modulate levels of arousal.

In this particular case, involving Noelle, the student discussed earlier, it was determined that this procedure was not effective at decreasing the frequency of maladaptive behaviors. Given that this finding was

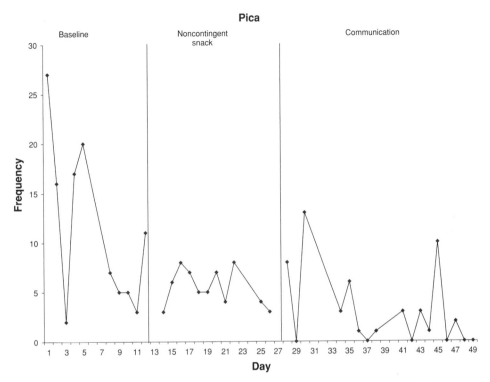

Figure 5.7. An example of the use of behavior analysis to evaluate the effects of communication training.

inconsistent with the outcome anticipated by the use of such a procedure, it was determined that this intervention should be discontinued. Additional procedures to target this behavior were explored and therapist time was freed to allow continued consultation with the classroom regarding the student's other OT needs.

CONCLUSIONS

In this chapter we have attempted to shed some light on the complicated and yet potentially manageable consequences of ABI in children. When viewed demographically, one clearly sees a large number of these children and adolescents in need of services and the potential for life-long problems if they are unable to obtain them (Lash, Russo, Navalta, & Baryza, 1995).

While children now routinely survive their brain injuries, many are unable to identify treatment programs or professionals specifically trained to address their deficits. As a society, we have been very successful in saving these children's lives and accommodating to the physical injuries of these children. We have not, however, been successful at building a cognitive

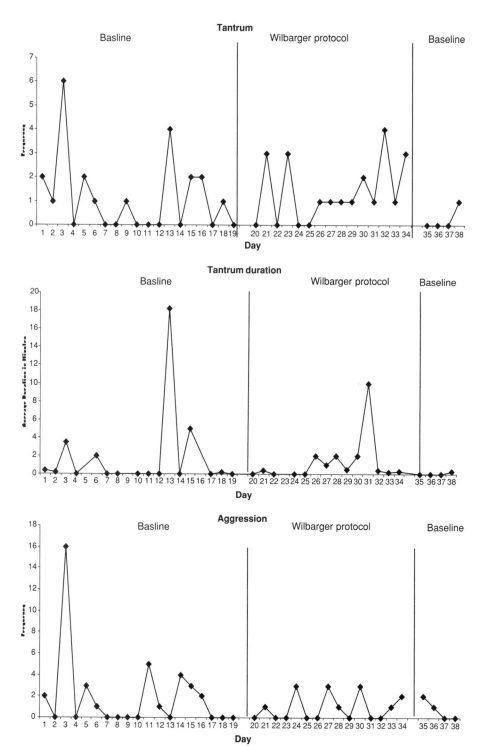

Figure 5.8. An example of the use of behavior analysis to evaluate the effects of OT interventions.

and behavioral ramp back to the community for large numbers of the ABI population (Russo, 1990). It is clear that we need to develop, as well, increasing knowledge of these children within the population of behavioral practitioners. While they may present with behaviors, which appear familiar, treatment must be based on thorough assessment of deficit rather than primarily topography.

There exists a significant body of literature identifying the utility of behavioral methods in ameliorating problems and enhancing skills in those with ABI. What is comforting is that the same benchmarks of definition, objective assessment, and consistency of implementation make well-designed behavior interventions particularly effective with these children.

REFERENCES

Academy for the Certification of Brain Injury Specialists. (2004). *Training manual for certified brain injury specialists* (3rd ed.). McLean, VA: Brain Injury Association of America.

Bergman, A. I. (2003). President's message. *Brain Injury Source, 6*, 4.

Brain Injury Association Website://www.BIAUSA.ORG/word.files.to.pdf/good.pdfs/2002. fact.sheet.tbi.incidence.pdf

Carnevale, G. J., Amselmi, V., Busichio, K., & Millis, S. R. (2002). Changes in ratings of caregiver burden following a community-based behavior management program for persons with traumatic brain injury. *Journal of Head Trauma Rehabilitation, 17*, 83–95.

Centers for Disease Control. (1997a). Traumatic brain injury—Colorado, Missouri, Oklahoma, and Utah, 1990–1993. *Morbidity and Mortality Weekly Reports, 46*, 8–11.

Iwata, B. A., Dorsey, M. F., Slifer, K. J., Bauman, K. E., & Richman, G. S. (1982). Toward a functional analysis of self-injury. *Analysis and Intervention in Developmental Disabilities, 2*, 3–20.

Kraus, J. F., Rock, A., & Hemyari, P. (1990). Brain injuries among infants, children, adolescents, and young adults. *American Journal of Disabled Children, 144*, 684–691.

Lash, M., Navalta, C., Kahn, P., Osberg, J. S., Russo, D. C., & Savage, R. C. (1996). *A Manual for families of children with acquired brain injuries.* Boston, MA: Research and Training Center in Rehabilitation and Childhood Trauma.

Lash, M., Russo, D. C., Navalta, C. P., & Baryza, M. J. (1995). Families of children with injuries identify needs for research and training. *NeuroRehabilitation: An Interdisciplinary Journal, 5*, 331–346.

Luiselli, J. K., Gardner, R., Arons, M., McDonald, H., Madigan, C., Marchese, N., et al. (1998). Comprehensive community-based education neurorehabilitation for children and adolescents with traumatic brain injury. *Behavioral Interventions, 13*, 181–200.

Luiselli, J. K., Pace, G. M., & Dunn, E. K. (2003). Antecedent analysis of therapeutic restraint in children and adolescents with acquired brain injury: A descriptive study of four cases. *Brain Injury, 17*, 255–264.

Miltenberger, R. G. (1997). *Behavior modification: Principles and procedures.* Pacific Grove, CA: Brooks/Cole.

National Institute of Child Health and Human Development. (1999). *Report of the consensus development conference on the rehabilitation of persons with traumatic brain injury.* Washington, DC: Government Printing Office.

O'Neill, R. E., Horner, R. H., Albin, R. W., Sprague, J. R., Storey, K., & Newton, J. S. (1997). *Functional assessment and program development for problem behavior* (2nd ed.). Pacific Groove, CA: Brooks/Cole.

Pace, G. M., Ivancic, M. T., & Jefferson, G. (1994). Stimulus fading as treatment for obscenity in a brain-injured adult. *Journal of Applied Behavior Analysis, 24*, 301–304.

Pace, G. M., & Nau, P. (1993). Behavior analysis in brain injury rehabilitation: Training staff to develop, implement, and evaluate behavior change programs. In C. J. Durgin, N. D.

Schmidt, & L. J. Fryer (Eds.), *Staff development and clinical interventions in brain injury rehabilitation* (pp. 105–128). Gaithersburg, MD: Aspen.

Russo, D. C. (1990). Specialized rehab needs for head injured children. *Continuing Care, 9*(2), 28–32.

Russo, D. C., & Navalta, C. P. (1995). Some new dimensions of behaviour analysis and therapy. In H. van Bilsen, P. C. Kendall, & J. H. Slavenburg (Eds.), *Behavioural approaches for children and adolescents: Challenges for the Next Century* (pp. 19–39). New York: Plenum.

Savage, R. C., Russo, D. C., & Gardner, R. (1997). Brain injuries in children: Coming back to school. In J. Leon-Carrion (Ed.), *Neuropsychological rehabilitation: Fundamentals, innovations, and directions* (pp. 499–512). Delray Beach, FL: St. Lucie.

Savage, R. C., & Wolcott, G. F. (1988). *An educator's manual: What educators need to know about students with traumatic brain injury.* Washington, DC: National Brain Injury Association.

Schlund, M. W., & Pace, G. M. (1999). Relations between traumatic brain injury and the environment: Feedback reduces maladaptive behavior by three persons with traumatic brain injury. *Brain Injury, 13*, 889–897.

Shinn, M. R. (Ed.). (1989). *Curriculum-based measurement: Assessing special children.* New York: Guilford.

Smith, R. G., & Iwata, B. A. (1997). Antecedent influences on behavior disorders. *Journal of Applied Behavior Analysis, 30*, 343–375.

The University of the State of New York. (1995). *Traumatic brain injury: A guidebook for educators.* Albany, NY: New York State Education.

Ylvisaker, M., Szekeres, S. F., & Hartwick, P. (1994). A framework for cognitive intervention. In R. C. Savage & G. F. Wolcott (Eds.), *Educational dimensions of acquired brain injury* (pp. 35–67). Austin, TX: Pro-Ed.

6

Behavioral Effects of Genetic Mental Retardation Disorders

ROBERT M. HODAPP and ELISABETH M. DYKENS

In the humanities and in the social sciences, it is almost a truism to say that one cannot escape the influence of one's own historical time. Certain novelists of the past, for example, are highly valued during one historical period, "lost" to another, only to be reembraced at a later time. Similarly in a field like history, we see changes over the decades in how society views the accomplishments of certain individuals. Are Jefferson, Adams, Franklin, and other of America's "Founding Fathers" omniscient visionaries, as portrayed in many recent books, or instead should they be criticized for leaving unresolved such basic national issues as slavery (Brands, 2003)? Fields, like people, reflect the times in which they exist.

So too with the field of intellectual disabilities and its relation to genetics and other biomedical sciences. Consider Norman Ellis' (1969) statement that "Rarely have behavioral differences characterized different etiological groups" (p. 561). Such a statement may have been an accurate description of intellectual disability (ID) research 35 years ago, when few genetic disorders were identified and few etiology-based studies existed outside of Down syndrome. In contrast, such a statement seems dated today. At last count, geneticists have identified over 1000 genetic disorders associated with ID, and the field of "behavioral phenotypes" has taught us that behavioral differences do indeed characterize many of these disorders (see Barnard, Pearson, Rippon, & O'Brien, 2002 for brief reviews). Each day brings us closer to understanding how genes, brain, and behavior go together, and

ROBERT M. HODAPP and ELISABETH M. DYKENS • John F. Kennedy Center and Peabody College, Vanderbilt University, Nashville, Tennessee.

the study of behavioral outcomes of various genetic disorders is critical to these efforts.

One preliminary way to assess the growing interest in etiology-related behaviors is to tally behavioral studies on different genetic ID syndromes over time. Consider the number of empirical articles on behavior in a few genetic disorders during the 1980s compared to the 1990s. In fragile X syndrome, the numbers over these decades rose from 60 to 149; in Williams syndrome, from 10 to 81; in Prader–Willi syndrome, from 24 to 86. Even in Down syndrome, the sole etiology featuring a long tradition of behavioral research, the numbers of behavioral studies nearly doubled—from 607 to 1140 articles—from the 1980s to the 1990s (Hodapp & Dykens, 2004). More recent years have continued such trends, particularly in disorders such as Williams, Rett, fragile X, and Prader–Willi syndromes (Einfeld, 2004).

Almost as a side-benefit, we see increasing connections between those interested in the behaviors of persons with ID and those interested in genetic and biomedical issues. Clinical, developmental, behaviorist, and other psychologists now routinely work with geneticists, neurologists, and pediatricians. The "behavior people" have begun to join with the "biomedical people," and what we earlier (Hodapp & Dykens, 1994) identified as IDs two separate cultures of behavioral research have begun to merge. Almost by necessity, behavioral research in the field of ID has become more integrated, more interdisciplinary.

This chapter provides a sense of that more integrated, interdisciplinary field by examining behavioral research in genetic ID syndromes. Although we cannot do justice to the explosion of new knowledge generated even over the past 5–10 years, our goal is to provide some highlights of this approach. To this end, we begin by defining "behavioral phenotype," a widely used—but not always clear—term within this area of research. We then consider two classes of examples, before ending with some issues that remain for research and intervention.

BEHAVIORAL PHENOTYPES: DEFINITION AND EXAMPLES

In considering the behavioral effects of genetic ID syndromes, many researchers and clinicians use the term "behavioral phenotypes." Although variously defined, most recent workers would agree to some variant of a definition first proposed by Dykens (1995). According to this definition, a behavioral phenotype involves "...the heightened probability or likelihood that people with a given syndrome will exhibit certain behavioral and developmental sequelae relative to those without the syndrome" (p. 523).

This definition emphasizes several issues. First, and contrary to several earlier proposed definitions (e.g., Flint & Yule, 1994), behavioral phenotypes are considered to be probabilistic. That is, although many persons with a particular disorder will show the behavior (or behaviors) that characterize a particular syndrome, some will not. To quote O'Brien (2002a), "Behavioral phenotypes are here defined as *consistently* associated with a biological disorder, but *not universally*" (p. 3; italics in original). This "consistency question" leads to the idea that, within every syndrome, there is a certain amount of within-syndrome variability (Pennington, O'Connor, & Sudhalter, 1991).

Although seen in virtually every etiology, such within-syndrome variability can be shown strikingly in Down syndrome. For many years, studies have found that, even compared to their overall mental ages, children and adults with Down syndrome generally show deficits in several areas of language. Fowler (1990; see also Chapman & Hesketh, 2000) noted such greater-than-mental age-level deficits in linguistic grammar, and Miller (1999) showed similar deficits in expressive language. In addition, approximately 95% of mothers of children with Down syndrome report that others have difficulty in understanding their child's articulation of words and phrases (Kumin, 1994).

And yet, even if most persons with Down syndrome show specific deficits in grammar, expressive language, and articulation, such is not the case with every person with this disorder. For example, Rondal provided an in-depth examination of the language of Francoise, a 32-year-old woman whose IQ is 64. Although Francoise has trisomy 21, she nevertheless utters sentences such as (translated), "And that does not surprise me because dogs are always too warm when they go outside" ("Et ca m'etonne pas parce que les chiens ont toujours trop chaud quand ils vont a la port"; Rondal, 1995, p. 117). Such complicated sentences, though common in Francoise's speech, rarely occur in the speech of most other adults with Down syndrome.

A second issue relates to the specificity of behavioral effects. Do genetic syndromes lead to behavioral outcomes that are unique to one and only one syndrome (so-called "total specificity"), or instead might several syndromes lead to identical behavioral outcomes ("partial specificity")? Surveying the available studies, both possibilities seem supported (Hodapp, 1997). Although no good numbers exist concerning how often each occurs, we suspect that there are only a few instances of total specificity, many more of partial specificity.

To begin with total specificity, a few genetic syndromes predispose affected individuals to a particular outcome that is not seen in other genetic disorders. At present, the following behaviors seem unique to one and only one syndrome:

- extreme hyperphagia (overeating; Dykens, 1999) in Prader–Willi syndrome;
- extreme self-mutilation (Anderson & Ernst, 1994) in Lesch–Nyhan syndrome;
- stereotypic "hand washing" or "hand wringing" (Van Acker, 1991) in Rett syndrome;
- the "cat cry" (Gersh et al., 1995) in 5p- (Cri du Chat) syndrome; and
- body "self-hugging" (Finucane, Konar, Haas-Givler, Kurtz, & Scott, 1994) and putting objects into bodily orifices (Greenberg et al., 1996) in Smith–Magenis syndrome.

Although a few other examples might yet be discovered in which a particular behavior is unique to one syndrome, such 1:1 relationships seem relatively rare.

In contrast, many more etiology-related behaviors will likely involve partial specificity. To give but a few examples, a particular advantage in simultaneous (i.e., holistic, Gestalt-like) processing compared to sequential (step-by-step) processing has now been found in boys with fragile X syndrome (Dykens, Hodapp, & Leckman, 1987; Kemper, Hagerman, & Altshul-Stark, 1988) and in children with Prader–Willi syndrome (Dykens, Hodapp, Walsh, & Nash, 1992). Similarly, compared to groups with ID in general, hyperactivity is more frequently found in children with 5p-syndrome (Dykens & Clarke, 1997) and in boys with fragile X syndrome (Baumgardner, Reiss, Freund, & Abrams, 1995). In both instances, a pattern of strengths–weaknesses or a particular type of maladaptive behavior-psychopathology is found in a few genetic disorders to much greater degrees (or in higher percentages of individuals) than is commonly noted among others with ID.

As these examples also demonstrate, the situation is further complicated in that both totally specific and partially specific behaviors often coexist within the same syndrome. Groups with Prader–Willi syndrome are unique in that most individuals display hyperphagia, but persons with Prader–Willi syndrome join boys with fragile X syndrome in showing a profile of higher simultaneous compared to sequential processing abilities, which is not seen in groups with ID due to heterogeneous causes (Naglieri, 1985; Obrzut, Nelson, & Obrzut, 1987).

Finally, partially specific behavioral effects seem more in line with many areas of genetics, child psychiatry, and psychiatry. Across these different disciplines, researchers are discussing the many pathways—both genetic and environmental—by which one comes to have one or another psychiatric disorder. The clinical geneticist John Opitz (1985) put it well when he noted, "The causes are many, but the common developmental pathways are few" (p. 9).

TWO EXAMPLES OF BEHAVIORAL PHENOTYPES

When considering the effects of genetic ID syndromes on behavior, one could cite many, possibly even hundreds of, examples. Considered together, however, most etiology-based behavioral studies involve either profiles or maladaptive behavior. In the first instance, researchers examine relative strengths and weaknesses, broadly conceived, across and within particular behavioral domains. In the second, researchers examine whether a particular etiological group shows more maladaptive behavior-psychopathology compared to others with ID.

Profiles of Abilities

To efficiently present as much information as possible, Table 6.1 provides an overview of findings from many studies that examine cognitive and

Table 6.1. Cognitive and Language Profiles for Several Genetic Intellectual Disability Syndromes

Syndrome	Findings	Representative studies
Williams syndrome	Verbal abilities > visual–spatial abilities	Jarrold et al. (2001); Jarrold, Hartley, Phillips and Baddeley (2000)
	Verbal > performance IQ	Don, Schellenberg, and Rourke (1999)
	Verbal memory > visuospatial skills	Klein and Mervis (1999)
	Facial recognition/memory > mental age (MA)	Pezzini, Vicari, Volterra, Milani, and Osella (1999)
Down syndrome	Receptive vocabulary > verbal short-term memory	Jarrold, Baddeley, and Phillips (2002), Jarrold, Baddeley, and Hewes (2000)
	Visual short-term memory > verbal short-term memory	Hodapp, Evans, and Gray (1999)
	Long-term (hippocampal) memory < MA controls	Pennington et al. (2003)
	Visuospatial skills > verbal memory	Klein and Mervis (1999), Miller (1999)
	Receptive > expressive language	
Fragile X syndrome	Simultaneous > sequential processing	Dykens et al. (1987)
	Expressive and receptive language > short-term memory	Hodapp, Dykens, Ort, Zelinsky, and Leckman (1991)
		Crowe and Hay (1990)
Prader–Willi syndrome	Simultaneous > sequential processing	Dykens (2002)
	Long-term memory > short-term memory	Dykens et al. (1992)
	Visual/spatial skills, e.g., puzzles > overall MA	Conners, Rosenquist, Atwell, and Klinger (2000)

linguistic profiles. Other domains of functioning obviously exist, but Table 6.1's organization touches on the main findings across several syndromes.

Many of Table 6.1's findings have now been fairly well established. Children with Williams syndrome show relative strengths in linguistic abilities (although usually not at chronological age levels) and relative weaknesses in various visual–spatial tasks. Similarly, boys with fragile X syndrome and children with Prader–Willi syndrome both show a profile of "simultaneous over sequential processing" on such tests as the Kaufman Assessment Battery for Children (K-ABC) (Kaufman & Kaufman, 1983), and children with Down syndrome show particular difficulties in linguistic grammar and expressive language. Each of these findings has been obtained by several different research groups.

But in addition to the findings themselves, Table 6.1 also highlights several other issues. A first involves the design of studies. As in many other areas of ID behavioral research, no consensus exists about how best to perform etiology-based behavioral studies. Within the field of behavioral phenotypes, some studies compare individuals to others with mixed or heterogeneous causes for their ID. Other studies compare individuals to themselves—hence, the many studies comparing individuals' performance against themselves on one versus another psychometric test or subtests. Still others compare children or adults with a particular genetic syndrome to mental age-matched typically developing controls. With the interest in "spared" or "age-level" functioning (e.g., are individuals with Williams syndrome spared in their linguistic abilities?), comparisons to chronological age-matched typically developing children have also become common (for evaluations of each, see Hodapp & Dykens, 2001).

Second, Table 6.1's etiology-related profiles were discovered through the use of a variety of different types of assessment. Many studies that compare across domains use different psychometric tests. Some of the "within-domain" examinations compare functioning on different subtests (e.g., hand movements vs. number recall on the K-ABC), whereas others compare across different experimental measures. Still other areas use more naturalistic, observational measures, as for example the use of the child's conversational speech to determine the child's mean length of utterance (MLU), index of productive syntax (IPSyn), or other measure of level of grammar.

A third issue concerns how these lines of work develop. Over time, profile studies usually move from general to specific. Early studies present a more general finding, for example, the observation that children with Williams syndrome seem high functioning in language. Later studies then test this idea, usually employing psychometric instruments. Later still, more specialized studies come along, systematically examining particular subareas of language, cognition, or visual–spatial abilities. Such later, more specialized studies are often performed by developmental psycholinguists, cognitive neuropsychologists, or other professionals with intimate knowledge of how one particular aspect of human cognitive or linguistic functioning is differentiated within typically developing individuals (and how this pattern does or does not hold in the specific etiological group). Finally, researchers begin to examine within-syndrome variability due to any number of factors (e.g., age, molecular genetic status, environment, gender).

Maladaptive Behavior-Psychopathology

Table 6.2 presents similar information for the second class of etiology-based behavioral studies, those focusing on maladaptive behavior-psychopathology. As before, several of these findings have now been shown several times. Thus, we now appreciate the high prevalence rates of hyperphagia (i.e., overeating), temper tantrums and obsessions–compulsions in Prader–Willi syndrome, of anxieties and fears in Williams syndrome, and of autism or autistic-like behaviors in both fragile X and Rett syndromes.

Again, though, several issues are hidden in the table itself. First, as in the wider field of ID, these studies struggle with how one measures and conceptualizes maladaptive behavior in persons with ID. How, for example, does one assess depression, or even depressed mood, in individuals who may be less able to reflect on or talk about their feelings? Such issues have

Table 6.2. Salient Maladaptive Behaviors in Different Genetic Syndromes

Syndrome	Findings	Reported %
Prader–Willi	Hyperphagia	82
	Temper tantrums	77–88
	Compulsivity	45–80
	Skin picking	66–97
Williams	Hypersociability	73–79
	Inattention	91–96
	Sleep problems	24–50
	Generalized anxiety/specific phobias	18–33
Fragile X	Hyperactivity/inattention	90–100
	Social anxiety/anxiety	50
	Autism-like behaviors	33
Rett	Unusual hand movements	89
	Sleep/wake disturbances	60–80
	Autism-like behaviors	40
5p-	Hyperactivity	85–90
	Self-stimulatory behavior	96
	Self-injury	70
	Cat cry (of those with specific deletion)	100
Smith–Magenis	Self-injury	92–100
	Stereotypies	100
	Sleep disturbances	94
Velocardiofacial	Inattention	24
	Psychosis-adult onset	29
Down	Depression in adults	6–11
	Dementia in adults (behavioral)	4–6

Note. Percentages reported in Bregman, Leckman, and Ort (1988), Collacott (1992), Meyers and Pueschel (1991), Cornish and Pigram (1996), Dimitropoulos et al. (2001), Dykens (2003), Dykens, Finucane, and Gayley (1997), Dykens and Clarke (1997), Carlin (1990), Dykens and Kasari (1997), Dykens et al. (1996), Dykens and Rosner (1999), Dykens and Smith (1998), Finucane, Dirrigl, and Simon (2001), Finucane et al. (1994), Gosch and Pankau (1994), Hagerman (1996), Mount, Charman, Hastings, Reilly, and Cass (2002, 2003), Papolos et al. (1996), Pulver et al. (1994), Rogers, Wehner, and Hagerman (2001), Udwin (1990), Udwin, Yule, and Martin (1987), Wigren and Heimann (2001).

partially been addressed by the flurry of new measures normed especially on persons with ID (*Aberrant Behavior Checklist*, Aman & Singh, 1994; *Developmental Behavioural Checklist*, Einfeld & Tonge, 1992; *Reiss Screen for Maladaptive Behavior*, Reiss, 1988). In addition, researchers have adopted (modified) behavioral criteria to diagnose psychiatric disorders and informants to tell about individuals' problems. Nevertheless, measurement issues remain a challenge in this line of work (see Dykens, 2000).

Second, we again note the issue of control or contrast groups. For the most part, studies of maladaptive behavior have compared individuals with a particular genetic disorder to a "mixed" or "heterogeneous" group of individuals with ID (Dykens & Hodapp, 2001). Possibly more than in the profile studies, however, studies of maladaptive behavior-psychopathology have sometimes gone beyond the usual mixed-ID comparisons. Thus, Dykens and Rosner (1999) compared individuals with Prader–Willi syndrome to those with Williams syndrome, the rationale being to examine how anxiety-related problems might manifest themselves differently in the two groups.

Other studies compared groups with a particular ID etiology to nonretarded persons who have a particular psychiatric disorder, as in Dykens, Leckman, and Cassidy's (1996) comparison of the obsessions and compulsions of individuals with Prader–Willi syndrome with those seen in nonretarded persons with OCD.

Finally, several recent studies have examined changes in maladaptive behavior-psychopathology as children and adults get older. Dykens, Shah, Sagun, Beck, and King (2002) noted that adolescents with Down syndrome may become more "inward" during the adolescent years, in addition to showing lesser amounts of stubbornness and other externalizing problems (see also Meyers & Pueschel, 1991; Tonge & Einfeld, 2003). Similar changes with age have also been shown in the maladaptive behavior-psychopathology of children or adults with Prader–Willi syndrome (Dimitropoulos et al., 2000; Dimitropoulos, Feurer, Butler, & Thompson, 2001; Dykens, 2004), and Williams syndrome (Dykens, 2003). The issue of change with age promises to concern etiology-oriented researchers examining a variety of syndrome groups, as it increases the importance of age as a variable meriting study, and may, in part, be a surrogate for not only biological, but also environmental influences on development.

NEW AREAS, REMAINING CHALLENGES

Although we have so far mostly defined and exemplified research on behavioral phenotypes, this subfield involves more than documenting etiology-related profiles or maladaptive behaviors. Instead, etiology-based researchers are tackling larger questions that, as they are answered over the next 10–20 years, promise to inform us about both basic and applied issues. We now turn to five of these larger issues.

Within-Syndrome Variability

Faced with an initial task of showing whether various genetic etiologies differentially affected behavior, many etiology-based behavioral studies adopted a group-difference approach. But why do only most—not all— persons with one or another disorder show a disorder's "characteristic" behavior or behaviors? Although studies in this area are only beginning, a few preliminary answers are emerging. In some cases, within-syndrome variability occurs due to genetic variants of particular syndromes. Compare persons who have Prader–Willi syndrome due to a deletion (i.e., missing material from the paternally derived chromosome 15) versus a uniparental disomy (i.e., two chromosome 15's from the mother). Long thought to be identical in their behaviors, these two subtypes may differ both in maladaptive behavior-psychopathology (Dykens, Cassidy, & King, 1999; Vogels et al., 2004) and in intellectual profiles (Roof et al., 2000). More recently, Butler, Bittel, Kibiryeva, Talebizadeh, and Thompson (2004) noted that, even among those individuals with the deletion subtype, one can have either large (TI or Type I) or smaller (T2 or Type II) deletions. Behaviorally, individuals with Type I deletions showed lower adaptive behavior scores and several specific obsessive-compulsive behaviors. In addition to differences in genetic subtypes, within-syndrome differences in behavior may also result from the individual's gender, background genetics of the family, everyday activities chosen by the child, degree of stimulation provided to the child, or even the family's communication styles or parents' problem-solving styles.

Development Over Time

A special case of within-syndrome variability relates to changes over the course of development. Discussed above in relation to how maladaptive behavior changes with age, age-related changes may also occur in profiles of cognitive-linguistic strength and weakness. In one study, Jarrold, Baddeley, Hewes, and Phillips (2001) tested children with Williams syndrome six times over a 4-year period as they developed in both receptive vocabulary and visual–spatial skills. They found that, over time, vocabulary skills developed at a much faster rate than did visual–spatial skills. As children got older, the two domains therefore became increasingly out of synch, such that relative strengths became stronger compared to relative weaknesses.

The question of why, exactly, increasing dissynchrony occurs is more difficult to answer. One possibility may involve as yet unknown genetic or neurological factors that change across development. Another may involve the specific everyday, leisure-time activities chosen by children with different genetic syndromes. Rosner, Hodapp, Fidler, Sagun, and Dykens (2004) found that, compared to children with Down syndrome or Prader–Willi syndrome, children with Williams syndrome generally avoid performing arts and crafts, puzzles, and other everyday visuo-spatial tasks. Compared to participation rates of roughly one-third among children with either Prader–Willi syndrome or Down syndrome (30% and 35%, respectively), only 5% of children with Williams syndrome participated in any arts-and-crafts activities. It is almost as if children with Williams syndrome (or their parents) are shying away from these children's areas of weakness, possibly exacerbating already existing weaknesses as time goes on.

Gene-Brain-Behavior Links

Although of interest to researchers from many different disciplines, the examination of gene-brain-behavior links is only beginning. But even today, some studies tie these three together. Consider Pennington, Moon, Edgin, Stedron, and Nadel's (2003) study comparing children with Down syndrome to mental age-matched typically developing children on two sets of tasks. The first set related to functioning of the prefrontal cortex, which involves holding information in active or working memory. The second set examined hippocampal functioning, which relates to the storage of episodic information into long-term memory. As predicted, children with Down syndrome performed more poorly than their matches on tasks involving the hippocampus, but equally well on tasks relating to the prefrontal cortex.

Pennington et al. (2003) began with a clear neurological hypothesis: Children with Down syndrome will perform worse on tasks related to the hippocampus, while tasks related to the prefrontal cortex will more closely conform to the child's overall mental age. The authors then grouped together two sets of otherwise disparate tasks. Hippocampal measures, all of which require long-term memory, included the long-term recall of a list of 15 words presented five times, learning a visual map, learning visual patterns, and learning paired associates (linking an abstract visual pattern and its location). Prefrontal tasks included planning, "stopping" (i.e., inhibiting one's actions), verbal and nonverbal fluency, and spatial and verbal working memory. Through functional magnetic resonance imaging (MRI), positron emission tomography (PET), or computer tomographic (CT) scans, these tasks had previously been linked to either the hippocampus or prefrontal cortex. Children with Down syndrome then showed relative weaknesses in hippocampal tasks, illustrating one of the first etiology-related deficits to be so tightly tied to neurological functioning and localization.

Indirect Effects

In most discussions of behavioral phenotypes, the focus has been on the outcome behaviors of the person with the genetic disorder. But, in line with Bell (1968) and other developmental psychologists, we now know that children's behaviors affect adults. Within genetic disorders, this effect has been called a genetic disorder's "indirect effects" (Hodapp, 1997, 1999). The idea has been that a particular genetic disorder predisposes affected individuals to show one or more characteristic behaviors; these behaviors, in turn, may elicit particular types of reactions and behaviors from mothers, fathers, siblings, teachers, and others in the surrounding environment, including differences in parenting and instructional behavior.

Although the idea of genetic disorders' indirect effects is relatively new, several preliminary findings are intriguing. The first concerns what various researchers have referred to as the "Down syndrome advantage." This advantage involves the finding that parents of children with Down syndrome generally cope better than do parents of children with other disabilities. This advantage seems to hold when parents of children with Down syndrome are compared to parents of children with autism (Kasari & Sigman, 1997), with psychiatric disorders (Thomas & Olsen, 1993), with different genetic forms of ID (Fidler, Hodapp, & Dykens, 2000), and with mixed or heterogeneous ID (Hodapp, Ricci, Ly, & Fidler, 2003). Although not found in every study, compared to parents of other children with disabilities, parents of children with Down syndrome usually cope better; these parents also often judge their children as happy, sociable, and more rewarding to the parent (Carr, 1995; Hodapp, Ly, Fidler, & Ricci, 2001; Hornby, 1995).

Granted, one could argue that, apart from the child's behavior per se, parents of children with Down syndrome already differ from parents of children with other disabilities. Parents of children with Down syndrome are more likely to be older, to have access to a greater number of (often more active) parent groups, to be aware of their child's disability from birth or near-birth, and to be raising children with a more well-known disorder. Cahill and Glidden (1996) have pointed to such other-than-behavior characteristics as the reason why the Down syndrome advantage exists. At this point the question remains unresolved, but we would argue that a more pleasant, outgoing personality (Hodapp et al., 2003) and relatively low levels of maladaptive behavior-psychopathology (Dykens & Kasari, 1997) play at least some role in parent–family coping in relation to their child with Down syndrome.

The Leap from Basic Findings to Clinical Interventions

A final line of work has begun to ask how etiology-related findings can be used to enhance intervention efforts. To date, etiology-related suggestions, though seemingly helpful, have not been rigorously assessed. Dykens et al. (2000), for example, have made clinical recommendations for individuals with Williams, Prader–Willi, and fragile X syndromes (see also Dykens & Hodapp, 1997; O'Brien, 2002b). One suggestion was that interventionists might capitalize on the verbal and sociable nature of many persons with Williams syndrome by having them participate in group or verbal therapies; another, to get persons with Prader–Willi syndrome "unstuck," involved giving extra warnings about changes in routine or upcoming transitions. Similar recommendations, mostly based on cognitive-linguistic strengths and weaknesses, have also been made in educational approaches for children with Prader–Willi syndrome (Dorn & Goff, 2003; Levine & Wharton, 1993), Williams syndrome (Levine, 1994; Udwin & Yule, 2001), and other genetic etiologies (Finucane, 1996; Hodapp & Fidler, 1999).

What remains to be shown are whether such recommendations actually work and how, exactly, one should conceptualize etiology-based interventions. To date, few studies have been performed to assess the efficacy of almost any type of etiology-based intervention. We do not know, for example, whether interventions that should be effective based on any etiology-related cognitive-linguistic profiles do indeed work better than other, more generic techniques. Even in the area of psychopharmacology, few studies yet exist on the efficacy of anxiety-reducing medications for individuals with Williams syndrome, or of medications that reduce compulsions for individuals with Prader–Willi syndrome (Dykens & Shah, 2003; Hagerman, 1999).

Beyond this lack of studies, other issues loom. In the area of educational interventions, it remains unclear about how, exactly, one should use any etiology-based profile. Should one play to strengths or ameliorate weaknesses? Should, for example, one use more visual methods to teach children with Prader–Willi syndrome and more auditory-linguistic methods to teach children with Williams syndrome? Although our general sense has been that it is usually better to play to strengths as opposed to ameliorating weaknesses, others have legitimately questioned why etiology-based profiles necessarily lead to such a recommendation (Abbeduto & Keller-Bell, 2002). Despite such questions, etiology-related profiles and maladaptive behaviors have set the stage for outcome research that evaluates etiology-specific treatments.

CONCLUSION

Until as few as 20 years ago, most behavioral researchers in ID did not feel that genetics, neurosciences, or any biomedical areas had much to do with their work. But as this chapter illustrates, we have come a very long way in a very short time.

Bringing about greater change in future years will be both exciting and difficult. It will be exciting in that behavioral phenotype work now occupies an important, some might even say a central, role in understanding how different domains of complex human functioning operate. But we are also struck by just how many different professionals will need to come together to achieve progress. Fortunately, such collaborations increasingly occur both within such individual disciplines as psychology, as well as across diverse disciplines (e.g., psychology, neurosciences, genetics).

In some sense, we end this chapter with many more questions than answers, but the recent progress makes us hopeful. And although we cannot know how our generation of researchers—and the explosion of work they have produced—will be judged by future generations, our hope is that our generation will have begun a process that resulted in better, multidisciplinary understandings of behavior and more targeted interventions for persons with different genetic ID disorders.

REFERENCES

Abbeduto, L., & Keller-Bell, Y. (2002). Review of genetics and mental retardation syndromes: A new look at behavior and interventions. *American Journal on Mental Retardation, 107,* 412–414.

Aman, M. G., & Singh, N. N. (1994). *Aberrant Behavior Checklist—community supplementary manual.* East Aurora, NY: Slosson Educational.

Anderson, L., & Ernst, M. (1994). Self-injury in Lesch–Nyhan disease. *Journal of Autism and Developmental Disorders, 24,* 67–81.

Barnard, L., Pearson, J., Rippon, L., & O'Brien, G. (2002). Behavioural phenotypes of genetic syndromes: Summaries, including notes on management and therapy. In G. O'Brien (Ed.), *Behavioural phenotypes in clinical practice* (pp. 169–227). London, England: Mac Keith.

Baumgardner, T. L., Reiss, A. L., Freund, L. S., & Abrams, M. T. (1995). Specification of the neurobehavioral phenotype in males with fragile X syndrome. *Pediatrics, 95,* 744–752.

Bell, R. Q. (1968). A reinterpretation of direction of effects in studies of socialization. *Psychological Review, 75,* 81–95.

Brands, H. W. (2003). Founders chic. *The Atlantic, 292*(2), 101–110.

Bregman, J. D., Leckman, J. F., & Ort, S. I. (1988). Fragile X syndrome: Genetic predisposition onto psychopathology. *Journal of Autism and Developmental Disorders, 18,* 343–354.

Butler, M. G., Bittel, D. C., Kibiryeva, N., Talebizadeh, Z., & Thompson, T. (2004). Behavioral differences among subjects with Prader–Willi syndrome and type I or type II deletion and maternal disomy. *Pediatrics, 113,* 565–573.

Cahill, B. M., & Glidden, L. M. (1996). Influence of child diagnosis on family and parent functioning: Down syndrome versus other disabilities. *American Journal on Mental Retardation, 101,* 149–160.

Carlin, M. E. (1990). The improved prognosis in cri du chat (5p-) syndrome. In W. I. Fraser (Ed.), *Proceedings of the 8th Congress of the International Association of the Scientific Study of Mental Deficiency* (pp. 64–73). Edinburgh, UK: Blackwell.

Carr, J. (1995). Down's syndrome: Children growing up. Cambridge, UK: Cambridge University Press.

Chapman, R. S., & Hesketh, L. J. (2000). Behavioral phenotype of individuals with Down syndrome. *Mental Retardation and Developmental Disabilities Research Reviews, 6,* 84–95.

Collacott, R. A. (1992). The effect of age and residential placement on adaptive behavior of adults with Down's syndrome. *British Journal of Psychiatry, 161,* 675–679.

Conners, F. A., Rosenquist, C. J., Atwell, J. A., & Klinger, L. G. (2000). Cognitive strengths and weaknesses associated with Prader–Willi syndrome. *Education and Training in Mental Retardation and Developmental Disabilities, 35,* 441–448.

Cornish, K. M., & Pigram, J. (1996). Developmental and behavioural characteristics of cri du chat syndrome. *Archives of Diseases in Childhood, 75,* 448–450.

Crowe, S., & Hay, D. (1990). Neuropsychological dimensions of the fragile X syndrome: Support for a non-dominant hemisphere dysfunction hypothesis. *Neuropsychologia, 28,* 9–16.

Dimitropoulos, A., Feurer, I. D., Butler, M. G., & Thompson, T. (2001). Emergence of compulsive behavior and tantrums in children with Prader–Willi syndrome. *American Journal on Mental Retardation, 106,* 39–51.

Dimitropoulos, A., Feurer, I. D., Roof, E., Stone, W., Butler, M. G., Sutcliffer, J., et al. (2000). Appetitive behavior, compulsivity, and neurochemistry in Prader–Willi syndrome. *Mental Retardation and Developmental Disabilities Research Reviews, 6,* 125–130.

Don, A. J., Schellenberg, E. G., & Rourke, B. P. (1999). Music and language skills of children with Williams syndrome. *Child Neuropsychology, 5,* 154–170.

Dorn, B., & Goff, B. J. (2003). The student with Prader–Willi syndrome: Information for educators. Sarasota, FL: Prader–Willi Syndrome Association (USA); Retrieved July 17, 2006 from www.pwsausa.org

Dykens, E. M. (1995). Measuring behavioral phenotypes: Provocations from the "new genetics." *American Journal on Mental Retardation, 99,* 522–532.

Dykens, E. M. (1999). Prader–Willi syndrome. In H. Tager-Flusberg (Ed.), *Neurodevelopmental disorders* (pp. 137–154). Cambridge, MA: MIT Press.

Dykens, E. M. (2000). Psychopathology in children with intellectual disability. *Journal of Child Psychology and Psychiatry, 41,* 407–417.

Dykens, E. M. (2002). Are jigsaw puzzle skills "spared" in persons with Prader-Willi syndrome? *Journal of Child Psychology and Psychiatry, 43,* 343–352.

Dykens, E. M. (2003). Anxiety, fears, and phobias in persons with Williams syndrome. *Developmental Neuropsychology, 23,* 291–316.

Dykens, E. M. (2004). Maladaptive behaviors and compulsions in Prader–Willi syndrome: New insights from older adults. *American Journal on Mental Retardation, 109,* 142–153.

Dykens, E. M., Cassidy, S. B., & King, B. H. (1999). Maladaptive behavior differences in Prader–Willi syndrome due to paternal deletion versus maternal uniparental disomy. *American Journal on Mental Retardation, 104,* 67–77.

Dykens, E. M., & Clarke, D. J. (1997). Correlates of maladaptive behavior in individuals with 5p- (cri du chat) syndrome. *Developmental Medicine and Child Neurology, 39,* 752–756.

Dykens, E. M., Finucane, B. M., & Gayley, C. (1997). Brief report: Cognitive and behavioral profiles in persons with Smith–Magenis syndrome. *Journal of Autism and Developmental Disorders, 27,* 203–211.

Dykens, E. M., & Hodapp, R. M. (1997). Treatment issues in genetic mental retardation syndromes. *Professional Psychology: Research and Practice, 28,* 263–270.

Dykens, E. M., & Hodapp, R. M. (2001). Research in mental retardation: Toward an etiologic approach. *Journal of Child Psychology and Psychiatry, 42*, 49–71.

Dykens, E. M., Hodapp, R. M., & Leckman, J. F. (1987). Strengths and weaknesses in intellectual functioning of males with fragile X syndrome. *American Journal of Mental Deficiency, 92*, 234–236.

Dykens, E. M., Hodapp, R. M., Walsh, K. K., & Nash, L. (1992). Profiles, correlates, and trajectories of intelligence in Prader–Willi syndrome. *Journal of the American Academy of Child and Adolescent Psychiatry, 31*, 1125–1130.

Dykens, E. M., & Kasari, C. (1997). Maladaptive behavior in children with Prader–Willi syndrome, Down syndrome, and non-specific mental retardation. *American Journal on Mental Retardation, 102*, 228–237.

Dykens, E. M., Leckman, J. F., & Cassidy, S. B. (1996). Obsessions and compulsions in Prader–Willi syndrome. *Journal of Child Psychology and Psychiatry, 37*, 995–1002.

Dykens, E. M., & Rosner, B. A. (1999). Refining behavioral phenotypes: Personality-motivation in Williams and Prader–Willi syndromes. *American Journal on Mental Retardation, 104*, 158–169.

Dykens, E. M., Hodapp, R. M., & Finucane, B. M. (2000). Genetics and mental retardation syndromes: A new look at behavior and genetics. Baltimore, MD: Paul H. Brookes Publishing Company.

Dykens, E. M., & Shah, B. (2003). Psychiatric disorders in Prader–Willi syndrome: Epidemiology and treatment. *CNS Drugs, 17*, 167–178.

Dykens, E. M., Shah, B., Sagun, J., Beck, T., & King, B. Y. (2002). Maladaptive behaviour in children and adolescents with Down's syndrome. *Journal of Intellectual Disability Research, 46*, 484–492.

Dykens, E. M., & Smith, A. C. M. (1998). Distinctiveness and correlates of maladaptive behaviour in children and adolescents with Smith–Magenis syndrome. *Journal of Intellectual Disability Research, 42*, 481–489.

Einfeld, S. L. (2004). Behaviour phenotypes of genetic disorders. *Current Opinion in Psychiatry, 17*, 343–349.

Einfeld, S. L., & Tonge, B. J. (1992). *Manual for the Developmental Behaviour Checklist: Primary carer version.* Australia: School of Psychiatry, University of New South Wales.

Ellis, N. R. (1969). A behavioral research strategy in mental retardation: Defense and critique. *American Journal on Mental Deficiency, 73*, 557–566.

Fidler, D. J., Hodapp, R. M., & Dykens, E. M. (2000). Stress in families of young children with Down syndrome, Williams syndrome, and Smith–Magenis syndrome. *Early Education and Development, 11*, 395–406.

Finucane, B., Dirrigl, K. H., & Simon, E. W. (2001). Characterization of self-injurious behaviors in children and adults with Smith–Magenis syndrome. *American Journal on Mental Retardation, 106*, 52–58.

Finucane, B. M. (1996). *What's so special about genetics? A guide for special educators.* Elwyn, PA: Elwyn.

Finucane, B. M., Konar, D., Haas-Givler, B., Kurtz, M. D., & Scott, L. I. (1994). The spasmodic upper-body squeeze: A characteristic behavior in Smith–Magenis syndrome. *Developmental Medicine and Child Neurology, 36*, 78–83.

Flint, J., & Yule, W. (1994). Behavioural phenotypes. In M. Rutter, E. Taylor, & L. Hersov (Eds.), *Child and adolescent psychiatry: Modern approaches* (3rd ed., pp. 666–687). London: Blackwell Scientific.

Fowler, A. E. (1990). Language abilities in children with Down Syndrome: Evidence for a specific syntactic delay. In D. Cicchetti & M. Beeghly (Eds.), *Children with Down syndrome: A developmental approach* (pp. 302–328). New York: Cambridge University Press.

Gersh, M., Goodart, S. A., Pasztor, L. M., Harris, D. J., Weiss, L., & Overhauser, J. (1995). Evidence for a distinct region causing a cat-like cry in patients with 5p- deletions. *American Journal of Human Genetics, 56*, 1404–1410.

Gosch, A., & Pankau, R. (1994). Social–emotional and behavioral adjustment in children with Williams syndrome. *American Journal of Medical Genetics, 53*, 335–339.

Greenberg, F., Lewis, R. A., Potocki, L., Glaze, D., Parke, J., Killian, J. (1996). Multidisciplinary clinical study of Smith–Magenis syndrome: Deletion 17p11.2. *American Journal of Medical Genetics, 62*, 247–254.

Hagerman, R. J. (1996). Fragile X syndrome. *Child and Adolescent Psychiatric Clinics of North America, 5,* 895–911.

Hagerman, R. J. (1999). Psychopharmacological interventions in fragile X syndrome, fetal alcohol syndrome, Prader–Willi syndrome, Angelman syndrome, Smith–Magenis syndrome, and velocardiofacial syndrome. *Mental Retardation and Developmental Disabilities Research Reviews, 5,* 305–313.

Hodapp, R. M. (1997). Direct and indirect behavioral effects of different genetic disorders of mental retardation. *American Journal on Mental Retardation, 102,* 67–79.

Hodapp, R. M. (1999). Indirect effects of genetic mental retardation disorders: Theoretical and methodological issues. *International Review of Research in Mental Retardation, 22,* 27–50.

Hodapp, R. M., & Dykens, E. M. (1994). Mental retardation's two cultures of behavioral research. *American Journal on Mental Retardation, 98,* 675–687.

Hodapp, R. M., & Dykens, E. M. (2001). Strengthening behavioral research on genetic mental retardation disorders. *American Journal on Mental Retardation, 106,* 4–15.

Hodapp, R. M., & Dykens, E. M. (2004). Studying behavioral phenotypes: Issues, benefits, challenges. In E. Emerson, C. Hatton, T. Parmenter, & T. Thompson (Eds.), *International handbook of applied research in intellectual disabilities* (pp. 203–220). New York: Wiley.

Hodapp, R. M., Dykens, E. M., Ort, S. I., Zelinsky, D. G., & Leckman, J. F. (1991). Changing patterns of intellectual strengths and weaknesses in males with fragile X syndrome. *Journal of Autism and Developmental Disorders, 21,* 503–516.

Hodapp, R. M., Evans, D. W., & Gray, F. L. (1999). Intellectual development in children with Down syndrome. In J. Rondal, J. Perera, & L. Nadel (Eds.), *Down syndrome: A review of current knowledge* (pp. 124–132). London: Whurr.

Hodapp, R. M., & Fidler, D. J. (1999). Special education and genetics: Connections for the 21st century. *The Journal of Special Education, 33,* 130–137.

Hodapp, R. M., Ly, T. M., Fidler, D. J., & Ricci, L. A. (2001). Less stress, more rewarding: Parenting children with Down syndrome. *Parenting: Science and Practice, 1,* 317–337.

Hodapp, R. M., Ricci, L. A., Ly, T. M., & Fidler, D. J. (2003). The effects of the child with Down syndrome on maternal stress. *British Journal of Developmental Psychology, 22,* 137–151.

Hornby, G. (1995). Fathers' views of the effects on their families of children with Down syndrome. *Journal of Child and Family Studies, 4,* 103–117.

Jarrold, C., Baddeley, A. D., & Hewes, A. K. (2000). Verbal short-term memory deficits in Down syndrome: A consequence of problems in rehearsal? *Journal of Child Psychology and Psychiatry and Allied Disciplines, 41,* 223–244.

Jarrold, C., Baddeley, A. D., Hewes, A. K., & Phillips, C. (2001). A longitudinal assessment of diverging verbal and non-verbal abilities in the Williams syndrome phenotype. *Cortex, 37,* 423–431.

Jarrold, C., Baddeley, A. D., & Phillips, C. E. (2002). Verbal short-term memory in Down syndrome: A problem of memory, audition, or speech? *Journal of Speech, Language, and Hearing Research, 45,* 531–544.

Jarrold, C., Hartley, S. J., Phillips, C., & Baddeley, A. D. (2000). Word fluency in Williams syndrome: Evidence for unusual semantic organization? *Cognitive Neuropsychiatry, 5,* 292–319.

Kasari, C., & Sigman, M. (1997). Linking parental perceptions to interactions in young children with autism. *Journal of Autism and Developmental Disorders, 27,* 39–57.

Kaufman, A. S., & Kaufman, N. L. (1983). *Kaufman Assessment Battery for children.* Circle Pines, MN: American Guidance Service.

Kemper, M. B., Hagerman, R. J., & Altshul-Stark, D. (1988). Cognitive profiles of boys with fragile X syndrome. *American Journal of Medical Genetics, 30,* 191–200.

Klein, B. P., & Mervis, C. B. (1999). Contrasting patterns of cognitive abilities of 9- and 10-year-olds with Williams syndrome or Down syndrome. *Developmental Neuropsychology, 16,* 177–196.

Kumin, L. (1994). Intelligibility of speech in children with Down syndrome in natural settings: Parents' perspective. *Perceptual and Motor Skills, 78,* 307–313.

Levine, K. (1994). *Williams syndrome: Information for teachers.* Clawson, MI: The Williams Syndrome Association.

Levine, K., & Wharton, R. H. (1993). *Children with Prader–Willi syndrome: Information for school staff*. Roslyn Heights, NY: Visible Ink (available through the Prader–Willi Syndrome Association, US; Retrieved July 17, 2006 from www.pwsausa.org).

Meyers, B. A., & Pueschel, S. M. (1991). Psychiatric disorders in persons with Down syndrome. *Journal of Nervous and Mental Disease, 179*, 609–613.

Miller, J. F. (1999). Profiles of language development in children with Down syndrome. In J. F. Miller, M. Leddy, & L. A. Leavitt (Eds.), *Improving the communication of people with Down syndrome* (pp. 11–39). Baltimore, MD: Paul H. Brookes.

Mount, R. H., Charman, T., Hastings, R. P., Reilly, S., & Cass, H. (2002). The Rett Syndrome Behavior Questionnaire (RSBQ): Refining the behavioral phenotype of Rett syndrome. *Journal of Child Psychology and Psychiatry, 43*, 1099–1110.

Mount, R. H., Charman, T., Hastings, R. P., Reilly, S., & Cass, H. (2003). Features of autism in Rett syndrome and severe mental retardation. *Journal of Autism and Developmental Disorders, 33*, 435–442.

Naglieri, J. A. (1985). Assessment of mentally retarded children with the Kaufman Assessment Battery for Children. *American Journal of Mental Deficiency, 89*, 367–371.

O'Brien, G. (2002a). The clinical practice of behavioural phenotypes. In G. O'Brien (Ed.), *Behavioural phenotypes in clinical practice* (pp. 1–12). London, England: Mac Keith.

O'Brien, G. (Ed.). (2002b). *Behavioural phenotypes in clinical practice*. London, England: Mac Keith.

Obrzut, A., Nelson, R. B., & Obrzut, J. E. (1987). Construct validity of the Kaufman Assessment Battery for Children with mildly mentally retarded students. *American Journal of Mental Deficiency, 92*, 74–77.

Opitz, J. M. (1985). Editorial comment: The developmental field concept. *American Journal of Medical Genetics, 21*, 1–11.

Papolos, D. F., Faedda, G. L., Veit, S., Goldberg, R., Morrow, B., et al. (1996). Bipolar spectrum disorders in patients diagnosed with velo-cardio-facial syndrome: Does a hemizygous deletion on chromosome 22q11 result in bipolar affective disorder? *American Journal of Psychiatry, 153*, 1541–1547.

Pennington, B. F., Moon, J., Edgin, J., Stedron, J., & Nadel, L. (2003). The neuropsychology of DS: Evidence for hippocampal dysfunction. *Child Development, 74*, 75–93.

Pennington, B. F., O'Connor, B., & Sudhalter, V. (1991). Toward a neuropsychology of fragile X syndrome. In R. J. Hagerman & A. C. Silverman (Eds.), *Fragile X syndrome: Diagnosis, treatment, and research* (pp. 173–201). Baltimore, MD: The Johns Hopkins.

Pezzini, G., Vicari, S., Volterra, V., Milani, L., & Osella, M. T (1999). Children with Williams syndrome: Is there a single neuropsychological profile? *Developmental Neuropsychology, 15*, 141–155.

Pulver, A. E., Nestadt, G., Shpritzen, R. J., Lamacz, M., Wolyniec, P. S., Morrow, B., et al. (1994). Psychotic illness in patients diagnosed with velo-cardio-facial syndrome and their relatives. *Journal of Nervous and Mental Disease, 182*, 476–478.

Reiss, S. (1988). *The Reiss screen for maladaptive behavior*. Worthington, OH: IDS.

Rogers, S. J., Wehner, E. A., & Hagerman, R. (2001). The behavioral phenotype of fragile X: Symptoms of autism in very young children with fragile X syndrome, idiopathic autism, and other developmental disorders. *Journal of Developmental and Behavioral Pediatrics, 22*, 409–417.

Rondal, J. (1995). *Exceptional language development in Down syndrome*. New York: Cambridge University Press.

Roof, E., Stone, W., MacLean, W., Feurer, I. D., Thompson, T., et al. (2000). Intellectual characteristics of Prader–Willi syndrome: Comparison of genetic subtypes. *Journal of Intellectual Disability Research, 44*, 25–30.

Rosner, B. A., Hodapp, R. M., Fidler, D. J., Sagun, J. N., & Dykens, E. M. (2004). Social competence in persons with Prader–Willi, Williams, and Down syndromes. *Journal of Applied Research in Intellectual Disabilities, 17*, 209–217.

Thomas, V., & Olsen, D. H. (1993). Problem families and the circumplex model: Observational assessment using the clinical rating scale (CRS). *Journal of Marital and Family Therapy, 19*, 159–175.

Tonge, B. J., & Einfeld, S. L. (2003). Psychopathology and intellectual disability: The Australian child to adult longitudinal study. *International Review of Research in Mental Retardation, 26,* 61–91.

Udwin, O. (1990). A survey of adults with Williams syndrome and idiopathic infantile hypercalcaemia. *Developmental Medicine and Child Neurology, 32,* 129–141.

Udwin, O., & Yule, W. (2001). Guidelines for teachers. [On-line]. Retrieved July 17, 2006 from: www.wsf.org

Udwin, O., Yule, W., & Martin, N. (1987). Cognitive abilities and behavioural characteristics of children with idiopathic infantile hypercalcaemia. *Journal of Child Psychology and Psychiatry and Allied Disciplines, 28,* 297–309.

Van Acker, R. (1991). Rett syndrome: A review of current knowledge. *Journal of Autism and Developmental Disorders, 21,* 381–406.

Vogels, A., De Hert, M., Descheemaeker, M. J., Govers, V., Devriendt, K., Legius, E., et al. (2004). Psychotic disorders in Prader–Willi syndrome. *American Journal of Medical Genetics, 127A*(Pt. A), 238–243.

Wigren, M., & Heimann, M. (2001). Excessive picking in Prader–Willi syndrome: A pilot study of phenomenological aspects and comorbid symptoms. *International Journal of Disability, Development and Education, 48,* 129–142.

7

Social Acceptance and Attitude Change

Fifty Years of Research

GARY N. SIPERSTEIN, JENNIFER NORINS, and AMANDA MOHLER

Fifty years ago, people with intellectual disability (ID) were "out of the sight and mind of the general public" (Perske, 2003). Little attention was given to this group in popular culture or in scientific research. However, following on the heels of the civil rights movement, and with strong parent advocacy, the doors of the public arena began to open to this once isolated group. Previously, few would have imagined that children with ID would be going to their neighborhood school and sitting in regular classrooms with their peers, or that adults with ID would be working next to their fellow, nondisabled employees. As the movement toward inclusion gained momentum, research in the field of ID began to focus on societal attitudes that act as implicit and often explicit barriers to success. In fact, over the past 50 years, well over 500 studies have been carried out to examine the attitudes of children, teachers, service providers, employers, and the general pubic toward people with ID. Given that the inclusion movement has been most evident in the schools, researchers have focused most of their attention on children and teachers. Therefore, this chapter will provide a review of research that specifically addresses the attitudes of children and teachers toward children with ID and the interventions designed to influence those attitudes.

GARY N. SIPERSTEIN, JENNIFER NORINS, and AMANDA MOHLER • Center for Social Development and Education, University of Massachusetts Boston, Boston, Massachusetts 02125.

CHILDREN'S ATTITUDES

Historically, studies of children's attitudes toward ID have generally taken two forms, those that focus on documenting the presence or absence of negative attitudes and those that intervene to change children's attitudes. Both types of studies began to emerge in the 1950s, and became quite prominent in the 1960s and 1970s. Because the expectation that the inclusion of children with disabilities in regular classrooms would promote more understanding and acceptance among nondisabled children, much of the research during this time was motivated by the societal question, "Does inclusion work?" The initial answer to this question was not one that parent advocates and educators wanted to hear.

Prior to the legislation that mandated the inclusion of children with ID in regular classrooms, it was well documented that these children were either socially rejected or neglected by their nondisabled peers (Baldwin, 1958, 1962; Bruininks, Rynders, & Gross, 1974; Dentler & Mackler, 1961; Heber, 1956; Johnson, 1950; Lapp, 1957; Miller, 1956; Rucker, Howe, & Snider, 1969). In fact, it was found that children with ID were more rejected when they were integrated into regular education classrooms than when they remained in segregated classrooms (Goodman, Gottlieb, & Harrison, 1972). Subsequent studies have found similar results (Brewer & Smith, 1989; Hughes et al., 1999; Iano, 1974; Margalit, 1993; Sabornie & Kauffman, 1987; Wolfberg, Zercher, & Lieber, 1999). These findings are dramatic in that children with ID were found to be rejected significantly more often than their nondisabled peers in *both* integrated and segregated settings.

The social rejection experienced by children with ID can be traced, in part, to the negative attitudes of their nondisabled peers. Over the years, studies have consistently demonstrated that children hold negative attitudes toward their peers with ID (Bak & Siperstein, 1987b; Clark, 1964a, 1964b; Graffi & Minnes, 1988; Renz & Simensen, 1969; Siperstein & Bak, 1980; Stainback & Stainback, 1982; Whalen, Henker, Dotemoto, & Hinshaw, 1983; Willey & McCandless, 1973). In many of these studies, children tended to ascribe negative traits to children with ID, such as being academically and socially "deviant," and were less inclined to interact with them than with others. Siperstein, Bak, and O'Keefe (1988) took these findings a step further and were able to document a strong connection between the negative attitudes of nondisabled children toward children with ID and their actual social rejection of these children.

These negative attitudes are further documented by studies that directly compared and contrasted children's attitudes toward different disability groups. Most of these studies have found a clear social preference hierarchy in children's attitudes toward different disabilities, in which children with ID consistently ranked lowest in acceptability compared to those with orthopedic or sensory disabilities (Jones, Gottfried, & Owens, 1966; Karnilowicz, Sparrow, & Shinkfield, 1994; Kennedy & Thurman, 1982; Peach, Hood, & Branton, 1982; Siperstein & Bak, 1985b; Wisely & Morgan, 1981). However, children with ID are not always *perceived* the most negatively. When compared to children who exhibit antisocial behaviors, such as those with behavioral problems or emotional disturbance, children with ID were often seen as deviant, but not *as* deviant as this other group. Reasons for the existence of such a hierarchy can be found when examining the norms of the classroom. For example, academic competence is valued highly in the classroom and children with significant academic problems are recognized by their peers as being "different." Furthermore, inappropriate social behavior in which children with ID often engage within the classroom can be disruptive to positive interpersonal interactions with nondisabled peers (Siperstein & Leffert, 1997).

One must also recognize that the observed differences in children's attitudes toward different disability groups are somewhat clouded by the fact that children often confuse ID with other disabilities, particularly orthopedic and sensorial disabilities, as well as emotional disturbance (Budoff, Siperstein, & Conant, 1979; Gottlieb & Siperstein, 1976; Payne, 1985; Siperstein & Bak, 1980, 1985b). For example, Siperstein and Bak (1980) found that when asked, "What does it mean if a boy or girl is mentally retarded?" children often confused ID with these other disability groups. Furthermore, the image they held of a child with mental retardation was often one of a severely impaired child with Down syndrome, which is also an image generally held by adults (Gottlieb & Siperstein, 1976; Siperstein & Gottlieb, 1977).

To fully understand children's negative attitudes toward children with ID, one has to consider the various contextual factors that influence these attitudes. Researchers have examined such factors as exposure to children with disabilities, the presence of labels, and the behavioral characteristics of the individual with ID.

One of the main assumptions maintained by proponents of inclusion is that exposure to peers with ID will promote more positive attitudes among nondisabled children. Jaffe (1967), who was the first to address the role of exposure in student's attitudes, found that exposure had a positive effect solely on the cognitive component of attitudes (i.e., children's knowledge or misinformation about ID). Subsequent studies have shown that there is in fact some positive effect on children's attitudes as a result of having contact with students with ID in their classrooms or schools (Esposito & Reed, 1986; Gash & Coffey, 1995; Slininger, Sherrill, & Jankowski, 2000; Strauch, 1970; Townsend, Wilton, & Vakilirad, 1993; Voeltz, 1980). Krajewski took a unique approach to studying the effects of exposure on student attitudes by comparing the attitudes of high school students over an 11-year period, spanning from 1987 to 1998. Focusing on a high school that underwent a transformation from separate classrooms to inclusive classrooms during this period, Krajewski observed a positive shift in attitudes, strongly suggesting that the inclusion movement had been a factor (Krajewski & Hyde, 2000; Krajewski, Hyde, & O'Keefe, 2002). These researchers believed that the more positive attitudes among the newer cohort of students were due to their exposure to peers with ID.

However, while the above studies show promising results with regard to the positive effects of exposure, the causal relationship between contact and attitudes is not conclusive. In fact, several studies have reported contradictory results about the role of exposure. For example, Goodman et al. (1972) found that the more exposure that elementary school students had with their peers with ID, the more negative their attitudes became. Similarly, subsequent studies of elementary students show that inclusion in regular classrooms does not promote more positive attitudes or greater social acceptance (Brewer & Smith, 1989; Manetti, Schneider, & Siperstein, 2001; Stager & Young, 1981). The possible reasons for the maintenance of negative attitudes are because, irrespective of any new knowledge, unstructured interactions between nondisabled children and their peers with ID are not socially rewarding or what the nondisabled children observe of their peers with ID reinforces their existing stereotypes and fosters a perception of "dissimilarity" (e.g., Strauch, 1970). Further, in speculating why middle school students "exposed" to children with mental retardation did not change their negative attitudes, Strauch (1970) suggested that the social contact that took place between the different groups of children possibly served to confirm existing negative stereotypes held by students without disabilities.

It is worth noting that, while a number of studies have shown that inclusion of students with ID does not always bring about positive attitudes, two studies, in particular, have shown that it can effect how adolescents view the policy of inclusion. High school students believe that inclusion brings about an added dimension of diversity to their school and increases their tolerance of other people (Fisher, 1999; Helmstetter, Peck, & Giangreco, 1994; Peck, Donaldson, & Pezzoli, 1990).

In the above review of studies, it is evident that exposure to children with ID is an important contextual factor that moderates nondisabled children's attitudes. It is not clear, however, why in certain circumstances "exposure" has a positive influence and in others, a negative influence. We can only speculate that the observed negative effects occur when there is contact between children with and without ID who *do not* share equal status and whose similarities are overshadowed by differences in academic behavior, social behavior, and even physical appearance. In fact, it is these differing characteristics that may serve to reinforce existing misconceptions.

Another important contextual variable that influences attitudes are the labels that clinicians and educators assign to children with ID. Yet, like exposure, the direction of the influence is equivocal. As mentioned with regard to exposure, Jaffe (1966) was also one of the first to conduct research into the significance of labels, beginning a line of programmatic research that continues to this day. By presenting children with different target peers who were either labeled or not labeled "mentally retarded," he found that children responded more negatively to the label than to a "retarded sketch," i.e., a written description of a target child's behavior.

However, a number of studies since then have demonstrated that the label "mental retardation" has sometimes been shown to have a positive influence on attitudes, particularly in the presence of academic incompetence or inappropriate social behavior. For example, children have been found to express neutral to positive attitudes toward a target child who exhibits poor academic or social behavior *and* is labeled "mentally retarded" (Bak & Siperstein, 1986; Budoff & Siperstein, 1978; Elam & Sigelman, 1983; Hemphill & Siperstein, 1990). The authors speculate that the presence of a label allows students to provide special dispensation to the child with ID. In addition, the label is also seen as providing children with an understanding of, and explanation for, the incompetent and inappropriate behaviors that they observe. Such an interpretation is supported by the early work by Towne and Joiner (1968), who, in describing their "sick role hypothesis" suggest that people use a different set of criteria when judging a labeled person than when judging a person not labeled. This distinct set of standards refers to the often-used term "special dispensation."

While the label "mental retardation" may serve as a protective factor when a target child exhibits incompetent or inappropriate behavior, it is not a factor when the child exhibits competent behavior. In one study, middle school students were more apt to select an actual peer with ID than a nondisabled peer as a team member when the peer with ID was perceived to be highly competent (Aloia, Beaver, & Pettus, 1978). The study was replicated by Bak and Siperstein (1987a), who found that children selected a peer with ID as a playing partner in a competitive game when the peer exhibited competence in that area. Taken together, both studies demonstrate the power of competent behavior in children's decision making as to whether or not they would play with a peer labeled as "mentally retarded." Further, they show that children do not need to, and tend not to, provide special dispensation to a peer with ID when the peer performs competently.

The clinical label "mental retardation" has not been the only term examined in past studies of attitudes. Siperstein, Budoff, and Bak (1980) found that the pejorative term "retard" elicited strong negative attitudes in contrast to the clinical label "mental retardation." Further, de facto labels, which characterize a child as being educated in separate classrooms, have also been found to influence children's attitudes. For example, when target children were described as being from a "special class for the retarded" (Van Bourgondien, 1987) or from a "special classroom" (Bak, Cooper, Dobroth, & Siperstein, 1987), children expressed more negative attitudes than when presented with a target child who exhibited the same types of academic or social behavior but was said to be from a regular class.

It is interesting to note that the social characteristics of the child with ID may also serve as a "de facto" label. Siperstein and Bak (1985a) found that elementary students exhibited strong negative attitudes toward a target child who demonstrated inappropriate social behavior. This confirmed the early work by Johnson (1950) and Kirk and Johnson (1951), who found that when children with ID were rejected, inappropriate or antisocial behavior was most often given as the reason for that rejection.

Overall, it is apparent that the clinical label "mental retardation" can serve as a protective factor, while the pejorative label, de facto labels, or inappropriate social behavior displayed by the child may reinforce existing stereotypes and further stigmatize children with ID.

Given the existence of negative attitudes among nondisabled children, researchers began to consider whether children with intellectual disabilities also stigmatize their fellow disabled peers. In an early study, Johnson and Ferreira (1958) observed that up to 90% of students in special education classrooms held negative attitudes toward their special class placement. These negative attitudes were a result, in part, of over 40% of the children reporting that they had been called names because of their special class placement. In a more rigorously controlled study wherein children with ID were randomly assigned to special or regular education classrooms, Meyerowitz (1962) found that children in special classes were significantly more self-derogatory than those who were in the regular education classrooms. More recently researchers have shown that children with ID hold negative stereotypes about other children with academic problems, similar to the stereotypes held by their nondisabled peers, (Altman & Lewis, 1990; Lewis & Altman, 1987; Miller et al., 1989) but are not negatively affected by the label "mentally retarded" (Budoff & Siperstein, 1982; Gibbons, 1985; Johnson, Sigelman, & Falkenberg, 1986). It is apparent that children with and without ID share similar attitudes toward peers who are academically or socially different. It is not clear, however, whether the pathway to children's negative attitudes are the same or different for the two groups.

CHANGING CHILDREN'S ATTITUDES

While there have been numerous studies that have documented children's negative attitudes toward their peers with ID, there is even more research that focuses on *changing* children's attitudes. In fact, there has been a general decline in the number of studies focusing on documenting attitudes, and a substantial increase in research on attitude change over time. The reason is obvious. Irrespective of the few studies that have documented positive attitudes, there is a general consensus that children react negatively to those who are different, and children with ID exhibit academic and social characteristics that place them most saliently in the "different" group. Therefore, as the move for greater inclusion of children with ID has gained momentum, researchers have shifted their focus from documenting children's negative attitudes to identifying ways to promote positive attitudes.

Several different approaches to changing attitudes have been employed with children. One of the most common approaches involves teacher-directed instruction about ID, which may include video presentations about people with disabilities, in person presentations by an individual with a disability, role playing or simulation activities, and related activities. Another major approach to attitude change involves structured contact through third-party facilitation, such as cooperative groupings, peer tutoring, and peer buddy programs. Some interventions even combine instruction with structured contact. In addition, attitude change interventions have been implemented as part of after-school programs, often utilizing community resources. Taken together, the landscape of attitude change interventions represents a rich array of creative approaches that have achieved varying levels of success.

The most common approach to improving children's attitudes involves utilizing direct instruction, based on the belief that improvement of children's knowledge and familiarity with ID will moderate cognitive aspects of their attitudes, i.e., misconceptions. Methods within this approach vary greatly. Implementation of an extensive curriculum (Perske, 1990; SO Get Into It™, 2001; Sullivan & Brightman, 1979; Voeltz et al., 1983), problem solving training using hypothetical situations (Salend & Knops, 1984), storytelling with question and answer activities (Reis, 1988), and computer-mediated instruction (Hammond, Zucker, Burstein, & DiGangi, 1997) have all been used with school-aged children with some success. Further, information about ID has been conveyed through tours of state facilities (Cleland & Chambers, 1959; Cleland & Cochran, 1961), puppet shows (Gilfoyle & Gilner, 1985), disability simulation activities (e.g., "what it would be like to be . . .") (Clunies-Ross & O'Meara, 1989; Hazzard & Baker, 1982), role playing (McConkey, McCormack, & Naughton, 1983; Simpson, Parrish, & Cook, 1976), experiential exercises (Shortridge, 1982), or a combination of these activities (Clunies-Ross & O'Meara, 1989; Favazza, Phillipsen, & Kumar, 2000: Hunt, Alwell, Farron-Davis, & Goetz, 1996). All of these approaches have resulted in different levels of success. One study, in particular, showed that positive change in attitudes could occur from "kids-teaching-kids about mental retardation" (Turnbull & Bronicki, 1986, 1987). While several of these studies demonstrated that the positive effects of direct instruction are sustainable (Clunies-Ross & O'Meara, 1989; Favazza et al, 2000; Salend & Knops, 1984; Turnbull & Bronicki, 1987), a few studies have shown a fading of intervention effects as early as 1 month after the treatment conclusion (Hazzard & Baker, 1982; McConkey et al., 1983).

The second major approach to changing children's attitudes involves structured contact, which is assumed to foster equality of status, recognition of similarities, cooperative interdependence, tolerance for diversity, and the opportunity for developing friendships. Despite the expectation that exposure per se would have an ameliorating effect on the attitudes of children toward their peers with ID, studies that looked at in situ exposure provided no consistent results. Therefore, researchers designed interventions to structure the level and type of contact between children with and without ID. Several structured contact interventions that have been studied include cooperative learning, peer-tutoring, peer buddy programs, and after-school programs.

Drawing from the extensive literature on the academic benefits of cooperative grouping, researchers have been successful in applying cooperative learning techniques to improve peer relationships of children with ID. Chennault (1967) was one of the first to demonstrate the social benefits of cooperative group activities among children with ID. She observed significant improvements in the social status of children with ID as a result of their participation in out of class cooperative group activities. Since then, educators have successfully applied cooperative grouping and cooperative goal structures with children with and without ID in the regular classroom at the preschool level (Piercy, Wilton, & Townsend, 2002), at the elementary school level (Acton & Zarbatany, 1988; Ballard, Corman, Gottlieb, &

Kaufman, 1977; Eichinger, 1990; Jacques, Wilton, & Townsend, 1998; Madden & Slavin, 1983), and at the middle and high school levels (Johnson, 1979). Many of these studies directly compared and contrasted cooperative learning and individual learning, or cooperative goal structure and individualistic goal structure. In all of the comparisons, cooperative grouping brought about positive attitudes or improved social interactions among children with and without ID, in contrast to the noncooperative conditions, which had little or no effect.

Allport (1954), in his discussion of contact, stated that for contact to be successful, it must ". . . reach below the surface in order to be effective in altering prejudice. Only the type of contact that leads people to do things is likely to result in changed attitudes. It is the cooperative striving for a goal that engenders solidarity" (Allport, 1954, p. 264). Applying Allport's contention to the results of the above intervention studies with children, it is easy to understand why cooperative grouping has been successful in promoting more positive attitudes among nondisabled children toward their peers with ID. It fosters participation around a common goal structure or purpose, thus creating a stronger bridge of similarity, and perhaps disconfirming some stereotypes of differences, than exposure per se.

In the same way that educators recognized the potential social benefits of cooperative learning, educators and researchers have applied peer tutoring as a means of changing children's attitudes and acceptance of their peers with disabilities. However, the effects of peer tutoring on children's attitudes are not as consistent or strong as the effects of cooperative grouping. In a major review of the literature on peer tutoring, Cook, Scruggs, Mastropieri, and Casto (1986) found that while children in peer tutoring programs improved academically, there were varied and small changes in social relationships between the tutor and tutees. There have been several studies, however, that did show significant changes in children's interpersonal interactions and social relationships. For example, Costa (1983), Fenrick and Petersen (1984), and Osguthorpe and colleagues (Osguthorpe, Eiserman, & Shisler, 1985; Shisler, Osguthorpe, & Eiserman, 1987) all found positive changes in nondisabled children's attitudes toward their peers with disabilities as well as greater social acceptance. In fact, Osguthorpe et al. (1985), along with Mortweet (1999), found that the improved social interactions observed in the tutoring situation generalized to other social situations.

In addition to cooperative grouping and peer tutoring, another type of structured contact involves adult facilitated and directed "peer buddy" activities. While peer tutoring is seen by many as an effective means of improving attitudes, Voeltz (1980) believes that it may have a reverse effect on what is intended because it reinforces a hierarchical relationship between the child with and without a disability. In contrast, the peer buddy experiences emphasize reciprocal interactions. Voeltz's contention is supported, in part, by Siperstein, Leffert, and Wenz-Gross (1997), who found that naturally-forming friendships between children with and without ID are not reciprocal, but rather are hierarchical. Friendships between children with and without ID resemble acquaintanceships. Thus, a number of studies have attempted to directly intervene to facilitate friendship between children with and without ID.

Interventions such as peer buddy programs began with the *Special Friends* program (Voeltz et al., 1983). Voeltz (1982) observed changes in nondisabled students' social interactions with their disabled peers as a result of participation in the program. In a follow up to the study, Kishi and Meyer (1994) found that high school students who had participated in the *Special Friends* program 6 years earlier showed greater social acceptance of their peers with ID than a comparison group. Since then, similar programs have been carried out at the high school level and involve students with severe disabilities. For example, Hughes and colleagues (Hughes et al., 2001; Hughes, Carter, Hughes, Bradford, & Copeland, 2002) gave verbal directions on how students with and without ID should interact, and provided an environment to foster positive social relationships. Not only did the peer buddy activities result in a significant increase in positive attitudes, but there was also an increase in social interactions involving reciprocal interchanges between the adolescents with and without disabilities. Similar results were found by Haring and Breen (1992), also with high school students, and by Cole, Vandercook, and Rynders (1988) and Cole, Meyer, Vandercook, and McQuarter (1986) with elementary level students. Interestingly, in the latter study, teachers' verbal directives were found to facilitate positive social interaction, although positive effects diminished over time.

Although all of the above interventions take place in schools and classrooms, structured contact interventions have also been embedded within after-school and community programs. Most of these programs provide recreational or cultural activities in which children with ID have the opportunity to demonstrate competent behavior, and children without disabilities have the opportunity to see their fellow peers as similar and of equal status. The after-school intervention programs have been highly diverse and have included integrated after-school clubs and athletic activities at the high school level (McDaniel, 1971; Sheare, 1974), integrated Boy Scout and Girl Scout activities (Newberry & Parish, 1987), integrated recreational summer programs (Hamre-Nietupski, Hendrickson, Nietupski, & Sasso, 1993), and integrated cultural programs such as visits to museums (Schleien, Ray, Soderman-Olson, & McMahon, 1987). All of these type of programs resulted in an increase in positive attitudes among children and adolescents toward their peers with ID, and, in a few cases, improved social interaction between the children with and without disabilities.

Organized competitive sports have also been a focus of interventions to improve child and adolescent attitudes. Building upon earlier work in laboratory situations in which children were found to exhibit positive behavioral intentions toward peers with ID who exhibited competent athletic abilities, researchers have examined effects when children with and without ID compete on the same team. Using Special Olympics as the venue, Gibbons and Bushakra (1989), Ninot, Bilard, Delignieres, and Sokolowski (2000), and Castagno (2001) found that participation of adolescents in Special Olympics and Special Olympics Unified Sports programs improved nondisabled athletes' attitudes toward people with ID. It is worth noting, that when nondisabled students participated in Special Olympics as volunteers, rather than as athletes on the same playing team, their attitudes either stayed the same or became more negative (Roper, 1990). The role of a volunteer is one that often excludes or discourages reciprocal interaction and the perception of equal status.

Each of these intervention approaches have resulted in differing levels of success in creating more positive attitudes toward, and greater social acceptance of, peers with ID. While most changes occurred in the children's knowledge and understanding of ID, there were some observed changes in children's social interactions with their peers with disabilities. As is evident in the field of ID, prepost treatment designs, with or without a control group, have continually shown that cognitive attitudes are more amenable to change (e.g., ratings, trait inferences, etc.) than established social relationships. Furthermore, only a few studies have looked at the long-term effects of attitude change interventions, and those that have found that observed change in attitudes was often transitory.

TEACHERS' ATTITUDES

Up until now, we have focused on student attitudes as barriers to the inclusion of children with intellectual disabilities in the regular classroom. Students, however, make up only one component of the classroom context. Teachers play a tantamount, if not paramount, role in the success of inclusion (Forlin, Hattie, & Douglas, 1996; Scruggs & Mastropieri, 1996; Semmel, Abernathy, & Butera, 1991). Because teacher attitudes can, in part, determine the academic and social success of children with ID in their classroom, many researchers have focused on teachers' attitudes toward students with disabilities, and in many cases, students with ID.

Studies of teacher attitudes have focused on their beliefs about inclusion, their feelings about teaching children with intellectual disabilities, and their judgments of these children's academic and social behavior. In addition, as in studies of student attitudes, researchers have focused on contextual factors involving "exposure" and "labels," as moderators of teacher attitudes. Lastly, a number of teacher characteristics have been examined as predictors of teacher attitude, in particular, teachers' past experience with inclusion, and teachers' perceived competence and sense of efficacy in teaching children with ID.

In the last two decades, there have been a number of literature reviews that focused on teachers' beliefs about and acceptance of inclusion (Hannah, 1988; Jamieson, 1984; Yanito, Quintero, Killoran, & Striefel, 1987; Siperstein & Gottlieb, 1977). The most comprehensive literature review was recently carried out by Scruggs and Mastropieri (1996), who synthesized the results of 28 studies involving the perceptions of over 8500 teachers. The results are quite dramatic. First, the authors found a significant relationship between the nature and severity level of the disability and teachers' support for inclusion. Teachers were less inclined to support inclusion when it involved children with ID than other disability groups. Second, teachers' support for inclusion also was related to their perception of the level of responsibility they had for the student with a disability. The more responsibility they were given, the less they favored inclusion. Third, only a small percentage of teachers believed that inclusion results in significant academic or social benefits for the student with a disability. Most importantly, Scruggs and Mastropieri observed that over the 35 years (1958–1995) in which the studies took place, teachers' perceptions of inclusion and their specific attitudes toward the inclusion of children with ID did not appear to change.

There are a number of reasons why teachers have steadfastly maintained these negative perceptions of the inclusion of children with ID. For example, several studies point to teachers' general feeling of "uneasiness" in teaching children with ID. Kvaraceus (1956) found that teachers think they know less about children with ID, and when given the choice, prefer not to teach children with ID. Further, more than 20 years later, Guerin (1979) found that teachers felt less comfortable having children with ID in their classroom than other disability groups, such as children who are "educationally handicapped" (learning disabled). In fact, teachers felt more comfortable both instructionally and interpersonally working with children with physical disabilities than those with ID (Ashman, 1984). The only students, other than students with ID, that teachers felt less able of teaching were students with emotional and behavioral problems (Hastings & Oakford, 2003). It is evident, then, that teachers demonstrate a preferential hierarchy that mirrors the one observed in children's attitudes. Teachers' lack of comfort in teaching children with ID may, in part, be due to their perception that these children pose a threat to the instructional atmosphere of the classroom, impeding their ability to successfully teach the nondisabled students (Feldman & Altman, 1985).

Turning our attention from teachers' beliefs about the inclusion of children with ID to their specific attitudes toward students with ID, we find that the same contextual factors that influence student attitudes influence teacher attitudes. Teachers' exposure to students with disabilities and the presence of labels (i.e., educational classifications) are the two most critical contextual factors.

With regard to exposure, a number of studies have demonstrated that increased experience in teaching students with ID can positively impact teacher attitudes. For example, preschool teachers became more positive toward children with ID after a child with ID was placed in his or her classroom (Clark, 1976), while elementary school teachers with previous experience and contact with children and adults with ID, exhibited more positive attitudes than did teachers with little experience (Kennon & Sandoval, 1978). Not surprisingly, Hanrahan and Rapagna (1987) found that teachers with academic training in special education and experience teaching children with disabilities expressed more positive attitudes than teachers with little or no training or experience and further, numerous studies indicate that teachers who have had several years of experience implementing inclusive programs exhibit more positive attitudes than teachers with no experience with inclusion (Avramidis, Bayliss, & Burden, 2000; Balboni & Pedrabissi, 2000).

Labeling children also has an impact on teachers as it does on children, except in the opposite direction. Teachers have been found to judge a student's academic performance and social behavior more negatively in the presence of the label "mental retardation" (McEvoy, Nonquidst, & Cunningham, 1984; Moberg, 1995; Semmel & Gao, 1992; Taylor, Smiley, & Ziegler, 1983). Not only does the label have a negative influence on how teachers judge behavior, but it also negatively impacts their expectations for the child's ability to learn in the inclusive classroom (Minner, 1982; Rolison & Medway, 1985). In contrast, Combs and Harper (1967) found that in the absence of the label "mental retardation," teachers responded more negatively to the characterization of a child as having intellectual disabilities than in the presence of the label. This was one of the few studies that has lent support to the notion that the label "mental retardation" helps a person understand and place in context incompetent or inappropriate behavior and allows for special dispensation to be given.[1] The overall findings clearly document, however, that the label "mental retardation" negatively impacts how teachers not only perceive students with intellectual disabilities, but how they judge them.

Contextual factors involving teachers' experience with inclusion and the presence or absence of labels are only one of several factors found to influence their attitudes. Teacher characteristics also play an influential role in their attitudes toward children with disabilities. One teacher characteristic that has been shown to be the most influential is perceived competence in being able to respond to the specific and unique needs of children with ID. At the preschool level, teachers who perceived themselves as less competent to teach severely impaired children were more negative toward inclusion (Avramidis et al., 2000). At the elementary level teachers' perceived competence was most predictive of teachers' positive attitudes toward teaching children with ID (Zanandrea & Rizzo, 1998; i.e., more so than age, years teaching, and experience with inclusion); and finally, at both the elementary and secondary levels, teachers who perceived themselves as more competent in selecting appropriate methods for teaching children with ID were more supportive of inclusion (Thomas, 1985). Even among physical education teachers, those who perceived themselves as more competent to teach children with disabilities were more positive in their attitudes toward children with ID (Rizzo & Kirkendall, 1995; Rizzo & Vispoel, 1992). An indirect approach to examining perceived competence in teachers is assessing their expressed need for curriculum and personal support, in teaching children with ID. McNally, Cole, and Waugh (2001) found that to teach children with severe intellectual disabilities, teachers felt they needed more personal support than curriculum support.

When the above findings are considered within the context that teachers have identified inadequate resources and less than adequate teacher

---

[1]As was mentioned previously, this is an explanation that is often given to explain children's responses to the label "mental retardation."

preparation as factors that contribute to their lack of support for inclusion (Vaughn et al., 1996), one can appreciate why regular education teachers do not have confidence in their ability to teach children with ID. In fact, many of the studies that identified teachers' perceived competence as a major factor in teacher attitudes concluded that better teacher preservice training and in-service interventions were needed to improve teacher attitudes and their sense of self-efficacy.

CHANGING TEACHERS' ATTITUDES

To implement inclusion, teachers who have little or no training in special education or experience with children with disabilities are called upon to involve these children in their instructional practices. It is no wonder, then, that teachers have not been quick to embrace the philosophy of inclusion. Because, as we have previously stated, teachers' attitudes toward inclusion can serve to facilitate or hinder its success (Semmel et al., 1991), researchers have focused on ways to change teacher attitudes. Interventions to change teacher attitudes, again similar to interventions for children, focus on increasing teachers' knowledge of students with disabilities. Often, direct instruction at the preservice and in-service levels is accompanied by structured exposure through practica involving inclusive educational sites.

Intervention programs to improve prospective teacher's attitudes toward children with ID and general attitudes toward the inclusion of these children have met with mixed results. Introductory courses on disabilities alone have not shown to be effective in altering prospective teachers' attitudes (Parish, Eads, Reece, & Piscitello, 1977), but when direct instruction is combined with videotape portrayals of people with disabilities (Beattie, Anderson, & Antonak, 1997), direct contact with children with intellectual disabilities and vicarious experience (Rizzo & Vispoel, 1992), and placement in special education classrooms (Rowe & Stutts, 1987; Stainback & Stainback, 1982), positive changes have been observed in either teachers' attitudes toward children with ID or general beliefs about inclusion. In a recent study (Hodge, Davis, Woodard, & Sherrill, 2002), the combination of direct instruction with a practicum experience in inclusive classrooms also had a positive affect on future teachers' perceived competence to teach children with ID.

Of the few studies that have focused on practicing teachers' attitudes, interventions that involve direct instruction (on-site courses and workshops) have had some success. Positive change has occurred in teachers' knowledge of ID and their attitudes toward the inclusion of children with intellectual disabilities (Aldridge & Clayton, 1987; Harasymiw & Horne, 1976). It is important to note that although there are many studies that have attempted to intervene and improve teacher attitudes, most have focused on attitudes toward disabilities in general, and not teachers' specific attitudes toward children with ID. Because teachers have shown a clear preferential hierarchy for teaching children with different types of disabilities, we cannot readily extrapolate from the findings about teachers' general attitudes toward disabilities to their specific attitudes toward children with ID.

Overall, as has been found concerning interventions to improve children's attitudes, the most successful interventions to improve teachers' attitudes seem to be those that combine direct instruction with different variations of contact, particularly for preservice teachers. Most importantly, the evidence seems clear that in the absence of constructive interventions for both children and teachers, students with ID are at risk for being socially rejected and receiving less than effective instruction in the regular classroom.

CONCLUSION

Over the past 50 years, we have witnessed a change process that is unprecedented in the history of education. Where once children with ID were barely being educated in state facilities, they are now included in all aspects of public education. What is startling, however, is that the attitudes of students and teachers toward children with ID have not kept pace with the philosophic shift that has occurred in special education. The negative attitudes of students and teachers that were observed at the beginning of the inclusion movement still exist today, although more muted. Children still hold negative attitudes and are less inclined to accept their peers with ID in regular classrooms, and similarly, teachers still do not believe in inclusion and would prefer not to teach children with ID in their classrooms. Moreover, both demonstrate similar preferential hierarchies with regard to students with disabilities. Simply stated, students less prefer to socially interact with, and teachers less prefer to teach, children with ID.

Given this reality, researchers have shifted their emphasis from documenting negative attitudes to developing interventions to change these attitudes. While the results of attitude change interventions have been encouraging, indicating positive impacts on children's and teachers' understanding of ID and in certain instances improvements in children's and teachers' interactions with children with ID, there is presently no one best approach. However, what is patently clear is that we cannot rely on exposure per se to alter children's or teachers' attitudes. Merely placing children with ID into the regular classroom has not sufficed. To successfully change attitudes, well-planned and structured contact is critical.

Although change interventions implemented up until now have not been consistently successful, future research should continue to design such interventions based upon existing attitude models, beginning with Ajzen and Fishbein (1980), Allport (1954), Triandis (1971), and others. Researchers should continue to look for ways to adapt instructional strategies with proven academic benefits that can potentially have social benefits, such as has been seen with the use of cooperative grouping and peer tutoring. Furthermore, in documenting the efficacy of conceptually driven attitude change interventions, researchers need to continue to employ rigorous research designs. At minimum, a good design should focus on not only whether attitudes improve, but the degree to which the change in attitudes can be sustained over time and can translate into changes in behavior.

The current reality is that we are asking teachers to follow policy, that is, to accept inclusion irrespective of whether they are prepared to accept, and believe that they are able to instruct, a child with ID into their classroom. As a result, teachers, in their own words, feel that educational leaders and decision-makers are "out of touch" with the reality of the classroom (Vaughn et al., 1996). While physical integration has taken place and instructional integration through the adaptation of instruction and assessment strategies is beginning to occur, social integration, perhaps the most difficult to achieve, has not taken place and remains stagnant.

Two pioneers in the field of special education (Johnson, 1950; Kirk & Johnson, 1951) alerted us to the fact that children with ID faced significant barriers in the regular classroom. More than 50 years later, these barriers still exist. This literature review, if nothing else, points to the very real fact that we, as educators, still have a way to go to insure that students with ID are not just physically *in* the regular classroom, but socially a *part of* the regular classroom.

REFERENCES

Acton, H. M., & Zarbatany, L. (1988). Interaction and performance within cooperative groups: Effects on nonhandicapped students' attitudes toward their mildly mentally retarded peers. *American Journal on Mental Retardation, 93*, 16–23.

Ajzen, I., & Fishbein, M. (1980). *Understanding attitude and predicting social behavior.* Englewood Cliffs, NJ: Prentice-Hall.

Aldridge, J. T., & Clayton, G. A. (1987). Elementary teachers' cognitive and affective perceptions of exceptional children. *Psychological Reports, 61*, 91–94.

Allport, G. W. (1954). *The nature of prejudice.* Cambridge, MA: Addison-Wesley.

Aloia, G. F., Beaver, R. J., & Pettus, W. F. (1978). Increasing initial interactions among integrated EMR students and their nonretarded peers in a game-playing situation. *American Journal of Mental Deficiency, 82*, 573–579.

Altman, R., & Lewis, T. J. (1990). Social judgments of integrated and segregated students with mental retardation toward their same-age peers. *Education and Training in Mental Retardation, 25*, 107–112.

Ashman, A. F. (1984). Assessing student teachers' attitudes toward mentally retarded and physically handicapped persons. *International Journal of Rehabilitation Research, 7*, 434–438.

Avramidis, E., Bayliss, P., & Burden, R. (2000). A survey into mainstream teachers' attitudes towards the inclusion of children with special educational needs in the ordinary school in one local education authority. *Educational Psychology, 20*, 191–211.

Bak, J. J., Cooper, E. M., Dobroth, K. M., & Siperstein, G. N. (1987). Special class placements as labels: Effects of different placements on children's attitudes toward learning handicapped peers. *Exceptional Children, 54*, 151–155.

Bak, J. J., & Siperstein, G. N. (1986). Protective effects of the label "mentally retarded" on children's attitudes toward their mentally retarded peers. *American Journal of Mental Deficiency, 91*, 95–97.

Bak, J. J., & Siperstein, G. N. (1987a). Effects of mentally retarded children's behavioral competence on nonretarded peers' behaviors and attitudes: Toward establishing ecological validity in attitude research. *American Journal of Mental Deficiency, 92*, 31–39.

Bak, J. J., & Siperstein, G. N. (1987b). Similarity as a factor effecting change in children's attitudes toward mentally retarded peers. *American Journal of Mental Deficiency, 91*, 524–531.

Balboni, G., & Pedrabissi, L. (2000). Attitudes of Italian teachers and parents toward school inclusion of students with mental retardation: The role of experience. *Education and Training in Mental Retardation and Developmental Disabilities, 35*, 148–159.

Baldwin, W. K. (1958). The social position of the educable mentally retarded child in the regular grades in the public schools. *Exceptional Children, 25*, 106–108, 112.

Baldwin, W. K. (1962). The social position of the educable mentally retarded in the regular grades in the public schools. *Exceptional Children, 29*, 106–112.

Ballard, M., Corman, L., Gottlieb, J., & Kaufman, M. J. (1977). Improving the social status of mainstreamed retarded children. *Journal of Educational Psychology, 69*, 605–611.

Beattie, J. R., Anderson, R. J., & Antonak, R. F. (1997). Modifying attitudes of prospective educators toward students with disabilities and their integration into regular classrooms. *Journal of Psychology, 13*, 245–259.

Brewer, N., & Smith, J. M. (1989). Social acceptance of mentally retarded children in regular schools in relation to years mainstreamed. *Psychological Reports, 64*, 375–380.

Bruininks, R. H., Rynders, J. E., & Gross, J. C. (1974). Social acceptance of mildly retarded pupils in resource rooms and regular classes. *American Journal of Mental Deficiency, 78*, 377–383.

Budoff, M., & Siperstein, G. N. (1978). Low income children's attitudes toward mentally retarded children: Effects of labeling and academic behavior. *American Journal of Mental Deficiency, 82*, 474–479.

Budoff, M., & Siperstein, G. N. (1982). Judgements of EMR students toward their peers: Effects of label and academic competence. *American Journal of Mental Deficiency, 86*, 367–371.

Budoff, M., Siperstein, G. N., & Conant, S. (1979). Children's knowledge of mental retardation. *Education and Training of the Mentally Retarded, 14*, 277–281.

Castagno, K. S. (2001). Special Olympics Unified Sports: Changes in male athletes during a basketball season. *Adapted Physically Activity Quarterly, 18*, 193–206.

Chennault, M. (1967). Improving the social acceptance of unpopular educable mentally retarded pupils in special classes. *American Journal of Mental Deficiency, 72*, 455–458.

Clark, B. A. (1976). Teacher attitudes toward integration of children with handicaps. *Education and Training of the Mentally Retarded, 11*, 333–335.

Clark, E. T. (1964a). Children's perception of a special class for educable mentally retarded children. *Exceptional Children, 30*, 289–295.

Clark, E. T. (1964b). Children's perception of educable mentally retarded children. *American Journal of Mental Deficiency, 68*, 602–610.

Cleland, C. C., & Chambers, W. R. (1959). Experimental modification of attitudes as a function of an institutional tour. *American Journal of Mental Deficiency, 64*, 124–130.

Cleland, C. C., & Cochran, I. L. (1961). The effect of institutional tours on attitudes of high school seniors. *American Journal of Mental Deficiency, 65*, 473–479.

Clunies-Ross, G., & O'Meara, K. (1989). Changing the attitudes of students towards peers with disabilities. *Australian Psychologist, 24*, 273–284.

Cole, D. A., Meyer, L. M., Vandercook, T., & McQuarter, R. (1986). Interactions between severely handicapped and nonhandicapped children: Dynamics of teacher intervention. *American Journal of Mental Deficiency, 91*, 160–169.

Cole, D. A., Vandercook, T., & Rynders, J. (1988). Comparison of two peer interaction programs: Children with and without severe disabilities. *American Education Research Journal, 25*, 415–439.

Combs, R. H., & Harper, J. L. (1967). Effects of labels on attitudes of educators toward handicapped children. *Exceptional Children, 33*, 399–403.

Cook, S. B., Scruggs, T. E., Mastropieri, M. A., & Casto, G. C. (1986). Handicapped students as tutors. *The Journal of Special Education, 19*, 483–492.

Costa, F. M. (1983). Friendship patterns in young adulthood: A social psychological approach. *Dissertation Abstracts International, 44*(4-B), 1277.

Dentler, R. A., & Mackler, B. (1961). The socialization of retarded children in an institution. *Journal of Health and Human Behavior, 2,* 243–252.

Eichinger, J. (1990). Goal structure effects on social interaction: Nondisabled and disabled elementary students. *Exceptional Children, 56,* 408–416.

Elam, J. J., & Sigelman, C. K. (1983). Developmental differences in reactions to children labeled mentally retarded. *Journal of Applied Developmental Psychology, 4,* 303–315.

Esposito, B. G., & Reed, T. M. (1986). The effects of contact with handicapped persons on young children's attitudes. *Exceptional Children, 53,* 224–229.

Favazza, P. C., Phillipsen, L., & Kumar, P. (2000). Measuring and promoting acceptance of young children with disabilities. *Exceptional Children, 66,* 491–508.

Feldman, D., & Altman, R. (1985). Conceptual systems and teacher attitudes toward regular classroom placement of mildly mentally retarded students. *American Journal of Mental Deficiency, 89,* 345–351.

Fenrick, N. J., & Peterson, T. K. (1984). Developing positive changes in attitudes towards moderately/severely handicapped students through a peer tutoring program. *Education and Training of the Mentally Retarded, 19,* 83–90.

Fisher, D. (1999). According to their peers: Inclusion as high school students see it. *Mental Retardation, 37,* 458–467.

Forlin, C., Hattie, J., & Douglas, G. (1996). Inclusion: Is it stressful for teachers? *Journal of Intellectual and Developmental Disability, 21,* 199–217.

Gash, H., & Coffey, D. (1995). Influences on attitudes towards children with mental handicap. *European Journal of Special Needs Education, 10,* 1–16.

Gibbons, F. X. (1985). Stigma perception: Social comparison among mentally retarded persons. *American Journal of Mental Deficiency, 90,* 98–106.

Gibbons, S. L., & Bushakra, F. B. (1989). Effects of Special Olympics participation on the perceived competence and social acceptance of mentally retarded children. *Adapted Physical Activity Quarterly, 6,* 40–51.

Gilfoyle, E. M., & Gilner, J. A. (1985). Attitudes toward handicapped children: Impact of an educational program. *Physical and Occupational Therapy in Pediatrics, 5,* 27–41.

Goodman, H., Gottlieb, J., & Harrison, R. H. (1972). Social acceptance of EMRs integrated into a nongraded elementary school. *American Journal of Mental Deficiency, 76,* 412–417.

Gottlieb, J., & Siperstein, G. N. (1976). Attitudes toward mentally retarded persons: Effects of attitude referent specificity. *American Journal of Mental Deficiency, 80,* 376–381.

Graffi, S., & Minnes, P. M. (1988). Attitudes of primary school children toward the physical appearance and labels associated with Down syndrome. *American Journal on Mental Retardation, 93,* 28–35.

Guerin, G. R. (1979). Regular teacher concerns with mainstreamed learning handicapped children. *Psychology in the Schools, 16,* 543–545.

Hammond, D. G., Zucker, S. H., Burstein, K. S., & DiGangi, S. A. (1997). Computer-mediated instruction for increasing regular education students' acceptance of students with mental retardation. *Education and Training in Mental Retardation and Developmental Disabilities, 32,* 313–320.

Hamre-Nietupski, S., Hendrickson, J., Nietupski, J., & Sasso, J. (1993). Perceptions of teachers of students with moderate, severe, or profound disabilities on facilitating friendships with nondisabled peers. *Education and Training in Mental Retardation and Developmental Disabilities, 28,* 111–127.

Hannah, M. E. (1988). Teacher attitudes toward children with disabilities: An ecological analysis. In H. E. Yuker (Ed.), *Attitudes toward persons with disabilities* (pp. 154–170). New York: Springer.

Hanrahan, J., & Rapagna, S. (1987). The effects of information and exposure variables on teachers' willingness to mainstream mentally handicapped children into their classrooms. *Mental Retardation and Learning Disability Bulletin, 15,* 1–6.

Harasymiw, S. J., & Horne, M. D. (1976). Teacher attitudes toward handicapped children and regular class integration. *Journal of Special Education, 10,* 393–400.

Haring, T. G., & Breen, C. (1992). A peer-mediated social network intervention to enhance the social integration of persons with moderate and severe disabilities. *Journal of Applied Behavior Analysis, 25,* 319–333.

Hastings, R. P., & Oakford, S. (2003). Student teachers' attitudes towards the inclusion of children with special needs. *Educational Psychology, 23,* 87–94.

Hazzard, A. P., & Baker, B. L. (1982). Enhancing children's attitudes toward disabled peers using a multi-media intervention. *Journal of Applied Developmental Psychology, 3,* 247–262.

Heber, R. F. (1956). The relation of intelligence and physical maturity to social status. *Journal of Educational Psychology, 47,* 158–162.

Helmstetter, E., Peck, C. A., & Giangreco, M. F. (1994). Outcomes of interactions with peers with moderate or severe disabilities: A statewide survey of high school students. *Journal of the Association of Persons with Severe Handicaps, 19,* 263–276.

Hemphill, L. E., & Siperstein, G. N. (1990). Conversational competence and peer response to mildly retarded children. *Journal of Educational Psychology, 82,* 128–134.

Hodge, S. R., Davis, R., Woodard, R., & Sherrill, C. (2002). Comparison of practicum types in changing preservice teachers' attitudes and perceived competence. *Adapted Physical Activity Quarterly, 19,* 155–171.

Hughes, C., Carter, E. W., Hughes, T., Bradford, E., & Copeland, S. R. (2002). Effects of instructional versus non-instructional roles on the social interactions of high school students. *Education and Training in Mental Retardation and Developmental Disabilities, 37,* 146–162.

Hughes, C., Copeland, S. R., Guth, C., Rung, L. L., Hwang, B., Kleeb, G., & Strong, M. (2001). General education students' perspectives on their involvement in a high school peer buddy program. *Education and Training in Mental Retardation and Developmental Disabilities, 36,* 343–356.

Hughes, C., Rodi, M. S., Lorden, S. W., Pitkin, S. E., Derer, K. R., Hwang, B., & Cai, X. (1999). Social interactions of high school students with mental retardation and their general education peers. *American Journal of Mental Retardation, 104,* 533–544.

Hunt, P., Alwell, M., Farron-Davis, F., & Goetz, L. (1996). Creating socially supportive environments for fully included students who experience multiple disabilities. *Journal for the Association for Persons with Severe Handicaps, 21,* 53–71.

Iano, R. P. (1974). Sociometric status of retarded children in an integrative program. *Exceptional Children, 40,* 267–271.

Jacques, N., Wilton, K., & Townsend, M. (1998). Cooperative learning and social acceptance of children with mild intellectual disability. *Journal of Intellectual Disability Research, 42,* 29–36.

Jaffe, J. (1966). Attitudes of adolescents toward the mentally retarded. *American Journal of Mental Deficiency, 70,* 907–912.

Jaffe, J. (1967). Attitudes and interpersonal contact: Relationships between contact with the mentally retarded and dimensions of attitude. *Journal of Counseling Psychology, 14,* 482–484.

Jamieson, J. D. (1984). Attitudes of educators toward the handicapped. In R. L. Jones (Ed.), *Attitude and attitude change in special education: Theory and practice* (pp. 206–222). Reston, VA: Council for Exceptional Children.

Johnson, C. G., Sigelman, C. K., & Falkenberg, V. F. (1986). Impacts of labeling and competence on peers' perceptions: Mentally retarded versus nonretarded perceivers. *American Journal of Mental Deficiency, 90,* 663–668.

Johnson, C. J., & Ferreira, J. R. (1958). School attitudes of children in special classes for mentally retarded. *California Journal of Educational Research, 9,* 33–37.

Johnson, G. O. (1950). A study of the social position of mentally-handicapped children in the regular grades. *American Journal of Mental Deficiency, 55,* 60–89.

Johnson, R. T. (1979). Interaction between handicapped and nonhandicapped teenagers as a function of situational goal structuring: Implications for mainstreaming. *American Educational Research Journal, 16,* 161–167.

Jones, R. L., Gottfried, N. W., & Owens, A. (1966). The social distance of the exceptional: A study at the high school level. *Exceptional Children, 32,* 551–556.

Karnilowicz, W., Sparrow, W. A., & Shinkfield, A. J. (1994). High school students' attitudes toward performing social behaviors with mentally retarded and physically disabled peers. *Journal of Social Behavior and Personality, 9,* 65–80.

Kennedy, A. B., & Thurman, S. K. (1982). Inclinations of nonhandicapped children to help their handicapped peers. *Journal of Special Education, 16*, 319–327.

Kennon, A. F., & Sandoval, J. (1978). Teacher attitudes toward the educable mentally retarded. *Education and Training of the Mentally Retarded, 13*, 139–145.

Kirk, S. A., & Johnson, G. O. (1951). *Educating the retarded child.* Oxford, UK: Houghton-Mifflin.

Kishi, G. S., & Meyer, L. H. (1994). What children report and remember: A six-year follow-up of the effects of social contact between peers with and without severe disabilities. *Journal of the Association for Persons with Severe Handicaps, 19*, 277–288.

Krajewski, J. J., & Hyde, M. S. (2000). Comparison of teen attitudes toward individuals with mental retardation between 1987 and 1998: Has inclusion made a difference? *Education and Training in Mental Retardation and Developmental Disabilities, 35*, 284–293.

Krajewski, J. J., Hyde, M. S., & O'Keefe, M. K. (2002). Teen attitudes toward individuals with mental retardation from 1987 to 1998: Impact of respondent gender and school variables. *Education and Training in Mental Retardation and Developmental Disabilities, 37*, 27–39.

Kvaraceus, W. C. (1956). Acceptance, rejection, and exceptionality. *Exceptional Children, 22*, 328–331.

Lapp, E. R. (1957). A study of the social adjustment of slow-learning children who were assigned part-time to regular classes. *American Journal of Mental Deficiency, 62*, 254–262.

Lewis, T. J., & Altman, R. (1987). Attitudes of students with mental retardation toward their handicapped and non-handicapped peers. *Education and Training in Mental Retardation, 22*, 256–261.

Madden, N. A., & Slavin, R. E. (1983). Effects of cooperative learning on the social acceptance of mainstreamed academically handicapped students. *Journal of Special Education, 17*, 171–182.

Manetti, M., Schneider, B. H., & Siperstein, G. N. (2001). Social acceptance of children with mental retardation: Testing the contact hypothesis with an Italian sample. *International Journal of Behavioral Development, 25*, 279–286.

Margalit, M. (1993). Social skills and classroom behavior among adolescents with mild mental retardation. *American Journal on Mental Retardation, 97*, 685–691.

McConkey, R., McCormack, B., & Naughton, M. (1983). Changing young people's perceptions of mentally handicapped adults. *Journal of Mental Deficiency Research, 27*, 279–290.

McDaniel, C. O. (1971). Extra-curricular activities as a factor in social acceptance among EMR students. *Mental Retardation, 9*, 26–28.

McEvoy, M. A., Nordquist, V. M., & Cunningham, J. L. (1984). Regular and special education teachers' judgments about mentally retarded children in an integrated setting. *American Journal of Mental Deficiency, 89*, 167–173.

McNally, R. D., Cole, P. G., & Waugh, R. F. (2001). Regular teachers' attitudes to the need for additional classroom support for the inclusion of students with intellectual disability. *Journal of Intellectual and Developmental Disability, 26*, 257–273.

Meyerowitz, J. H. (1962). Self-derogations in young retardates and special class placement. *Child Development, 33*, 433–451.

Miller, C. T., Malcarne, V. L., Clarke, R. T., Lobato, D., Fitzgerald, M. D., & Brand, P. A. (1989). What mentally retarded and nonretarded children expect of one another. *American Journal on Mental Retardation, 93*, 396–405.

Miller, R. V. (1956). Social status and socioempathic differences among mentally superior, mentally typical and mentally retarded children. *Exceptional Children, 23*, 114–119.

Minner, S. (1982). Expectations for vocational teachers for handicapped students. *Exceptional Children, 48*, 451–453.

Moberg, S. (1995). Impact of teachers' dogmatism and pessimistic stereotype on the effect of EMR-class label on teachers' judgments in Finland. *Education and Training in Mental Retardation and Developmental Disabilities, 30*, 141–150.

Mortweet, S. L., Utley, C. A., Iwalker, D., Dawson, H. L., Delquadri, J. C., Reddy, S. S., et al. (1999). Classwide peer tutoring: Teaching students with mild mental retardation in inclusive classrooms. *Exceptional Children, 65*(4), 524–536.

Newberry, M. K., & Parish, T. S. (1987). Enhancement of attitudes toward handicapped children through social interactions. *Journal of Social Psychology, 127*, 59–62.

Ninot, G., Bilard, J., Delignieres, D., & Sokolowski, M. (2000). Effects of integrated sport participation on perceived competence for adolescents with mental retardation. *Adapted Physical Activity Quarterly, 17*, 208–221.

Osguthorpe, R. T., Eiserman, W. D., & Shisler, L. (1985). Increasing social acceptance: Mentally retarded students tutoring regular class peers. *Education and Training of the Mentally Retarded, 20*, 235–240.

Parish, T. S., Eads, G. M., Reece, N. H., & Piscitello, M. A. (1977). Assessment and attempted modification of future teachers' attitudes toward handicapped children. *Perceptual and Motor Skills, 44*, 540–542.

Payne, M. A. (1985). Barbadian children's understanding of mental retardation. *Applied Research in Mental Retardation, 6*, 185–198.

Peach, W. J., Hood, J. M., & Branton, J. R. (1982). Peer acceptance of the handicapped: A categorical survey. *Journal of Instructional Psychology, 9*, 88–90.

Peck, C. A., Donaldson, J., & Pezzoli, M. (1990). Some benefits non-handicapped adolescents perceive for themselves from their social relationships with peers who have severe handicaps. *Journal of the Association for Persons with Severe Handicaps, 15*, 241–249.

Perske, R. (1990). *Circle of Friends.* Nashville, TN: Abingdon

Perske, R. (2003). Parents who moved against the tide. *Mental Retardation, 41*, 133–134.

Piercy, M., Wilton, K., & Townsend, M. (2002). Promoting the social acceptance of young children with moderate-severe intellectual disabilities using cooperative-learning techniques. *American Journal on Mental Retardation, 107*, 352–360.

Reis, E. M. (1988). Improving attitudes of nonretarded fourth graders toward people who are mildly mentally retarded: Implications for mainstreaming. *Education and Training in Mental Retardation, 23*, 85–91.

Renz, P., & Simensen, R. J. (1969). The social perception of normals toward their EMR grademates. *American Journal of Mental Deficiency, 74*, 405–408.

Rizzo, T. L., & Kirkendall, D. R. (1995). Teaching students with mild disabilities: What affects attitudes of future physical educators? *Adapted Physical Activity Quarterly, 12*, 205–216.

Rizzo, T. L., & Vispoel, W. P. (1992). Changing attitudes about teaching students with handicaps. *Adapted Physical Activity Quarterly, 9*, 54–63.

Rolison, M. A., & Medway, F. J. (1985). Teachers' expectations and attributions for student achievements: Effects of label, performance pattern, and special education intervention. *American Educational Research Journal, 22*, 561–573.

Roper, P. (1990). Changing perceptions through contact. *Disability, Hardships and Society, 5*, 243–255.

Rowe, J., & Stutts, R. M. (1987). Effects of practica type, experience, and gender on attitudes of undergraduate physical education majors toward disabled persons. *Adapted Physical Activity Quarterly, 4*, 268–277.

Rucker, C. N., Howe, C. E., & Snider, B. (1969). The participation of retarded children in junior high academic and nonacademic regular classes. *Exceptional Children, 35*, 617–623.

Sabornie, E. J., & Kauffman, J. M. (1987). Assigned, received, and reciprocal social status of adolescents with and without mild mental retardation. *Education and Training in Mental Retardation, 22*, 139–149.

Salend, S. J., & Knops, B. (1984). Hypothetical examples: A cognitive approach to changing attitudes toward the handicapped. *Elementary School Journal, 85*, 229–235.

Schleien, S. J., Ray, M. T., Soderman-Olson, M. L., & McMahon, K. T. (1987). Integrating children with moderate to severe cognitive deficits into a community museum program. *Education and Training in Mental Retardation, 22*, 112–120.

Scruggs, T. E., & Mastropieri, M. A. (1996). Teacher perceptions of mainstreaming/inclusion, 1958–1995: A research synthesis. *Exceptional Children, 63*, 59–74.

Semmel, M. I., Abernathy, T. V., & Butera, G. (1991). Teacher perceptions of the regular education initiative. *Exceptional Children, 58*, 9–24.

Semmel, M. I., & Gao, X. (1992). Teacher perceptions of the classroom behaviors of nominated handicapped and nonhandicapped students in China. *Journal of Special Education, 25*, 415–430.

Sheare, J. B. (1974). Social acceptance of EMR adolescents in integrated programs. *American Journal of Mental Deficiency, 78*, 678–682.

Shisler, L., Osguthorpe, R. T., & Eiserman, W. D. (1987). The effects of reverse-role tutoring on the social acceptance of students with behavioral disorders. *Behavioral Disorders, 13*, 35–44.

Shortridge, S. D. (1982). Facilitating attitude change toward the handicapped. *American Journal of Occupational Therapy, 36*, 456–460.

Simpson, R. L., Parrish, N. E., & Cook, J. J. (1976). Modification of attitudes of regular class children towards the handicapped for the purpose of achieving integration. *Contemporary Educational Psychology, 1*, 46–51.

Siperstein, G. N., & Bak, J. J. (1980). Students' and teachers' perceptions of the mentally retarded child. In J. Gottlieb (Ed.), *Educating mentally retarded persons in the mainstream* (pp. 207–230). Baltimore, MD: University Park.

Siperstein, G. N., & Bak, J. J. (1985a). Effects of social behavior on children's attitudes toward their mildly and moderately mentally retarded peers. *American Journal of Mental Deficiency, 90*, 319–327.

Siperstein, G. N., & Bak, J. J. (1985b). Understanding factors that affect children's attitudes toward mentally retarded peers. In C. J. Meisel (Ed.), *Mainstreaming handicapped children: Outcomes, controversies, and new discoveries* (pp. 55–75). Hillsdale, NJ: Erlbaum.

Siperstein, G. N., Bak, J. J., & O'Keefe, P. (1988). Relationship between children's attitudes toward and their social acceptance of mentally retarded peers. *American Journal on Mental Retardation, 93*, 24–27.

Siperstein, G. N., Budoff, M., & Bak, J. J. (1980). Effects of the labels "mentally retarded" and "retard" on the social acceptability of mentally retarded children. *American Journal of Mental Deficiency, 84*, 596–601.

Siperstein, G. N., Leffert, J. S., & Wenz-Gross, M. (1997). The quality of friendships between children with and without mental retardation. *American Journal on Mental Retardation, 102*, 55–70.

Slininger, D., Sherrill, C., & Jankowski, C. M. (2000). Children's attitudes toward peers with severe disabilities: Revisiting contact theory. *Adapted Physical Activity Quarterly, 17*, 176–196.

SO Get Into It™. (2001). Special Olympics, Inc. Washington, DC: Author.

Stager, S. F., & Young, R. D. (1981). Intergroup contact and social outcomes for mainstreamed EMR adolescents. *American Journal of Mental Deficiency, 85*, 497–503.

Stainback, W. C., & Stainback, S. B. (1982). Nonhandicapped students' perceptions of severely handicapped students. *Education and Training of the Mentally Retarded, 17*, 177–182.

Strauch, J. D. (1970). Social contact as a variable in the expressed attitudes of normal adolescents toward EMR pupils. *Exceptional Children, 36*, 495–500.

Sullivan, M. B., & Brightman, A. J. (1979). *Feeling free.* Reading, MA: Addison-Wesley.

Taylor, R. L., Smiley, L. R., & Ziegler, E. W. (1983). The effects of labels and assigned attributes on teacher perceptions of academic and social behavior. *Education and Training of the Mentally Retarded, 18*, 45–51.

Thomas, D. (1985). The determinants of teachers' attitudes to integrating the intellectually handicapped. *British Journal of Educational Psychology, 55*, 251–263.

Towne, R. C., & Joiner, L. M. (1968). Some negative implications of special placement for children with learning disabilities. *Journal of Special Education, 2*, 217–222.

Townsend, M. A., Wilton, K. M., & Vakilirad, T. (1993). Children's attitudes toward peers with intellectual disability. *Journal of Intellectual Disability Research, 37*, 405–411.

Triandis, H. (1971). *Attitude and attitude change.* New York: Wiley.

Turnbull, A., & Bronicki, G. J. (1986). Changing second graders' attitudes toward people with mental retardation: Using kid power. *Mental Retardation, 24*, 44–45.

Turnbull, A., & Bronicki, G. J. (1987). Using kid power to teach kids about mental retardation: A long-term follow up. *Journal of the Association for Persons with Severe Handicaps, 12*, 216–217.

Van Bourgondien, M. E. (1987). Children's responses to retarded peers as a function of social behaviors, labeling, and age. *Exceptional Children, 53*, 432–439.

Vaughn, S., Schumm, J. S., Jallad, B., & Slusher, J. (1996). Teachers' views of inclusion. *Learning Disabilities Research and Practice, 11,* 96–106.

Voeltz, L. M. (1980). Children's attitudes toward handicapped peers. *American Journal of Mental Deficiency, 84,* 455–464.

Voeltz, L. M. (1982). Effects of structured interactions with severely handicapped peers on children's attitudes. *American Journal of Mental Deficiency, 86,* 380–390.

Voeltz, L. M., Hemphill, N. M., Brown, S., Kishi, G., & Klein, R. (1983). *The Special Friends program: A trainer's manual for integrated school settings* (rev. ed.). Honolulu, HI: University of Hawaii, Department of Special Education.

Whalen, C. K., Henker, B., Dotemoto, S., & Hinshaw, S. P. (1983). Child and adolescent perceptions of normal and atypical peers. *Child Development, 54,* 1588–1598.

Willey, N. R., & McCandless, B. R. (1973). Social stereotypes for normal, educable mentally retarded, and orthopedically handicapped children. *Journal of Special Education, 7,* 283–288.

Wisely, D. W., & Morgan, S. B. (1981). Children's ratings of peers presented as mentally retarded and physically handicapped. *American Journal of Mental Deficiency, 86,* 281–286.

Wolfberg, P. J., Zercher, C., & Lieber, J. (1999). "Can I play with you?" Peer culture in inclusive preschool programs. *Journal of the Association for Persons with Severe Handicaps, 24,* 69–84.

Yanito, T., Quintero, M. C., Killoran, V. C., & Striefel, S. (1987). *Teacher attitudes toward mainstreaming: A literature review.* ERIC Document #290290.

Zanandrea, M., & Rizzo, T. (1998). Attitudes of undergraduate physical education majors in Brazil toward teaching students with disabilities. *Perceptual and Motor Skills, 86,* 699–706.

II

Disability Services

The focus of this section is on broad practice issues and professional functions within the field of developmental disabilities, with a primary focus on psychological and behavioral practice, and emphasizing parameters of effective practice.

8

Evaluating Developmental Disabilities Services

JOHN W. JACOBSON[†]

This chapter focuses on contemporary program evaluation activities in adult developmental disabilities (DD) services. Program evaluation is best understood as a:

> tool through which management seeks to understand the operational elements of a social program and the processes through which beneficial impacts are achieved. Critical issues confronting administrators involve (1) the degree to which an individual's needs and abilities mesh with the programmatic and social characteristics of his or her residential situation; (b) responsiveness to constituent demands and resource limitations related to changing care philosophies, new legislation, and regulation; and (c) the determination of relative program benefits and costs.... (Jacobson & Schwartz, 1991, pp. 35–36)

This definition is similar in its focus and overt parameters to services research (Jacobson & Holburn, in press, 2004, based on Newman, Howard, Windle, & Hohmann, 1994), which also similarly encompasses

> epidemiology (including risk factors) and demographics of service and of services distribution..., the development of improved measures of disability..., the efficacy and effectiveness of treatment for specific disorders..., rehabilitative and habilitative features parameters of service delivery programs or classes of services, and assessment of outcomes of treatment with respect to alleviation of disorders, alleviations of symptoms

JOHN W. JACOBSON • Sage Colleges Center for Applied Behavior Analysis, Troy, New York 12180.

[†] Deceased.

of disorders, and social, family, and vocational functioning, as
well as personal well-being and quality of life.

There are both critical and not-so-critical distinctions between program evaluation and services research. Some of the critical distinctions lie
in considerations of breadth, application of findings, and generalizability
of findings, whereas some of the less-critical distinctions involve focus of
studies (where considerable overlap is apparent between these activities),
and the initial goals of evaluative or research projects. While evaluative
studies are generally intended to produce findings and services research
often addresses administrative or systemic concerns, and hence are structured for application of findings at these differing areas of emphasis, the
methods used in some evaluative studies may permit broad applicability
of findings that transcend individual service organizations. Critically, depending on the breadth and clarity of definition of measured independent
and dependent variables, and parameters such as single-site or multisite
data collection and measurement, ensuing recommendations that are developed for management application may also demonstrate suitability for
more pervasive generalization.

COMPLEMENTARY EVALUATION REVIEWS

The primary focus of this chapter is on considerations of individualization and implementation of specialized interventions in contemporary
DD services. This focus was selected because substantive summaries of
other aspects of past and present services have encompassed numerous
other aspects of service operations (e.g., Jacobson & Holburn, in press,
2004; Jacobson & Schwartz, 1983, 1991), including foci on implementing evaluation activities (Jacobson & Regula, 1988) and training personnel or transferring technology (Jacobson & Holburn, 2004). Jacobson
and Schwartz (1983), during a very active period of deinstitutionalization
activity, focused their review on analysis of community residences and
their impact on people served, and offered a general model for evaluation
based on primary dimensions of developmental progress, quality of life,
and home-like environments. Later, as community services had become
well-developed, more diverse in form, and as barriers to effective coordination and cross-organizational collaboration had become more evident,
Jacobson and Schwartz (1991) broadened their review of evaluative findings to include family living, supportive residential foster care, and medical
and behavioral services, heightened emphasis on organizational and management issues such as staff turnover, and slightly increased attention to
consumer and family. These reviews also identified instruments or measures suitable for application in evaluation of a range of settings.

Although it can be suggested that the primary concerns of program
evaluation in developmental services have changed over the past 20 years
(Schalock, 2000), in fact a substantive shift in the purposes of research
is not so much apparent as a shift in the variables of interest. Whereas

20 years ago it was common to include measures used to assess the presence of noninstitutional and normalizing practices in evaluation efforts, today the types of measures used tend to be more narrowly focused on particular aspects of normalizing and noninstitutional practices, such as choice, self-determination, variation among individuals in lifestyle characteristics and routines, or receipt of clinical services. But individualization and responsiveness of services and supports (the latter referring to the activities of paraprofessionals in most instances, or to actions undertaken on behalf of, or to assist an individual) has remained a foundational aspect of evaluative activity throughout this period into the present.

EVALUATIVE METHODOLOGIES

Over the past decade or so it has become fashionable to distinguish between quantitative and qualitative approaches to program evaluation and services research. This distinction has emerged both as a consequence of reassessment of the parameters and purposes of program evaluation by evaluation specialists (Fishman, 1992) and as a manifestation of blending of ideology, constructs, and methodologies of special education research and evaluation into adult DD services research (Bogdan & Biklen, 1982). Whether the distinction between these methods is meaningful, and whether purely quantitative or qualitative methods are possible, can be challenged on rational grounds. Nonetheless, concerns for potential generalization of findings render purely qualitative methods and derivative findings impossible to assess for their utility, and it is reasonable to conclude that quantitative methods complemented by qualitative methods provide a reasonably sound basis for analysis, inference, and conclusions. Unfortunately, although purely qualitative studies can illuminate nuances of services and supports, and suggest valuable relationships among phenomena or events that merit further study and analysis, procedures recommended to reconcile and interpret the voluminous qualitative data collected in many studies and to enhance internal validity of conclusions, are fraught with potential shared researcher biases, and, unfortunately, the procedures used in many qualitative studies within special education and DD services research do not approach the rigor of kindred or model procedures for high-precision qualitative research, for example, as applied in anthropological research (Edgerton, 1993).

Many qualitative studies in the special education and DD sectors focus on descriptive analysis of implementation methods for practice that may themselves have an uncertain foundation with respect to efficacy and effectiveness. Further limitations of qualitative research in DD services reflect ideological rather than theoretical grounds for interpretation of findings, selection of narrow samples, use of extreme or index cases as exemplars, and conclusions of cause and effect relationships based on methods that do not permit these types of inferences to be made (e.g., Biklen, 1993). Because of these limitations, the primary focus of this chapter is on recent findings that have emerged from studies that included use of quantitative methods (see Jacobson & Schwartz, 1991, p. 50 for features of evaluative activities that permit and enhance generalization of findings).

CONTEMPORARY EVALUATION RESEARCH

Impacts of Progressive Practices

Contemporary research on semi-independent or group living includes some reports that are quite comprehensive in scope. Extensive evaluations in recent years, resulting in multiple reports of different aspects of the evaluations, have been reported by several groups in the past decade, mainly in the United Kingdom (e.g., Emerson et al., 2000; Smith, Felce, Jones, & Lowe, 2002) and in the United States (e.g., Burchard, 1999; Stancliffe, Hayden, & Lakin, 1999a,b,c). An example of this type of research is a study by Stancliffe and Keane (2000), who compared 27 matched pairs of adults in Australia living in group homes or semi-independent settings. They note that

> Available research comparing outcomes for individuals living in group homes or semi-independently (i.e., with drop-in staff support) suggests better outcomes for semi-independent living services in a number of domains: quality of life, choice, self-determination, autonomy, satisfaction, self-esteem, independence, lifestyle normalisation, physical and social integration, compatibility with living companions, participation in preferred activities, and personal well being.... On the other hand, loneliness, self-care, domestic management, personal safety, money management and health can be areas of concern [in] semi-independent [living].... Problems may arise in these areas because of insufficient support... or inappropriate housing. (p. 282)

In their study they assessed social networks and use of mainstream community services, community participation, participation in domestic tasks, stability of place of residence, living companion turnover, and natural supports. They examined outcomes entailing quality of life, safety, aloneness, social dissatisfaction, personal care, domestic management, health care, money management, social network, use of mainstream community services, community participation, domestic participation, stability of place of residence, living companion turnover, and natural support. Outcomes tended not to differ between semi-independent and group-home settings, although better outcomes were found in semi-independent settings reflecting "less social dissatisfaction, more frequent and independent use of community facilities, more participation in domestic tasks, and greater empowerment" (p. 281).

Stancliffe and Keane suggested that the findings indicated that people living in semi-independent settings were provided sufficient support to enable them to attain outcomes similar to those for their peers in group homes, and that, because of differences in staff availability in these two

types of settings, "the semi-independent living environment not only provided *opportunities* for independent participation, it *demanded* independent participation," (p. 300), and that this, at least in part, accounted for
some of the observed differences. Limitations to interpretation and generalization of findings included the considerations that comparisons were not
made to nondisabled peers with respect to outcomes (e.g., findings did not
indicate that outcomes were "satisfactory"; "they could have been equally
poor," pp. 299–300) and that data on services used or service processes
were not gathered to place the findings in context. These are common limitations of studies that assess outcomes of settings or services like those
addressed in this study (e.g., Holburn, Jacobson, Schwartz, Flori, & Vietze,
2004; Holburn, Jacobson, Vietze, Schwartz, & Sersen, 2000). Moreover,
studies of service utilization in various settings seldom place their findings in context through measures of individualization or autonomy in the
manner embodied by the Stancliffe and Keane study (e.g., Jacobson, 1987;
Stancliffe & Lakin, 1999), despite the desirability of enhancing interpretation in this manner.

In a separate study of 74 adults living independently or in group
residences operated by seven organizations, Stancliffe, Avery, and Smith
(2000) investigated factors that were associated with increased personal
control (of lifestyle and activity) by participants. Greater personal control
was found in semi-independent settings, compared to group residences,
and among living situations ranging from one to five persons in size.
In a path analysis, greater adaptive behavior skills were associated with
greater self-determination skills, policies, and practices that were more
supportive of autonomy, greater individualization, and greater availability
of money for discretionary use. In turn, these latter factors were associated with greater personal control. Given these findings, and as noted by
the authors, unambiguous interpretation of differences in personal control
among types of settings and those differing in size is compromised to some
degree by the presence of differences in participant skills among the types
of settings. Studies such as this one suggest possible factors for intervention that may support greater self-determination. However, as Algozzine,
Browder, Karvonen, Test, & Wood (2001) have noted, few studies of instruction in choice-making and self-determination have focused on outcomes in terms of quality of life (including personal control, autonomy, or
self-determination, which may be largely interchangeable constructs) and
convincing demonstrations that self-determination can be taught, learned,
and makes a difference in the lives of people with disabilities are still
needed.

Social Networks

Robertson et al. (2001) studied the social networks of 500 adults with
intellectual disabilities (ID) living in a variety of residential settings. From
their literature review they concluded that the social networks of people
with ID are often restricted in number of friendships, and involve few reciprocal relationships with others who do not have ID, or are not relatives

or staff. Further, relationships do not necessarily develop spontaneously or over the course of time as the result of community living or of deinstitutionalization, and do not necessarily entail frequent contacts with family members. Findings from prior research also suggested that living near family and in smaller residences, and personal characteristics such as being younger, having a disability that is not highly visible, and being more responsive socially were factors associated with increased contact with family.

Robertson et al. (2001) found that about 50% of participants had three or fewer people in their social networks, disregarding staff, and only 4% had a nondisabled neighbor in their social network. As in previous research, participants were seldom found to be engaged in reciprocal relationships with nondisabled people, although reciprocal relationships with other people with ID were far more common. Relationships with other people with ID tended to be lasting, with 75% of such relationship enduring more than 5 years. People living in smaller residences and supported housing had larger and more diverse networks, as did younger individuals. Those with autism or lower adaptive skills or with more severe problem behaviors tended to have smaller networks. The authors concluded that many of these individuals were socially isolated, at least with respect to the structure of social networks.

Another study that compared community use by people with ID and a staff control group (Baker, 2000) found that those with disabilities had a smaller range of activities, engaged in fewer frequent activities, and were less likely to use community resources alone with friends. Although tangible and meaningful differences in community use were identified, the extent that community access patterns "alone" reflected concerns for safeguarding and well-being, rather than restrictions upon access, were not addressed and are not well-addressed in most social network analyses.

Whether conclusions that social networks are coarsely deficient among people with ID is a broadly accurate characterization is less than certain. Exclusions of staff as legitimate members of social networks, and of peers or others with disabilities as members of networks are largely ideological exclusions, as such adjustments as to social network estimates are typically made in the absence of measures of individual preference for social engagement with particular staff or peers, or satisfaction with present social networks. Although such measures may be difficult or impossible to apply for people with few communication skills, they could be readily applied with those individuals with the requisite skills. Among people without disabilities, assortive formation of friendships reflecting educational levels and personal interests are common, as are social networks dominated by relatives, housemates or cohabitants, and longstanding coworkers. The question of possible relationships between satisfaction and social networks was investigated as part of a study by Gregory, Robertson, Kessissglou, Emerson, and Hatton (2001). In interviews of 95 people with ID living in "village communities" or community situations, those living in village communities expressed greater satisfaction with friendships and relationships. Extent of day services was associated with satisfaction with weekly hours of scheduled activity, including those involving friendships and relationships, as was implementation of active support (see, e.g., Mansell, Elliott, Beadle-Brown, Ashman, & Macdonald, 2002). Relationships noted here between friendships and relationships and life satisfactions suggest that network size, at least, and possibly other aspects of networks merit improvement as a means to increase general life satisfactions.

In a few instances, community presence and participation of people with DD and of peers without disabilities has been assessed, without remarkable differences in some dimensions of networks being noted between disabled and nondisabled individuals in the extent of participation (Pretty, Rapley, & Bramston, 2002; Rosen & Burchard, 1990), although subjectively the extent of participation by those with disabilities might be characterized as low. Such findings underscore the importance of community norms for interpretation of findings regarding the lifestyle qualities of community living for people with DD.

Individualized Planning of Services

One enduring aspect of DD services is utilization of a process of individualized planning, usually embodied in a plan of services and supports. Planning processes have not been studied in adult or child DD services (e.g., Jacobson, 1987), to the extent that they have in special education, but as these processes have changed over the years from multidisciplinary or interdisciplinary in form to those characterized as person-centered, and public agencies have adopted policies encouraging or requiring these latter processes, efforts to evaluate the impact of planning on service and support delivery have increased (e.g., Holburn & Jacobson, 2004; Stancliffe et al., 1999).

In their study, Stancliffe et al. (1999) followed a cohort of 157 people with mild to profound ID in Minnesota who moved from institutional living to community settings over the course of 3 years. Individual plan objectives developed for these individuals were assessed on dimensions of quality (e.g., specification of community focus, teaching methods, and related data collection) and objectives were assessed further as predictors of outcomes such as social inclusion, community participation, or self-determination, as well as adaptive behavior change. Goals in individual plans focused, from most frequently to least frequently, on: self-care, household chores, communication, leisure and recreation, and community participation. Presence of leisure and recreation goals was applied as a predictor of social activities in the last 30 days. Neither the "five [goal] quality domain scores nor number of objectives were significant predictors" (p. 110) of social activities. Furthermore, from their analyses, the authors concluded:

> This study provided no evidence to support expectations that the presence or quality of IHP objectives contributes to the increase of desired behaviors, skills, or participation among persons with mental retardation nor was there evidence that the

presence of IHP objectives is important in maintaining such outcomes.... These findings...cast significant doubt on the contribution of IHP objectives to developmental and lifestyle gains by adults with mental retardation in residential service settings (Stancliffe et al., 1999, p. 110).

The authors noted some potential restrictions on generalization of their findings: (1) the outcome measures may not have been sufficiently sensitive to detect changes associated with objectives; (2) the abbreviated adaptive behavior scale they used may not have been sufficiently sensitive (although their findings converge with comparable direct measures in other research, citing Felce, de Kock, Mansell, & Jenkins, 1984); and (3) they did not measure whether objectives were achieved (e.g., objectives were implemented and completed, but did not contribute to the broad outcomes assessed). It seems plausible that an abbreviated adaptive behavior measure might well be too insensitive to capture adaptive behavior changes in adults over the course of even 3 years. Of greater concern in this study, and a common limitation in large-scale DD sector evaluations, is that neither implementation of objectives nor outcomes assessed through completion of scales or report forms were confirmed by direct observation. Because this is a common limitation of large-scale evaluations, and the presence of close correspondence between scales and actual events is seldom confirmed during scale development, in this instance, and other studies relying principally on scaled measures (e.g., Holburn et al., 2004), whether findings of such studies should be regarded as relatively conclusive or suggestive in nature, warranting study using direct observation and measures, can be unclear.

DUAL DIAGNOSIS OR CO-OCCURRING BEHAVIOR PROBLEMS: AN INCREASING FOCUS

Developing and maintaining responsive community services for people with ID and either severe chronic health problems (including frailty) or persistent mental illness or severe and disruptive behavior problems have come to be one of the most difficult undertakings in operation of fully community based and highly individualized services. Adams and Allen (2001) conducted a retrospective study of aggressive behavior in a group of children referred for specialist services, and found that about 60% engaged in aggressive acts. Physical interventions were used in 56% of cases but were generally improvized by caregivers. Nottestad and Linaker (1999) followed 109 people with ID from institutions to community living and found persistence of psychiatric problems and a significant increase in behavior problems (including disruptive and aggressive acts), as well as reduced access to psychological and psychiatric services.

Joyce, Ditchfield, and Harris (2001) identified 482 people with ID and behavior problems in London and found that 24% had experienced a placement breakdown (moved from family or among community settings), 24% had come to the attention of the police, and 29% had been excluded from day services at least once. Tonge and Einfeld (2000) followed a sample of children with ID ages 4–19 years over 4 years and found that 40% had psychiatric disorders that persisted over this period, in all likelihood because less than 10% of those in need received specialist services (see also Kiernan & Alborz, 1996). Varying and inconsistently available expertise in dual diagnosis and behavioral treatment, structural features of services, and difficulties in cross-sector collaboration and cooperation in service delivery have been identified broadly as barriers to effective services for people living in the community with ID and either mental or behavioral conditions (e.g., Alexander, Piachaud, & Singh, 2001; Davidson et al., 1994; Linhorst, McCutchen, & Bennett, 2003; Lohrer, Greene, Browning, & Lesser, 2002; Ward, Trigler, & Pfeiffer, 2001).

Recent Relevant Evaluations

Three recent evaluations (Emerson & Forrest, 1996; Stancliffe, Hayden, & Lakin, 1999a, 1999b) and one literature review (Ager & O'May, 2001) are especially relevant to appraisal of services for people with ID and either dual diagnosis or severe problem behavior. As a further aspect of the community living follow-along study conducted by Stancliffe and Keane (2000), Stancliffe et al. (1999a, 1999b) reported on the impact of IHP objectives entailing behavioral intervention (1999a) and their relationship to maladaptive behavior scores, and sought to predict the extent of behavioral intervention (1999b). Stancliffe et al. (1999a), found that, in this sample of predominantly people with severe to profound ID, 99 of 157 participants retained same status of having or not having a challenging behavior objective across three annual reviews. Moreover, there was no significant change in problem behavior across three annual assessments, or in the frequency of crisis intervention. Stancliffe et al. concluded that "These findings suggest that most challenging behavior IHP objectives are ineffective in reducing challenging behavior" (p. 482). They also suggested that the extant behavioral objectives may have been directed at behavior management rather than behavior change, as such.

However, the authors did note some possible reasons to qualify their findings: (1) the sample consisted primarily of people with severe or profound ID and long histories of institutionalization; and (2) although some data were collected on implementation, analyses were based on presence or absence of behavioral objectives rather than quality and implementation, and (3) discontinuation of an objective could reflect completion or discontinuation of an ineffective intervention. The use of maladaptive behavior scales rather than direct measures of behavior occurrence or magnitude might also have masked effects in this study, because it has not been established previously that the measures they used are sensitive to psychiatric or behavioral intervention effects. Overall, although such findings raise important questions regarding the quality and effectiveness of behavioral interventions in community living situations, because direct observational measures and records of intervention outcomes were not used, further evaluations of behavioral intervention in community settings should use these methods in order to more exhaustively identify the consistency and parameters of implementation of these services.

As already noted, Stancliffe et al. (1999b) sought to predict behavioral intervention within the same study cohort (but including both those who stayed in an institutional setting and those who moved to communities). Presence of individual objectives and magnitude of maladaptive behavior was used to predict one-to-one crisis intervention during the past 30 days and services by behavior management professionals during the past 6 months. Less than 25% of participants received services from psychiatrists, psychologists, or behavior analysts, although as noted above, a majority had behavioral objectives in their plans. The researchers found that 68% of participants with behavioral objectives received professional services, as compared with 16% of those with no behavioral objectives. Participants were more likely to receive psychiatric or behavioral services if they evidenced more externalized behavior (see also, Rudolph, Lakin, Oslund, & Larson, 1998), were stayers (i.e., in an institution), and had greater adaptive behavior skills (i.e., because those with greater skills evidenced more difficult behavior).

Taken together with the findings from Stancliffe et al. (1999a) these findings suggest that presence of behavioral objectives did not effectively predict utilization of mental health or behavioral specialists, or referral to such practitioners; again, these findings suggest the need for service processes in community settings that entail behavioral intervention to be studied more closely.

Current research findings within the field of behavior analysis indicate that implementation fidelity and duration of behavioral interventions is improved by organizational provisions focused on maintaining interventions, as well as by ongoing involvement of a behavioral consultant (see Jacobson & Holburn, 2004).

Implementation of faithful and durable behavioral interventions within community living situations or day services requires sufficient training of staff in behavioral intervention competencies, supervisory practices that systematically encourage implementation. When staff and clinician competencies are not sufficient to conduct appropriate assessments, design corresponding interventions, and effectively monitor and alter interventions based on individual effects, efficient utilization of consultants and community practitioners (Ager & O'May, 2001; Jacobson & Holburn, 2004, in press, 2004; Parsons, Cash, & Reid, 1989; Reid, 1992). As noted by Stancliffe et al. (1999a), "specialist community behavior support teams are of limited effectiveness if nonspecialist ID services are ineffective in day-to-day management of challenging behavior" (p. 482). Research on the impact of specialist teams, which exist in the United Kingdom and to some (unknown) extent in the United States, has been mixed, variable across teams, and not entirely encouraging (Emerson & Forrest, 1996; Lowe, Felce, & Blackman, 1996).

Emerson and Forrest (1996) conducted a survey of community support teams for people with ID and problem behaviors in England and Wales, which they estimated to employ about 450 staff, at a cost of £10 million to serve about 2000 people yearly. There were 65 of these teams in operation, 46 of which returned survey forms. Teams generally reported operating with a general behavioral orientation and allocating the greatest amount of consultation time to working with direct care staff. Only 1% of team members were reported to be psychiatrists and 24% were reported to be psychologists or assistant psychologists. Half (50%) of the team members were nurses.

Data collected on caseloads suggested that 48% of the estimated people with severe problem behavior in the localities served by teams were carried within current caseload. Other estimates indicated that annually case closures occurred for 19% of estimated local need, and successful closure for 13%. A majority of the teams required placement jeopardy as a specific criterion for consultative engagement.

Teams reported spending more time working with direct care staff on interventions for specific individuals than any other activity, followed by advice and consultation to caregivers (family members and staff) and direct intervention with specific individuals. People with less severe ID were less likely to receive direct intervention by specialist team members.

Many of the cases that were reported to be "successfully closed" were found to be considered successful by respondents based on acceptance of recommendations for referral to another service or the completion of assessments, not as the result of interventions that were effective in reducing problem behavior. This finding suggested that teams might not be effectively monitoring interventions, or following-up sufficiently.

Emerson and Forrest concluded from their findings that team engagement was often insufficient to achieve substantive impact on the treatment concerns for which assistance had been sought and posed the question of whether specialist teams not affiliated with programs or services "effectively influence their management and operation when this is needed" (p. 403). Conclusions offered by Ager and O'May (2001) as "best practices" in community behavioral intervention in DD services, based on review of the recent research base are compatible with the conclusions reached by Emerson and Forrest (1996) and Stancliffe et al. (1999a, 1999b) regarding the need for the development of more sufficient behavioral competencies among personnel in DD service and support settings, rather than primary reliance upon consultative involvement as a means to compensate for inadequate staff and clinician expertise within community agencies.

The conclusions reached by Ager and O'May (2001, pp. 253–254) merit consideration here, due to their foundation in empirical studies of implementation, and are closely paraphrased below:

> Empirical evidence supports the effectiveness of interventions, particularly those that address socially disruptive and internally maladaptive behavior, involve manipulation of response contingencies, and are based upon prior functional analysis.

> "Only one in four studies reports follow-up data to 12 months post-intervention; the general durability of change subsequent to intervention is thus uncertain.

Where details are given, researchers external to the service setting are responsible for assessment, analysis and design in
about half of reported interventions . . . the recruitment of such
external expertise, or the development of appropriate competences within existing staff, is a major challenge for services
seeking to institute "best practice" in intervention.

In terms of developing such competence, Training to develop
such competence has little impact on staff performance in service settings without additional emphasis on organizational processes.

Formalized procedures of feedback, supervision and support do
have an established impact on staff behavior.

Staff training targeting reappraisal of assumptions and expectations may play an important role in shaping staff
behavior . . . intervention protocols may be implemented with
greater fidelity if they are coherent with staff attitudes and
beliefs although this direct relationship has not been demonstrated.

Formal review mechanisms, where intervention strategies and
protocols are explicitly defended on the basis of evidence of empirical support, may usefully foster accountability.

SUMMARY

There is a rich and diverse research literature focusing on program
evaluation in DD services and in this chapter it has been possible to indicate some exemplars and key concerns of contemporary studies. One of
the most important concerns not addressed in this chapter include organizational factors that are associated with individualization and responsiveness of services and supports (e.g., Hatton et al., 1999; Hatton & Emerson,
1993; Holburn et al., 2000; Schwartz, Jacobson, & Holburn, 2000). As previously indicated, this literature is discussed in greater detail elsewhere
(e.g., Jacobson & Holburn, in press, 2004).

Despite the wealth of applied research undertaken for evaluative and
administrative purposes, there remain important research questions that
have not been addressed with the needed precision of measurement and
breadth of sampled settings needed to draw suitably compelling conclusions or to assure generalizability of findings. Medium to large-scale studies continue to rely, as in past decades, on rated indicators of key desirable
features and outcomes of services, and to eschew more direct observation,
even if limited to a subsample of programs with highly divergent ratings.
Exemplars of substantive observational studies remain largely historical
(e.g., Landesman-Dwyer, Sackett, & Kleinman, 1980; Romer & Berkson,
1980, 1981), with some very notable exceptions (e.g., Felce et al., 1999).
Evaluation efforts that collect direct observational data tend to remain
confined to approaches that focus on only one or several service settings. Finally, as evaluative efforts have continued to hone in on more

specific aspects of individualization of services or outcomes, such as self-determination, choice, autonomy, independence, lifestyle normalization, participation, and integration, because of the subtleties that differentiate many of these constructs, investigators need to further verify that the aspects of services they are measuring are (at least relatively) independent attributes of settings and services, and are not conflated by overlap of measures; as these distinctions become more subtle studies need to verify the suitability of planned analyses through such procedures as combined factor analyses of measures (e.g., Holburn et al., 2000).

Notwithstanding changes in the character of dominant rationales for services over time, some philosophical and others ideological, or even empirically founded, evaluators have continued to focus on factors that contribute to a varied lifestyle, individualization, and responsiveness of services, supports, and communities to people with developmental disabilities, although contemporary service systems remain largely unevaluated with respect to key concerns about the quality of services, or of impacts of often complex management and administrative procedures in unambiguous terms. These considerations point to the continued need to expand both the breadth and depth of medium to large-scale studies and to more effectively study key issues through independent replication of high-profile service issues that have been addressed by only one or two research groups.

REFERENCES

Adams, D., & Allen, D. (2001). Assessing the need for reactive behaviour management strategies in children with intellectual disability and severe challenging behaviour. *Journal of Intellectual Disability Research, 45,* 335–343.

Ager, A., & O'May, F. (2001). Issues in the definition and implementation of "best practice" for staff delivery of interventions for challenging behaviour. *Journal of Intellectual and Developmental Disability, 26,* 243–256,

Alexander, R. T., Piachaud, J., & Singh, I. (2001). Two districts, two models: In-patient care in the psychiatry of learning disability. *The British Journal of Developmental Disabilities, 47*(93), 105–110.

Algozzine, B., Browder, D., Karvonen, M., Test., D. W., & Wood, W. M. (2001). Effects of interventions to promote self-determination for individuals with disabilities. *Review of Educational Research, 71,* 219–277.

Baker, P. A. (2000). Measurement of community participation and use of leisure by service users with intellectual disabilities: The Guernsey Community Participation and Leisure Assessment (GCPLA). *Journal of Applied Research in Intellectual Disabilities, 13,* 169–185.

Biklen, D. (1993). *Communication unbound: How facilitated communication is challenging traditional views of autism and ability/disability.* New York: Teacher's College Press, Columbia University.

Bogdan, R., & Biklen, S. K. (1982). *Qualitative research for education: An introduction to theory and methods.* Boston: Allyn and Bacon.

Burchard, S. N. (1999). Normalization and residential services: The Vermont studies. In R. J. Flynn & R. A. Lemay (Eds.), *A quarter-century of normalization and social role valorization: Evolution and impact* (pp. 241–270). Ottawa, Canada: University of Ottawa.

Davidson, P. W., Cain, N. N., Sloane-Reeves, J. E., Van Speybroech, A., Segel, J., Gutkin, J., Quijano, L. E., & Kramer, B. M. (1994). Characteristics of community-based individuals with mental retardation and aggressive behavioral disorders. *American Journal on Mental Retardation, 98,* 704–716.

Edgerton, R. B. (1993). *The cloak of competence* (2nd ed.). Berkeley, CA: University of California Press.

Emerson, E., & Forrest, J. (1996). Community support teams for people with learning disabilities and challenging behaviours: Results of a national survey. *Journal of Mental Health, 5*, 395–404.

Emerson, E., Robertson, J., Gregory, N., Hatton, C., & Kessissoglou, S., Hallam, A. (2000). Quality and costs of community-based residential supports, village communities, and residential campuses in the United Kingdom. *American Journal on Mental Retardation, 105*, 81–102.

Felce, D., de Kock, U., Mansell, J., & Jenkins, J. (1984). Providing systematic individual teaching for severely disturbed and profoundly mentally-handicapped adults in residential care. *Behaviour Research and Therapy, 22*, 299–309.

Felce, D., Lowe, K., Perry, J., Jones, E., & Baxter, H., Baxter, H. (1999). The quality of residential and day services for adults with intellectual disabilities in eight local authorities in England: Objective data gained in support of a social services inspectorate inspection. *Journal of Applied Research in Intellectual Disabilities, 12*, 273–293.

Fishman, D. B. (1992). Postmodernism comes to program evaluation: A critical review of Guba and Lincoln's fourth generation evaluation. *Evaluation and Program Planning, 15*, 263–270.

Gregory, N., Robertson, J., Kessissglou, S., Emerson, E., & Hatton, C. (2001). Factors associated with expressed satisfaction among people with intellectual disability receiving residential supports. *Journal of Intellectual Disability Research, 45*, 279–291.

Hatton, C., & Emerson, E. (1993). Organizational predictors of staff stress, satisfaction, and intended turnover in a service for people with multiple disabilities. *Mental Retardation, 31*, 388–395.

Hatton, C., Rivers, M., Mason, H., Mason, L., & Emerson, E., Kiernan, C. (1999). Organizational culture and staff outcomes in services for people with intellectual disabilities. *Journal of Intellectual Disability Research, 43*, 206–218.

Holburn, C. S., Jacobson, J. W., Schwartz, A., Flori, M., & Vietze, P. (2004). The Willowbrook Futures Project: A longitudinal analysis of person-centered planning. *American Journal of Mental Retardation, 109*, 63–76.

Holburn, S., & Jacobson, J. W. (2004). Implementing and researching person-centered planning. In L. Williams (Ed.), *Developmental disabilities: Advances in scientific understanding, clinical treatments, and community integration* (pp. 315–330). Reno, NV: Context.

Holburn, S., & Jacobson, J. W. (2004). Implementing and researching person-centered planning. In L. Williams (Ed.), *Developmental disabilities: Advances in scientific understanding, clinical treatments and community integration* (pp. 315–330). Reno, NV: Context press.

Holburn, S., Jacobson, J. W., Schwartz, A. A., Flory, M. J., & Vietze, P. M. (in press). The Willowbrook Futures Project: A longitudinal analysis of person-centered planning. *American Journal on Mental Retardation.*

Holburn, S., Jacobson, J. W., Vietze, P. M., Schwartz, A. A., & Sersen, E. (2000). Quantifying the process and outcomes of person-centered planning. *American Journal on Mental Retardation, 105*, 402–416.

Jacobson, J., & Holburn, S. (2004). Research to practice: Management, staff training, and improvement of service in technology transfer. In L. Williams (Ed.), *Developmental disabilities: Advances in scientific understanding, clinical treatments, and community integration* (pp. 331–363). Reno, NV: Context.

Jacobson, J. W. (1987). Individual program plan goal content in developmental disabilities programs. *Mental Retardation, 3*, 157–164.

Jacobson, J. W., & Holburn, S. (in press). Residential services research in the developmental disabilities sector. In L. Glidden (Ed.), *International review of research in mental retardation.* San Diego, Academic Press.

Jacobson, J. W., & Holburn, S. (2004). Research to practice: Management, staff training, and improvement of services. In W. L. Williams (Ed.), *Developmental disabilities: Advances in scientific understanding, clinical treatments and community integration* (pp. 331–363). Reno, NV: Context press.

Jacobson, J. W., & Regula, C. R. (1988). Evaluation issues and resources for community living situations. In M. P. Janicki, M. W. Krauss, & M. M. Seltzer (Eds.), *Community residences for people with developmental disabilities: Here to stay* (pp. 85–101). Baltimore: Brookes.

Jacobson, J. W., & Schwartz, A. A. (1983). Evaluation of community living alternatives. In J. L. Matson & J. A. Mulick (Eds.), *Handbook of mental retardation* (pp. 39–66). Elmsford, NY: Pergamon.

Jacobson, J. W., & Schwartz, A. A. (1991). Evaluating the living situations of persons with developmental disabilities. In J. L. Matson & J. A. Mulick (Eds.), *Handbook of mental retardation* (2nd ed., pp. 35–62). Elmsford, NY: Pergamon.

Joyce, T., Ditchfield, H., & Harris, P. (2001). Challenging behaviour in community services. *Journal of Intellectual Disability Research, 45,* 130–138.

Kiernan, C., & Alborz, A. (1996). Persistence and change in challenging and problem behaviours of young adults with intellectual disability living in the family home. *Journal of Applied Research in Intellectual Disabilities, 9,* 181–193.

Landesman-Dwyer, S., Sackett, G. P., & Kleinman, J. S. (1980). Relationship of size to resident and staff behavior in small community residences. *American Journal of Mental Deficiency, 85,* 6–17.

Linhorst, D. M., McCutchen, T. A., & Bennett, L. (2003). Recidivism among offenders with developmental disabilities participating in a case management program. *Research in Developmental Disabilities, 24,* 210–230.

Lohrer, S. P., Greene, E., Browning, C. J., & Lesser, M. S. (2002). Dual diagnosis: Examination of service use and length of stay during psychiatric hospitalization. *Journal of Developmental and Physical Disabilities, 14,* 143–158.

Lowe, K., Felce, D., & Blackman, D. (1996). Challenging behaviour: The effectiveness of specialist support teams. *Journal of Intellectual Disability Research, 40,* 336–347.

Mansell, J., Elliott, T., Beadle-Brown, J., Ashman, B., & Macdonald, S. (2002). Engagement in meaningful activity and "active support" of people with intellectual disabilities in residential care. *Research in Developmental Disabilities, 23,* 342–352.

Newman, F. L., Howard, K. I., Windle, C. D., & Hohmann, A. A. (1994). Introduction to the special section on seeking new methods in mental health services research. *Journal of Consulting and Clinical Psychology, 62,* 667–669.

Nottestad, J. A., & Linaker, O. M. (1999). Psychiatric health needs and services before and after complete deinstitutionalization of people with intellectual disability. *Journal of Intellectual Disability Research, 43,* 523–530.

Parsons, M. B., Cash, V. B., & Reid, D. H. (1989). Improving residential treatment services: Implementation and norm-referenced evaluation of a comprehensive management system. *Journal of Applied Behavior Analysis, 22,* 143–156.

Pretty, G., Rapley, M., & Bramston, P. (2002). Neighbourhood and community experience, and the quality of life of rural adolescents with and without an intellectual disability. *Journal of Intellectual and Developmental Disability, 27,* 106-116.

Reid, D. H. (1992). Recent developments in treating severe behavior disorders: Advances or impediments for residential services? *Behavioral Residential Treatment, 7,* 181–197.

Robertson, J., Emerson, E., Gregory, N., Hatton, C., Kessissoglou, S., Hallam, A., et al. (2001). Social networks of people with mental retardation in residential settings. *Mental Retardation, 39,* 201–214.

Romer, D., & Berkson, G. (1980). Social ecology of supervised communal facilities for mentally disabled adults: III. Predictors of social choice. *American Journal of Mental Deficiency, 85,* 243–252.

Romer, D., & Berkson, G. (1981). Social ecology of supervised communal facilities for mentally disabled adults: IV. Characteristics of social behavior. *American Journal of Mental Deficiency, 86,* 28–38.

Rosen, J. W., & Burchard, S. N. (1990). Community activities and social support networks: A social comparison of adults with and adults without mental retardation. *Education and Training in Mental Retardation, 25,* 193–204.

Rudolph, C., Lakin, K. C., Oslund, J. M., & Larson, W. (1998). Evaluation of outcomes and cost effectiveness of a community behavioral support and crisis response demonstration project. *Mental Retardation, 36,* 187–197.

Schalock, R. L. (2000). Three decades of quality of life. *Focus on Autism and Other Developmental Disabilities, 15,* 116–127.

Schwartz, A. A., Jacobson, J. W., & Holburn, S. C. (2000). Defining person centeredness: Results of two consensus methods. *Education and Training in Mental Retardation and Developmental Disabilities, 35,* 235–249.

Smith, C., Felce, D., Jones, E., & Lowe, K. (2002). Responsiveness to staff support: Evaluating the impact of individual characteristics on the effectiveness of active support training using a conditional probability approach. *Journal of Intellectual Disability Research, 46,* 594–604.

Stancliffe, R. J., Avery, B. H., & Smith, J. (2000). Personal control and the ecology of community living settings: Beyond living-unit size and type. *American Journal on Mental Retardation, 105,* 431–454.

Stancliffe, R. J., Hayden, M. F., & Lakin, K. C. (1999a). Effectiveness and quality of individual planning in residential settings: An analysis of outcomes. *Mental Retardation, 37,* 104–116.

Stancliffe, R. J., Hayden, M. F., & Lakin, K. C. (1999b). Effectiveness of challenging behavior IHP objectives in residential settings: A longitudinal study. *Mental Retardation, 37,* 482–493.

Stancliffe, R. J., Hayden, M. F., & Lakin, K. C. (1999c). Interventions for challenging behavior in residential settings. *American Journal on Mental Retardation, 104,* 364–375.

Stancliffe, R. J., & Keane, S. (2000). Outcomes and costs of community living: A matched comparison of group homes and semi-independent living. *Journal of Intellectual and Developmental Disability, 25,* 281–305.

Stancliffe, R. J., & Lakin, K. C. (1999). A longitudinal comparison of day services and outcomes of people who left institutions and those who stayed. *The Journal of the Association for Persons with Severe Handicaps, 24,* 44–57.

Tonge, B., & Einfeld, S. (2000). The trajectory of psychiatric disorders in young people with intellectual disabilities. *Australia and New Zealand Journal of Psychiatry, 34,* 80–84.

Ward, K. M., Trigler, J. S., & Pfeiffer, K. T. (2001). Community services, issues, and service gaps for individuals with developmental disabilities who exhibit inappropriate sexual behaviors. *Mental Retardation, 39,* 11–19.

9

Educational Service Interventions and Reforms

JAMES M. KAUFFMAN and
TIMOTHY J. LANDRUM

Education—more specifically, special education—plays a unique and central role in addressing the problems of students with developmental disabilities. Proposed reforms of general and special education are thus critically important issues for developmental disabilities. Failure at school is tantamount to failure at life for children and youths, as school is the occupation of the young. The primary purpose of educational service interventions is to help youngsters with developmental disabilities have a successful school experience. Reforms that advance this purpose are beneficial; those that undermine or preclude it are misguided at best. We explain the central role of education in children's lives, the necessity of special education and the nature of it, popular but misanthropic proposals for reform, and needed improvements in special education.

CENTRALITY OF ACADEMIC COMPETENCE

Helping students achieve academic competence is the central role of schools. Competence in basic academic skills is not the only goal of schooling, but schools are derelict if they do not do all they can to help students achieve such competence (Kauffman, 2002; Kauffman & Hallahan, 2005a; Kauffman, McGee, & Brigham, 2004).

Academic failure is one of the first signs of developmental disability in the context of school. Furthermore, remediation of academic deficits is one of the first lines of prevention of additional difficulties in school

JAMES M. KAUFFMAN and TIMOTHY J. LANDRUM • Department of Curriculum, Instruction, and Special Education, University of Virginia, Charlottesville, Virginia 22904-4273.

(e.g., Forness & Kavale, 2001; Lane, 1999; Manset-Williamson, St. John, Hu, & Gordon, 2002; Redden et al., 1999; Walker, Ramsey, & Gresham, 2004). Despite strong evidence that prevention of further academic failure and the emotional or behavioral difficulties that often follow depends on responding to the first indications of school failure, the response of schools has been slow. In current practice, academic and social failures are often allowed to become protracted and severe before intervention is mandated (Kauffman, 1999a, 2003a, 2003b, 2004, 2005a, 2005b).

School failure is undoubtedly linked to a variety of developmental disabilities, some of which may be a cause of and some of which occur as sequelae of academic failure. Despite this obvious link, effective instruction is often not the focus of schooling, or even the focus of special education (Kauffman, 1999b). Effective teaching often requires something that many contemporary reformers find objectionable—homogeneous grouping for instruction (Kauffman, Landrum, Mock, Sayeski, & Sayeski, 2005). Moreover, socialization and other appearances of normalization, such as inclusion in regular schools and classrooms, sometimes may be seen as more important than instruction. But our literature base is unequivocal; effective instruction should be the first consideration in the management of problem behavior, and relative homogeneity of learners is essential for the most effective instruction. Nevertheless, poor instruction is often overlooked as the breeding ground for behavior problems (Kauffman, Mostert, Trent, & Pullen, 2006), and heterogeneous grouping for instruction is often recommended in the face of evidence and logic to the contrary (Kauffman et al., 2005).

A cloak or appearance of academic competence fools few or none (Edgerton, 1967, 1993; Kauffman, 2003a). Actual literacy and numeracy are the essential foundation for independence and success in the social mainstream. If such academic competencies are not achievable even when our most powerful and sustained interventions are brought to bear, then actual competence (as opposed to an appearance or cloak) in daily living skills becomes all the more critical.

In short, the importance of competency in basic academic skills cannot be overstated. Helping students with developmental disabilities acquire such competence requires extraordinary (special) education, which is neither possible nor desirable for all students. Teaching children with developmental disabilities requires helping them learn social problem-solving skills in addition to academics, which in turn helps in solving one of the critical problems of society—youngsters who lack both academic skills and socially acceptable ways of solving their problems (Hune & Nelson, 2002; Kauffman, 2005a; Walker et al., 1998, 2004).

DIMENSIONS OF INSTRUCTION FOR STATISTICAL OUTLIERS

Special education is designed for students who are atypical in development, who are statistical outliers in a distribution of educational abilities.

Without it, some students are inevitably badly served (cf. Kauffman, 2002; Kauffman & Hallahan, 2005a). Education may be described as special because it differs from typical education in one or more of the following: (a) pacing or rate, (b) intensity, (c), relentlessness, (d) structure, (e) reinforcement, (f) pupil–teacher ratio, (g) curriculum, or (h) monitoring or assessment. These dimensions of teaching are continuously distributed. Therefore, the distinction between general and special education is somewhat indistinct, meaning that education can be "sort of" special, or "somewhat" special—indeed, education can be on the border between general and special. Although the line between general and special education is arbitrary and arguable (as is the line between having and not having a developmental disability), refusal to draw a line means abandonment of a critically important distinction. If we presume that special education does not really exist or cannot be distinguished from good general education, then many students will be poorly served.

Kauffman and Hallahan (2005a) point out that the distinction between general and special education is in fact a matter of degree. The degree of difference matters a great deal, just as does the degree of difference in student characteristics defining developmental disability. For some students, education that is "sort of" special is sufficient to help them achieve success, but for most students with disabilities, it is not. The following description of the dimensions of special education's specialness is based on the work of Kauffman and Hallahan (2005a).

Pacing or Rate

Rate of instruction may refer to either the pace with which a given lesson proceeds (i.e., the speed with which tasks are presented and responses are demanded) or the pace with which a student is lead through a body of knowledge (i.e., the speed with which the teacher builds concepts, discriminations, or competencies). Most students learn well with a typical pace of both types. Some students learn little or nothing unless the teacher alters the pace significantly.

Good instruction is paced at a proper rate for the child's ability to learn whatever is being taught (i.e., good instruction is relatively fast-paced *for learners with particular characteristics*). Students are presented tasks at what is, for them, a rapid rate, and they have frequent opportunities to respond. "Down time," in which no response is expected, is minimized. The pace is fast enough that the student is challenged and does not get bored, yet slow enough that the student can keep up. For some, "wait time" (i.e., allowable latency in responding) must be longer than for typical students. Special education for students with disabilities often must proceed more slowly through a given curriculum than is optimal for typical students.

Typical teachers are not taught to accommodate the extremes of pacing. Furthermore, typical teachers are not able to make such accommodations in the context of the regular classroom without jeopardizing the learning of typical students (see Berninger et al., 2002, and Zigmond, 2003).

Intensity

Typical students should perceive general education as intensely demanding, although many do not. Furthermore, many typical students have relatively few opportunities to respond. Regardless of attempts to reform general education by increasing its intensity for all students, some students with developmental disabilities require greater intensity than can be offered in regular classrooms. They may need additional trials, more practice or review, a longer period of instruction, and a more "fine-grained" curriculum (one with smaller steps or skills broken down further into components) than is appropriate for general education students, even those who are relatively low performers but do not have disabilities (see Foorman & Torgesen, 2001; Fuchs & Fuchs, 2001; Moody, Vaughn, Hughes, & Fischer, 2000).

Relentlessness

Good teachers give students as many repeated trials and as much review as they need. In good general education, the teacher moves on in the curriculum when most or all of the students have learned the concept or skill being taught. Sometimes, low performers are left behind because they have not mastered the idea or skill or not become competent in the subject matter. It cannot be otherwise in general education, else the majority of students would be held back in achievement.

Special education involves giving learners with developmental disabilities even more trials, more opportunities, more attention, and more instructional time. A teacher may eventually decide that trying to teach a given student a particular skill is useless and decide to teach something else. However, the tenacity, persistence, and relentlessness of the special education teacher go beyond what can be offered in general education. The teacher may try a variety of instructional approaches that the general education teacher does not know or cannot implement in the context of teaching a larger, general class of students. Moreover, the special education teacher does not abandon teaching a concept or skill to the student for the sake of the larger group that must move on (see Horner, Sugai, & Horner, 2000; Lewis, Colvin, & Sugai, 2000; Zigmond, 2003).

Structure

Structure refers to the (a) explicitness of rules and expectations, (b) regularity and predictability of routines, (c) amount of teacher direction, (d) tolerance for misbehavior or its precursors, and (e) immediacy, frequency, and explicitness of positive consequences for desirable behavior and negative consequences for unacceptable behavior. Most students do not need structure that is as "tight" as necessary for many students with developmental disabilities. There are limits to the amount of differentiation in structure that a teacher and class can manage. A given environment can no more be structured appropriately for every possible student than a given commercial outlet can meet the needs and desires of every possible customer. Special education teachers need special training in how to structure the learning environment for students who do not respond well to the structure of good general education classrooms (see Boyda, Zentall, & Feiko, 2002; Kauffman et al., 2006; Swanson & Hoskyn, 2001; Troia & Graham, 2002; Walker et al., 2004).

Reinforcement

Negative consequences (punishment) that are expertly used may have an important role in teaching and child rearing, but the key to a positive and supportive classroom environment is positive reinforcement (Landrum & Kauffman, 2006). Evidence obtained from decades of research has suggested that the general education classroom does not provide sufficient or effective reinforcement for the learning and appropriate behavior of children with disabilities (e.g., Strain, Lambert, Kerr, Stagg, & Lenkner, 1983). Well-trained special education teachers are skilled in finding and using positive reinforcement to support the learning and behavior of students who have special difficulty in school. They know that the following characteristics of reinforcement make it effective, and they modulate such reinforcement so that it is effective for the individual student: Immediacy, frequency, enthusiasm, eye contact, description of precisely what is being reinforced, anticipation of reward, and variety of reward (Rhode, Jenson, & Reavis, 1992; see also Boyda et al., 2002; Horner, Sugai, Todd, & Lewis-Palmer, 1999–2000; Kauffman et al., 2006; Shores & Wehby, 1999; Sutherland, Wehby, & Yoder, 2002). The typical general education classroom is not characterized by frequent positive reinforcement. Furthermore, the idea that rewarding good conduct is counterproductive has become popular among many general educators (see Kohn, 1993).

Pupil–Teacher Ratio

Special education has benefits in part because the teacher is responsible for a relatively small number of students. Special education is labor-intensive, demanding more adults per child than does general education. Reducing class size in general education or having two teachers in classes with students who have developmental disabilities may produce good results in some cases. However, in other cases, it is extremely unlikely that students will be well-taught except in a special class in which the number of students per adult is dramatically fewer than in general education (see Foorman & Torgesen, 2001; Rashotte, MacPhee, & Torgesen, 2001; Vaughn, Gersten, & Chard, 2000).

Curriculum

Some students with developmental disabilities can be successful in the general education curriculum, but many cannot be. However, even many of those who can successfully pursue the regular curriculum may need especially precise teaching (special education) in order to benefit from the regular curriculum. For some students with developmental disabilities, the general education curriculum is either inappropriate or does not contain all the subjects or features they need (Bouck, 2004). For example, some students need intensive, explicit instruction in social skills or basic academic skills. Students with severe mental retardation may require intensive and explicit teaching in skills that most students would find demeaning—basic communication, dressing, toileting, self-feeding or chewing and swallowing, and other self-care or daily living skills. The general education curriculum may be appropriate for most students, even for many students with developmental disabilities. However, some students with milder disabilities require curricula not needed by most students, or they may need additional curricula if they are to be able to understand and respond correctly to the standard curriculum (see Bouck, 2004; Coyne, Kameenui, & Simmons, 2001; Hallahan & Kauffman, 2006; Troia & Graham, 2002).

Monitoring or Assessment

Good teachers check frequently on students' progress, but it is neither necessary nor feasible to monitor and assess the performance of most students as frequently or closely as is required for teaching those with developmental disabilities. Adequate training of special education teachers includes instruction in how to monitor students' progress daily. Although not essential for typical students, this intense level of monitoring is necessary for those with special problems in learning. Progress is often slow when special education is initiated, and both students with developmental disabilities and their teachers need to be aware of progress, even if it is far below that of average students. Another hallmark of good special education—adapting instruction (altering materials, strategies, contingencies, etc.) when progress is deemed insufficient—depends entirely on continuous monitoring of student performance (see Espin, Busch, Shin, & Kruschwitz, 2001; Fletcher, Foorman, & Boudousquie, 2002; Walker & Sprague, 1999).

Education can be sort of special in structure (for example) or very special along all the dimensions of instruction (Kauffman & Hallahan, 2005a). That is, specialness in instruction is continuously distributed; it is not a discrete variable, not all-or-nothing, not on-or-off, 0-or-1. The degree of specialness possibly may depend on three primary factors: (a) a teacher who has special training and is truly expert in implementing teaching procedures with extraordinary precision, (b) a small and relatively homogeneous group of students, and (c) a place in which teacher and students can work without undue interference or demands from others and in which their work does not compete with or impede the education of other students. One researcher and teacher educator has stated,

> Special education was once worth receiving; it could be again. In many schools, it is not now. Here is where practitioners, policymakers, advocates, and researchers in special education need

to focus—on defining the nature of special education and the competencies of the teachers who will deliver it (Zigmond, 1997, p. 389).

The focus on instruction has been downplayed in the movement toward full inclusion of students with developmental disabilities in regular schools and classrooms (Hall, 2002; Mock & Kauffman, 2002, 2005). The emphasis on consultation between special education and general education teachers rather than direct service to students with developmental disabilities by special educators has exacerbated this lack of focus on specialized instruction and training. Making special education reliably what it should be awaits the rediscovery of this focus.

It is unfortunate that statements about the strengths of special education and calls for its renewal may connote for some a criticism of general education and its teachers. We have described the ways that special education is special, and some critics might infer from this argument that we mean to cast general education as something of less value or less effective than special education. In fact, general education is often quite effective in fulfilling its mission to serve a large subset of all students, with curriculum and methods designed to meet their needs and teachers trained to teach them well. Special education is nothing more than *different* education— different methods and materials, provided by differently trained educators, sometimes using different curriculum and sometimes using the general curriculum—designed to meet the different needs of a smaller subset of students. Special education is not inherently superior to general education, and special education teachers are not inherently better teachers than the general education teachers. But data seem to suggest that special education is superior to general education *for many students with developmental disabilities*, just as general education should be superior to special education for most students without disabilities (for further discussion of evidence of special education's effectiveness for students with disabilities, see Hallahan & Kauffman, 2006; Hanushek, Kain, & Rivkin, 2002; Zigmond, 1997). The argument that one form of education can serve all students (i.e., each and every student) well is specious.

POPULAR SPECIAL EDUCATION REFORM PROPOSALS

The central issue in proposals for reforming special education has been place, not instruction (Crockett & Kauffman, 1999; Kauffman & Hallahan, 1995, 2005b; Mock & Kauffman, 2005). Smith (2002) refers to "place-based education" without reference to special education reform per se. However, many proposals for reforming special education have made place the implicit issue, and some have explicitly defined the issue as the place of instruction, not instruction itself:

> "Place" is the issue... *There is nothing pervasively wrong with special education.* What is being questioned is not the interventions and knowledge that have been acquired through special

education training and research. Rather, what is being challenged is the location where these supports are being provided
to students (Blackman, 1992, p. 29, italics in original).

Others have suggested a very similar view, that student placement—
specifically, in regular classrooms—is the critical change that will reform
special education (e.g., Lipsky & Gartner, 1996; Stainback & Stainback,
1991). However, the idea that placement in general education, better
known as "inclusion," is the key has been challenged (see Crockett &
Kauffman, 2001; Hall, 2002; Kauffman, 1995, 2002; Kauffman, Bantz, &
McCullough, 2002; Kauffman & Hallahan, 1995, 1997, 2005b; Zigmond,
2003):

> The idea that place or location is prepotent over the details of in-
> struction is a particularly noxious delusion when special educa-
> tion is under attack. The delusion is especially noxious because
> it distracts attention from important issues and holds out the
> false hope that the [full inclusion movement] will result in bet-
> ter instruction for students with disabilities while undercutting
> fiscal support for special education (Mock & Kauffman, 2005,
> p. 114).

Special education is under attack. It has been referred to in the popular press as a "the gold-plated garbage can of American schooling" (Fisher,
2001; see also Bolick, 2001; Cottle, 2001). It is also said by some to be
defective in concept and structure, sometimes with reference to the superiority of a "postmodern" view of disabilities (e.g., Danforth, 2004; Danforth &
Rhodes, 1997; Gallagher, 2004). But postmodernism in education (special
education in particular) is a prescription for reform disaster (see Kauffman,
2002; Sasso, 2001). As one psychologist critic said of postmodernism,
"All it can offer, by its own admission, is word games—word games that
lead nowhere and achieve nothing. Like anthrax of the intellect, if allowed
into mainstream psychology, postmodernism will poison the field" (Locke,
2002, p. 458).

The rationale for restructuring for inclusion is based on presumptive
moral values, not research data showing that one model is superior to another in outcomes. But the presumed moral values are not connected to
realities, rendering them meaningless (see Kauffman, 2003a, 2003b). Inclusion is motivated by the observation that an equitable society demands
equal access—including the equal access of children with developmental
disabilities to schools, classrooms, and curricula. The ideology of full inclusion suggests that this equal access can be achieved only when *all* children
(each and every one), including those with developmental disabilities, are
included in neighborhood schools and regular classes, taking their rightful
places alongside their neighbors and peers who have not been identified
as having disabilities. Unfortunately, it ignores the considerable evidence
that children and adults need affiliation, for at least some of the time, with
others like themselves (Hall, 2002).

However, neither research nor parental reflections on full inclusion for
their children with developmental disabilities supports the idea of reform

for full inclusion (e.g., Kauffman & Hallahan, 2005b; Mock & Kauffman, 2005; Palmer, Fuller, Arora, & Nelson, 2001). First, teachers simply cannot teach a general education class effectively and at the same time offer the intensive, focused, relentless instruction that many children with disabilities require if they are to make reasonable progress (Zigmond, 2003). Second, although data do suggest that *some* students with developmental disabilities can be included in general education, no data suggest that *all* students can be included successfully. Palmer et al. reviewed the pros and cons of full inclusion and reported one parent's observations as follows:

> I have two children with disabilities; this survey is about one. He is uncomfortable around other children and in close spaces. He expresses dislikes of normal students. He is also disliked by them and they tell me about his behavior when I'm on campus. Mainstreaming to a large extent would not do anyone service in this case.

> My other son has been fully and successfully mainstreamed for years. I know the downfalls, I know the up side. I consider mainstreaming as something that *must be decided on a case-by-case basis*. Like any other fad, it is being evangelized as a cure-all. It isn't. It is terrific in some cases. In others, it is child abuse (p. 482).

Such arguments make obvious on purely pragmatic grounds the problems inherent in educating *all* students in the general classroom. Others and we have argued elsewhere that neither logical analyses nor empirical data support the notion of full inclusion (e.g., Crockett & Kauffman, 1999, 2001; Hall, 2002; Kauffman & Hallahan, 1993, 1997, 2005b; Landrum, Tankersley, & Kauffman, 2003; MacMillan, Gresham, & Forness, 1996; Mock & Kauffman, 2005; Simpson, 2004).

Arguments invoking "equal access" probably provide unnecessary fuel to already incendiary debates about reform. For example, we have suggested that the general curriculum may not be "accessible" to all students, and particularly to those with more severe developmental disabilities. Does this mean that students are not "allowed" to be involved in the general curriculum, are "denied access," or that barriers are set up (or not removed) that prevent them from accessing this curriculum? Certainly not. Accessibility implies appropriate, cognitive access that results in observable learning in domains that are appropriate to a given student's needs and capabilities. Merely exposing students to a particular curriculum through simple physical arrangement does not necessarily provide access. Nor does the pretense of "parallel" work provide true access. Such pretense is analogous to interpreting parallel play as social interaction.

Current criticisms of special education also include the observation that it does not produce student achievement comparable to that of general education and that only a small percentage of students are decertified and exit special education during their school years. Thus, special education is said to have unacceptably low and disappointing outcomes (see Bolick, 2001; Cottle, 2001; Lipsky & Gartner, 1996). Apparently, current reform proponents have bought into Deno's (1970) notion that special education should work itself out of business by (a) turning over to general educators the instructional techniques developed by special educators and (b) improving students' performance in the general education curriculum to the point at which they are no longer considered to have disabilities. We see this as somewhat like the suggestion that cardiac surgeons could turn over their practice to general medical practitioners (or to general surgeons) and, hence, work themselves out of business. Kauffman (2002) has pointed out that most of the disabilities that result in students receiving special education are *developmental* disabilities—they are life-long conditions that can be treated competently but have no cure. Indeed, an ironic corollary to arguments toward reform and full inclusion may be a shrinking of sentiment that people with disabilities need and deserve sustained application of the best interventions and supports that special education has to offer.

Although the popular reform rhetoric of full inclusion (sometimes argued under the guise of the "integration" of special and general education) finds little or no support in empirical data, it seems obvious to us (and to most observers) that special education is in need of improvement. Moreover, the recent reauthorization of the Individuals with Disabilities Education Act (i.e., the Individuals with Disabilities Education Improvement Act of 2004), particularly its attempt to align special education with the No Child Left Behind Act of 2002 (NCLB), promises no substantive improvement in special education. Indeed, the report of the President's Commission on Excellence in Special Education and the expectation of NCLB that averages for students with disabilities match those of students without disabilities is nothing short of farce (see Kauffman, 2004, 2005c).

Special education often is not and frequently has not been what it should be. It must become again the specialized instruction that it was conceptualized to be at the time of its origin (Kauffman & Hallahan, 2005a).

NEEDED IMPROVEMENTS IN SPECIAL EDUCATION

The needed improvements in special education include conceptual changes as well as changes in practice. However, the conceptual and practical changes are not those highlighted in historical or current reform rhetoric (Kauffman & Landrum, 2006).

One conceptual change is that improved instruction, not place, must become the central issue. That is, special education must come to mean special instruction along the dimensions we discussed earlier. A second conceptual change involves outcomes. Neither the expectation that the achievement of special education students will approximate that of general education students nor the expectation that a high percentage of students with disabilities will be decertified or lose their identity as having a disability is rational. A third needed conceptual change is that special education must be distinctively different from general education. Although education can be "sort of" or marginally special, if a line separating special from general education is not drawn, then special education's distinctiveness or identity will be lost, and with it the possibility of its viability.

Instruction

Special education can be no better than the instruction it entails. The instruction entails special expertise in the dimensions we discussed earlier. It cannot be delivered primarily by instructional aides. Paraprofessionals are important components of both general and special education, but their role is to carry out activities at the direction of a fully trained professional who understands and selects curriculum and instructional strategies and carefully monitors their work with students.

Turning special education toward the special instruction that Zigmond (1997, 2003) and Kauffman and Hallahan (2005a) describe will not be easy, and it cannot be accomplished quickly. It will demand better training of teacher educators, who will train a cadre of teachers who value evidence-based practice (see Forness, Kavale, Blum, & Lloyd, 1997; Landrum et al., 2003; Lloyd, Forness, & Kavale, 1998). Thus, the improvement of instruction in special education is a long-term project, and it will require the adoption of more direct, explicit, teacher-controlled, and content-oriented instruction than is currently popular.

Outcomes

Expectations of the outcomes of special education must be reasonable. The value of special education is not determined by the extent to which the achievement of students receiving it approximate the achievement of those not receiving it, but the extent to which the achievement of students receiving it is higher than it would have been had they not received it (see Hanushek et al., 2002). Research of the value of special education leaves much to be desired. Comparisons of various service delivery options have been seriously compromised, as random assignment of students or schools to options differing along known dimensions has not been possible (see Hallahan & Kauffman, 1994, 2006; Kauffman & Hallahan, 1993; Simpson, 2004).

The research question needing an answer is not whether differences in achievement attributable to disabilities can be made to disappear but whether special education produces better achievement than no special education for students with disabilities. Anecdotal evidence (e.g., Palmer et al., 2001) and statistical evidence (e.g., Hanushek et al., 2002) seem to suggest that special education is better than no special education for students with developmental disabilities. Experimental data on outcomes are needed, but it is important that research addresses the pertinent question. It is absolutely predictable that "The outcomes used to judge the effectiveness of general education are not always appropriate as criteria for judging the effectiveness of special education" (Kauffman & Hallahan, 1993, p. 94).

Distinctiveness

Much of the current reform rhetoric recommends merging or integrating general and special education. We contend that special education is already an integral part of public education and that the loss of its identity or distinctiveness can only result in its demise or ineffectiveness (see Kauffman, 1999–2000). Goodlad (1990) describes how teacher education requires distinctiveness if it is to be viable in the context of a university. He argues that teacher education requires a clear focus, identity, and authority, including special personnel dedicated to the task and its own budget. Kauffman and Hallahan (1993) argue that the same is true for special education—that without its clear and distinctive focus, identity, authority, personnel, and budget it becomes a derelict enterprise.

Special education needs to be both separate from and better than general education *for the students it serves* (Kauffman et al., 2002). Our contention is that special education needs to be unapologetically and clearly special—*different* from general education (Kauffman & Hallahan, 2005a; Landrum et al., 2003). It can be such a distinctive and invaluable part of public education in America. Just as any subunits of a larger entity, be it military, commercial, or educational, it will require the same distinctions needed by teacher education described so eloquently by Goodlad (1990).

SUMMARY

The education of students with developmental disabilities requires that schools do what they do at peak capacity. We have argued that it is the role of schools to ensure the achievement of the students they serve. But the most efficient model for adequately schooling students whose abilities fall in a typical range (i.e., regular education) is clearly not the most efficient or effective model for ensuring the achievement of students with developmental disabilities—at least not *all* of them. Some students with developmental disabilities can and should benefit from the general curriculum. Moreover, some can benefit from that curriculum with the general instruction provided to all students by general education teachers, but others will need more intensive, specialized instruction and support to benefit meaningfully from the general curriculum. We think such special instruction is currently available only from special education teachers and that it is not feasible for general education teachers to offer such special education. Finally, for students with more significant developmental disabilities, the general curriculum is not only inaccessible but represents a misguided goal that in practice can prevent students from learning the more necessary basic academic, social, self-care, and daily living skills they need to maximize their achievement in school and their independence beyond school.

We have not argued that special education is perfect or even close to it, and we have delineated several reforms that are necessary if special education is to improve and fulfill its original intent. Most important among these improvements may be the need for special education to reclaim its identity by unabashedly focusing on the uniqueness of its methods and procedures, and, in turn, highlighting the clear benefits it provides to students with developmental disabilities beyond what they may experience from general education alone.

REFERENCES

Berninger, V. W., Abbott, R. D., Vermeulen, K., Ogier, S., Brooksher, R., Zook, D., et al. (2002). Comparison of faster and slower responders to early intervention in reading: Differentiating features of their language profiles. *Learning Disability Quarterly, 25,* 59–76.

Blackman, H. P. (1992). Surmounting the disability of isolation. *The School Administrator, 49*(2), 28–29.

Bolick, C. (2001, September 5). A bad IDEA is disabling public schools. *Education Week, 21*(1), 56–63.

Bouck, E. C. (2004). Exploring secondary special education for mild mental impairment. *Remedial and Special Education, 25,* 367–382.

Boyda, S. D., Zentall, S. S., & Feiko, D. J. K. (2002). The relationship between teacher practices and the task-appropriate and social behavior of students with behavioral disorders. *Behavioral Disorders, 27,* 236–255.

Cottle, M. (2001, June 18). Reform school: Jeffords kills special ed. *The New Republic,* pp. 14–15.

Coyne, M. D., Kameenui, E. J., & Simmons, D. C. (2001). Prevention and intervention in beginning reading: Two complex systems. *Learning Disabilities Research and Practice, 16,* 62–73.

Crockett, J. B., & Kauffman, J. M. (1999). *The least restrictive environment: Its origins and interpretations in special education.* Mahwah, NJ: Erlbaum.

Crockett, J. B., & Kauffman, J. M. (2001). The concept of the least restrictive environment and learning disabilities: Least restrictive of what? Reflections on Cruickshank's 1977 guest editorial for the *Journal of Learning Disabilitie*s. In D. P. Hallahan & B. K. Keogh (Eds.), *Research and global perspectives in learning disabilities* (pp. 147–166). Mahwah, NJ: Erlbaum.

Danforth, S. (2004). The "postmodern" heresy in special education: A sociological analysis. *Mental Retardation, 42,* 445–458.

Danforth, S., & Rhodes, W. C. (1997). Deconstructing disability: A philosophy for inclusion. *Remedial and Special Education, 18,* 357–366.

Deno, E. (1970). Special education as developmental capital. *Exceptional Children, 37,* 229–237.

Edgerton, R. B. (1967). *The cloak of competence: Stigma in the lives of the mentally retarded.* Berkeley: University of California Press.

Edgerton, R. B. (1993). *The cloak of competence* (revised and updated). Berkeley: University of California Press.

Espin, C. A., Busch, T. W., Shin, J., & Kruschwitz, R. (2001). Curriculum-based measurement in the content areas: Validity of vocabulary-matching as an indicator of performance in social studies. *Learning Disabilities Research and Practice, 16,* 142–151.

Fisher, M. (2001, December 13). Students still taking the fall for DC schools. *The Washington Post,* pp. B1–B4.

Fletcher, J. M., Foorman, B. R., & Boudousquie, A. (2002). Assessment of reading and learning disabilities: A research-based intervention-oriented approach. *Journal of School Psychology, 40,* 27–63.

Foorman, B. R., & Torgesen, J. (2001). Critical elements of classroom and small group instruction to promote reading success in all children. *Learning Disabilities Research and Practice, 16,* 203–212.

Forness, S. R., & Kavale, K. A. (2001). Reflections on the future of prevention. *Preventing School Failure, 45,* 75–81.

Forness, S. R., Kavale, K. A., Blum, I. M., & Lloyd, J. W. (1997). What works in special education and related services: Using meta-analysis to guide practice. *Teaching Exceptional Children, 29*(6), 4–9.

Fuchs, L. S., & Fuchs, D. (2001). Principles for the prevention and intervention of mathematics difficulties. *Learning Disabilities Research and Practice, 16,* 85–95.

Gallagher, D. J. (Ed.). (2004). *Challenging orthodoxy in special education: Disserting voices.* Denver, CO: Love.

Goodlad, J. I. (1990). *Teachers for our nation's schools.* San Francisco: Jossey-Bass.

Hall, J. P. (2002). Narrowing the breach: Can disability culture and full educational inclusion be reconciled? *Journal of Disability Policy Studies, 13,* 144–152.

Hallahan, D. P., & Kauffman, J. M. (1994). Toward a culture of disability in the aftermath of Deno and Dunn. *Journal of Special Education, 27,* 496–508.

Hallahan, D. P., & Kauffman, J. M. (2006). *Exceptional learners: Introduction to special education* (10th ed.). Boston: Allyn & Bacon.

Hanushek, E. A., Kain, J. F., & Rivkin, S. G. (2002). Inferring program effects for special populations: Does special education raise achievement for students with disabilities? *Review of Economics and Statistics, 84,* 584–599.

Horner, R. H., Sugai, G., & Horner, H. F. (2000). A schoolwide approach to student discipline. *School Administrator, 57,* 20–23.

Horner, R. H., Sugai, G., Todd, A. W., & Lewis-Palmer, T. (1999–2000). Elements of behavior support plans: A technical brief. *Exceptionality, 8,* 205–215.

Hune, J. B., & Nelson, C. M. (2002). Effects of teaching a problem-solving strategy on preschool children with problem behavior. *Behavioral Disorders, 27,* 185–207.

Kauffman, J. M. (1995). Why we must celebrate a diversity of restrictive environments. *Learning Disabilities Research and Practice, 10,* 225–232.

Kauffman, J. M. (1999a). How we prevent the prevention of emotional and behavioral disorders. *Exceptional Children, 65,* 448–468.

Kauffman, J. M. (1999b). Today's special education and its messages for tomorrow. *Journal of Special Education, 32,* 244–254.

Kauffman, J. M. (1999–2000). The special education story: Obituary, accident report, conversion experience, reincarnation, or none of the above? *Exceptionality, 8*(1), 61–71.

Kauffman, J. M. (2002). *Education deform: Bright people sometimes say stupid things about education.* Lanham, MD: Scarecrow Education.

Kauffman, J. M. (2003a). Perspectives: Appearances, stigma, and prevention. *Remedial and Special Education, 24,* 195–198.

Kauffman, J. M. (2003b). Reflections on the field. *Behavioral Disorders, 28,* 205–208.

Kauffman, J. M. (2004). The president's commission and the devaluation of special education. *Education and Treatment of Children, 27,* 307–324.

Kauffman, J. M. (2005a). *Characteristics of emotional and behavioral disorders of children and youth* (8th ed.). Upper Saddle River, NJ: Prentice-Hall.

Kauffman, J. M. (2005b). How we prevent the prevention of emotional and behavioural difficulties in education. In P. Clough, P. Garner, J. T. Pardeck, & F. K. O. Yuen (Eds.), *Handbook of emotional and behavioural difficulties* (pp. 429–440). London: Sage.

Kauffman, J. M. (2005c). Waving to Ray Charles: Missing the meaning of disability. *Phi Delta Kappan, 86,* 520–521, 524.

Kauffman, J. M., Bantz, J., & McCullough, J. (2002). Separate and better: A special public school class for students with emotional and behavioral disorders. *Exceptionality, 10,* 149–170.

Kauffman, J. M., & Hallahan, D. P. (1993). Toward a comprehensive delivery system for special education. In J. I. Goodlad & T. C. Lovitt (Eds.), *Integrating general and special education* (pp. 73-102). Columbus, OH: Merrill/Macmillan.

Kauffman, J. M., & Hallahan, D. P. (Eds.). (1995). *The illusion of full inclusion: A comprehensive critique of a current special education bandwagon.* Austin, TX: Pro-Ed.

Kauffman, J. M., & Hallahan, D. P. (1997). A diversity of restrictive environments: Placement as a problem of social ecology. In J. W. Lloyd, E. J. Kameenui, & D. Chard (Eds.), *Issues in educating students with disabilities* (pp. 325–342). Hillsdale, NJ: Erlbaum.

Kauffman, J. M., & Hallahan, D. P. (2005a). S*pecial education: What it is and why we need it.* Boston: Allyn & Bacon.

Kauffman, J. M., & Hallahan, D. P. (Eds.). (2005b). *The illusion of full inclusion: A comprehensive critique of a current special education bandwagon* (2nd ed.). Austin, TX: Pro-Ed.

Kauffman, J. M., & Landrum, T. J. (2006). *Children and youth with emotional and behavioral disorders: A history of their education.* Austin, TX: Pro-Ed.

Kauffman, J. M., Landrum, T. J., Mock, D. R., Sayeski, B., & Sayeski, K. L. (2005). Diverse knowledge and skills require a diversity of instructional groups: A position statement. *Remedial and Special Education, 26,* 2–6.

Kauffman, J. M., McGee, K., & Brigham, M. (2004). Enabling or disabling? Observations on changes in the purposes and outcomes of special education. *Phi Delta Kappan, 85,* 613–620.

Kauffman, J. M., Mostert, M. P., Trent, S. C., & Pullen, P. L. (2006). *Managing classroom behavior: A reflective case-based approach* (4th ed.). Boston: Allyn & Bacon.

Kohn, A. (1993). *Punished by rewards.* Boston: Houghton Mifflin.

Landrum, T. J., & Kauffman, J. M. (2006). Behavioral approaches to classroom management. In C. M. Evertson & C. S. Weinstein (Eds.), *Handbook of classroom management: Research, practice, and contemporary issues* (pp. 47–71). Mahwah, NJ: Erlbaum.

Landrum, J. T., Tankersley, M., & Kauffman, J. M. (2003). What's special about special education for students with emotional and behavioral disorders? *Journal of Special Education, 37,* 148–156.

Lane, K. L. (1999). Young students at risk for antisocial behavior: The utility of academic and social skills interventions. *Journal of Emotional and Behavioral Disorders, 7,* 211–223.

Lewis, T. J., Colvin, G., & Sugai, G. (2000). The effects of pre-correction and active supervision on the recess behavior of elementary students. *Education and Treatment of Children, 23,* 109–121.

Lipsky, D. K., & Gartner, A. (1996). Equity requires inclusion: The future for all students with disabilities. In C. Christensen & F. Rizvi (Eds.), *Disability and the dilemmas of education and justice* (pp. 144–155). Philadelphia: Open University Press.

Lloyd, J. W., Forness, S. R., & Kavale, K. A. (1998). Some methods are more effective. *Intervention in School and Clinic, 33*(1), 195–200.

Locke, E. A. (2002). The dead end of postmodernism. *American Psychologist, 57,* 458.

MacMillan, D. L., Gresham, F. M., & Forness, S. R. (1996). Full inclusion: An empirical perspective. *Behavioral Disorders, 21,* 154–159.

Manset-Williamson, G., St. John, E., Hu, S., & Gordon, D. (2002). Early literacy practices as predictors of reading related outcomes: Test scores, test passing rates, retention, and special education referral. *Exceptionality, 10,* 11–28.

Mock, D., & Kauffman, J. M. (2002). Preparing teachers for full inclusion: Is it possible? *Teacher Educator, 37,* 202–215.

Mock, D. R., & Kauffman, J. M. (2005). Controversial therapies for developmental disabilities: Fad, fashion, and science in professional practice. In J. W. Jacobson, J. A. Mulick, & R. M. Foxx (Eds.), *Fads: Dubious and improbable treatments for developmental disabilities* (pp. 113–128). Mahwah, NJ: Erlbaum.

Moody, S. W., Vaughn, S., Hughes, M. T., & Fischer, M. (2000). Reading instruction in the resource room: Set up for failure. *Exceptional Children, 66,* 305–316.

Palmer, D. S., Fuller, K., Arora, T., & Nelson, M. (2001). Taking sides: Parent views on inclusion for their children with severe disabilities. *Exceptional Children, 67,* 467–484.

Rashotte, C. A., MacPhee, K., & Torgesen, J. K. (2001). The effectiveness of a group reading instruction program with poor readers in multiple grades. *Learning Disability Quarterly, 24,* 119–134.

Redden, S. C., Forness, S. R., Ramey, S. L., Ramey, C. T., Zima, B. T., Brezausek, C. M., et al. (1999). Head Start children at third grade: Preliminary special education identification and placement of children with emotional, learning, and related disabilities. *Journal of Child and Family Studies, 8,* 285–303.

Rhode, G., Jenson, W. R., & Reavis, H. K. (1992). *The tough kid book: Practical classroom management strategies.* Longmont, CA: Sopris West.

Sasso, G. M. (2001). The retreat from inquiry and knowledge in special education. *Journal of Special Education, 34,* 178–193.

Shores, R. E, & Wehby, J. H. (1999). Analyzing the classroom social behavior of students with EBD. *Journal of Emotional and Behavioral Disorders, 7,* 194–199.

Simpson, R. L. (2004). Inclusion of students with behavior disorders in general education settings: Research and measurement issues. *Behavioral Disorders, 30,* 19–31.

Smith, G. A. (2002). Place-based education: Learning to be where we are. *Phi Delta Kappan, 83,* 584–594.

Stainback, W., & Stainback, S. (1991). A rational for integration and restructuring: A synopsis. In J. W. Lloyd, N. N. Singh, & A. C. Repp (Eds.), *The regular education initiative: Alternative perspectives on concepts, issues, and models* (pp. 225–239). Sycamore, IL: Sycamore.

Strain, P. S., Lambert, D. L., Kerr, M. M., Stagg, V., & Lenkner, D. A. (1983). Naturalistic assessment of children's compliance to teachers' requests and consequences for compliance. *Journal of Applied Behavior Analysis, 16,* 243–249.

Sutherland, K. S., Wehby, J. H., & Yoder, P. J. (2002). Examination of the relationship between teacher praise and opportunities for students with EBD to respond to academic requests. *Journal of Emotional and Behavioral Disorders, 10,* 5–13.

Swanson, H. L., & Hoskyn, M. (2001). Instructing adolescents with learning disabilities: A component and composite analysis. *Learning Disabilities Research and Practice, 16,* 109–119.

Troia, G. A., & Graham, S. (2002). The effectiveness of a highly explicit, teacher directed strategy instruction routine: Changing the writing performance of students with learning disabilities. *Journal of Learning Disabilities, 35,* 290–305.

Vaughn, S., Gersten, R., & Chard, D. J. (2000). The underlying message in LD intervention research: Findings from research syntheses. *Exceptional Children, 67,* 99–114.

Walker, H. M., Forness, S. R., Kauffman, J. M., Epstein, M. H., Gresham, F. M., Nelson, C. M., et al. (1998). Macro-social validation: Referencing outcomes in behavioral disorders to societal issues and problems. *Behavioral Disorders, 24,* 7–18.

Walker, H. M., Ramsey, E., & Gresham, F. M. (2004). *Antisocial behavior in school: Strategies and best practices* (2nd ed.). Pacific Grove, CA: Brooks/Cole.

Walker, H. M., & Sprague, J. R. (1999) Longitudinal research and functional behavioral assessment issues. *Behavioral Disorders, 24,* 335–337.

Zigmond, N. (1997). Educating students with disabilities: The future of special education. In J. W. Lloyd, E. J. Kameenui, & D. Chard (Eds.), *Issues in educating students with disabilities* (pp. 377–390). Mahwah, NJ: Erlbaum.

Zigmond, N. (2003). Where should students with disabilities receive special education services? Is one place better than another? *Journal of Special Education, 37,* 193–199.

10

Psychological Services for Older Adults with Intellectual Disabilities

JAMES P. ACQUILANO, PHILIP W. DAVIDSON, and MATTHEW P. JANICKI[1]

In this chapter, we review the psychological needs and service provisions for older adults with an intellectual disability (ID). The reader will be directed toward research that identifies an increasing longevity, concomitant increases in aging-related morbidities, and psychosocial factors. Specific aging-related conditions will be discussed, along with their impact on functional status and mental health, including a discussion of the complexity of differential diagnosis and the usefulness of comprehensive assessment.

BACKGROUND

Aging in Persons with ID: General Trends

There has been a general trend toward an increasing longevity for individuals with ID. For example, Yang, Rasmussen, and Friedman (2002) studied mortality associated with Down syndrome (DS) in the United States from 1983 to 1997 and identified an increase in the median age at death

JAMES P. ACQUILANO • Comprehensive Geriatric Assessment Clinic, Finger Lakes Developmental Disabilities Service Office, Rochester, New York 14620. **PHILIP W. DAVIDSON** • Strong Center for Developmental Disabilities, Golisano Children's Hospital at Strong, Rochester, New York 14642. **MATTHEW P. JANICKI** • RRTC on Aging and Developmental Disabilities, University of Illinois at Chicago, Chicago, Illinois 60608.

[1] This chapter is dedicated to John W. Jacobson, Ph.D., a colleague, collaborator and good friend of the second and third authors for over three decades. His tragic, untimely death is an immeasurable loss to our entire field.

during this time frame. The median age at death increased from 25 to 49 years during that period, an average increase of 1.7 years per year of the study. This increase was eight times greater than the increase in the median age at death for the general population during the same time period. Individuals with DS have enjoyed an increase in health care utilization during this time frame, as well as the interventions to address congenital heart conditions, thereby allowing for this increase (Yang et al., 2002). It is expected that individuals with ID, but not DS, will have similar life expectancies as people without ID (Doka & Lavin, 2003).

The concept of what constitutes being "older" is arbitrary and varies depending on the population and social factors. Individuals with intellectual disabilities (ID) may be more predisposed to the development of early onset aging (Doka & Lavin, 2003). The authors also suggest that estimating the number of older individuals with ID becomes complicated due to the arbitrariness of the concept. Also, some older individuals have never accessed the developmental disability service systems and therefore are not included in prevalence estimates. The deinstitutionalization process has contributed to this increased longevity through removal of factors that contributed to a decreased life span.

This increased longevity provides an additional stress to service delivery systems that had not previously encountered such an increase in longevity (Bigby, 2002).

Psychological Needs of Older Persons with ID

The psychological needs of persons with ID vary with age. Concepts such as retirement, bereavement, and acceptance of mortality are of more concern for older individuals than for a younger cohort (Thorpe, Davidson, & Janicki, 2001). Older adults with ID who have had a lifetime of routinization and limited resources may perceive a minor change brought on by typical late onset aging conditions, such as arthritis, as a crisis (Doka & Lavin, 2003).

Differences Between Older Persons with and Without ID and the Need for Specialized Services

Older individuals with ID experience the same age-related physiological changes as older adults without ID. These aging-related changes may be complicated by limited social and environmental experiences and communication skills. Individuals with ID are more likely to have lived in congregate settings. These settings are typically designed to meet the needs of the typical person with ID and may not be specific to the individual needs of a given individual (Hutchings, Olsen, & Ehrenkrantz, 2000). Limitations in social experiences may restrict the availability of social supports that the typical person without ID has access to. The diagnosis of medical conditions is complicated by communication skills; in addition the presence of comorbid conditions diminishes the ability to diagnose psychiatric conditions (Thorpe, 1999).

GAPS IN PSYCHOLOGICAL SERVICES

As people with ID age their needs change from a striving for independence to an increased reliance on caregivers for support. This change in needs requires a concomitant change in service delivery. Systems, however, are slower to change than are individuals and it is incumbent upon them to adjust the provision of services to meet this aging population (Ansello & Janicki, 2000). In the midst of this process, it is imperative that these individuals who are experiencing aging-related influences are included in the identification of these additional supports. The need for self-direction and a person-centered approach do not diminish with age. In fact, these older individuals may be more in need of a person-centered approach as they were more likely to have experienced the dehumanization of congregate care.

Functional Decline and its Effects on Healthy Aging

It is suspected that dementia is being over-diagnosed and other age-related diagnoses and mental health factors are either not being diagnosed or discounted as contributing to functional decline (Henderson & Davidson, 2000; Tsiouris & Patti, 1997). Dementia is one of a multitude of aging-related conditions that can cause functional decline in individuals with ID. Others include congenital heart conditions, hypothyroidism, hearing and visual impairments, cerebral palsy, gastric disorders, depression, and other mental health issues (Burt, 1999; Burt et al., 1998; Burt, Loveland, & Lewis, 1992; Evenhuis, 1995a, 1995b, 1997; Prasher & Chung, 1996; Prasher & Hall, 1996; Roeden & Zitman, 1995; Sung et al., 1997; van Schrojenstein Lantman-deValk et al., 1997). Increasing visual and hearing impairments with age has been identified (Evenhuis, 1995a, 1995b; Roeden & Zitman, 1995) and these conditions can result in functional impairment. An individual with a sensory deficit can become confused and overwhelmed by the environment. An increase in organ system morbidity (OSM) has been identified with age (Evenhuis, 1997; Janicki et al., 2002) and absence of OSM has been correlated with functional independence in ADL skills (Roeden & Zitman, 1995).

Traditional primary care models encounter difficulty in establishing medical diagnoses for individuals with ID. The gold standard for identification of physical conditions is self-report; in many situations individuals with ID have a compromised ability to effectively communicate physical symptoms or complaints. This difficulty with communication may be a factor contributing to an increased risk for undiagnosed medical conditions (Chicoine, McGuire, Hebein, & Gilly, 1994; Henderson & Davidson, 2000), increased use of psychopharmacological interventions and potential for adverse side effects and delirium (Henderson & Davidson, 2000), and over-diagnosis of dementia (Acquilano, 2002). Doka and Lavin (2003) identify two factors that may contribute to detrimental effects of medical conditions. The first being the person with ID not being able to readily recognize or report symptoms, secondly due to the fine balance between their abilities and environmental demands, and a diminished capacity to compensate, a small decline may have a dramatic effect. If an individual with poor verbal expressive skills is experiencing pain or discomfort, they may resort to utilizing overt behavior that has proven to be successful in the past in other situations. This behavior may be maladaptive and subsequently they receive treatment for the maladaptive behavior and not the underlying medical condition.

Many primary care providers have not received extensive training regarding ID and the difficulties encountered in assessing individuals with potentially limited expressive and receptive language skills. Those who may have had some exposure to individuals with ID in their training curriculums typically are pediatricians, and are therefore somewhat limited in an understanding of aging-related conditions. The complexity of diagnosis with this population requires the use of a team approach. Each member brings a certain level of understanding and skill to bear upon the assessment process based on their expertise. In this manner, a more holistic view of the person within their environment(s) may increase the likelihood of accurate diagnosis.

Comprehensive Geriatric Assessment (CGA)

Several models have been developed to deliver specialized geriatric assessment for individuals with ID (Carlsen, Galluzzi, Foreman, & Cavalieri, 1994; Chicoine et al., 1994; Henderson & Davidson, 2000; Tsiouris & Patti, 1997). These geriatric clinics developed out of a need to provide more accurate assessment of aging-related conditions to a population that was not fully understood by practitioners. The design of these clinics varied, with most including a gerontologist, nurse, and a social worker (Carlsen et al., 1994; Chicoine et al., 1994; Henderson & Davidson, 2000); the George A. Gervis Clinic included a psychiatrist, nurse, and psychologist (Tsiouris & Patti, 1997). These clinics utilized other team members as available. Typically, at least one team member had previous experience and knowledge of ID. The focus of these clinics was to provide assessment of aging-related conditions.

Henderson and Davidson (2000) concluded that CGA can accomplish several important goals, which include

- to provide comprehensive interdisciplinary clinical service;
- to serve as an education and training setting;
- to bring a different perspective to adults with ID who are utilizing mental health services; and
- to serve as a point of intersection between the intellectual disability and general aging services systems.

Change from Work to Retirement

Competing forces come to play when older adults with ID approach retirement age. The desire to slow down and attain the same goals of people without ID is counterbalanced by the need for meaningful activities and structure. Social support systems may become disrupted with retirement. It is incumbent upon carers to identify and promote the development of new social support systems as an older person begins the transition from work to retirement. Anxiety concerning ones future can develop during this time. The transition needs to be gradual providing information concerning retirement options so that each person feels empowered in the decision-making process, rather than a passive participant of an overpowering system. Training may be required to develop decision-making abilities due to a historical lack of opportunity to be involved in decisions of any magnitude.

Concerns may evolve out of an uncertain financial future. Retirement means the loss of income that may not be recovered. Persons may work beyond the time at which they would have liked to retire out of fear that they will lack the necessary finances to survive (Doka & Levin, 2003). Given the lifelong involvement with public funding for many individuals, the opportunity for a typical retirement account may be limited. Planning for this transition and setting aside retirement funds may alleviate this concern.

Modifying the Service System to Accommodate Retirement

Current service systems are in a transitional phase as they seek to accommodate a growing population. As the system addresses these needs it is important to include the older individual with ID in that process. A person-centered approach will empower the person and increase the opportunity for success (Sterns, Kennedy, Sed, & Heller, 2000). In the United States each state addresses the needs of its constituents on an individual basis. Some states, such as Ohio, have legislated that individuals with ID may retire at the age of 55 years, whereas others have not established an official retirement age (Sterns et al., 2000).

MENTAL HEALTH

Age-Related Prevalence Rates

It has been identified that prevalence rates of psychiatric conditions increase with age until old age, at which time prevalence rates decrease (Janicki et al., 2002). With that in mind, it has also been identified that depression is under-diagnosed in elderly people without ID (Fischer, Wei, Solberg, Rush, & Heinrich, 2003), and with ID (Tsiouris & Patti, 1997).

Behavioral Changes

As with the general population, with increasing age the incidence of actual physical aggression decreases and may be replaced by verbal aggression. Although physical aggression may decrease, an older person tends to be more resistive to changes in routine and rigid due to declining memory skills. Typical aging-related declines in sensory modalities may cause the person to have difficulty performing simple daily routines, especially those requiring fine detail, and this can lead to frustration or depressive symptomatology.

A variety of studies have targeted the identification of psychiatric diagnoses in this population. The validity of using traditional DSM III/IV or ICD 10 diagnostic criteria has been studied. There is variability in the results of the current research and therefore the need for further research is warranted. Finlay and Lyons (2001) suggest caution in utilizing self-reports and interviews when diagnosing psychiatric conditions in people with ID. Factors that need to be taken into account include difficulty with time frames, direct comparisons, questions pertaining to feelings, generalized judgments (e.g., usually), sensitive topics, negatively worded questions, subject–object confusion, and multiple choice or open-ended questions. Additionally, yes–no questions can be problematic due to acquiescence and therefore questions using this format should be counterbalanced. This is especially true of instruments normed on individuals without ID; the importance of this will be further discussed in the section on dementia assessments. Despite the questionable validity of findings, ultimately an assessment must occur or else mental health conditions will not be addressed. Psychopharmacological or behavioral interventions should not occur in the absence of a psychiatric diagnosis.

Cain et al. (2003) evaluated the validity of identifying bipolar disorders in individuals with ID utilizing DSM IV criteria. Blind reviewers adhered to DSM IV criteria for the diagnosis of bipolar disorder and retrospectively reviewed the charts of a convenience sample of 166 participants that had been seen at an outpatient clinic for adults with ID. The intent was to determine if individuals with bipolar disorder could be differentiated from individuals with other mood disorders or thought disorders whose behavioral symptoms frequently overlap those of bipolar disorder. Kappa values for interrater reliability ranged from 0.68 to 1.00. Participants with bipolar disorder were found to have a significantly higher average number of symptoms (mood and nonmood). Mood symptoms included irritability, elevated mood, lability, and euphoric mood. In addition, participants with bipolar disorder displayed significantly more behaviors that impaired social functioning, such as difficulty with peer interactions, staff interactions, lower activities of daily living (ADL) skills, and work skills. The authors concluded that DSM IV criteria could be accurately used to diagnose bipolar disorders in adults with ID.

Pawlarcyzk and Beckwith (1987) provide support for the use of DSM criteria with individuals whose ID resides in the mild or moderate range. The authors suggested that for persons with ID in the severe to profound range DSM III criteria might not adequately identify depression. They suggested the use of behavioral equivalents.

Clarke and Gomez (1999) evaluated utilizing ICD 10 criteria in the diagnosis of depression. Whereas Cain and colleagues used standard DSM IV criteria, this study utilized modified ICD 10 criteria. The modification was limited to the addition of items that were considered to be behavioral equivalents of depression. This study is limited by the small sample size (11), and because success was determined by response to antidepressant treatment. There were no behavioral or psychotherapeutic interventions referenced. Pharmacological treatment in lieu of psychological interventions should not be considered the norm.

The results of research in this area have been mixed, with some studies supporting the use of standard diagnostic procedures (Kazdin, Matson, & Senatore, 1983), and others suggesting the use of modified criteria (Powell, 2003).

Assessment Tools and Their Applicability to Older Persons with ID

Attempts to assess mood disorders in individuals with ID have been an ongoing endeavor for more than 20 years. The use of assessment tools and adhering to diagnostic criteria are crucial to establishing a diagnosis of depression in this population. A variety of assessment tools normed on individuals without ID have been used in their original format or adapted for individuals with ID. Still others have developed assessment tools specific to individuals with ID. Kazdin et al. (1983) assessed the efficacy of administering the *Beck Depression Inventory* (Beck, Ward, Mendelson, Mock, & Erbaugh, 1961), *Zung Self-Rating Depression Scale* (Zung, 1965), the MMPI depression scale (Hathaway & McKinley, 1967), and the *Psychopathology Instrument for Mentally Retarded Adults* (PIMRA; Kazdin et al., 1983), which was developed for this study. *DSM III* criteria were adhered to in establishing a diagnosis of depression. It was identified that higher scores on the Zung and Beck were correlated with lower IQs. The Beck and Zung were found to differentiate between depressed and nondepressed participants. The PIMRA depression scale was not identified to have enough specificity for depression. The authors concluded that individuals with ID are capable of reporting symptoms of depression.

Powell (2003) evaluated the utility of administering the *Beck Depression Inventory* (Beck & Steer, 1993) and the Zung Self-Rating Depression Scale (Zung, 1965) with individuals with ID. This study utilized 120 participants and the level of ID was stated as 36% mild ID, 46% moderate ID, and 12% severe ID. Both measures were administered to all participants and the Pearson r correlation was significant. Cronbach's alpha yielded an internal consistency of .86 for the Beck Depression Scale. Factor analysis identified seven factors on the Beck that accounted for 65.7% of the sample variance. The author established that the Beck Depression Inventory has clinical validity with individuals with ID, but questioned the reliability of the Zung. The validity of using tests normed on a non-ID population was questioned by Glenn, Bihm, and Lammers (2003), even though they found that the Beck and the Reynolds Child Depression Scale (Reynolds, 1989) could be reliably used with adults with ID in assessing depression and anxiety. Although recognizing that scales normed on a non-ID population can be reliably utilized, the authors made a call for instruments normed on individuals with ID.

The Zung and Beck depression inventories have been well evaluated with this population. Adherence to standard administration has occurred (Prout & Schaefer, 1985), as well as studies using the standard version with questions read to the participants and/or modified Likert ratings (pictorial vs. numerical) in the administration (Matson, 1982; Nezu, Nezu, Rothenberg, DelliCarpini, & Groag, 1995). The overall consensus has been that the Beck is a reliable measure and consistently is rated as superior or equal to the Zung. The MMPI has received minimal evaluation (Kazdin et al., 1983; Matson, 1982) and this measure has questionable utility for individuals with ID. Although the studies reference reading the items to participants to offset the requirement of a sixth grade reading level, that still does not mitigate the required reading level. Incumbent within the prescribed reading level is a concomitant level of comprehension necessary to understand the question. In addition, the test is quite lengthy and may be too burdensome for older adults to reliably complete.

Impact of Age-Related Environmental Interactions and Their Relationship to Psychiatric Symptomatology

The diagnosis of psychiatric disorders, inclusive of dementia, must be tempered by a thorough understanding of the presence of sensory impairments for each individual and environmental influences. As we age gradual reductions occur in visual acuity, taste, tactile sensitivity, olfactory sensation, and hearing. Incidences of hearing and visual deficits have been reported to increase with age (Evenhuis, 1995a, 1995b). Superimposing this increased loss of sensory abilities over a preexisting developmental disability may result in increased confusion and disorientation. For example, an older individual with ID reporting visual hallucinations may not in actuality be hallucinating, but rather due to poor lighting and declining visual discrimination skills may be misinterpreting a fluttering curtain in a room. Recognition of environmental and age-related influences must occur at all junctures. When identifying precipitating factors to maladaptive behaviors it is important to identify such influences as background noise, lighting, and the ambient temperature. Depressive symptoms such as withdrawal and loss of interest in favored social activities may be the result of diminished capacity to filter background noises and ensuing confusion. It is important to reinforce the use of glasses and hearing aides.

FAMILY ISSUES

Changes in Family Involvement

As the person with ID ages, the likelihood of diminished family support systems increases. Unlike the population without ID, persons with ID are less likely to have children (Doka & Lavin, 2003). Children provide an important support system to their aging parents. During a time when these aging people are most in need of support systems, these systems are the most depleted. Surviving siblings may not be able to fully provide for the needs of the older person with ID, as they may need to allocate resources to deal with their own health concerns.

Loss and Bereavement

Issues pertaining to grieving and bereavement affect everyone to some degree. It has been suggested that individuals with ID routinely have mourning needs neglected and unrecognized and grief not adequately addressed (Kauffman, 1994). It is during older age that there is increased risk for loss and bereavement as parents, siblings, and friends begin to expire, and long-term relationships with specific service providers may end through staff retirements. The focus of service provision to older adults with ID involves skill training and behavior modification (Kauffman, 1994). Supporting the expression of feelings and concerns has not received a similar level of intervention. This is also complicated by the previously mentioned decrements in verbal expressive and receptive communication skills. Thus, people at the greatest risk for loss and bereavement may not be supported in understanding feelings and are less able to communicate what they are experiencing.

Stoddart, Burke, and Temple (2002) suggest that initially individual counseling should be the primary approach, as opposed to group, in that someone recently experiencing bereavement may not be comfortable sharing pain and feelings with others. In addition, some individuals may not benefit from group therapy due to individual factors, or psychiatric or behavioral influences may be disruptive to the group process. Individual therapy offers the opportunity for more close interpersonal connections between the therapist and participant, than does the group therapy.

The goal of group therapy is similar to individual in that the focus is information sharing, promoting awareness that the persons feelings and experiences are not unique, to assist in the mourning process, and to help the person move forward without the deceased. In addition, group therapy offers the additional benefit of enhancing the participants' ability to share experiences and emotions (Stoddart et al., 2002). Although these goals are with merit, the authors concluded that the therapy did not have an effect on knowledge and understanding of bereavement, but did result in a significant decrease of depressive symptomotology for individuals that were dually diagnosed (ID and psychiatric illness).

DEMENTIA

Diagnostic Issues

Depression is one of the first rule outs in diagnosing dementia (American Psychiatric Association, 1994). In a longitudinal study of an aging cohort of adults with ID (van Schrojenstein Lantman-deValk et al., 1997) a relatively high incidence of dementia was reported in individuals with DS aged 40 years and older, rates for ID adults with other etiologies aged 50 and older were much lower. Conversely, a very low incidence of affective disorders was diagnosed in this same cohort, most notably individuals diagnosed with DS. The authors questioned the accuracy of these diagnoses and postulated that the incidence of depression may have been artificially lowered due to the symptomatology resembling dementia. They concurred that depression is difficult to diagnose in people with poor verbal expressive skills.

Functional decline may not be readily apparent; individuals whose baseline functioning is diminished may not display readily recognizable declines as a person adjusts to internal and external changes. This makes it difficult to correlate the onset of decline with an identifiable precursor. A gradual onset decline may appear as sudden onset due to lack of early recognition, or even if identifiable as gradual may be so distant from the initial precursor that it is not attributed to that influence. This is further exacerbated by the presence of poor expressive or receptive language skills.

In evaluating functional decline an important delineation is required, that being screening versus assessment. Screening is a process in which individuals that may have risk factors, such as DS or age, are identified. Screening tools are not adequate to perform dementia assessments. These tools are not designed for differential diagnosis; the purpose for screening tools is to increase the likelihood of identifying a person that possesses a particular condition through over-inclusion. Assessment is a process that utilizes tools designed for specificity. Screening tools are not designed for differential diagnosis, but assessment tools are.

Assessment Tools

A battery of assessment tools for older adults with ID should include adaptive behavior, memory, cognitive changes, and mental health factors (Aylward, Burt, Thorpe, Lai, & Dalton, 1997). This section will focus on tools to assess cognitive, behavioral, and memory changes. Mental health factors will be discussed in a subsequent section. Some of these tests are rather encompassing in their scope (Dalton, Fedor, Patti, Tsiouris, & Mehta, 2002; Evenhuis, Kengen, & Eurilings, 1990; Gedye, 1995) and utilize a respondent, whereas others focus more on memory or cognitive skills (Dalton, 1996; Krinsky-McHale, Devenny, & Silverman, 2002; Patti, 1999) and rely on direct examination. A test battery should always include both types of measures. Practice guidelines for the assessment of dementia have been promulgated (Janicki, Heller, Seltzer, & Hogg, 1996) and support the framework for assessment delineated here within. The strengths and weaknesses of these various assessment tools will be discussed. Respondent-based assessments will be covered first, followed by direct measures of cognitive and memory skills.

The *Dementia Scale for Down Syndrome* (DSDS; Gedye, 1995) was standardized on a cohort of adults ($N = 70$) with DS aged 40 years or older that were followed for approximately 4 years. A control group of 37 adults >40 years of age without dementia were used as a comparison group.

Interrater reliability was assessed on 50 participants and yielded a kappa coefficient of .91. The DSDS has been identified as a valid assessment of dementia in adults with other etiologies of ID (Gedye, 1995). The scale utilizes an informant format and provides a list of specific behaviors that the respondent is required to respond to regarding presence or absence of the behavior. Presence of specific behaviors elicits further questioning pertaining to approximate date that the behavioral change was first observed. This mechanism of scoring is designed toward identifying the typical slow progression of decline present in Alzheimer's disease. This measure seeks to rule out treatable conditions, through specific questions, and the establishment of minimum scores required supporting a diagnosis of dementia. In addition, the scale should be readministered at least on an annual basis for individuals with a suspected dementia. The DSDS is sensitive for behavioral changes in the profound range of ID due to the manner of scoring. The individual is used as his or her own baseline, rather than being compared to other age and level of ID matched participants. The only requirement is that the respondent has known the individual for at least a year.

The DSDS derives two scores, a cognitive cutoff score (CCS) and an early and middle tally (EMT). The CCS is based on 12 items from the test that are correlated with cognitive decline consistent with dementia. The EMT is an aggregate score of all behavioral factors scored as present in the early stage dementia questions and the middle stage of dementia questions. A CCS ≥ 3 and an EMT ≥ 10 are required to substantiate a diagnosis of dementia. There is an elaborate diagnostic tree for ruling out differential diagnoses such as hypothyroidism, depression, and sensory deficits. Possibly due to the apparent all encompassing nature of this test, some clinicians have made the mistake of using it as the sole determinant for a diagnosis of dementia. This format places a clinician in the situation where they must be psychologist, physician, and nurse all in one. Very few professional would be competent wearing all those hats; therefore this tool should only be used as one aspect of a comprehensive assessment.

Another respondent-based assessment is the *Multidimensional Observation Scale for Elderly Subjects* (MOSES; Dalton, Fedor, & Patti, 1999). This tool differs from the DSDS in that it only requires the respondent only know the individual for 1 week prior to the assessment. The MOSES takes only 10–15 min to complete. The MOSES was normed on 100 individuals with DS. The mean age of the women was 36.5 years and the mean age for the men was 35.1 years. Dalton et al. (2002) report that intellectual levels of the participants ranged from mild-profound MR, although there were only 10 participants with profound MR. These scales include self-help skills, disorientation, depression, irritability, withdrawal, and an overall score. Interrater reliability was reported to be $r = .85$ for the three raters utilized in the sample of 14 individuals. Further longitudinal analysis of the MOSES using 138 individuals with DS over a 3-year period identified significant differences between the group < 40 years of age and the participants that were > 40 years of age. These significant differences occurred in self-help skills, disorientation, and the overall score. Dalton et al. (2002)

concluded that the changes evidenced were not due to comorbid medical conditions or normal aging, yet no statistical analysis occurred.

A further comparison occurred between individuals without ID who were diagnosed with Alzheimer's type dementia (DAT) and older individuals with DS. It was identified that the group without ID scored significantly worse than did the individuals with DS. Dalton and colleagues concluded that the individuals without ID were in the later stages of dementia and the individuals with DS were in an earlier stage of dementia.

In comparing individuals with DS and DAT and individuals with DS and other psychiatric diagnoses Dalton et al. (2002) found significant differences. The individuals with DS and DAT scored worse than did individuals with DS and other diagnoses on self-help skills, disorientation, and total score. There were no differences for depression, irritability, or withdrawal. One further comparison that did not occur would be between individuals with DS but not with DAT, and age-matched individuals with DS and DAT. A critique of the MOSES is that there are no cutoff criteria for the diagnosis of dementia (Deb & Braganza, 1999).

The *Dementia Questionnaire for Mentally Retarded Persons* (DMR; Evenhuis et al., 1990) contains 50 questions divided into eight categories. Administration of the DMR yields a sum of cognitive scores that is based on memory (short- and long-term) and spatial and temporal orientation. In addition, a sum of social scores is obtained. This score is derived from speech, practical skills, mood, activity and interest, and behavioral disturbances (Evenhuis, 1996). This test differs from the DSDS and MOSES in that no individuals with DS were included in the normative population. In addition, individuals with severe/profound ID were not included in the normative group and as such floor effects are noted. Thus, there is a lack of specificity for individuals that have severe/profound ID and a concomitant risk for over-diagnosis of dementia. As with the other measures, a diagnosis of dementia is obtained through repeated measures. Clinicians are cautioned that a diagnosis of dementia should not be identified on initial administration of any of these measures.

Deb and Braganza (1999) compared the DSDS, DMR, and *Mini Mental State Exam* (MMSE; Folstein, Folstein, & McHugh, 1975) against a clinical rating of dementia using ICD 10 criteria. A sample of 62 adults with ID participated in the study. No individuals with profound ID were included in the study. The DSDS and DMR were positively correlated and were also positively correlated with clinician diagnosis, although the degree of agreement was based on severity of dementia. Clinicians were more accurate in diagnosing late stage, versus early stage dementia. The MMSE did not yield adequate specificity due to floor effects, there was a tendency to over-diagnose dementia in individuals, 77% of the individuals that scored below 24 (the cutoff used for individuals without ID) did not attain criteria on the DSDS or DMR. The authors concluded that the use of a respondent-based assessment was more useful than direct neuropsychological tests. This is an overgeneralization for the following reasons. Respondent-based examinations have been shown to have moderate interrater reliability, and the neuropsychological exam used in this study was normed on a non-ID population. Direct exam as a rule has more specificity than utilizing a respondent to offer an opinion of a person's capability. Neuropsychological measures that have been normed on individuals with ID should be administered in conjunction with a respondent measure.

Selected memory tests have been chosen due to the normative populations being developmentally disabled (Dalton & McMurray, 1995; Krinsky-McHale et al., 2002; Patti, 1999), or including individuals with ID (Psychological Corporation, 2002). As with the MMSE, tests normed on the general population have been utilized with the ID with mixed results. Gibson, Groeneweg, Jerry, and Harris (1988) utilized the Wechsler Intelligence Scale for Children (WISC) to assess age-related intellectual decline comparing a group of adults with DS to a group of adults with ID with mixed etiologies other than DS. Both of these groups were separated into younger (average age = 23.9 years, $N = 18$) and older (average age = 35.5 years, $N = 18$) groupings. Significant differences in full-scale IQ scores between the DS and other etiology group as well as between age groups were identified. The decline in IQ scores with age was mostly related to decline in performance scaled scores. Although this study suggests declines in intellectual functioning with age, there are some procedural problems with the study. The WISC's normative group is children, with an upper age range of 16 years; the participants in this study well exceeded the normative group. The question arises pertaining to which age group the raw scores were compared. Were the scores matched for mental age or compared to the 16-year-old category? Either method has serious methodological implications. In addition, it was noted that the decline in IQ scores was most evident on the performance-based tests. Four of the five subtests on the performance scale of the WISC have either time limits or provide an increase in scaled score based on speed of response. It would be expected that comparing test results that have a timed factor for older adults with a normative group of teenagers would identify that the younger group had better fine-motor skills and speed of processing. Therefore, the older group would be at a disadvantage and resultant raw scores would present as a decline in scaled scores, and ultimately a decline in IQ.

As a rule, the use of mental age as a comparison should be avoided. A 65-year-old person with ID who has a mental age of 3 years 4 months is in no way comparable to a child without ID of that same age. The use of mental age may lead us to deny the actual physiological age of the person with ID and predisposes caregivers and clinicians to view the person in an infantile manner. In assessing functional decline in an older person with ID we must endeavor to view that person in the totality of their existence. Recognizing the history of that person, their highest level of functional independence, stability of social and emotional support systems, prior and current psychiatric diagnoses, and the current wants, needs, and desires of that person. Although measures seek to compare the individual being assessed against a normative group, ultimately what must occur to solidify a diagnosis of dementia is that the person is compared with their personal highest level of functioning. It is recognized that small decreases in memory may occur with age and are not indicative of dementia (Krinsky-McHale et al., 2002).

The *Memory for Objects* (Patti, 1999) test does not have established reliability and validity data; this is a shortcoming. *Memory for Objects* is an adaptation of the *Fuld Memory Test* (Buschke & Fuld, 1974). The test consists of three objects (cup, ball, comb) that are first introduced to the individual to ascertain their ability to name the objects. The cup is then placed in the bag, the other two objects are named, and the individual is prompted to state which object is in the bag. Next the ball is placed in the bag with the cup and the comb is named. The person is prompted to again name the objects in the bag. In the following sequence all three objects are placed in the bag, three other objects are introduced (spoon, scissors, and key), named, and then removed; then after the distraction the person is required to name the objects in the bag. The three objects are then placed back in the bag and set aside for 5 min during which other distracting events occur. After 5 min the individual is prompted to name the objects. This sequence is followed for a subsequent 5-min delay. The score is derived as a percentage of correct responses.

Devenny, Zimmerli, Kittler, and Krinsky-Mchale (2002) also developed a short-term memory scale based on the study by Fuld (Buschke & Fuld, 1974) and reported good results in identifying early memory loss in a cohort of adults with DS. The Fuld test has been validated as a test of short-term memory for adults without ID (Buschke & Fuld, 1974). This provides evidence that revisions of the Fuld can be successful with this population. The Devenny and colleagues test is limited, as it requires an IQ > 30 and the person has to recall three sets of 12 words utilizing a cued recall format.

Test–retest and interrater reliabilities for the Dalton McMurray *Visual Memory Test* (Dalton & McMurray, 1995) have both demonstrated good results. Validity was established via postmortem examination of the neuropathological signs of AD in seven individuals with DS, two persons with ID without DS, and through computerized transaxial tomography of seven individuals with DS.

The *Dyspraxia Test* (Dalton, 1996) is a test of physical performance, and to a smaller extent knowledge, that was normed on individuals with DS. The three areas assessed are apraxia, body parts/counting, and psychomotor skills. Test–retest reliability is good, z scores are provided. The initial administration establishes a baseline for the individual and subsequent administrations can gauge the rate of decline, if any, that exists. This measure is more sensitive to mid-to-later stage dementia. Declines in praxis have not been reported in early stage dementia and therefore this test should be combined with a test of short-term memory (Dalton, Mehta, Fedor, & Patti, 1999).

PERSONNEL AND TRAINING

Impact on Caregivers

As people with ID age, even in situations where successful aging is evidenced, there will be an increased burden upon carers. This burden may take many forms depending on the nature of the caregiving. If a person with ID is living with family, an additional variable will be the aging of the parents or siblings. As the caregivers age they become less able to assist with lifting or otherwise helping with physical assistance. Although an aging caregiver may be more understanding of the physical and psychological changes that the aging person with ID is experiencing, there may also be denial of those changes if the caregiver is having a difficult time adjusting to their own changes. Support groups and training modules should be offered to assist the caregiver and meet their needs. It is also important to work in conjunction with the caregiver and individual with ID to identify factors that would require additional support or the need for a residential change to provide the ability to maintain the current residence, or create a smooth transition to the next.

Staff working with an aging person will also require additional support. A philosophical change regarding programmatic activities occurs as the aging person transitions from middle age to older age. Rather than focusing on development of work-related skills, the individual may choose to decrease the amount of time working, and increase leisure time activities. In addition to the change from work to retirement, aging-related medical and sensory conditions might lead to additional stress for staff. In providing support, Harris and Rose (2002) point out that perceived support is more beneficial in reducing stress than is actual support. Staff requires a degree of social support from professionals and administrators to assist them in managing the stress of a changing population and focus.

One manner of assessing the degree of stress that staff may be experiencing is to administer a questionnaire. This information gathering should include data from two related areas, the difference in actual care activities performed in comparing an elderly population without dementia to those with dementia (McCarron, Gill, Lawlor, & Beagly, 2002), and the amount of perceived support that staff identifies (Harris & Rose, 2002). The Caregiver Activity Survey—Intellectual Disability (CAS-ID; McCarron et al., 2002) was developed as a means of determining the relative differences in providing care to adults with ID and dementia, versus age-matched controls without dementia. The authors recognize that as a person progresses through the process of dementia care needs change. This survey is reported to have good reliability and convergent validity, and measures the amount of time that staff spends providing typical day-to-day care.

RESEARCH ISSUES

Research drives practice and the field of aging and ID is ripe with opportunities for future research. These opportunities include validation of the comprehensive geriatric clinic model. The model has face validity, but has not been proven to be more reliable in assessing functional decline in older adults with ID as compared to the primary care model. Further studies examining the use of standard diagnostic criteria such as the *DSM IV* will benefit if accurate diagnosis of psychiatric conditions are based on sound clinical judgment supported by standard criteria. In accordance with the need for sound diagnostic criteria, is the requirement for assessment tools normed on a population with ID. There have been mixed results concerning the use of tools validated on individuals without ID. In addition to the development of tools normed on individuals with ID, further studies assessing the use of tools normed on a non-ID population are required.

In addition to the need for development of tools to assess psychiatric diagnoses, is the requirement for further development of assessment tools is designed toward measuring cognitive and memory abilities. The majority of the research within this realm has focused on individuals with DS and further studies are required to ascertain if the results of these earlier studies are transferable to individuals with ID, but not to individuals with DS. In addition, updated assessment tools of functional skills and decline are warranted. The tools currently in use (dementia scales) were normed approximately 10 years ago and as with any psychological measure, updated norms are required. As each generation ages, life experiences and base behavior change on the basis of cohort effects such as prior educational and social experiences. Assessment tools need to adapt to changing cohort effects as required.

CONCLUSIONS

As with individuals without ID, those with ID are living into old age on a much more regular basis. This movement into old age alters traditional service delivery systems. Retirement and bereavement issues need to be addressed, as well as recognition of what constitutes normal aging versus pathological aging. A systematic approach toward the assessment of functional decline is required. Medical comorbidities and psychiatric diagnoses can have an effect on functional capabilities.

REFERENCES

Acquilano, J. P. (2002, March). *A comprehensive geriatric assessment clinic for the intellectually disabled.* Paper presented at the 12th Annual Roundtable of the International Association for the Scientific Study of Intellectual Disabilities, Koriyama, Fukishima, Japan.

American Psychiatric Association. (1994). *Diagnostic and statistical manual of mental disorders* (4th ed.). Washington, DC: Author.

Ansello, E. F., & Janicki, M. P. (2000). The aging of nations. In M. P. Janicki & E. F. Ansello (Eds.), *Community supports for aging adults in lifelong disabilities* (pp. 3–18). Baltimore: Brookes.

Aylward, E. H., Burt, D. B., Thorpe, L. U., Lai, F., & Dalton, A. (1997). Diagnosis of dementia in individuals with intellectual disability. *Journal of Intellectual Disability Research, 41,* 152–164.

Beck, A. T., & Steer, R. A. (1993). *Beck Depression Inventory—Manual.* San Antonio, TX: Psychological Corp.

Beck, A. T., Ward, C. H., Mendelson, M., Mock, J., & Erbaugh, J. (1961). An inventory for measuring depression. *Archives of General Psychiatry, 4,* 53–63.

Bigby, C. (2002). Ageing people with a lifelong disability: Challenges for the aged care and disability sectors. *Journal of Intellectual and Developmental Disability, 27*(4), 231–241.

Burt, D. B. (1999). Dementia and depression. In M. P. Janicki & A. J. Dalton (Eds.), *Dementia, aging and intellectual disabilities: A handbook* (pp. 198–216). Philadelphia: Brunner/Mazel.

Burt, D. B., Loveland, K. A., & Lewis, K. (1992). Depression and the onset of dementia in adults with mental retardation. *American Journal on Mental Retardation, 96,* 502–511.

Burt, D. B., Loveland, K. A., Primeaux-Hart, S., Chen, Y., Phillips, N. B., Cleveland, L. A., et al. (1998). Dementia in adults with Down syndrome: Diagnostic challenges. *American Journal on Mental Retardation, 103*(2), 130–145.

Buschke, H., & Fuld, P. A. (1974). Evaluating storage, retention, and retrieval in disordered memory and learning. *Neurology, 24,* 1019–1025.

Cain, N. N., Davidson, P. W., Burhan, A. M., Andolsek, M. E., Baxter, J. T., Sullivan, L., et al. (2003). Identifying bipolar disorders in individuals with intellectual disability. *Journal of Intellectual Disability Research, 47*(1), 31–38.

Carlsen, W. R., Galluzzi, K. E., Foreman, L. F., & Cavalieri, T. A. (1994). Comprehensive geriatric assessment: Applications for community-residing, elderly people with mental retardation/developmental disabilities. *Mental Retardation, 32*(5), 334–340.

Chicoine, B., McGuire, D., Hebein, S., & Gilly, D. (1994). Development of a clinic for adults with Down syndrome. *Mental Retardation, 32*(2), 100–106.

Clarke, D. J., & Gomez, G. A. (1999). Utility of modified DCR-10 criteria in the diagnosis of depression associated with intellectual disability. *Journal of Intellectual Disability Research, 43*(5), 413–420.

Dalton, A. J. (1996). *Dyspraxia scale for adults with Down syndrome.* Staten Island, NY: Research Innovations.

Dalton, A. J., Fedor, B. L., & Patti, P. J. (1999). *Multi-Dimensional Observation Scale for Elderly Subjects: Adapted for persons with Down syndrome, 1999 Revision.* Staten Island, NY: Institute for Basic Research in Developmental Disabilities.

Dalton, A. J., Fedor, B. L., Patti, P. J., Tsiouris, J. A., & Mehta, P. D. (2002). The Multidimensional Observation Scale for Elderly Subjects (MOSES): Studies in adults with intellectual disability. *Journal of Intellectual and Developmental Disability, 27*(4), 310–324.

Dalton, A. J., & McMurray, K. (1995). *Dalton/McMurray Visual Memory Test.* Copyright 1984–1995 by A. J. Dalton and Bytecraft Inc., Waterloo, Ont., Canada.

Deb, S., & Braganza, J. (1999). Comparison of rating scales for the diagnosis of dementia in adults with Down's syndrome. *Journal of Intellectual Disability Research, 43*(5), 400–407.

Devenny, D. A., Zimmerli, E. J., Kittler, P., & Krinsky-Mchale, S. J. (2002). Cued recall in early-stage dementia in adults with Down's syndrome. *Journal of Intellectual Disability Research, 46,* 472–483.

Doka, K. J., & Lavin, C. (2003). The paradox of ageing with developmental disabilities: Increasing needs, declining resources. *Ageing International, 28*(2), 135–154.

Evenhuis, H. M. (1995a). Medical aspects of ageing in a population with intellectual disability: I. Visual impairment. *Journal of Intellectual Disability Research, 39,* 19–25.

Evenhuis, H. M. (1995b). Medical aspects of ageing in a population with intellectual disability: II. Hearing impairment. *Journal of Intellectual Disability Research, 39,* 27–33.

Evenhuis, H. M. (1996). Further evaluation of the dementia questionnaire for persons with mental retardation (DMR). *Journal of Intellectual Disability Research, 40,* 369–373.

Evenhuis, H. M. (1997). Medical aspects of ageing in a population with intellectual disabilities: III. Mobility, internal conditions and cancer. *Journal of Intellectual Disability Research, 41,* 8–18.

Evenhuis, H. M., Kengen, M. M. F., & Eurlings, H. A. L. (1990). *Dementia questionnaire for mentally retarded persons.* Swammerdam, The Netherlands: Hooche Burch Institute for Mentally Retarded People.

Finlay, W. M., & Lyons, E. (2001). Methodological issues in interviewing and using self-report questionnaires with people with mental retardation. *Psychological Assessment, 13,* 319–335.

Fischer, L. R., Wei, F., Solberg, L. I., Rush, W. A., & Heinrich, R. L. (2003). Treatment of elderly and other adult patients for depression in primary care. *Journal of the American Geriatric Society, 51*(11), 1554–1562.

Folstain, M. F., Folstain, S. E., & McHugh, P. R. (1975). "Mini-Mental State". A practical method for grading the cognitive state of patients for the clinician. *Journal of Psychiatric Research, 12,* 189–198.

Gedye, A. (1995). *Dementia scale for Down syndrome* (Manual). Vancouver, Canada: Gedye Research and Consulting.

Gibson, D., Groeneweg, G., Jerry, P., & Harris, A. (1988). Age and pattern of intellectual decline among Down syndrome and other mentally retarded adults. *International Journal of Rehabilitation Research, 11*(1), 47–55.

Glenn, E., Bihm, E. M., & Lammers, W. J. (2003). Depression, anxiety, and relevant cognitions in persons with mental retardation. *Journal of Autism and Developmental Disorders, 33*(1), 69–76.

Harris, P., & Rose, J. (2002). Measuring staff support in services for people with intellectual disability: The staff support and satisfaction questionnaire, version 2. *Journal of Intellectual Disability Research, 46*(2), 151–157.

Hathaway, S. R., & McKinley, J. C. (1967). *Minnesota Multiphasic Personality Inventory: Manual for administration and scoring.* New York: Psychological Corp.

Henderson, C. M., & Davidson, P. W. (2000). Comprehensive adult and geriatric assessment. In M. P. Janicki & E. F. Ansello (Eds.), *Community supports for aging adults with lifelong disabilities* (pp. 373–386). Baltimore: Brookes.

Hutchings, B. L., Olsen, R. V., & Ehrenkrantz, E. D. (2000). Modifying home environments. In M. P. Janicki & E. F. Ansello (Eds.), *Community supports for aging adults with lifelong disabilities* (pp. 243–256). Baltimore: Brookes.

Janicki, M. P., Davidson, P. W., Henderson, C. M., McCallion, P., Taets, J. D., Force, L. T., et al. (2002). Health characteristics and health services utilization in older adults with intellectual disability living in community residences. *Journal of Intellectual Disability Research, 46,* 287–298.

Janicki, M. P., Heller, T., Seltzer, G., & Hogg, J. (1996). Practice guidelines for the clinical assessment and care management of Alzheimer's disease and other dementias among adults with intellectual disability. *Journal of Intellectual Disability Research, 40,* 374–382.

Kauffman, J. (1994). Mourning and mental retardation. *Death Studies, 18,* 257–271.

Kazdin, A. E., Matson, J. L., & Senatore, V. (1983). Assessment of depression in mentally retarded adults. *American Journal of Psychiatry, 140,* 1040–1043.

Krinsky-McHale, S. J., Devenny, D. A., & Silverman, W. P. (2002). Changes in explicit memory associated with early dementia in adults with Down's syndrome. *Journal of Intellectual Disability Research, 46*(3), 198–208.

Matson, J. L. (1982). The treatment of behavioral characteristics of depression in the mentally retarded. *Behavior Therapy, 13,* 209–218.

McCarron, M., Gill, M., Lawlor, B., & Beagly, C. (2002). A pilot study of the reliability and validity of Caregiver Activity Survey—Intellectual Disability (CAS-ID). *Journal of Intellectual Disability Research, 46*(8), 605–612.

Nezu, C. M., Nezu, A. M., Rothenberg, J. L., DelliCarpini, L., & Groag, I. (1995). Depression in adults with mild mental retardation: Are cognitive variables involved? *Cognitive Therapy and Research, 19*(2), 227–239.

Patti, P. J. (1999). *Memory for Objects Test.* Unpublished data, Staten Island, New York.

Pawlarcyzk, D., & Beckwith, B. E. (1987). Depressive symptoms displayed by persons with mental retardation: A review. *Mental Retardation, 25,* 325–330.

Powell, R. (2003). Psychometric properties of the Beck Depression Inventory and the Zung Self-Rating Depression Scale in adults with mental retardation. *Mental Retardation, 41,* 88–95.

Prasher, V. P., & Chung, M. C. (1996). Causes of age-related decline in adaptive behavior of adults with Down syndrome: Differential diagnosis of dementia. *American Journal on Mental Retardation, 101*(2), 175–183.

Prasher, V. P., & Hall, W. (1996). Short-term prognosis of depression in adults with Down syndrome: Association with thyroid states and effects on adaptive behavior. *Journal of Intellectual Disability Research, 40,* 32–38.

Prout, H. T., & Schaefer, B. M. (1985). Self-reports of depression by community-based mildly mentally retarded adults. *American Journal of Mental Deficiency, 90*(2), 220–222.

The Psychological Corporation (2002). Wechsler memory scale-third edition, technical manual San Antonio TX: Harcourt Brace & Company: Anthos.

Reynolds, W. M. (1989). *Reynolds Child Depression Scale: Professional manual.* Odessa, FL: Psychological Assessment Resources.

Roeden, J. M., & Zitman, F. G. (1995). Ageing in adults with Down's syndrome in institutionally based and community-based residences. *Journal of Intellectual Disability Research, 39,* 399–407.

Sterns, H. L., Kennedy, E. A., Sed, C. H., & Heller, T. (2000). Later-life planning and retirement. In M. P. Janicki & E. F. Ansello (Eds.), *Community supports for aging adults with lifelong disabilities* (pp. 179–191). Baltimore: Brookes.

Stoddart, K. P., Burke, L., & Temple, V. (2002). Outcome evaluation for bereavement groups for adults with intellectual disabilities. *Journal of Applied Research in Intellectual Disabilities, 15,* 28–35.

Sung, H., Hawkins, B. A., Eklund, S., Kim, K., Foose, A., May, M., et al. (1997). Depression and dementia in aging adults with Down syndrome: A case study approach. *Mental Retardation, 35*(1), 27–38.

Thorpe, L., Davidson, P., & Janicki, M. (2001). Healthy ageing-adults with intellectual disabilities: biobehavioural issues. *Journal of Applied Research in Intellectual Disabilities, 14,* 218–228.

Thorpe, L. U. (1999). Psychiatric disorders. In M. P. Janicki & A. J. Dalton (Eds.), *Dementia, aging, and intellectual disabilities: A handbook* (pp. 217–231). Philadelphia: Brunner/Mazel.

Tsiouris, J. A., & Patti, P. J. (1997). Drug treatment of depression associated with dementia or presented as 'pseudodementia' in older adults with Down syndrome. *Journal of Applied Research in Intellectual Disabilities, 10,* 312–322.

van Schrojenstein Lantman-deValk, H. M. J., van den Akker, M., Maskaant, M. A., Haveman, M. J., Urlings, H. F. J., Kessels, A. G. H., et al. (1997). Prevalence and incidence of health problems in people with intellectual disability. *Journal of Intellectual Disability Research, 41*(Pt. 1), 42–51.

Yang, Q., Rasmussen, S. A., & Friedman, J. M. (2002). Mortality associated with Down's syndrome in the USA from 1983–1997: A population-based study. *Lancet, 359,* 1019–1025.

Zung, W. W. K. (1965). A Self-Rating Depression Scale. *Archives of General Psychiatry, 12,* 63–70.

11

Residential and Day Services

RICHARD R. SAUNDERS

Thinking about the current state of affairs in residential and day services for people with intellectual and developmental disabilities (ID/DD) prompted reflection first on the conditions and events that existed when I entered the field in 1965. My first experience was as an undergraduate assistant in a research project funded by the National Institutes of Health. The performance site for the grant was a ward in a large state residential facility. The ward provided residential and day services to at least 35 boys with severe or profound intellectual disability (ID) and diagnoses of mental illness. The setting consisted of a congregate bedroom, congregate bathroom, congregate dining room, a large "day" room, and a concrete "porch" with chain link "walls." My recollection is that aside from grant staff, three or four regular direct service workers supported the children during the morning and evening shifts.

Despite those comparatively bleak and unpromising conditions, it was a time of some considerable excitement and optimism. Applied behavior analysis was emerging in its earliest form and showing potential for developing effective means of educating people with ID/DD and for eliminating severely maladaptive behavior. For example, among my first responsibilities, and that of a couple of other student employees, was to use an emerging method, "modeling," to establish effective washing behaviors during shower time. My evenings on the job were spent in a bathing suit demonstrating underarm movements with a face cloth. Community alternatives to institutions were scarce at that time (less than 20,000 people were in homes of six or fewer by 1977, when statistical tracking began; Lakin & Stehly, 1990). I remember that more integrated residential options were emerging because of my next modeling assignment. Other students and

RICHARD R. SAUNDERS • Schiefelbusch Institute for Life Span Studies, University of Kansas, Lawrence, Kansas 66045

I were scheduled to take our lunches with residents of a ward for teenagers with mild ID. These young people were scheduled for placement in community settings. Appropriate social behavior was deemed "a must" if they were to succeed. I doubt any of those teenagers would ever be institutionalized today.

Concurrent with the emergence of behavioral training methods, medical science was continuing its advances in identifying the causes of particular syndromes and specific means of prevention and treatment. Robinson and Robinson (1965) catalogued many of these in a major text of that time, *The Mentally Retarded Child*. Many of their photos were taken in the same institution as my modeling assignments. Among us students, there was genuine excitement that we were entering a field where we were going to make a difference through a coupling of medical and behavioral interventions. We believed that science could accelerate and support the emerging social policy of integration. Thus, as Dickens (1892) puts it,

> "It was the best of times, it was the worst of times, it was the age of wisdom, it was the age of foolishness, it was the epoch of belief, it was the epoch of incredulity, it was the season of Light, it was the season of Darkness, it was the spring of hope, it was the winter of despair, we had everything before us, we had nothing before us, we were all going direct to Heaven, we were all going direct the other way—in short, the period was so far like the present period that some of its noisiest authorities insisted on its being received, for good or for evil, in the superlative degree of comparison only" (p. 1).

RESEARCH ON RESIDENTIAL AND DAY SERVICES

The purpose of this text is to provide an overview of the state of knowledge on the topics addressed in the respective chapters. The intent of the editors is to provide foundational conceptual information derived from historical and recent research on each topic, with emphasis on the most valuable studies. But in the case of residential and day services as unitary topics, scientific data are scant, except for the ongoing debate about institutional versus community care. A recent review of the literature on relative costs (Walsh, Kastner, & Green, 2003) reveals the history and scope of this type of research. This chapter is not going to address that type of research.

First, no one doubts that the vast majority of people with DD will be supported primarily in the community in the next century and that institutions will continue to close or downsize. Further, such reports nearly always engender multiple perspectives and commentaries already available to the reader (e.g., Eidelman, Pietrangelo, Gardner, Jesien, & Croser, 2003; Perske, 2003). Perhaps because the debate still lingers, little attention has been given to variables related to successfully operating residential and day programs. Further, there are little data on the relationship between characteristics such as size, location, staffing, and program approach on important administrative outcomes such as longevity, financial health, growth, and consumer satisfaction.

The lack of data on the working parts of service delivery is partly due to the "speeding target" nature of residential and day services (although what is rapid may be defined differently by those waiting for services and those studying service delivery systems). Clearly though, more change, innovation, and experimentation in these services is occurring now than at any time in history. Those changes are being driven by the voices of people with DD and the resulting changes in public awareness of important issues. The changes are being enabled by the exponential expansion of options fundable under Medicaid, options arising directly as a result of the Home and Community-Based Services (HCBS) Waiver program. The Center for Medicare and Medicaid Services (CMS), currently encourages "Promising Practices" in service delivery systems that will enable people with disabilities to

1. "Live in the most integrated community setting appropriate to their individual support requirements and preferences;
2. Exercise meaningful choices about their living environment, their service providers, the types of supports they receive, and the manner in which supportive services are provided; and
3. Obtain quality services in a manner consistent with their living preferences and priorities" (Retrieved June 5, 2003, from http:www.cms.hhs.gov/promisingpractices/overview.asp).

Although direct purchase of support services or direct employment of support staff is now possible for some individuals, most individuals with DD currently obtain community-based residential and day services from a provider agency that manages the facilities, personnel, and logistics of support services. From the provider perspective, there is likely to be general consensus that successful operation of a support system means that for the individuals served

1. person-centered planning is actualized;
2. personal preferences are enabled;
3. ongoing choice opportunities are essential features of daily activities;
4. maladaptive behaviors are minimized;
5. participation in adaptive routines is maximized;
6. personal independence is emphasized and rewarded;
7. good health is maintained
8. abuse and neglect are prevented;
9. activities, including employment, are as integrated as possible;
10. staff turnover is uncommon.

In addition, the agency is interested in insuring that

11. licensure or certification standards are met;
12. local social validity of their services is achieved;
13. costs do not exceed income.

When one considers the multiple goals of service providers embedded in a rapidly growing array of service permutations, it becomes clear why research on residential and day services per se is rare. That is, researchers tend to target the individual elements, such as the effects of choice opportunities on aberrant behavior, or the effects of a new drug on social behavior, rather than complexity of larger questions. (Several such elements are the foci of other chapters in this text.) A related obstacle of course is that the independent variables in residential and day services are numerous and interdependent as well (see Butterfield, 1987, and Robinson, 1987, for discussions of issues in research on residential services). Indeed, see several of the chapters in Landesman, Vietze, and Begab (1987) for research on residential services near the midpoint of the institution-to-community transition.

Thus, neither residential nor day services represent organized units for purposes of dissection and discussion. Further, there is no overarching professional organization unifying either service array. I am not aware of university degrees in DD community service administration; rather, DD services are usually under another umbrella, such as health care and nursing home administration. Neither service array is bonded by a single set of certifying standards, as individual state agencies, for example, create idiosyncratic rules and expectations. Likewise, neither is defined by a particular source of funds. Despite a majority dependence on Medicaid, most operate on some mixture of federal, state, local government, private pay, and charitable income. There is also no single approach to consumer assessment, personal service planning, program implementation, staff training, or outcome evaluation. Thus, what is notable or exceptional varies from agency to agency as does what plagues each agency's growth, refinement, financial success, and its consumers' satisfaction.

There are important basic and applied scientific questions, however, in need of investigation. The remainder of this chapter discusses three highly related areas that hopefully will engender consideration of others. The three presented here are staffing systems and their relation to effective supports, current issues in supports planning, and one example of a serious community health problem engulfing individuals and agencies. Research is envisioned that might result in integration of some of the best features of all the various support systems that we have experimented with over time, including institutions, group homes, sheltered workshops, integrated supported employment, work alternatives, supported apartments, and semi-independent living. If over the last 30 years, the goal has been to institutionalize the option to live, work, and recreate in the community, perhaps the next goal could be to institutionalize evidence-based best practices in the community from which individuals with DD can choose on the basis of sound data.

RESEARCH ON STAFFING MODELS

One enduring characteristic of all residential and day service settings is that people are employed to provide individualized supports to other people. That is, direct service employees provide support to consumers with DD. Today, we mostly see employees with limited postsecondary education, often earning wages in the lowest hourly wage quartile, providing social, psychological, physical, nutritional, behavioral, educational, recreational, and employment related supports. These supports often are provided to individuals who have complex patterns of learning and behavioral characteristics, sensory deficits, attention deficits, medical conditions, and physical impairments. Thus, all agencies providing residential and day services face a major ongoing challenge: staff training and supervision that translates into appropriate high-quality individualized supports. And as with most low-paying professions, the agencies also face the potential of high employee turnover.

In congregate care settings that do not qualify under the HCBS Waiver, Medicaid regulations require, "...a continuous active treatment program, which includes aggressive, consistent implementation of a program of specialized and generic training, treatment, health services..." (Federal Register, 1988). Because funding levels for such settings are relatively high, responding to these requirements can be met in part by employing full-time trained professionals, such as psychologists, speech therapists, and nurses who can assess for, design, and train support staff to implement these habilitative interventions. Training support staff and maintaining consistency of outcome, however, pose several problems unique to congregate settings that utilize multiple shifts of direct support staff each 24 h.

The problem is illustrated by this example: Suppose eight individuals with DD are supported in a group living arrangement wherein support staff are employed in an 8-h shift model for 7-day-per-week coverage. Given an intention to provide complete coverage with minimal paid overtime and a plan to have two staff on duty during the shift, four staff must be employed. Four is the appropriate round number to consider when vacation, sick leave, discretionary days, holidays, and turnover factors (recruitment interval, background screening, preservice training) are factored in. In most scheduling schemes, four staff filling two on-duty positions creates six staffing combinations—AB, BC, CD, AC, AD, BD—meaning each staff member will work with each of the other staff members on some occasions. Thus, six efficient, cooperative, compatible, and coordinated teams must emerge. If the facility operates with shift staffing for 16-bed residences, the 7–8 staff employed for each shift can comprise many more unique teams of 4 staff each. Adding staff for individuals with more intensive needs magnifies the downside of this model. For example, 5 staff employed to fill 3 on-duty positions for 8 individuals creates 10 combinations of 3 staff per shift. If the residence employs a lead-worker model, the lead worker can facilitate the teaming effort; when the lead worker is not on duty, the staff must coordinate their activities without supervisory guidance.

A downside to congregate shift staffing from the individual's perspective is that he or she must expect supports from several different individuals and many different teams of individuals, such as when two people are needed for lifts and transfers, or for protection from self-injurious behavior. A downside from the consulting professional's perspective is that many different support staff on each of at least two shifts must be trained in each habilitative intervention, presumably to competency, and then monitored for competency thereafter. Under active treatment regulations, each individual with DD may require as many as 10–12 different multielement interventions (e.g., a complex feeding program), not to mention many minor interventions (e.g., should sign for "more" at meals). It is not uncommon to interview staff members who report being responsible for knowing the details of more than 100 individualized programs or interventions. An upside from the direct support staff's perspective is that often the consulting professional or supervisor comes to the consumer and staff to provide the training and training comes consistently from the same individual(s). This model also has plusses and minuses for staff turnover issues. Existing staff members can train new employees, but teamwork will lag until the new staff member is trained and begins working compatibly with other personnel.

In contrast to congregate shift-staffed settings, many community-based residences are smaller and serve fewer people under one roof. For comparison purposes, consider an arrangement where one staff member supports two individuals with DD in an apartment during a particular shift or time period. Depending on the staff scheduling system, only 1–3 employees must be trained on each habilitative intervention, usually labeled "support plans" in community settings. For example, some agencies employ "split shifts" or 4-day, 10-h shifts to minimize the total number of required employees. Individuals with DD may see more consistency in delivery of their supports when fewer support staff are involved. Because the individual employees often do not work side-by-side, training new employees often falls to supervisors with no current day-to-day experience in providing the supports. Moreover, there may be a period of days or weeks when the individuals with DD are supported by a temporary replacement who is not familiar with the prescribed supports. Thus, staff turnover may have more serious consequences for program consistency in settings supporting small numbers of consumers.

Usually, only large community agencies can afford full-time professional staff to prescribe and prepare support plans. Part-time consultants appear to be the norm for many agencies and the array of consultants often is less inclusive than the array in institutions. For example, community practitioners selected by the individual with DD or family members and guardians usually provide medical, dental, and psychiatric services. Thus, staff in community residences often interact with different practitioners across the individuals they serve, may have less access to practitioners and consultants, may receive less training in implementing supports, may have to travel with the individual with DD to receive consultative services, and only one member of the staff from the setting may actually have contact with the practitioner or consultant.

The observed result of these differences between service settings is that individuals receiving supports in the community often have fewer formal habilitative interventions or supports prescribed, supports may be less comprehensive and less aggressively provided, supports may be developed by practitioners and consultants with less experience with individuals with

DD, supports may be provided by less well-trained staff, and coordination across staff with regard to supports may be somewhat inconsistent. In many rural areas of the country, persons with no formal training in assessment, diagnosis, or treatment may develop most supports. For example, it is not uncommon for behavioral supports to be developed without the advice of a psychologist or behavior analyst, or for supports for more effective communication to be developed without the advice of a speech pathologist.

Today in many community agencies, the reality is that support planning, often referred to as person-centered planning, places by design much less emphasis on active-treatment-type habilitative interventions. Most of the emphasis is on another class of outcomes, such as those offered by Kincaid (1996). These are as follows:

1. Being present and participating in community life.
2. Gaining and maintaining satisfying relationships.
3. Expressing preferences and making choices in everyday life.
4. Having opportunities to fulfill respected roles and to live with dignity.
5. Continuing to develop personal competence (p. 458).

Clearly, planning for Outcomes 1–4 may draw less on clinical knowledge from the disciplines that have historically guided treatment for people with DD and more from practical knowledge of the people closely associated with and personally interested in the individual. That is, supports are now likely to be developed by people who each "know" the individual holistically rather than by those who, from a professional standpoint, know some subset of his or her strengths and deficits. Consistent with this shift, such planning is touted as relying more heavily on the wishes of the person supported than in institutional models.

One key research question related to staffing, however, is not "who does the planning," nor "what plans have the highest priorities," but rather "how to achieve and sustain the results of planning with measurable effectiveness?" No matter whether a support plan is developed by a case manager working alone, a close-knit circle of friends, or a team of professional consultants, the plan is nothing if not implemented correctly and consistently. Thus, what are the best ways to actualize one individual's plan? Are these methods different if a single support person must actualize the plans for multiple individuals concurrently? Are the essential details of effective strategies to be found in the plan or in the acquired knowledge of the person implementing the plans? If the latter, how do we insure that such knowledge is passed from today's support staff to tomorrow's? One model for answering these questions, referred to as the "scenario system" (Saunders, Rast, & Saunders, 1988) arose in the institutional environment, but has found acceptance in some community supported-living settings. The "teaching family" model (Phillips, Phillips, Fixsen, & Wolf, 1971) arose in service to predelinquent children, but may be a good alternative to typical staffing patterns in community residences for people with DD (Strouse, 1996). Neither model has prompted formal research on its benefits relative to other approaches, until most recently (Strouse, Carroll-Hernandez, Sherman, & Sheldon, 2003). A relevant element in choosing what kind of staffing pattern or support model to use is understanding the programmatic implications of the supports planning model chosen.

RESEARCH ON APPROACHES TO PLANNING

Recently behavior analysts debated, across issues of their journal, *The Behavior Analyst*, the relative merits of person-centered planning (PCP) and its near relatives (lifestyle planning and action planning). Holburn's historical perspective on residential behavior analysis outlined ups and downs of the behavior analyst in residential settings across time and system changes (Holburn, 1997). Holburn sees residential behavior analysts as becoming increasingly disenfranchised over recent years. Optimistically, Holburn views the PCP process as radically behavioristic and ripe with opportunities for the behavior analyst to apply the craft effectively. In contrast, a response by Osborne describes PCP as the newest *faux fixe* (Osborne, 1999) in the DD field. The most relevant of Osborne's observations to the present discussion are that *faux fixes* (a) are constructed so as to preclude analysis of their effectiveness, (b) promise much and are therefore maintained by the feeling that something good is happening, (c) purport to accomplish amazing results with ease (see the first research question above), and (d) careful examination of the *fixe* is met with scorn by those who promote it because of epistemological differences with the potential examiner.

To date, there are little data on PCPs and their effectiveness (e.g., Everson and Zhang, 2000) and promulgation of the approach is often through "stories" (Wagner, 1999). Wagner notes, however, that planners often report that the use of a PCP reduces challenging behavior. He notes that the relationship could be a functional one if the PCP minimized evocative stimuli and maximized the likelihood of positive reinforcement, both common strategies for behavior analysts.

Risley (1996) states that his "Get a Life" approach to planning affects the order in which PCP and behavioral interventions should be applied. Risley states that formal, technically precise behavioral methods should be applied, if necessary, only after the individual has been enabled through new lifestyle arrangements and life coaching. Indeed, Risley believes these steps require little training or specialized knowledge. Risley says that

> "In general, there is a negative correlation between the flexibility of life arrangements available and the technical precision of the behavior programming needed. The wider the latitude available for modifying the life arrangements for a person with challenging behaviors, the less precise and technical the behavior programming needs to be. The opposite is also true in that the less flexible a person's life arrangements are, the more technical and precise the behavior programming must be" (p. 429).

Risley restates a notion that has been around in various forms for some time. Wetzel and Hoschouer (1984), for example, suggested that a basic assumption in the development of "residential teaching communities" was that one need not begin with the elimination of maladaptive behaviors. They suggested that environmental design alone could "crowd out" such behaviors. The implication is that if individuals can be engaged in adaptive behavior with practical, common sense environmental modification, formal interventions will be less necessary or even desirable.

Generally, people of all kinds remain adaptively engaged most readily when they are relatively competent or fluent in an activity. Greater competence and fluency are normally associated with more reinforcers than are incompetence and disfluency. If enabling competence is what today's PCP is about, then PCP strategies have been in development for some time. A brief exercise in connecting some interdisciplinary dots on enabling competence could start with Lindsley (1964):

> Although prosthetic devices and training have the advantage of permitting a behaviorally handicapped individual to function within an average environment, their design usually requires detailed knowledge of the variables controlling the deficits. Since at this stage we cannot precisely describe the higher-order behavioral deficits, the most practical immediate strategy would be to design prosthetic environments in which the deficient behavior is not needed, rather than attempting to provide prosthetic devices and training (p. 65).

And Wolfensberger (1972) on normalizing action on the person level:

> On the first level of the interaction dimension (i.e., the person level), the normalization principle would dictate that we provide services which maximize the behavioral competence of a (deviant) person. Indeed, much of the programming by human management fields and agencies would fall into this general category (pp. 32–33).

And Skinner (1978):

> [create] an environment in which people behave in reasonably effective ways in spite of deficiencies, in which they take an active interest in life and begin to do for themselves what the institution previously did for them (p. 41).

And Gilbert (1978/1996) on enabling valuable accomplishments:

> Because our purpose is to design a system of engineering, a useful behavioral engineering model will deal with events that we can manipulate. It cannot be useful if it points to conditions of competence over which we have no control. There may be a chemical somewhere that, when taken orally, inevitably results in exemplary performance. But until someone discovers, refines, and packages it, we shall have to be satisfied with what we do have to work with. Thus, we are not looking for a model that tells us about the ultimate causes of behavior. What we are

looking for is a simple and useful way to identify the kinds of behavioral conditions we can manipulate—and at a cost that is less than the value received (p. 80).

And on structured normalization in the community, Thompson and Carey (1980):

> Creative, structured normalization depends critically on carefully designing social and habilitative environments which engender independence and overcome deficits resulting from years of destructive institutional experience. Essential ingredients in this process are individualized behavioral assessment, reinforcement of independent and socially competent behavior, and on-going assessment of outcome. Through combining environmental relocation with behavior intervention principles, normalization becomes something more than an abstract ideal (p. 196).

And on goodness-of-fit between persons and their environments, Schalock and Jensen (1986):

> Recent studies have indicated that the successful adjustment of people with disabilities to their environments is related to both person-specific behavioral capabilities and setting-specific performance requirements...This article summarizes how one might assess the goodness-of-fit (congruence) between a person's behavioral capabilities and setting-specific performance requirements. Once assessed, these data can be used for a number of purposes, including providing an index of important matched and mismatched skills; quantifying the congruence for planning, monitoring, and evaluation purposes; and permitting discrepancy analysis to establish habilitation strategies including skill training, prosthetic utilization, and/or environmental modification (p. 103).

On the purpose of supported routines, Saunders and Spradlin (1991):

> "...the right to competence should not be a right that the individual must earn, nor a right that is deferred because of where the individual lives or because of retardation *per se*. If competence is a right that meets these criteria, then its expression should be enabled immediately just as other rights are enabled. We believe that honoring this right means that the goal of residential services must be to enable the individual to do things for him/herself *now* by learning what the individual can do and then creating the supports necessary for it to happen (pp. 34–35).

On assessment of quality of life for a woman observed to be awakened and lifted into her wheelchair after "lights-on" in the morning, Heal, Borthwick-Duffy, and Saunders (1996):

> In other words, an assessment is made of the discrepancy between the individual's current participation in a routine or

> situation and the individual's participation that would fully challenge her abilities, characteristics, and preferences. The presence of unnecessary supports that preempt the individual's consenting, independent performance indicates a need for (a) instructional programs to build new skills, (b) opportunities for greater participation, or (c) better adaptations or prostheses. Teaching the individual safer bed-to-wheelchair transfer sequences, providing the individual with an alarm clock, and creating a remote-controlled light switch are, respectively, examples of these types of changes (p. 208).

And most recently, Mansell, Elliott, Beadle-Brown, Ashman, and McDonald (2002), summarizing some components of "active support" [edited]:

> Staff pay particular attention to working as a team and to scheduling and coordinating the choices and opportunities they offer. This involves establishing routines ... for the carrying out of ordinary activities ... and regular ... planning of how they will systematically share themselves across clients to provide the high level of support needed, often by more than one person at a time, for meaningful participation. ... Staff focus on helping service users take part minute-by-minute ..., finding the parts of complicated tasks that even the most disabled person can do and doing the other parts of the task themselves, so that the person is almost guaranteed to succeed (pp. 343–344).

So, with such obvious consensus regarding enabling competencies, what are the questions? The first question is how to access knowledge useful for enabling competence. Useful knowledge is formal and informal assessment results translated by clinicians, parents, friends, and neighbors or transmogrified by experience into some situational importance. I will refer to these as the "secrets to success." An example of secrets to success can be taken from Saunders, Saunders, Brewer, and Roach (1996). We reported on the implementation of a supported dining room routine to eliminate hand biting and head hitting in a young adolescent with autism and profound mental retardation. During observation and assessment, we noted that the child often served himself (family style) with the stainless steel serving spoon and then began eating with that spoon. This action prompted teacher intervention, resulting in a delay in eating, and further resulting in the self-injurious behavior. This was just one of the evocative antecedents to self-injury identified during meals. Each such antecedent was modified similarly to the following example: Prior formal assessments coupled with observations in the dining room suggested that the child did not discriminate the slightly larger serving spoon from his own place-setting spoon. So, the stainless steel serving spoons were replaced with brightly colored plastic spoons, even larger than the steel serving spoons. Indeed, these spoons were so long that turning the bowl of the spoon into the mouth was nearly impossible when the spoon was held by the handle. This knowledge-to-practice secret to success in enabling competence (i.e., eating with the correct spoon and avoiding delay or correction in eating) was part of the overall solution to self-injury at meals.

Or consider Mary, a 60-year-old nonverbal participant in a sheltered workshop. She absolutely cherished the money she earned, but spent much of every day screaming. Following multiple behavior analytic intervention attempts (e.g., time out) and common socially correct intervention attempts (offering the possibility of nonwork day activities), a passing occupational therapist noticed that Mary was expected to sand the edges of her bird house components using a stabilizing vise. Mary had a relatively short torso, suffered from osteoporosis, and her work furniture was not adapted to her conditions. Nevertheless, she was sufficiently motivated to earn money that she persisted at sanding with her hand above her heart. The result was muscle pain within 15 min of beginning work. The subsequent secret to success was to raise Mary's chair height or lower the table.

Risley (1996) is correct that elements of the plan do not require trained clinicians, for example, but alas, as with so many other things, the devil is in the details. Not all secrets to success can be generated by untrained or unspecialized people. These solutions often come only from extensive professional experience with the characteristics of people with and without disabilities, the physical and behavioral effects of the responses in question, and experience in looking at the one in the context of the other. Each individual with DD in the examples above communicated his or her pain or frustration, but only people armed with certain experiences with others with DD, assessment data from which to generalize, or both, interpreted the communications well enough to derive a practical enabling solution. With respect to residential and day services yesterday and today, here are some data. In 1987, I surveyed by telephone 10 institutions for people with ID in the central Midwest. These institutions reported employing approximately one degreed, and often certified or licensed, professional with experience in ID/DD for each 10–12 individuals with DD served. I refer here not to administrators, but only to persons in a position to engage in quality assessments, consultations, and prescriptive services. Currently, my experience is that the ratio in community programs in this same region is about 1:50, with most agencies relying on services from a few community practitioners who never see the individual in the context of residential and day services and who may each serve only a few individuals with DD.

A second common finding in community programs is that the most recent comprehensive evaluation of an individual, if one exists in the agency records, is the one last completed before leaving an institution or special education services. This comparison should not be interpreted as advocacy for the institutional model. Rather, it is intended to echo the concern already raised regarding the longitudinal dissemination of important information across sequential direct support staff. We appear to be at serious risk of losing access to critical, potentially unrecoverable knowledge, both at the planning level and the delivery level. It is becoming all too common for knowledge recovery to emerge in the testimony of expert witnesses after some fateful event, rather than during PCP development.

How easy is it to lose knowledge important to individualized supports? During our study, described above, the lead teacher who implemented the modified routines was out for some time on extended leave (Saunders et al., 1996). A substitute teacher, employed during that leave, observed the dining room routine before assuming responsibility for the classroom. The substitute modified the routine, omitting many of the elements we had designed. Our results showed an increase in self-injury during meals until the substitute could be taught the details of our routine and their significance in the prevention of self-injury. This data-based example illustrates the necessity for having a reliable method for passing the secrets of success from one direct support person to the next, or from one professional to another. In our study, the certified substitute teacher did not immediately recognize the relationship between elements of the environment and the child's behavior. Untrained, unlicensed, and inexperienced direct support staff may be even less likely to independently recognize what works and what does not work and generalize to related situations.

Risley is correct in urging that appropriate life arrangements be implemented before more technical behavioral interventions are considered. Wagner is correct in concluding that certain life arrangements can have a functional relation to the prevention of challenging behavior and, thus, can be behavioral interventions themselves. But, Osborne is correct in observing that it is neither simple nor easy to get it right; production of amazing results is not common. Holburn searches for a new and functional role for residential behavior analysts within such settings. His concern is appropriate because a large percentage of behavior analysts find employment in residential and day service settings for people with DD. It would be appropriate, however, if his umbrella of concern also covered occupational therapists, physical therapists, speech pathologists, special educators, recreation therapists, assistive technologists, and nurses. Current planning approaches do not appear to value their contributions as significantly as previous methods. Risley (1996) even remarked that many professionals need to be "detrained."

Fortunately, for many classes of clinicians, and unfortunately for residential and day services for people with DD, there are often more positions available outside the DD field than can be filled by all the individuals certified or licensed to fill them. Often these employment sites also offer salaries higher than those paid by community DD agencies. How important is this loss? By analogy, should we take our scuba lessons from someone who knows us well (around the house, around the workplace), but has no knowledge of the relation between depth, time at depth, speed of ascent, and our ability to understand and act on those concepts? I do not believe that proponents of PCPs desire, expect, or intend for us to act so foolishly. I do believe, however, that many proponents are unaware of the scope and significance of knowledge that does not make it to the planning table in many community settings. This problem deserves serious evidence-based attention.

RESEARCH ON HEALTH-RELATED ISSUES

Let us examine one area in which the goals of PCP, individual choice, limited knowledge, employment limitations, and direct support staffing variables are combining in a dangerous way. Obesity is a chronic disease characterized by an excess accumulation of body fat. In adults, obesity is associated with various co-morbidities including heart disease (Hubert, Feinleib, McNamara, & Castelli, 1983), diabetes (Woloshin & Schwartz, 2002), hypertension (Dyer & Elliot, 1989), and some cancers (Chute, Willett, & Colditz, 1991). In the United States, adult obesity has doubted over the past 30 years (Centers for Disease Control, 2006) and thus now affects approximately 90 million Americans. Individuals with DD are an underserved minority that has obesity rates greater than that of the general population (Rimmer, Braddock, & Fujiura, 1993). Rimmer et al. reported that 40.9% of adults with ID living in group homes were obese compared with 55.3% living with their natural family, whereas only 16.5% of those living in an institution were obese. In a recent study, Draheim, Williams, and McCubbin (2002a) reported that 92% of adults with ID residing in community settings consume more than the recommended amounts of dietary fat. In a second study, Draheim, Williams, and McCubbin (2002b) reported that the average Body Mass Index (BMI; kg/m^2) for men and women living in community settings was 28 and 32.3, respectively. As an index of 30 or greater indicates obesity, at least 50% of those in Draheim et al.'s sample were obese. Thus, as individuals with DD leave institutional care, they appear to be adopting the energy intake characteristics of the general population and in turn, show increased rates of obesity. This is not a recent phenomenon that can be placed at the feet of current fast food restaurant advertising schemes. For example, Aninger, Growick, and Bolinsky (1979) noted that overeating was a problem for 40% of a group of adults transitioned into community living from 1974 to 1978.

In association with energy intake, the increase in obesity prevalence has been associated with lack of physical activity in the general population and in individuals with DD (Beange, McElduf, & Baker, 1995; Draheim, Williams, & McCubbin, 2002b; Rimmer, Braddock, & Marks, 1995). Individuals in residential supported living settings have less physical activity compared to their peers living in institutional settings (e.g., Rimmer et al., 1995). Physical inactivity while at work may further contribute to the problem.

Between 1984 and 1985, the types of jobs that individuals with DD were most often assigned included kitchen work, food and beverage preparation, janitor or housekeeper duties, fabrication and repair of products, and packaging (Kiernan, McGaughey, & Schalock, 1988). These latter two jobs require sitting for long periods and are thus sedentary. Sedentary jobs are most common in segregated or facility-based work programs where more than 242,102 individuals with DD were employed nationwide in 1988 (Kiernan Gilmore, & Butterworth, 1997). Although integrated or supported employment services increased 353% from 1988 to 1993 ($N = 77,294$; Kiernan et al., 1997), the use of facility-based work has remained high over the same period (Kiernan, 1996). Thus, for the majority of working individuals with DD, a sedentary job is likely to continue as their type of employment in the future. (See Rusch, 1990, for an early history of supported employment, procedures, and outcomes.)

In many community settings, menu planning, shopping, and meal preparation is accomplished primarily by staff. Of particular concern is that support staff often receives no systematic and formal training in nutrition and meal planning. Further, what to eat, where to eat, and even how much to eat are commonly seen components of PCPs. Kincaid (1996) lists "What to eat (home)" at the top of his sample list of "choices" for a child. It is not uncommon to hear that, despite essential knowledge about diet and nutrition, planners agree to diet concessions because restrictions on diet are observed to be evokers of maladaptive behavior. Because staff directly purchases the food, and often dines with the individuals with DD, the menu may reflect food preferences of the staff as often as those of the individuals with DD. Additionally, food variety, cooking technique, and portion size often are at staff discretion—staff drawn from the overall population that is showing increases in the prevalence of obesity. The support staff for individuals with DD frequently prepares three meals a day in these settings, including a sack lunch taken daily to work.

As with other aspects of residential supports, nutritional consultation may be available only for special problems or in response to a physician's recommendation. A further practical difficulty with dietary planning in residential supported-living settings is that only one individual in the setting may require a weight-management diet. Or worse, two or more individuals may be on different diets. Thus, preparing meals responsibly for all individuals in the setting is challenging, particularly for undertrained staff. Moreover, other individual characteristics and support needs (e.g., continuous supervision) of the individuals in a community residence may preclude regular exercise (e.g., walking around the block) by the one who needs it; that is, one staff member cannot be in two locations at once.

CONCLUDING REMARKS

As I write these remarks, funding for new community placements has ended or slowed across this country as a function of the severe economic downturn from 2000 to 2004. Waiting lists are swelling, probably beyond the 87,000 estimated in the late 1990s (Lakin, 1998). Thus, we are, and will be for some time, a long way from providing inclusionary and integrated supports for all adults with DD and those children who need them. It is an excellent time, however, to pursue research on what will lead to the highest quality outcomes. Research also should focus on keeping overall costs low; if the DD population is ravaged by diabetes and heart disease for example, the funds for service expansion can only shrink. I have suggested that issues regarding the direct service workforce, our planning approaches, and their impact on health are related areas needing attention, but there are others as well. As other chapters in this text document, we have and are continuing to develop excellent data-based practices in a number of important clinical or treatment areas. We need some similar research in the service delivery arena.

REFERENCES

Aninger, M., Growick, B., & Bolinsky, K. (1979). Individual community placement of deinstitutionalized mentally retarded adults: Some personal concerns. *Mental Retardation, 17,* 307–308.
Beange, H., McElduf, A., & Baker, W. (1995). Medical disorders of adults with mental retardation: A population study. *American Journal of Mental Retardation, 99,* 595–604.
Butterfield, E. C. (1987). Why and how to study the influence of living arrangements. In S. Landesman, P. M. Vietze, & M. J. Begab (Eds.), *Living environments and mental retardation* (pp. 43–59). Washington, DC: American Association on Mental Retardation.
Chute, C. G., Willett, W. C., & Colditz, G. A. (1991). A prospective study of body mass, height, and smoking on the risk of colorectal cancer in women. *Cancer Causes Control, 2,* 117–124.
Dickens, C. (1892). *A tale of two cities.* London: Chapman & Hall.
Draheim, C. C., Williams, D. P., & McCubbin, J. A. (2002a). Physical activity, dietary intake, and the insulin resistance syndrome in nondiabetic adults with mental retardation. *American Journal on Mental Retardation, 107,* 361–375.
Draheim, C. C., Williams, D. P., & McCubbin, J. A. (2002b). Prevalence of physical inactivity and recommended physical activity in community based adults with mental retardation. *Mental Retardation, 40,* 436–444.
Dyer, A. R., & Elliot, P. (1989). The INTERSALT study: Relations of body mass index to blood pressure: INTERSALT Cooperative Research Group. *Journal of Human Hypertension, 3,* 299–308.
Eidelman, S. M., Pietrangelo, R., Gardner, J. F., Jesien, G., & Croser, M. D. (2003). Let's focus on the real issues. *Mental Retardation, 41,* 126–129.
Everson, J. M., & Zhang, D. (2000). Person-centered planning: Characteristics, inhibitors, and supports. *Education and Training in Mental Retardation and Developmental Disabilities, 35,* 36–43.
Federal Register. 53, No. 107 (June 3, 1988), pp. 20498–20499.
Gilbert, T. F. (1978/1996). *Human competence: Engineering worthy performance.* New York: McGraw Hill. (Reprinted, 1978, Amherst, MA: HRD Press).
Heal, L. W., Borthwick-Duffy, S. A., & Saunders, R. R. (1996). Assessment of quality of life. In J. W. Jacobson & J. A. Mulick (Eds.), *Manual of diagnosis and professional practice in mental retardation* (pp. 199–209). Washington, DC: American Psychological Association.
Holburn, S. (1997). A renaissance in residential behavior analysis? A historical perspective and a better way to help people with challenging behavior. *Behavioral Analyst, 20,* 61–85.
Hubert, H. B., Feinleib, M., McNamara, P. M., & Castelli, W. P. (1983). Obesity as an independent risk factor for cardiovascular disease: A 26-year follow-up of participants in the Framingham Heart Study. *Circulation, 67,* 968–977.
Kiernan, W. E. (1996). *Integrated employment status, approaches and challenges.* Washington, DC: President's Committee on Mental Retardation.
Kiernan, W. E., Gilmore, D. S., & Butterworth, J. (1997). Integrated employment: Evolution of national practices. In W. E. Kiernan & R. L. Schalock (Eds.), *Integrated employment: Current status and future directions* (pp. 17–29). Washington, DC: American Association on Mental Retardation.
Kiernan, W. E., McGaughey, M. J., & Schalock, R. L. (1988). Employment environments and outcome for adults with developmental disabilities. *Mental Retardation, 26,* 279–288.
Kincaid, D. (1996). Person-centered planning. In L. K. Koegel, R. L Koegel, & G. Dunlap (Eds.), *Positive behavioral support: Including people with difficult behavior in the community* (pp. 439–465). Baltimore: Brookes.

Lakin, K. C. (1998). On the outside looking in: Attending to waiting lists in systems of services for people with developmental disabilities. *Mental Retardation, 36,* 157–162.

Lakin, K. C., & Stehly, C. (1990). Supported community living: From community facilities to homes in the community. *DD Network News, 3,* 1–3.

Landesman, S., Vietze, P. M., & Begab, M. J. (Eds.). (1987). *Living environments and mental retardation.* Washington, DC: American Association on Mental Retardation.

Lindsley, O. R. (1964). Direct measurement and prothesis of retarded behavior. *Journal of Education, 147,* 62–81.

Mansell, J., Elliott, T., Beadle-Brown, J., Ashman, B., & McDonald, S. (2002). Engagement in meaningful activity and "active support" of people with intellectual disabilities in residential care. *Research in Developmental Disabilities, 23,* 342–352.

Osborne, J. G. (1999). Renaissance or killer mutation? A response to Holburn. *The Behavior Analyst, 22,* 47–52.

Perske, R. (2003). Parents who moved against the tide. *Mental Retardation, 41,* 133–134.

Phillips, E. L., Phillips, E. A., Fixsen, D. L., & Wolf, M. M. (1971). Achievement place: Modification of the behaviors of predelinquent boys within a token economy. *Journal of Applied Behavior Analysis, 1*(4), 45–59.

Prevalence of overweight and obesity among adults: United States, 1999–2002. (2006). NCHS Health & Stats, National Center for Health Statistics, Centers for Disease Control. Downloaded May 30, 2006 from http://www.cdc.gov/nchs/products/pubs/pubd/hestats/obese/obse99.htm.

Rimmer, J. A., Braddock, D., & Marks, B. (1995). Health characteristics and behaviors of adults with mental retardation residing in three living arrangements. *Research in Developmental Disabilities, 16,* 489–499.

Rimmer, J. H., Braddock, D., & Fujiura, G. (1993). Prevalence of obesity in adults with mental retardation: Implications for health promotion and disease prevention. *Mental Retardation, 31,* 105–110.

Risley, T. (1996). Get a life! Positive behavioral intervention for challenging behavior through life arrangement and coaching. In L. K. Koegel, R. L. Koegel, & G. Dunlap (Eds.), *Positive behavioral support* (pp. 425–437). Baltimore: Brookes.

Robinson, H. B., & Robinson, N. M. (1965). *The mentally retarded child: A psychological approach.* New York: McGraw Hill.

Robinson, N. M. (1987). Directions for person–environment research in mental retardation. In S. Landesman, P. M. Vietze, & M. J. Begab (Eds.), *Living environments and mental retardation* (pp. 79–120). Washington, DC: American Association on Mental Retardation.

Rusch, F. R. (1990). *Supported employment: Methods, models, and issues.* Sycamore, IL: Sycamore.

Saunders, R. R., Rast, J., & Saunders, M. D. (1988). *A handbook for scenario-based active treatment.* Lawrence: University of Kansas.

Saunders, R. R., Saunders, M. D., Brewer, A., & Roach, T. (1996). The reduction of self-injury in two adolescents with profound retardation by the establishment of a supported routine. *Behavioral Interventions, 11,* 59–86.

Saunders, R. R., & Spradlin, J. E. (1991). A supported routines approach to active treatment for enhancing independence, competence, and self-worth. *Behavioral Residential Treatment, 6,* 11–37.

Schalock, R. L., & Jensen, C. M. (1986). Assessing the goodness-of-fit between persons and their environments. *Journal of the Association for Persons with Severe Handicaps, 11,* 103–109.

Skinner, B. F. (1978). *Reflections on behaviorism and society.* Englewood Cliffs, NJ: Prentice-Hall.

Strouse, M. C. (1996). Replicating and maintaining the Teaching Family Model adapted for persons with mental retardation. *Dissertation Abstracts International, 57*(3-B), 21–41.

Strouse, M. C., Carroll-Hernandez, T. A., Sherman, J. A., & Sheldon, J. (2003). Evaluation of a staff scheduling system. *Organizational Behavior Management, 23,* 45–63.

Thompson, T., & Carey, A. (1980). Structured normalization intellectual and adaptive behavior changes in a residential setting. *Mental Retardation, 18,* 193–197.

Wagner, G. A. (1999). Further comments on person-centered approaches. *Behavior Analyst, 22*, 53–54.

Walsh, K., Kastner, T. A., & Green, R. G. (2003). Cost comparisons of community and institutional residential settings: Historical review of selected research. *Mental Retardation, 41*, 103–122.

Wetzel, R. J., & Hoschouer, R. L. (1984). *Residential teaching communities*. Glenview, IL: Scott, Foresman and Co.

Wolfensberger, W. (1972). *The principle of normalization in human services*. Toronto, Ont.: National Institute on Mental Retardation through Leonard Crainford.

Woloshin, S., & Schwartz, L. M. (2002). Press releases—Translating research into news. *JAMA, 287*, 2856–2858.

12

Behavioral–Clinical Consultation in the Developmental Disabilities

Contemporary and Emerging Roles

JOSEPH N. RICCIARDI and JAMES K. LUISELLI

This past century has witnessed a major shift in the delivery of support services for people with developmental disabilities. In the first half of the most recent century, American society concerned itself with the proliferation of institutions for persons with developmental disabilities. Often in remote settings, a principle concern was to relocate individuals who were characterized as a "menace" to society (Brockley, 1999; Scheerenberger, 1983). Throughout the latter half of the century, many of the negative assumptions about people with developmental disabilities were challenged and human service ideology shifted toward normalization, least restriction, and the development of policies favoring community-based living arrangements (Brockley, 1999; Landesman & Butterfield, 1987).

As changes in attitudes and practices were emerging in the 1950s, the institutionalization of children with developmental disabilities may have increased. Once universal public education became widespread, communities began to focus on the compulsory education of all children thus drawing attention to those considered unsuitable for public education by virtue of their disability (Brockley, 1999). However, the reliance on institutional settings for special education soon abated as educational policies and indeed legislation mandated a free and appropriate public education (FAPE) for all children including those with disabilities (Baker,

JOSEPH N. RICCIARDI and JAMES K. LUISELLI • The May Institute, Randolph, Massachusetts 02368

1989). Consequently, children with developmental disabilities began to challenge the preparedness of public school systems to meet their needs. This gave rise to the emergence of "technical assistance," a predecessor to the broader, contemporary models of consultation (e.g., Luiselli & Diament, 2002).

The change from institution-based to community-based intensive services for children and adults with developmental disabilities created need for behavioral–clinical consultation to families, school systems, and communities (Jacobson & Knox, 1987; Schroeder, Schroeder, & Landesman, 1987), particularly for individuals with serious behavior disorders and other clinical complexities. Successful practices were identified and disseminated that, in turn, encouraged further federal support for community-based program development for persons with mental retardation (Jacobson & Knox, 1987). Indeed, school systems, human service agencies, and families now routinely look to the expertise of behavioral–clinical consultation to maximize the quality of life and well-being of persons with developmental disabilities (Carr et al., 1999).

The focus of this chapter is to review the contemporary role of consultation in various settings and to share guidelines for successful practice. In addition, we discuss the emerging role of behavioral–clinical consultation in improving the greater well-being of persons with developmental disabilities, the staff who serve them, and the service systems in which both operate.

CONSULTATION ACROSS CLIENTS AND SETTINGS

Family Consultation

It is now well documented that families caring for children with developmental disabilities encounter tremendous pressures beyond those experienced by parents of typically developing children (Baker, Blacher, Kopp, & Kraemer, 1997; Blacher & Baker, 2002), a factor that may adversely alter parenting style (Costigan, Floyd, Harter, & McClintock, 1997) and increase the risk for an out-of-home placement (Blacher & Hanneman, 1993). One variable specifically associated with heightened parental stress is the presence of significant problem behavior. Severe problem behavior has been identified as a primary reason for family referral to a specialty clinic serving individuals with mental retardation and psychiatric disorders (Petronko, Harris, & Kormann, 1994). Baker, Blacher, Crnic, and Edelbrock (2002) found that problem behavior was a stronger predictor of parental stress than was cognitive delay. Additionally, there is now wide agreement that skill acquisition and other developmental improvements are greater in children with developmental disabilities whose parents are trained to implement educational programs in the home setting (Anderson, 1989). Accordingly, behavior management and skill development are the primary foci of behavioral–clinical consultation to families of individuals with developmental disabilities.

Behavior management consultation to families takes a clinical and educative form. First, the clinician evaluates problem behavior using typical methods suggested by the clinical literature, notably, functional assessment using interview strategies combined with direct observation (O'Neill, Horner, Albin, Storey, & Sprague, 1997). Although analogue conditions functional analysis remains an important method for the assessment of function (Hanley, Iwata, & McCord, 2003), practical aspects such as available time and the service delivery setting limit its use in family consultation. However, viable strategies for brief functional analyses in outpatient settings, often as part of parent consultation, have been demonstrated (Derby et al., 1992; Wacker et al., 1994; Wacker & Steege, 1993). These protocols are time-efficient and show strong concordance with the results of lengthier functional analysis methods. Accordingly, clinicians should consider the use of brief functional analysis in the conduct of their assessment of problem behavior. A further extension of the method—also shown to be suitable in outpatient settings—includes the direct assessment of intervention components (Harding, Wacker, Cooper, Millard, & Jensen-Kovalan, 1994), and training parents in direct assessment methods including functional analysis (Najdowski, Wallace, Doney, & Ghezzi, 2003).

Behavior management consultation to families should include training caregivers to implement intervention recommendations. Involving families in all phases of assessment and intervention design, and including implementation training as part of the process, provides families with enduring and generalizable skills (Lucychyn, Albin, & Nixon, 1997; Vaughn, Clarke, & Dunlap, 1997). Recently, Kuhn, Lerman, and Vorndran (2003) demonstrated that training one family member in a behavioral procedure along with guidelines for training two other family members might be sufficient to "pyramid" training throughout a family system. This method would provide families with additional lifelong skills for meeting the clinical needs of their child as they learn not only the essential intervention skills but the skills needed to develop other effective caregivers within their family support network.

To a lesser degree, behavioral consultation to families has included training in the techniques for facilitating skill development in their child. Parent training has been widely used as a component of the education of children with autism (Anderson, 1989). Valuable techniques can be rapidly acquired and with specific programming can generalize to use outside the clinic setting (Koegel, Glahn, & Neiminen, 1978). Ideally, the consultant would teach family members how to replicate specific instructional strategies being used by their child's teachers and clinical staff (Anderson, 1989), plus additional guidance for applying behavioral learning techniques during natural teaching opportunities, such as communication junctures (Laski, Charlop, & Schreibman, 1988). Extensions of the approach include training siblings to implement similar procedures (Schreibman, O'Neill, & Koegel, 1983).

A detailed exemplar of behavioral–clinical consultation to a family was provided by Luiselli and Luiselli (1995). The participant was a 2.5-year-old girl with multiple developmental disabilities, medical problems, and sensory impairments. She was cared for by her parents in their home with assistance from a visiting nurse. The focus of intervention was the elimination of gastronomy-tube dependence and establishment of oral feeding. At baseline the child accepted on average 100 calories per day by mouth, and 1,500 per day via gastronomy tube. The intervention consisted of instructions to ensure consistent presentation of foods, quantity of food, the avoidance of forced-feedings, reinforcement of oral consumption, and fading of feeding tube delivered foods. Although under the guidance of a clinical consultant, the interventions were carried out by the family and a visiting nurse. The data depict a gradual increase in oral feedings during the intervention phase with elimination of the feeding tube by 30 weeks. The case is noteworthy for several reasons. First, the participant represents a degree of complexity that less than a generation earlier would likely have been served in an institutional setting. Second, although the consultant assessed behavioral–clinical features of the case and developed the intervention plan, the intervention itself was carried out by family members.

Recently, a conceptual development in behavioral–clinical consultation has emerged with particular applicability to families. Carr and Smith (1995) proposed a contextual model for problem behavior, hypothesizing that discriminative stimuli and setting events converged as a context for the exhibition of problem behavior. Theoretically, if the putative contexts were reliably identified, intervention could be specifically targeted toward these occasions (McAtee, Carr, & Schulte, 2004). McAtee et al. are developing the Contextual Assessment Inventory (CAI) specifically for this purpose and their preliminary data suggest good internal validity. The development of a valid and reliable instrument for the evaluation of discriminative stimuli and setting events that contribute to problem behavior in the home would be of immeasurable value to behavioral–clinical consultants.

In essence, the central role of the behavioral–clinical consultant working with families is to provide a direct service that has as its goal the resolution of the urgent presenting needs and the development of family care giving skills such that the family is capable of addressing their child's clinical needs into the future. These goals are consistent with the aims of consultation across other settings as well.

School Consultation

As described previously, the advent of policy and legislation mandating a free public education for all children during the past 35–40 years created the motivation for technical assistance and comprehensive behavioral–clinical consultation to public schools. The 1997 reauthorization of the Individuals with Disabilities Education Act (IDEA) increased the demand for such consultation. The reauthorization is quite specific in its language requiring under certain circumstances a functional behavior assessment (FBA), measurable goals, positive behavior supports, and social skills development (Luiselli, 2002). As has been noted, many public school districts will likely seek consultation in order to adhere to these new poli-cies (Luiselli, 2002).

Best practices in behavioral–clinical consultation, as well as the spe-cific language of the IDEA, suggest that consultation to schools should in-clude FBA; the development of specific, written guidelines that include pro-grams for increasing positive behaviors; and the development of objective data-collection methods. These practices are often conceptually grasped by nonspecialist educators, but they are technically sophisticated and usu-ally require specialized training and supervision. For this reason, the con-sultant ideally functions as both provider of these direct services and as trainer to school personnel with a goal of increasing the technical skills of educators during the course of consultation.

It is important for the school consultant to recognize the multiple pur-poses of conducting the FBA. There are three general reasons for conduct-ing an FBA, though often the consultant will learn of only the first—to ad-dress a problem behavior of concern. This is how the consultant is prepared for the case and it is usually the only focus on the school consultant's mind. However, a second purpose is the legal adherence to the requirements of IDEA. It is important for the behavioral–clinical school consultant to rec-ognize that their work has legal implications—special education cases are often the subject of litigation or careful scrutiny by other consultants possi-bly in preparation for litigation. For that reason, the consultant must take special care to ensure that the procedures are comprehensive, reflective of best practices, and clearly documented. The third reason for the functional analysis is to develop a hypothesis that will guide intervention decisions and lead to a better understanding of the person with a developmental disability.

The conduct of an FBA in school settings often begins with clinical in-terviews and direct observation. Although widely used, clinical interviewing generally has poor reliability and often amounts to nothing more than self-report—the recollections of the interviewee. The method is also hindered by limitations in the experience and training of the interviewer, making it likely that important questions will not be asked or will be asked in ways that "lead" the interviewee. These latter problems can be overcome by the use of structured clinical interviews where leading experts provide the com-prehensive questions and the order of questioning. One example designed specifically for school-based consultation is Steege and Watson (2003); an-other very popular structured interview is O'Neill et al. (1997), which can be modified for use in school settings as well. Although insufficient for the conduct of a functional assessment by itself, clinical interviewing is irreplaceable for beginning a collaborative dialogue with school personnel, setting the occasion to form mutual goals and expectations, and developing the positive exchange of information that is critical to successful consul-tation (Gutkin & Curtis, 1982).

More direct forms of assessment follow the clinical interview. In di-rect assessment, the student's behavior is recorded in vivo either through frequency count or other measurement strategy, or through event record-ings and narratives such as the ubiquitous "ABC" sheet method (Bijou, Peterson, & Ault, 1968) or the "Detailed Behavior Report" (DBR; Groden,

1989). In both cases, and in like systems, observers record details about what preceded and followed the behavior of concern and possibly other specified variables. By recording events as they occur or immediately following their occurrence, the problem of selective memory inherent in clinical interviewing is overcome.

Recently, researchers have demonstrated the feasibility of conducting analogue conditions functional analysis in school settings (Paige, McKerchar, & Thompson, 2004) and the practicality of using teachers as experimenters (Moore & Edwards, 2003; Moore et al., 2002). Training teachers to conduct functional analyses is consistent with the school-based consultant's role of building technical skills and also demonstrate in a profound way how typical environmental contingencies function as reinforcement. Other researchers have applied direct instruction and performance feedback to develop other advanced behavioral skills in teachers such as preference assessments (Lavie & Sturmey, 2002) and discrete trial instruction (LeBlanc, Ricciardi, & Luiselli, 2005). These studies provide school-consultants with a specific methodology for approaching the skills development component of their work.

One recent study illustrates an emerging role for clinical–behavioral consultants operating in school settings—the integration of school and home interventions. It is well accepted that generalization remains an imperative for behavioral intervention (Schindler & Horner, 2005). Indeed, the behavioral gains made by children with developmental disabilities in the school setting may not easily transfer to the home setting without specific programming or other interventions. Schindler and Horner (2005) demonstrated that a low-effort contextually based intervention applied in the home setting had little to no behavioral reductive effect until the participant acquired a functionally equivalent behavior in the school setting. The finding suggests the need for thoughtful coordination of home and school consultation, something that might be most expediently accomplished by having the school-based consultant coordinate home-based intervention as well. This model deserves to be explored further.

Finally, systems-oriented or "whole school" intervention has been addressed through behavioral consultation (Sugai & Horner, 2002). Consultation at this level targets the entire student population, is prevention-focused, emphasizes positive behavior support, and enlists the participation of all relevant stakeholders (students, teachers, administrators, and parents). A primary role for the consultant in developing "whole school" projects is facilitating an atmosphere of collaborative team building. With guidance from the consultant, in-school teams are taught how to identify behavior-change objectives, document dependent measures, formulate intervention plans, evaluate data, and make empirically derived decisions. In addition to showing large-scale positive outcomes, a critical objective of systems consultation is the sustainability of intervention across multiple academic years. Another goal is to ensure that schools maintain programming when consultation services are faded and ultimately eliminated (Luiselli, Putnam, Handler, & Feinberg, 2005; Putnam, Handler, Ramerez-Pratt, & Luiselli, 2003).

A detailed exemplar of a whole-school behavioral consultation approach, with 4-year longitudinal data is provided by Luiselli, Putnam, and Sunderland (2002). These authors describe the use of a system for reinforcing specific positive behaviors and academic achievements, plus a system for responding to discipline problems and increasing parent involvement with the same.

CONSULTATION WITHIN SERVICE PROVIDER AGENCIES

Human services agencies that serve individuals with developmental disabilities use expertise in behavioral–clinical psychology for several purposes. First, they design effective programming for increasing skills and independence in the individuals the agency serves. Second, many individuals served may display problem behavior (Eyman, Borthwick, & Miller, 1981) and behavioral–clinical consultants are asked to assess these problems and design effective interventions. Third, individuals with developmental disabilities may suffer from comorbid psychiatric conditions (Borthwick-Duffy, 1994; Einfeld & Tonge, 1996), and clinical consultants are asked to integrate behavioral approaches across disciplines and assist with addressing the complex relationship between psychiatric disorder and problem behaviors (Rojahn, Matson, Naglieri, & Mayville, 2004).

In addition, many human service agencies recognize the need to "professionalize" the direct support workforce. Accordingly, the infusion of advanced clinical expertise accessible to direct support staff in the form of consultation and training is one means for developing the professional skills and identity of this position. As seen in other consultation settings, clinical services are often integrated with staff development and training—successful consultation addresses the needs of the participant and the development of the staff that support her or him.

Often, the first step in behavioral–clinical consultation entails a review of existing supports and the contexts in which problem behaviors are observed to arise most frequently. Contextual assessment is especially important in community-based service settings given the fluctuation and change often noted in staffing patterns in such programs. The well-known "scatter-plot" method (Touchette, MacDonald, & Langer, 1985) is simple, and widely used. In this technique, the clinician devises data collection sheets to enable staff to record occurrences of targeted behaviors across times and in some cases settings. A modified version of the same has been provided by Steege and Watson (2003), who added opportunities for recording activities in 15-min intervals and qualitative ratings of participant's positive involvement with the same. The instrument is worth considering because for only a slight increase in effort more information is gathered to permit a clinician to identify patterns of stimulus control of positive behaviors as well.

Problem behaviors characterized by high intensity (thus worthy of clinical assessment and programming efforts) but low frequency are especially perplexing to clinicians. Their frequency is too low to quickly gather enough information to permit the detection of patterns of antecedents and consequences that is required for assessment-derived intervention, especially when simply reviewing frequency counts, ABC-sheets, or scatter-plot data. Groden (1989) developed the DBR with special utility for this problem. The DBR is similar to ABC-sheets in that it is completed immediately upon occurrence of defined targeted behaviors and that it requests the reporter to describe antecedent and consequent stimuli. However, the DBR is especially useful in that it includes very detailed questions and descriptors of such stimuli and definitions for the same. These conventions add precision and generate more detail. Accordingly, it is especially valuable for low-frequency target behaviors because it makes up for frequency by the depth of information captured upon each occurrence. We have used the DBR with specific instructions for program staff to "complete a report for five consecutive occurrences of the target behavior" and then bring to the consultant for review. Clearly, there is no "magic number" of reports. However, five often provides a substantial amount of information and may permit the consultant to generate a functional hypothesis and trial intervention. If not, then another five reports may be collected. Using this process, the effort to complete the DBR is short-term and reporting staff is spared the problem of interminable completion of incident reports, something that in our experience often leads to cursory completion of such reports rather than the careful attention to detail being requested.

Intervention design more often involves the development of a multicomponent plan than the provision of a single intervention. Interventions are combined to address a range of target behaviors, or to address multiple dimensions of a single target behavior. An example of the approach is shown by Bird, Dores, Moniz, and Robinson (1989), who address two cases of severe SIB and aggression using functional communication training, DRO, and stimulus (demand) fading procedures. This is typical of behavioral programming in community-based applied settings, where the consultant essentially engineers the behavioral environment. In this example, staff is instructed in procedures for removing eliciting stimuli (in this specific example, the density of work demands), prompting an alternative behavior (the functional and alternative communication "Break"), strategies for reinforcing the alternative behavior (immediate access to break during training sessions and at any time the emerging alternative behavior is exhibited), and reinforcing absence of targeted behaviors.

In some cases, recommendations are made for modifying the environment to maximize positive responding/minimize eliciting problem behaviors (Carr et al., 1999; Luiselli, 1998). In addition, specific strategies for increasing positive or adaptive behaviors that functionally compete with targeted behaviors and detailed guidelines for extinction are combined in a single support plan (Ricciardi, 2006). Generally, there will be three distinct intervention areas for the consultant to consider: (1) Controllable, environmental factors that influence expression of challenging and positive behaviors, (2) Behaviors to increase, particularly those believed to enhance quality of life, independence, well-being, and to compete with the function of problem behaviors, and (3) Behaviors to decrease, generally through a functionally suitable form of extinction or differential reinforcement.

Often the behavioral–clinical consultant functions as senior clinician in community-based agencies and as the first clinical resource for caregiving staff. Accordingly, the clinician must retain a broad perspective that incorporates an understanding of traditional behavior–environment relationships as well as an understanding of the influence of health and emotional well-being on behaviors of concern. Recently, Carr, Smith, Giacin, Whelan, and Pancari (2003) described their approach toward systematically identifying the effect of menstrual discomfort on problem behavior, functional assessment, and a multicomponent intervention for three participants. The intervention procedures were remarkably effective, yet simple and very much fitting a "normalized" approach to menstrual discomfort made possible by the provision of staff supports. Specifically, staff were trained to identify verbal and nonverbal indications of pain and discomfort, and then to respond to signs of pain by providing noncontingent access to reinforcement, incidental teaching of break requests, incidental teaching of requesting help or assistance with demands, choice making, and strategies to naturally reduce density of task demands. Accordingly, participants learned to take breaks or seek help when in pain, and to take it easy and spend time with the things they found most comforting when feeling uncomfortable. Through the work of consultation, staff learned *how and when* to teach these critical skills.

THE SUCCESSFUL PRACTICE OF CONSULTATION

The four-stage behavioral problem-solving sequence advocated by Bergan and Kratochwill (1990; Table 12.1) provides a framework for the implementation of consultation services. This approach integrates many

Table 12.1. Stages of Behavioral–Clinical Consultation

Stage 1: Problem identification
  Identify challenging behaviors and competencies
  Define target behaviors operationally
  Design baseline data collection procedures
  Initiate baseline assessment
Stage 2: Problem analysis
  Complete functional behavioral assessment
  Develop behavior hypotheses
  Formulate and design behavior support plan
Stage 3: Intervention plan implementation
  Implement behavior support plan
  Provide staff straining
  Refine and modify intervention
  Introduce maintenance facilitating strategies
Stage 4: Intervention plan evaluation
  Evaluate intervention effects
  Assess collateral behavior-change
  Gather social validity measures

---

steps linking assessment, case formulation, and intervention evaluation. To perform competently, a consultant should have knowledge of evidence-supported procedures, the ability to perform and interpret functional behavioral assessments, dexterity with single-case experimental designs, and solid communication skills to impart recommendations to service providers. Consultants also must adhere to ethical codes of conduct promulgated by state boards of registration and credentialing bodies such as the Behavior Analyst Certification Board (www.bacb.org).

The preceding discussion notwithstanding, delivering effective consultation services requires more than technical proficiency. As noted by Gutkin and Curtis (1982), "At its most basic level, consultation is an interpersonal exchange," such that "the consultant's success is going to hinge largely on his or her communication and relationship skills" (p. 822). Most professionals who function as consultants do not receive extensive training on the interpersonal elements of service delivery. Nonetheless, our experiences are that intervention success rests greatly on a particular "interactive style" between consultant and the consulted. Additionally, there are certain pragmatic considerations that predict a positive response from the recipients of consultation services. In this section, we review and expand upon some of these issues.

The Context of Service Settings

A consultant entering a developmental disability service setting has no administrative authority over employees. The consultant is present to evaluate one or more referral objectives, formulate strategies, and propose recommendations. Although the expectation is that consultation advice will be adopted, this outcome is not guaranteed and indeed, follow-through by practitioners may be inconsistent or absent entirely. These circumstances should alert consultants to a fundamental maxim: you are not in charge! Instead, a consultant is a visitor to an unfamiliar environment. Accommodating to that role is a first step toward building a successful alliance with staff.

As an "outsider" visiting a service setting, the consultant should be cognizant about organizational expectations. Whether consultation is being conducted at a residential facility for adults or a third-grade classroom at a public elementary school, learn the conventional protocol at the setting. This means knowing the "rules" of the surroundings and respective behaviors. For example, most public schools require visitors to wear an identification badge when on the premises. A school consultant should be diligent with this routine and other dictates such as singing in on the "visitors log" and remaining in designated locations within the building. Most service settings have similar guidelines.

A consultant also should be aware of the administrative hierarchy of a service setting. It is critical to know the people who make programmatic decisions and their scope of responsibility. Having this knowledge should enable a consultant to work more effectively. As an illustration, although the executive director of a habilitation service setting may have hired a consultant, the actual day-to-day operation usually falls to middle-tiered managers and supervisors. These individuals, as well as direct-care providers, will occupy most of the consultant's time and accordingly, be instrumental in eliciting support to carry out recommendations.

Another key to success is for the consultant to downplay the status of "expert." In actuality, a large measure of expertise can be found with the staff that regularly interacts with students and consumers. The consultant should enter the service setting recognizing this fact and demonstrate professional deference accordingly. Sensitivity to this mater would be shown by the consultant seeking the opinions of service providers, listening to divergent input, facilitating collaborative problem solving, and building consensus among participants (Hieneman & Dunlap, 2000).

It is good practice for a consultant to review her/his role with staff. Here, there should be an explanation of the circumstances culminating in a referral for consultation, the parameters involved, and expected outcomes. Information of this type usually is well received by staff that was not involved in the decision to seek consultation but is expected to comply with recommendations.

Understanding the Motivations of Service Providers

Understanding what practitioners want from consultation is a beneficial enterprise. Put succinctly, most staff looks for a consultant to solve a problem, make it go away, with the least amount of time and effort. Furthermore, the people responsible for instruction and habilitative care usually believe that they have too much to do and not enough time to do it. An astute professional must recognize these issues throughout the consultation process.

Identifying the motivations of service providers means that consultants must design "context-specific" interventions. That is, recommendations should fit with the practical exigencies of the setting including, but not limited to, personnel resource allocation, performance expectations, competing responsibilities, features of the physical environment, and administrative support. The challenge for the consultant is to propose behavior-change strategies that are consistent with evidence-based practices yet capable of being addressed by service providers. Thus, intervention plans should not be time-consuming or procedurally complex. Data recording should be simplified. Implementation should not require intensive supervision. By balancing clinical recommendations with "real-world" conditions, consultants can expect reasonable intervention integrity.

Staff motivation also is influenced by interpersonal perceptions of the consultation alliance. For example, how well staff "like" a consultant should not be overlooked. On one hand, "likeability" surely is dependent on the clinical expertise and problem-solving ability demonstrated by the consultant. Equally important is the style of interaction: is the consultant easy to talk to, considerate, and pleasant? Humor, when employed judiciously, often has a positive effect on deliberations. Considering the many interactions a consultant will have with staff, strong interpersonal skills are a requisite professional competency.

Language and Communication

On the topic of communication, Skinner (1957) advised selecting words for their effects on the listener, not the speaker. Paying close attention to language and the meaning of words is a defining attribute of the skillful consultant. Too often, professionals speak and write using a technical jargon that is accessible only to like-minded colleagues. Among a less sophisticated audience, communication should be "toned down" and free of arcane expressions and terminology. Failure to communicate simply and concisely confuses and alienates listeners.

Knowing your audience is critical for effective communication. In some cases, staff may have experience with certain assessment and intervention methods, or basic knowledge about a discipline such as applied behavior analysis. This background may enable the consultant to use technical terms that ease discussion. More often, however, staff is not experienced practitioners, with no to little education concerning developmental disabilities. In these circumstances, the consultant should choose words carefully, while studiously assessing the skill level and knowledge competencies of staff.

To improve communication consultants should not pontificate, lecture, or speak pedantically. It is important to be responsive to all questions and take time to clarify presentation whenever indicated. "Nit picking" over concepts and definitions also should be avoided. For example, if a staff person speaks about giving a "reward" to a consumer following appropriate behavior, there may be little to gain by offering correction (e.g., "You mean positive reinforcement."). A consultant also should deliberate carefully about posing counterarguments in the face of inaccurate discourse, such as a staff person referencing *negative reinforcement* instead of *punishment*. These caveats are particularly critical during the early phase of consultation when a collaborative relationship is being formed. Language that does not confuse or intimidate an audience leads to better acceptance and personal appeal, which we have found enhances the work to be done.

One additional communication recommendation is to converse with staff about general life events not integral to consultation. Inquiring about activities over the weekend, the local sports scene, and recent movie reviews are just a few acceptable topics. The simple intent is that brief, friendly exchanges establish the consultant as a "discriminative stimulus" for positive interactions that by extension should facilitate ongoing and future exchanges. Keep in mind that informal conversations always should be within the bounds of professional decorum.

Managing Consultation Services

Many professionals provide consultation to more than one service setting. Accordingly, consultants function best when they possess good time-management skills. Once financial obligations have been decided and a service contact arranged, a consultant should establish a visitation schedule. Ideally, weekly, biweekly, or monthly on-site consultation should be specified. Setting consultation on a particular day of the week and for a defined duration is advantageous because it allows staff to adjust their own schedules. Being the "outsider," a consultant should defer to the service setting when scheduling appointments.

Simple and basic protocol applies to consultation practice. The consultant should be punctual, respecting the many demands confronting service providers. Although cancellations are inevitable, they should be kept to a minimum so as not to interrupt service delivery. Each consultation visit should have an agenda delineating times for observation, meetings, data analysis, and related activities. Finally, we suggest that consultants prepare a brief report that captures the outcome of each encounter. The report would summarize discussion points, set forth recommended action plans, assign responsibilities, and specify the date of the next consultation.

Consultants must be open to communication between scheduled on-site visits. Staff at a service setting should have access to a consultant by telephone, e-mail, and pager. Consultants, in fact, should encourage such communication, particularly in situations where ongoing feedback is necessary or procedures are subject to rapid change. Any communication requests from staff should be answered in a timely manner. Delayed or ignored responses to inquiries are perceived poorly and undermine progress.

Your performance as a consultant can be improved by asking for feedback from service providers. We have found it advantageous to prepare abbreviated (1–2 pages) assessment forms that staff completes during and following the delivery of consultation services. The objectives of this assessment are to learn how staff judged the effectiveness of consultation and if they were satisfied with the outcomes. The same performance evaluation should be "self-managed" by the consultant. To illustrate, after each visit to a service setting, a consultant might ask, "Was I clear and concise in my communications?" or "How did I handle provoking questions during the staff meeting?" Self-evaluation, combined with more formal social validity assessment, builds continuous quality improvement into the fabric of consultation services.

Final Considerations

Clinical consultation is not static but evolves in response to the concerns of service providers, the achievement of therapeutic objectives, unanticipated events, and new knowledge disseminated to the professional community. Effective consultants start small, shaping behavior, and focusing on "strength-based" recommendations. Optimism, encouragement, and gentle persuasion are hallmarks of the successful professional. Consultants must be resourceful and willing to adapt to the variability that inevitably is associated with complex cases and systems issues. Concepts of "mindfulness and acceptance" are worth considerations in this regard

(Singh et al., 2004). As articulated in this section, one's technical skills as a consultant will have little impact unless other competencies are acquired and demonstrated fluently among the people and within the settings seeking your services.

SUMMARY

We have outlined salient issues in the practice of clinical–behavioral consultation to persons who have developmental disabilities. There is an increasing need for consultation-initiated intervention within families, schools, and human services agencies. Effective consultation requires fundamental knowledge of contemporary and evidence supported assessment and intervention procedures. Success also is determined by good interpersonal and communication skills. Our challenge is to ensure that these competencies are taught to young professionals and manifested proficiently by novice and seasoned consultants.

REFERENCES

Anderson, S. R. (1989). Autism. In B. L. Baker (Ed.), *Parent training and the developmental disabilities* (pp. 137–153). Washington, DC: American Association on Mental Retardation.

Baker, B. L. (1989). *Parent training and the developmental disabilities.* Washington, DC: American Association on Mental Retardation.

Baker, B. L., Blacher, J., Crnic, K. A., & Edelbrock, C. (2002). Behavior problems and parenting stress in families of three-year-old child with and without developmental delays. *American Journal on Mental Retardation, 107*, 433–444.

Baker, B. L., Blacher, J., Kopp, C. B., & Kraemer, B. (1997). Parenting children with mental retardation. *International Review of Research in Mental Retardation, 20*, 1–45.

Bergan, J. R., & Kratochwill, T. R. (1990). *Behavioral consultation and therapy.* New York: Plenum.

Bijou, S. W., Peterson, R. F., & Ault, M. H. (1968). A method to integrate descriptive and experimental field studies at the level of data and empirical concepts. *Journal of Applied Behavior Analysis, 1*, 175–191.

Bird, F., Dores, P. A., Moniz, D., & Robinson, J. (1989). Reducing severe aggression and self-injurious behavior with functional communication training. *American Journal on Mental Retardation, 94*, 37–48.

Blacher, J., & Baker, B. (2002). *Families and mental retardation.* Washington, DC: American Association on Mental Retardation.

Blacher, J., & Hanneman, R. (1993). Out-of-home placement of children and adolescents with severe handicaps: Behavioral interventions and behavior. *Research in Developmental Disabilities, 14*, 145–160.

Borthwick-Duffy, S. A. (1994). Epidemiology and prevalence of psychopathology in people with mental retardation. *Journal of Consulting and Clinical Psychology, 62*, 17–27.

Brockley, J. A. (1999). History of mental retardation: An essay review. *History of Psychology, 2*, 25–36.

Carr, E. G., Horner, R. H., Turnbull, A. P., Marquis, J. G., Magito-McLaughlin, D., McAtee, M. L., et al. (1999). *Positive behavior supports for dealing with problem behavior in people with developmental disabilities: A research synthesis.* Washington, DC: American Association on Mental Retardation.

Carr, E. G., & Smith, C. E. (1995). Biological setting events for self-injury. *Mental Retardation and Developmental Disabilities Research Reviews, 1*, 94–98.

Carr, E. G., Smith, C. E., Giacin, T. A., Whelan, B. M., & Pancari, J. (2003). Menstrual discomfort as a biological setting event for severe problem behavior: Assessment and intervention. *American Journal on Mental Retardation, 108*, 117–133.

Costigan, C. L., Floyd, F. J., Harter, K. S. M., & McClintock, J. C. (1997). Family process and adaptation to children with mental retardation: Disruption and resilience in family problem-solving interactions. *Journal of Family Psychology, 11*, 515–529.

Derby, K. M., Wacker, D. P., Sasso, G., Steege, M., Northup, J., Cigrand, K., et al. (1992). Brief functional assessments techniques to evaluate aberrant behavior in an outpatient setting: A summary of 79 cases. *Journal of Applied Behavior Analysis, 25*, 713–721.

Einfeld, S. L., & Tonge, B. J. (1996). Population prevalence of psychopathology in children and adolescents with intellectual disability. *Journal of Intellectual Disability Research, 40*, 91–109.

Eyman, R. K., Borthwick, S. A., & Miller, C. (1981). Trends in maladaptive behavior of mentally retarded persons placed in community and institutional settings. *American Journal on Mental Retardation, 85*, 473–477.

Groden, G. (1989). A guide for conducting a comprehensive behavior analysis of a target behavior. *Journal of Behavior Therapy and Experimental Psychiatry, 20*, 163–169.

Gutkin, T. B., & Curtis, M. J. (1982). School-based consultation: Theory and techniques. In C. R. Reynolds & T. B. Gutkin (Eds.), *The handbook of school psychology* (pp. 796–828). New York: Wiley.

Hanley, G. P., Iwata, B. A., & McCord, B. E. (2003). Functional analysis of problem behavior: A review. *Journal of Applied Behavior Analysis, 36*, 147–185.

Harding, J., Wacker, D. P., Cooper, L. J., Millard, T., & Jensen-Kovalan, P. (1994). Brief hierarchical assessment of potential treatment components with children in an outpatient clinic. *Journal of Applied Behavior Analysis, 27*, 291–300.

Hieneman, M., & Dunlap, G. (2000). Factors affecting the outcomes of community-based behavioral support: I. Identification and description of factor categories. *Journal of Positive Behavior Interventions, 2*, 161–169.

Jacobson, J. W., & Knox, L. A. (1987). Professional and technical opportunities for psychologists in mental retardation. *American Psychologist, 42*, 449–451.

Koegel, R. L., Glahn, T. J., & Neiminen, G. S. (1978). Generalization of parent training results. *Journal of Applied Behavior Analysis, 11*, 95–109.

Kuhn, S. A. C., Lerman, D. C., & Vorndran, C. M. (2003). Pyramidal training for families of children with problem behavior. *Journal of Applied Behavior Analysis, 36*, 77–88.

Landesman, S., & Butterfield, E. C. (1987). Normalization and deinstitutionalization of mentally retarded persons. Controversy and facts. *American Psychologist, 42*, 809–816.

Laski, K. E., Charlop, M. H., & Schreibman, L. (1988). Training parents to use the natural language paradigm to increase their autistic children's speech. *Journal of Applied Behavior Analysis, 21*, 391–400.

Lavie, T., & Sturmey, P. (2002). Training staff to conduct paired-stimulus preference assessment. *Journal of Applied Behavior Analysis, 35*, 209–211.

Leblanc, M.-P., Ricciardi, J. N., & Luiselli, J. K. (2005). Improving discrete trial instruction in paraprofessional staff through an abbreviated performance feedback intervention. *Education and Treatment of Children, 28*, 76–82.

Lucychyn, J. M., Albin, R. W., & Nixon, C. D. (1997). Embedding comprehensive behavioral support in family ecology: An experimental, single-case analysis. *Journal of Consulting and Clinical Psychology, 65*, 241–251.

Luiselli, J. K. (1998). Intervention conceptualization and formulation. In J. K. Luiselli & M. J. Cameron (Eds.), *Antecedent control: Innovative approaches to behavioral support* (pp. 29–44). Baltimore: Brookes.

Luiselli, J. K. (2002). Focus, scope, and practice of behavioral consultation to public schools. In J. K. Luiselli & C. Diament (Eds.), *Behavior psychology in the schools: Innovations in evaluation, support, and consultation* (pp. 5–21). New York: Hawthorn. *Child and Family Behavior Therapy, 24*(1/2), 2002.

Luiselli, J. K., & Diament, C. (Eds.). (2002). *Behavior psychology in the schools: Innovations in evaluation, support, and consultation*. New York: Hawthorn. *Child and Family Behavior Therapy, 24*(1/2), 2002.

Luiselli, J. K., & Luiselli, T. E. (1995). A behavior analysis approach toward chronic food refusal in children with gastronomy-tube dependency. *Topics in Early Childhood Special Education, 15,* 1–18.

Luiselli, J. K., Putnam, R. F., Handler, M. W., & Feinberg, A. B. (2005). Whole-school positive behavior support: Effects on student discipline problems and academic performance. *Educational Psychology, 25,* 183–198.

Luiselli, J. K., Putnam, R. F., & Sunderland, M. (2002). Longitudinal evaluation of behavior support intervention in a public middle-school. *Journal of Positive Behavior Support, 4,* 182–188.

McAtee, M., Carr, E. G., & Schulte, C. (2004). A contextual assessment inventory for problem behavior: Initial development. *Journal of Positive Behavior Interventions, 6,* 148–165.

Moore, J. W., & Edwards, R. P. (2003). An analysis of aversive stimuli in classroom demand contexts. *Journal of Applied Behavior Analysis, 36,* 339–348.

Moore, J. W., Edwards, R. P., Sterling-Turner, H. E., Riley, J., DuBard, M., & McGeorge, A. (2002). Teacher acquisition of functional analysis methodology. *Journal of Applied Behavior Analysis, 35,* 73–77.

Najdowski, A. C., Wallace, M. D., Doney, J. K., & Ghezzi, P. M. (2003). Parental assessment and treatment of food selectivity in natural settings. *Journal of Applied Behavior Analysis, 36,* 383–386.

O'Neill, R. E., Horner, R. H., Albin, R. W., Storey, K., & Sprague, J. R. (1997). *Functional assessment and program development for problem behavior.* Pacific Grove, CA: Brooks/Cole.

Paige, M., McKerchar, M., & Thompson, R. H. (2004). A descriptive analysis of potential reinforcement contingencies in the preschool classroom. *Journal of Applied Behavior Analysis, 37,* 431–444.

Petronko, M. R., Harris, S. L., & Kormann, R. J. (1994). Community-based behavioral training approaches for people with mental retardation and mental illness. *Journal of Consulting and Clinical Psychology, 62,* 49–54.

Putnam, R. F., Handler, M. W., Ramirez-Platt, C., & Luiselli, J. K. (2003). Improving student bus riding behavior through a whole-school intervention. *Journal of Consulting and Clinical Psychology, 36,* 583–589.

Ricciardi, J. (2006). Combining antecedent and consequence procedures in multicomponent behavior support plans: A guide to writing plans with functional efficacy. In J. K. Luiselli (Ed.), *Antecedent intervention: Recent developments in community focused behavior support* (pp. 227–245). Baltimore: Brookes.

Rojahn , J., Matson, J. L., Naglieri, J. A., & Mayville, E. (2004). Relationships between psychiatric conditions and behavior problems among adults with mental retardation. *American Journal on Mental Retardation, 109,* 21–33.

Scheerenberger, R. C. (1983). *A history of mental retardation.* Baltimore: Brookes.

Schindler, H. R., & Horner, R. H. (2005). Generalized reduction of problem behavior of young children with autism: Building transituational interventions. *American Journal on Mental Retardation, 110,* 36–47.

Schreibman, L., O'Neill, R. E., & Koegel, R. L. (1983). Behavioral training for siblings of autistic children. *Journal of Applied Behavior Analysis, 16,* 129–138.

Schroeder, S. R., Schroeder, C. S., & Landesman, S. (1987). Psychological services in educational settings to persons with mental retardation. *American Psychologist, 42,* 805–808.

Singh, N. N., Lancioni, G. E., Winton, S. W., Wahler, R. G., Singh, J., & Sage, M. (2004). Mindful caregiving increases happiness among individuals with profound multiple disabilities. *Research in Developmental Disabilities, 25,* 207–218.

Skinner, B. F. (1957). *Verbal behavior.* New York: Prentice-Hall.

Steege, M. W., & Watson, T. S. (2003). *Conducting school-based functional behavior assessments: A practitioners guide.* New York: Guilford.

Sugai, G., & Horner, R. (2002). The evolution of discipline practices: School-wide positive behavior supports. In J. K. Luiselli & C. Diament (Eds.), *Behavior psychology in the schools: Innovations in evaluation, support, and consultation* (pp. 23–50). New York: Hawthorn. *Child and Family Behavior Therapy, 24*(1/2), 2002.

Touchette, P. E., MacDonald, R. E., & Langer, S. N. (1985). A scatter plot for identifying stimulus control of problem behavior. *Journal of Applied Behavior Analysis, 18,* 343–351.

Vaughn, B. J., Clarke, S., & Dunlap, G. (1997). Assessment-based intervention for severe behavior problems in a natural family context. *Journal of Applied Behavior Analysis, 30,* 713–716.

Wacker, D. P., Berg, W. K., Cooper, L. J., Derby, K. M., Steege, M. W., Northup, J., et al. (1994). The impact of functional analysis methodology on outpatient clinic services. *Journal of Applied Behavior Analysis, 27,* 405–407.

Wacker, D. P., & Steege, M. W. (1993). Providing outclinic services: Evaluating treatment and social validity. In R. Van Houten & S. Axelrod (Eds.), *Behavior analysis and treatment* (pp. 297–319). New York: Plenum.

13

Advocacy and Litigation in Professional Practice

RICHARD J. LANDAU

On June 20, 2002, the Supreme Court of the United States overruled years of settled legal precedent when it declared that the execution of individuals with intellectual disabilities (ID) violated the United States Constitution's Eighth Amendment prohibition against cruel and unusual punishment (*Atkins v. Virginia*, 2002). This decision is the most recent in a line of cases that have been decided over the past 20 years that have changed the legal framework within which professionals who work with individuals with ID must function. As has been the case with most of these legal landmarks, *Atkins* represented the culmination of decades of legal and legislative advocacy on behalf of criminal defendants with ID seeking to bar the imposition of the death penalty in such cases. It had been a long and rocky road in reaching this watershed legal event. Indeed, only 13 years earlier the Supreme Court had ruled that the Eighth Amendment did *not* bar the execution of criminal defendants with ID (*Penry v. Lynaugh*, 1989). What had changed in those intervening years?

THE ROAD FROM *PENRY* TO *ATKINS*

Although 13 years may seem like a long time in the era of the 24 hour news cycle, within the rarified world of Supreme Court jurisprudence, 13 years is tantamount to the blink of an eye. The Supreme Court's decision in *Penry* was a 5 to 4 decision. Of the four dissenters in *Penry*, only Justice Stevens remained on the Court by the time *Atkins* was decided. The two most pro-civil liberties Justices in the dissenting minority, Justices Brennan and Marshall, had long since retired by the time of the *Atkins* decision. Assembling the 6 to 3 *Atkins* majority thus required not simply that

RICHARD J. LANDAU • Dykema Gossett PLLC, Ann Arbor, Michigan 48104.

Justice Stevens maintain his opposition to the death penalty on Eighth Amendment grounds, but also that two Justices from the *Penry* majority—Justices Kennedy and O'Connor—take the extraordinary step of reversing their positions and joining the *Atkins* majority. No one would argue that the Supreme Court had become more liberal, or more favorably disposed toward criminal defendants in the 13 years between *Penry* and *Atkins*—indeed most commentators would argue that the trend was in the opposite direction. What accounts for this change is not simply the vagaries of political appointments and coalition building among Supreme Court Justices. Rather, legal advocates on behalf of criminal defendants with ID, undaunted by their setback in *Penry*, did not relent in their advocacy in the intervening years. Instead, they cannily crafted the legal arguments and the support for those arguments that ultimately carried the day and yielded this landmark victory.

Daryl Atkins was convicted of abduction, armed robbery, and capital murder. The facts of his crime were not in dispute. In the summer of 1997 Atkins and another man, armed with a semi-automatic handgun, abducted a man, robbed him, drove him to an automatic teller machine where they were photographed withdrawing additional money, and then took him to an isolated location where he was shot eight times and killed. The forensic psychologist who testified for the defense concluded that Atkins was mildly mentally retarded, with a full scale IQ of 59. Atkins was sentenced to death, a penalty that was ultimately affirmed by the Virginia Supreme Court.

In justifying its decision to reverse the imposition of the death penalty in Atkins' case, the Supreme Court was compelled to explain what had changed in the 13 years since its decision in *Penry*. Certainly, it was not the plain language of the Eighth Amendment, which had remained unchanged for over 200 years, "Excessive bail shall not be required, nor excessive fines imposed, nor cruel and unusual punishments inflicted." What had changed, in the view of the Court, was the consensus of the American people as reflected in the deliberations of legislators, scholars, and judges. Of particular importance was the fact that in 1989 only two states had expressly prohibited the execution of defendants with ID. By 2002, in contrast, attorneys for Atkins were able to point to 17 states that had enacted such prohibitions. Moreover, even in those states that preserved the practice, only five had executed a defendant with a known IQ of less than 70 in the years since the Court had decided *Penry*. As a result, the Court concluded that "the practice has become truly unusual, and it is fair to say a national consensus has developed against it" (*Atkins v. Virginia*, 2002, p. 316).

Moreover, Atkins' counsel was able to cite significant clinical research that had been published in the years since *Penry* was decided. Indeed, *Atkins* is an object lesson in how the influence between litigation and professional practice is a two-way street. The Supreme Court in *Atkins* cited studies from the field of ID in the areas of self-control, understanding, and suggestibility to bolster their conclusions. This research suggested that the two principal justifications that are typically given in support of capital punishment—retribution and deterrence—were not applicable to criminal defendants with ID.

The Supreme Court summarized their conclusions in *Atkins* as follows: "Construing and applying the Eighth Amendment in the light of our 'evolving standards of decency,' we therefore conclude that such punishment is excessive and that the Constitution 'places a substantive restriction on the State's power to take the life' of a mentally retarded offender" (*Atkins v. Virginia*, 2002, p. 321). Thus, the legal advocates, citing clinical research, had convinced the Supreme Court to conclude that standards of decency had "evolved," and the resulting interpretation of the Constitution has forever changed the lives of individuals with ID who become entangled in the criminal justice system.

Throughout recent legal history, professional advocacy and litigation have served to open doors for people with ID, as well as providing them with a measure of legal protection that has set them apart from other groups of individuals with disabilities. In *Atkins* this advocacy meant the difference, literally, between life and death for one subgroup of individuals with ID. Yet the *Atkins* decision is simply one very recent and compelling example of the impact litigation can have on the lives of people with ID and the professionals who address their treatment needs. *Atkins* serves as a fascinating case example of the strategies employed by attorneys in persuading the judicial system to take special note of the challenges faced by individuals with ID in American society. These changes can have profound implications for the lives of people with ID, their families, and those who provide services to them.

YOUNGBERG V. ROMEO AND THE RIGHT TO HABILITATION

Although *Atkins* represents a landmark case in the long history of judicial responses to people with ID, its application is, thankfully, limited to a select group of individuals in the criminal justice system. But although *Atkins* is significant in setting limits regarding what government cannot do to people with ID, other cases set the stage for the legal victory enjoyed by criminal defendants with ID in that case. One of the most significant cases in recent years that impacted the rights of people with ID in an institutional setting was *Youngberg v. Romeo* (1982). *Youngberg* established the minimum level of care to which people with ID confined to state institutions are entitled, that is, a standard that must be met or exceeded.

The Youngberg case arose out of a very protracted piece of civil rights litigation brought by people with ID housed at what was then known as the Pennhurst State School in Pennsylvania. Nicholas Romeo was a 33-year-old man with an IQ estimated to be between 8 and 10. He was committed to Pennhurst at the age of 26 years, after his father died. His mother petitioned for Romeo's commitment because she was unable to control his occasionally violent behavior. While at Pennhurst, Romeo was injured on numerous occasions. His mother filed suit on his behalf, claiming that officials at Pennhurst knew or should have known that he was sustaining these injuries and that they had failed to institute appropriate preventive measures. This failure was characterized as a violation of Romeo's constitutional rights under the Eighth and Fourteenth Amendments. The Eighth Amendment, as we saw in *Atkins*, prohibits cruel and unusual punishment, whereas the Fourteenth Amendment protects an individual's right to personal liberty. In the course of the lawsuit Romeo was transferred from his ward to the infirmary for treatment of a broken arm. While in the infirmary, he was physically restrained on a daily basis. This development resulted in an amendment to the lawsuit, which was revised to allege that Romeo's constitutional rights were violated by the defendants' failure to provide him with appropriate treatment for his mental retardation.

The case was tried to a jury, and Romeo lost. On appeal his lawyers argued that the trial court judge had committed reversible error based on the instructions given to the jury. The appeal ultimately reached the Supreme Court of the United States, which addressed for the first time the rights of individuals with ID confined to state custody. The Supreme Court addressed three issues of historic importance to individuals with ID confined to state custody. First, Romeo claimed that he had the right to safe conditions. Second, Romeo argued that he had the right to freedom from bodily restraint. The third issue, which the Court described as "more troubling," was whether Romeo had the right to adequate habilitation, which the Court defined as the training and development of needed skills. The training Romeo sought was characterized as "minimal" and he left the type and extent of the training mandated by the Constitution to be determined on a case-by-case basis, in light of present medical or other scientific knowledge.

In analyzing these claims the Court began with what it characterized as "established principles." Specifically, citing prior Supreme Court precedent, the Court accepted the proposition that when a person is institutionalized and dependent on the State for his or her care, the State has a duty to provide certain services and care, although the State necessarily has considerable discretion in determining the nature and scope of its responsibilities. In Romeo's case, moreover, his lawyers conceded that no amount of training would have made possible his release from State custody. His needs were described as those for bodily safety and a minimum of bodily restraint. These needs the Court immediately characterized as constitutionally protected liberty interests. The Court then proceeded to dispose of the first two issues presented by the case by concluding that Romeo, and by implication other persons with ID confined to state institutions, had a constitutionally protected liberty interest in having the State provide for him "minimally adequate or reasonable training to ensure safety and freedom from undue restraint" (*Youngberg v. Romeo*, 1982, p. 319).

The Court then proceeded to address how these principles should be applied with regard to the habilitative needs of people with ID confined to state custody in general. It noted that the rights of such individuals to safety from freedom and bodily restraint were not absolute. Rather, these rights must be balanced by certain rights held by the state, such as the need to protect the individual, as well as others, from violence. The Court therefore stressed that restraint per se was not unconstitutional, and that in order to determine whether an individual's liberty interests had been violated one must determine whether the extent or nature of the restraint or lack of absolute safety was such as to violate the individual's constitutional right to due process.

The Court then proceeded to articulate a test applicable to both Romeo's case, as well as generally to institutionalized individuals with ID:

> [W]e agree that [Romeo] is entitled to minimally adequate train-ing. In this case, the minimally adequate training required by the Constitution is such training as may be reasonable in light of respondent's liberty interests in safety and freedom from unrea-sonable restraints. In determining what is 'reasonable'—in this and in any case presenting a claim for training by a State—we emphasize that courts must show deference to the judgment ex-ercised by a qualified professional. By so limiting judicial review of challenges to conditions in state institutions, interference by the federal judiciary with the internal operations of these in-stitutions should be minimized. Moreover, there certainly is no reason to think judges or juries are better qualified than appro-priate professionals in making such decisions. For these rea-sons, the decision, if made by a professional, is presumptively valid; liability may be imposed only when the decision by the professional is such a substantial departure from accepted pro-fessional judgment, practice, or standards as to demonstrate that the person responsible actually did not base the decision on such a judgment. In an action for damages against a pro-fessional in his individual capacity, however, the professional will not be liable if he was unable to satisfy his normal profes-sional standards because of budgetary constraints; in such a situation, good-faith immunity would bar liability (*Youngberg v. Romeo*, 1982, p. 322).

The Court also decided who ordinarily would be qualified to serve in the role of "professional decision-maker." Generally speaking, such profession-als should be individuals competent, whether by education, training, or experience, to make the particular decision at issue. Typically, such deci-sions should be made by individuals with degrees in medicine or nursing, or individuals with appropriate training in psychology, physical therapy, or the care and training of people with ID.

Although *Youngberg* is an important case in setting the constitutional minimum level of habilitation that a person with ID confined to state cus-tody is entitled to, the Court was careful to limit its holding to the facts before it. It did not, for example, address whether, by accepting Romeo for care and treatment, the State could then constitutionally refuse to provide him with "treatment" as that term was defined under State law, rather than simply "habilitation." In addition, the Court brushed upon, but did not expressly decide, the question of whether the "habilitation" to which an individual with ID was entitled required such training as was neces-sary to preserve the self-care skills he possessed when he first entered

State custody. By addressing the right to habilitation for the first time in its opinion, however, the Court at least set a constitutional limit to the level of neglect the State could permit to exist in its institutions for individuals with ID. As it was doing so, however, forces were at work in society that would render *Youngberg* less relevant to individuals with ID, because fewer and fewer of them would find themselves confined to state custody in institutions.

CITY OF CLEBURNE V. CLEBURNE LIVING CENTER AND THE EQUAL PROTECTION CLAUSE

The conditions at state facilities such as Pennhurst, and legal decisions such as *Youngberg* that effectively criticized these institutions, gave rise to changes in the law through legislation rather than litigation. In 1984, Congress passed the Developmental Disabilities Act (1984). This federal law required the establishment of watchdog organizations in each state that were responsible for protecting the rights of individuals with ID. The Act made it the policy of the federal government to promote the transition of individuals with ID from state run facilities into community settings:

> [T]he goals of the Nation properly include the goal of providing individuals with developmental disabilities with the opportunities and support to (A) make informed choices and decisions; (B) live in homes and communities in which such individuals can exercise their full rights and responsibilities as citizens; (C) pursue meaningful and productive lives; (D) contribute to their family, community, State, and Nation; (E) have interdependent friendships and relationships with others; and (F) achieve full integration and inclusion in society, in an individualized manner, consistent with unique strengths, resources, priorities, concerns, abilities, and capabilities of each individual (Developmental Disabilities Act of 1984, 42 U.S.C. § 6000 (a)(10)).

Although laudable in its effort to set the national agenda for people with ID, much of the language in the Developmental Disabilities Act regarding the goals for people with ID can be described in legalese as "precatory"—words that suggest action, but that lack the "teeth" of an enforcement mechanism. Whatever rights people with ID were entitled to enforce, as of the mid 1980s, arose either out of state law or the language of the U.S. Constitution itself.

As deinstitutionalization took hold as a state policy and practice expedited by federal financing initiatives, however, individuals with ID gradually moved out of institutions and into neighborhoods. As they did so, however, they encountered resistance among local communities. Because a broad statutory mandate prohibiting discrimination against individuals with disabilities by municipalities and private entities did not exist, advocates were once again forced to rely on the somewhat vaguer requirements of the U.S. Constitution. The constitutional bulwark against arbitrary discrimination by governmental entities is set forth in the Equal Protection Clause of the Fourteenth Amendment, which commands that no State shall "deny to any person within its jurisdiction the equal protection of the laws," and is thus essentially a direction that all persons similarly situated should be treated alike. It was the Equal Protection Clause to which the Cleburne Living Center, which wanted to lease a building for a group home for individuals with ID, had to resort when the City of Cleburne, Texas refused to issue it a special use permit that would allow it to operate (*Cleburne Living Center v. City of Cleburne*, 1985).

In 1980, the Cleburne Living Center (CLC) sought to lease a building for use as a group home for women with ID. CLC planned to house 13 women who would be under the constant supervision of CLC staff. CLC planned to comply with all applicable federal and state regulations. The city informed the CLC that it would have to apply for a special use permit. The city explained to CLC that under the applicable zoning regulations for the site, the proposed group home should be classified as a "hospital for the feeble-minded." Other multiple residence dwellings, such as apartment houses, boarding houses fraternities, and sororities, were not required to apply for such permits. A public hearing was held after which the City Council voted 3 to 1 to deny the special use permit. CLC filed suit in federal court, arguing that the zoning regulation was unconstitutional because it discriminated against people with ID. The trial court ruled in favor of the city. CLC then appealed to the United States Court of Appeals for the Fifth Circuit, which held that the zoning regulation was unconstitutional. As was the case in *Atkins* and *Youngberg*, the matter was then appealed to the United States Supreme Court.

The Supreme Court noted at the outset that without controlling statutory authority from Congress, the Equal Protection Clause itself is a fairly weak weapon against discrimination. Generally, any statute, ordinance, or regulation can survive an Equal Protection challenge if it is "rationally related to a legitimate governmental purpose." Applying this standard, most legislation is found to be constitutional. This general rule gives way only where a statute attempts to classify individuals by such factors as race and national origin. Under these circumstances, the presumption of validity gives way, and the legislation in question will be found constitutional under the Equal Protection Clause only if it is "suitably tailored to serve a compelling state interest." Under this latter test, most challenged legislation is found to be unconstitutional. Thus, unless a person challenging a law can claim that the law perpetuates racial or national origin discrimination, their chances of prevailing in an Equal Protection challenge are very slim.

Other ways of classifying individuals had also been considered by the Court in developing the law of Equal Protection. Gender, for example, was given a special status that fell somewhere between the heightened level of statutory scrutiny applied where laws divided people along racial lines, and the deferential standard applied when race was not an issue. Where a law sought to classify people by gender, the Court had previously held that such laws would violate the Equal Protection Clause unless the gender classification was "substantially related to a sufficiently important governmental interest." Other classifications, such as age, had been denied any protected status under Equal Protection analysis. Lawyers had come to characterize the three levels of Equal Protection analysis as "strict scrutiny" (race and national origin), "intermediate scrutiny" (gender), and presumptively valid (no protected class at issue).

The question before the *Cleburne* court had never been previously addressed—could an individual's ID status be sufficiently "suspect" that the increased scrutiny applied to legislation that discriminated on the basis race or national origin could be applied, was it more analogous to gender where an intermediate level of scrutiny would be applied, or was it analogous to neither, in which case the government could freely impose this classification with minimal scrutiny? In other words, could people with ID be granted the same protected constitutional status as individuals who were the victims of racial or gender-based discrimination? The determination of whether the City of Cleburne had discriminated against the CLC by requiring it to apply for a special use permit, and then denying the application, hinged upon which level of scrutiny the Court would apply in cases involving laws that treated people with ID distinctly from people without ID.

The Court concluded that classifying people by their ID status could not be considered irrational discrimination akin to racial classifications. Nor could it be deemed a "quasi-suspect" classification such as gender. Rather, the Court held laws that classified people by their ID status were subject to no more protection under the Equal Protection Clause than were laws that classified people by such factors as age. Having reached this conclusion, the Court then easily concluded that the special use permit ordinance was not unconstitutional on its face. But that did not end the inquiry.

The Court also had to consider whether the reasons given by the city in denying the permit were in fact rationally related to a legitimate governmental interest. It easily concluded that in the case of the CLC group home, this minimal standard had not been met. For example, the city argued that the permit should be denied because of the negative attitudes of property owners who lived within 200 feet of the proposed facility. But the Court concluded that irrational fears and prejudices could never support governmental action. Similarly, the city argued that the proposed facility was across the street from a junior high school. But the Court observed that the school itself was attended by 30 students with ID, thus suggesting that this fear too was irrational and not related to a legitimate governmental purpose. The Court thus concluded that the city's action was based on irrational prejudice against people with ID, and that the denial of the application for the special use permit violated the residents' rights under the Equal Protection Clause.

OLMSTEAD V. L.C. AND THE RIGHT TO BE FREE FROM INSTITUTIONAL CONFINEMENT

As the *Cleburne* case clearly illustrates, people with ID could not rely upon the strong constitutional mandate against discrimination enjoyed by racial minorities and women. By 1990, however, a new statutory enactment, one with "teeth" appeared on the national stage. The Americans with Disabilities Act of 1990 (ADA) was enacted with widespread fanfare as a historic milestone in establishing and enforcing the rights of people with disabilities. Similar legislation had appeared in the past, principally Section 504 of the Rehabilitation Act (1973), but that legislation applied only to programs receiving federal financial assistance. The ADA applied to public and private settings, and included specific commands to administrative agencies to enact regulations that would allow its broad mandate of nondiscrimination to be applied across a wide range of activities in American life. The ADA also provided legal avenues for addressing claims of discrimination both through enforcement by administrative agencies, as well as through private litigation.

Pursuant to the ADA's command, the Attorney General of the United States issued regulations seeking to implement the provisions of Title II, which applied to any "public entity." These regulations included what was called the "integration regulation," which read "A public entity shall administer services, programs and activities in the most integrated setting appropriate to the needs of qualified individuals with disabilities" (28 C.F.R. § 35.130(d)). The "most integrated setting" language was further defined as "a setting that enables individuals with disabilities to interact with nondisabled persons to the fullest extent possible" (35 C.F.R. pt. 35, App. A, p. 450). Public entities were required to make "reasonable modifications in policies, practices, or procedures" where necessary to avoid discrimination, unless the public entity could demonstrate that making such modifications would "fundamentally alter the nature of the service, program, or activity" (28 C.F.R. § 35.130(b)(7)).

It was against this legislative backdrop that the Court was required to address a controversy involving two women with ID who went by the pseudonyms L.C. and E.W. (*Olmstead v. L.C.*, 1999). L.C., who had mental illness as well as ID, had been voluntarily admitted to the Georgia Regional Hospital (GRH) in Atlanta in 1992. By May 1993, her condition had stabilized and her treatment team agreed that her needs could be met in community-based programs. She remained hospitalized until February 1996 when she was placed in a community program. E.W. was similarly voluntarily admitted to a psychiatric unit at GRH in 1995. After first trying to discharge her to a homeless shelter (her attorney complained and the plan was abandoned), her treatment team agreed in 1996 that she was ready to be treated in a community-based setting. She remained institutionalized at GRH until 1997.

In May 1995, L.C. brought suit in federal court. She alleged that her rights under the ADA to be placed in an integrated, community-based setting had been violated. E.W. intervened in the lawsuit with an identical claim. The State argued that its failure to place these women in a community-based setting was not discrimination by reason of their disabilities, but, rather that it was unable to implement such placements because of a lack of funding. The State also argued that requiring immediate transfers of patients whose treatment teams had concluded that the patients were ready for such transfers would "fundamentally alter" their activities, in violation of the public entity's rights under the ADA. The trial court rejected both these arguments and ruled in favor of L.C. and E.W.

The inevitable appeal ensued, and the Eleventh Circuit United States Court of Appeals reversed the trial court's rejection of the State's cost-based defense. It concluded that such a defense may be justified where the expenditure of funds to provide community-based services was so unreasonable, given the demands of the State's mental health budget, that it would fundamentally alter the services the State provides. Once again, the Supreme Court was required to weigh in on this dispute.

Unanimous Supreme Court decisions are relatively rare in hotly contested cases such as *Olmstead*. Generally speaking, a decision is not binding on the parties unless one side can muster five of the Justices to its position. It is not uncommon for some portions of a Supreme Court decision to command the required five votes, and thus become the law of the land, whereas others command less than five, thus becoming little more than miniature law review articles for the enjoyment and befuddlement of legal scholars. The Court's decision in *Olmstead* was thus broken into parts, only three of which commanded a majority of the Court.

The Court was first required to consider whether "undue institutionalization," that is the State's maintaining an individual with ID in an institutional setting where the individual's treating professionals believe that transition to a community-based setting is appropriate, qualifies as discrimination by reason of disability. The Court concluded, with some qualifications, that undue institutionalization was prohibited by the ADA. Its decision reflected "two evident judgments." The first was that institutional placements of individuals who could benefit from community settings perpetuates unwarranted assumptions that such persons are unworthy of participating in community life. Second, confinement in an institution precluded the individual with ID from enjoying everyday life activities, such as family life, social contacts, work options, economic independence, educational advancement, and cultural enrichment.

The Court noted, however, that nothing in the ADA or its underlying regulations mandates the deinstitutionalization of individuals unable to handle or benefit from community settings. The rule ultimately adopted by the Court was reminiscent of its ruling in *Youngberg*, which demonstrated a willingness to defer to professional judgment in matters involving individuals with ID.

> [T]he State generally may rely on the reasonable assessments of its own professionals in determining whether an individual 'meets the essential eligibility requirements' for habilitation in a community-based program. Absent such qualification, it would be inappropriate to remove a patient from the more restrictive setting. Nor is there any federal requirement that community-based treatment be imposed on patients who do not desire it (*Olmstead v. L.C.*, 1999, p. 602).

The Court was unable, however, to give clear direction to the lower courts regarding the manner in which courts should address the State's argument that cost limitations could serve as a defense to the ADA's deinstitution-alization mandate. Four Justices voted in favor of a standard that would have required the lower courts to consider the resources available to the State for individuals with ID, while also considering the needs of others with mental disabilities. A majority of the Justices appeared to believe that the State was entitled to raise as a defense that the expenditure of funds required for deinstitutionalization could represent a prohibited "fundamental alteration" of the State's programs under the ADA. The precise contours of this argument, however, did not command a majority of the Justices, leaving this issue for another case to definitively decide.

THE INDIVIDUALS WITH DISABILITIES EDUCATION ACT—BEYOND HABILITATION

As the discussion of the preceding cases demonstrates, progress for protected populations such as individuals with ID takes time in the world of constitutional jurisprudence. Moreover, the courts appear reluctant to grant this population rights beyond vague references to "minimal progress," "habilitation," and "reasonable accommodation"—all of which depend on the subjective discretion of professionals. The one area where Congress and the courts have required a more particularized effort to enhance the functioning of individuals with ID, and something more than subjective standards of accountability, has been in the area of the education of students from birth to the age of 18. The Individuals with Disabilities Education Act (IDEA) mandates not only that school districts locate and educate students with disabilities, but also requires that these students must make measurable educational progress no matter how severely impaired they may be. Like the ADA, IDEA provides for enforcement of the individual with ID's rights. Unlike the ADA, IDEA sets the standard to which the State is held at a level above that of simple "habilitation."

One of the bedrock principles underlying IDEA is that of "zero reject." Zero reject describes the policy shift toward the view that an appropriate education is the right of all students, regardless of disability status. Thus, students may not be categorically excluded on the basis of a disability. Instead, students eligible for special education services must be provided with appropriate services and aids. The broad scope of special education law is illustrated by the case of *Timothy W. v. Rochester, New Hampshire School Dist.* (1989). That case concerned a severely handicapped child with, among other conditions, severe metal retardation, complex developmental disabilities, spastic quadriplegia, cerebral palsy, and hydrocephalus, which had destroyed a large part of his brain. All of this combined to leave the child in a vegetative state, although there was testimony that he could see bright light, could smile, and responded to touching and talking.

In response to the severe nature to the child's disability, the school district refused to provide any special education services based upon its conclusion that he would not be able to benefit from such services. When the child's parents brought suit, the federal court held that a child with disabilities did not need to be able to demonstrate an ability to benefit from special education services in order to be eligible. Instead, the school had a duty to provide special education services to every such child, regardless of the severity of the disability or the level of achievement possible for the child. This case illustrates starkly that no child, regardless of the severity of his or her disability, may be denied services under IDEA. Under IDEA all eligible students are entitled to a free appropriate public education (FAPE), which must be composed of a written statement of goals and objectives, as well as the special education and ancillary services needed to help the student attain these goals. This plan is known as an Individualized Education Program (IEP).

Virtually all students with ID are likely to be eligible under the definition set forth under the regulations implementing IDEA. To qualify as a student with "mental retardation" under IDEA requires that the student have "significantly subaverage general intellectual functioning, existing concurrently with deficits in adaptive behavior and manifested during the developmental period, that adversely affects a child's educational performance" (34 CFR § 300.7(c)(6)). Similarly, IDEA makes it clear that all students with ID, not simply those likely to benefit from instruction, must be integrated with nondisabled students to the maximum extent possible. This is called the Least Restrictive Environment (LRE) requirement of IDEA. It sets a much higher standard than the one articulated by the ADA and interpreted by the Supreme Court in *Olmstead*. To the maximum extent appropriate, children with disabilities, including children in public or private institutions or other care facilities, are to be educated with children who are not disabled. Special classes, separate schooling, or other removal of children with disabilities from the regular educational environment should occur only when the nature or severity of the disability of a child is such that education in regular classes with the use of supplementary aids and services cannot be achieved satisfactorily (20 U.S.C. § 1412(a)(5)).

The power of the LRE concept is frequently illustrated in the cases that have arisen under IDEA. Neil Roncker was a 9-year-old student classified as trainable mentally impaired ("TMI") (*Roncker v. Walter*, 1983). Neil also had seizures, although his seizures were nonconvulsive and were controlled by medication. Both the parents and the school district recognized that Neil would require some type of restrictive placement but disagreed on the level of restrictiveness. The parents wanted Neil educated in a placement that would expose Neil to his nondisabled peers during gym, lunch, and recess. The district wanted to place Neil in a county school for children with ID.

The court framed the LRE issue under IDEA as follows:

> In a case where the segregated facility is considered superior, the court should determine whether the services which make that placement superior could be feasibly provided in a nonsegregated setting. If they can, the placement in the segregated school would be inappropriate under the Act. Framing the issue in this manner accords the proper respect for the strong preference in favor of mainstreaming while still realizing the

> possibility that some handicapped children simply must be educated in segregated facilities either because the handicapped child would not benefit from mainstreaming, because any marginal benefits received from mainstreaming are far outweighed by the benefits gained from services which could not feasibly be provided in the nonsegregated setting, or because the handicapped child is a disruptive force in the nonsegregated setting (*Roncker v. Walter*, 1983, p. 1063).

The approach to services under IDEA is thus much more hostile to institutional placements than that employed using either constitutional principles or the ADA. It is *presumed* that students with ID should be treated in a mainstream setting unless it can be *proven* that they cannot benefit from such a setting.

Unlike the approach to these issues under the principles of constitutional law, or even those of the ADA, cost is rarely recognized as a defense to providing services for students eligible under IDEA. If a particular program or service is required to provide a disabled child with FAPE, it must be provided, regardless of cost: The Supreme Court has specifically rejected cost as a defense to the provision of services. An illustrative case, *Cedar Rapids v. Garret* (1999), involved a student who was injured when his spinal cord was severed in a motorcycle accident, was ventilator-dependent and required continuous care, including urinary bladder catheterization once a day, suctioning of his tracheotomy tube as needed, being placed in a reclining position for 5 minutes per hour, ambu bagging occasionally while his ventilator equipment was tested, assistance in case of ventilator malfunction, and emergency services in the event he experienced autonomic hyperflexia.

The student's family personally attended to him during kindergarten and used settlement proceeds, insurance and other resources to employ a nurse for the next 4 years. When these funds ran out, the family asked the district to accept financial responsibility for his needs during the school day. The Supreme Court rejected the district's claim that the continuous care required by the student was too costly. Although recognizing that the District may have legitimate financial concerns, the Court concluded that the necessary services were required to provide the student with meaningful access to the public schools. Thus, the District was required to fund the services.

CONCLUSIONS

Although the injustices of the past will continue to linger, litigation by attorneys and advocacy by professionals in the field of ID, working together, have produced much to be proud of in terms of accomplishments over the past three decades. Presumptions in favor of institutionalization are being gradually transformed into presumptions in favor of integration into the community. The execution of criminal defendants with ID has been declared unconstitutional. Although the legal rights of adults with

ID continue to evolve, litigation under IDEA has established that young people with ID, and with other disabilities, have a statutory entitlement to a free appropriate education in the least restrictive environment. This progress will, no doubt, continue. Although the broad contours of the rights of people with ID have been drawn, much remains to be filled in. Issues of cost/benefit in treatment and education will continue to occupy the courts for some time to come. What constitutes adequate progress toward clinical goals remains a hotly debated topic within the legal, educational and clinical communities. As long as people of good may continue to differ on these points, and cannot come to consensus, litigation will remain one avenue of addressing and resolving these disputes.

REFERENCES

Americans with Disabilities Act of 1990, 42 U.S.C. § 12101 *et seq.*
Atkins v. Virginia, 536 U.S. 304 (2002).
Cedar Rapids v. Garret, 526 US 66 (1999).
Cleburne Living Center v. City of Cleburne, 473 U.S. 432 (1985).
Developmental Disabilities Act of 1984, 42 U.S.C. § 6000 *et seq.*
Individuals with Disabilities Education Improvement Act of 2004 (IDEA), 20 U.S.C. § 1400 *et seq.*
Olmstead v. L.C., 527 U.S. 581 (1999).
Penry v. Lynaugh, 492 U.S. 302 (1989).
Rehabilitation Act of 1973, Section 504, 29 U.S.C. § 794.
Roncker v. Walter, 700 F.2d 1058 (6th Cir. 1983).
Timothy W. v. Rochester, New Hampshire School Dist. 875 F.2d 954 (1st Cir. 1989).
Youngberg v. Romeo, 457 U.S. 307 (1982).

III

Assessment and Diagnosis

The focus of this section is on the state of knowledge, and to the extent that it has been ascertained, application of that knowledge with respect to specific aspects of assessment. The content includes consideration of definition of the topic area, the identification of and selection of well-validated measures, explanation of concerns regarding validity and reliability, and clarification of the relationship of assessment findings to the development of interventions.

14

Intellectual Assessment and Intellectual Disability

JOHN G. BORKOWSKI, SHANNON S. CAROTHERS, KIMBERLY HOWARD, JULIE SCHATZ, and JAELYN R. FARRIS

Three decades ago, the American Association on Mental Deficiency (AAMD) proposed a definition of intellectual disability (ID) that not only emphasized the academic side of intelligence but also considered two other important factors—adaptive behavior and the time of occurrence of the disabling condition: "Mental Retardation refers to significantly subaverage general intellectual functioning existing concurrently with deficits in adaptive behavior and manifested during the developmental period" (Grossman, 1983, p. 1).

Since that time, the definition of who should, and who should not, be classified as mentally retarded has been debated extensively but revised only slightly in two more recent editions of the AAMD's manual (Luckasson et al., 1992, 2002). The importance of intellectual functioning—as indexed through existing instruments such as the Binet, Wechsler, or Kaufman tests—has remained the first, and most salient, criterion in the definition of ID. What has changed in the most recent definitional modifications is the ideological and theoretical context in which intelligence is embedded.

Although the newest manual (Luckasson et al., 2002) gives lip service to planning, reasoning, problem solving, abstract thinking, speed of learning, and profiting from experience, it falls back on traditional IQ tests in order to diagnose and classify. The practice of IQ-based subgrouping (forming mild, moderate, severe, and profound categories)

JOHN G. BORKOWSKI, SHANNON S. CAROTHERS, KIMBERLY HOWARD, JULIE SCHATZ and JAELYN R. FARRIS • Department of Psychology, University of Notre Dame, Notre Dame, Indiana 46556.

has been dropped and, in its place, professionals are urged "to accompany diagnosis with descriptions of need supports" (Luckasson et al., 2002, p. 27) and to search for coexisting strengths in other psychological and social domains, in addition to identifying deficits. Although the field of ID is essentially left with traditional IQ tests that yield "objective" scores necessary to meet a specific diagnostic criterion, there is a sense, in both the 1992 and 2002 AAMR revisions, that "something more" is needed in order to both *identify* and *educate* children and adolescents with ID. In this chapter, we review intellectual assessment from past, present, and future perspectives, with the aim of suggesting new perspectives on intellectual assessment that have remedial and educational merit.

This chapter discusses traditional tests of intelligence, the potential of dynamic assessment, contemporary perspectives on intellectual assessments and ID, and the importance of integrating metacognitive skills—especially self-regulation—into a dynamic assessment framework. We contend that an increased emphasis on the contextualized assessment of cognitive, social, and emotional self-regulation is not only consistent with AAMR's underlying philosophy and assumptions about the proper role of intelligence in the definition of ID but also, more importantly, provides a fresh perspective on how a focus on self-regulation, in the context of dynamic assessment, can serve as a bridge between assessment, education, and contextualized learning.

HISTORY OF INTELLIGENCE TESTING

The first intelligence test was developed in 1904 by Alfred Binet and Theodore Simon for use in screening children for ID in the French public schools (Hunt, 1993). Their goal was to develop a test that could separate those who were performing poorly in school because of ID from those who were performing poorly for other reasons, namely lack of effort (Thorndike, 1997). Around 1910, Henry Goddard brought the Binet–Simon Scale to the United States, translated it to English, and began administering it to school children. In 1916, Lewis Terman produced the Stanford revision of the Binet–Simon Scale, and in its 1937 revision, the scale officially became known as the Stanford–Binet (Thorndike).

Several others were also working on development of tests to measure intelligence around this time. A pioneer in the American intelligence testing movement was David Wechsler who published the first version of the Wechsler–Bellevue in 1939, a scale for use with adults (Thorndike, 1997). The middle of the twentieth century was a time of relative stagnation in the area of test development. Later in the century, there would be changes in the theory behind intelligence testing that would yield new tests based on these underlying theories. Alan Kaufman, who had been influential in critiquing previous intelligence tests, published his own test in 1983, the Kaufman assessment battery for children (KABC; Lichtenberger,

Broadbooks, & Kaufman, 2000; Thorndike, 1997). In the following section, we review these tests of intelligence.

PROMINENT INTELLIGENCE TESTS

Stanford–Binet

Although the Stanford–Binet remains one of the most popular intelligence tests since Terman introduced it in the United States, it has undergone several revisions with the two most recent, the Stanford–Binet IV and V (Roid, 2003; Thorndike, Hagan, & Sattler, 1986). Although earlier versions of the Stanford–Binet lacked a specific theoretical framework, the fourth edition makes use of the latest advances in psychometric theory. This places the Stanford–Binet IV clearly within what Kamphaus, Petoskey, and Morgan (1997) refer to as the fourth wave of intelligence testing, set apart from the first three waves because of its strong theoretical framework. The Binet IV is used from the age of 2 years to adulthood. It contains 15 tests in four areas (verbal reasoning, abstract/visual reasoning, quantitative reasoning, and short-term memory), yielding four subscores as well as a composite score. The composite score represents the best estimate of general intelligence.

In contrast to many other popular intelligence tests, the Stanford–Binet IV is unique in that a single test can be used to assess individuals at any meaningful point in the lifespan. Although the Binet has been widely used to assess mental deficiency, some studies have also raised concern that the Binet IV may not be sensitive enough to detect developmental delays in very young children (Saylor, Boyce, Peagler, & Callahan, 2000). The fifth edition of the Stanford–Binet, which was released in 2003, includes five factors (fluid reasoning, knowledge, quantitative reasoning, visual-spatial processing, and working memory) and both verbal and nonverbal domains. This new version provides a better assessment of the strengths and weaknesses of individuals at the extremes of the intelligence distribution making it more sensitive in measuring younger children and high-risk individuals (Riverside Publishing Company, 2002).

The original Wechsler–Bellevue Scale was a measure of adult intelligence (Wechsler, 1939). Although it technically was designed to assess people between the ages of 7 and 69, it was not until the 1949 publication of the Wechsler Intelligence Scale for Children (WISC) that the Wechsler scales became appropriate for children (Kaufman & Lichtenberger, 2000). This extension placed the WISC in direct competition with the Stanford–Binet. In 1967, the Wechsler tests were scaled so as to be appropriate for even younger children, with the development of the Wechsler Preschool and Primary Scale of Intelligence (WPPSI; Wechsler, 1967). Since its first introduction, the original Wechsler–Bellevue has been revised three times, culminating in the 1997 version of the Wechsler adult intelligence scale—third edition (WAIS-III; Wechsler, 1997); the WPPSI is also in its third edition (Wechsler, 2002) and is appropriate for children from ages 2.5 to 7.5. The

WISC has recently been revised (WISC-IV; Wechsler, 2003) for children aged between 6 and 16 years.

The Wechsler scales are currently the most widely used IQ tests, even surpassing the Stanford–Binet in popularity. They are preferred because of their age appropriateness to specific groups of people as well as their stability and reliability over time. The Wechsler tests consist of two sub-scales, verbal and performance, each of which can be used in interpreting strengths and weaknesses. Originally, the Wechsler scales led the way in clinical profile analysis (Flanagan, McGrew, & Ortiz, 2000; Kamphaus et al., 1997), which aims to understand the overall clinical picture of the individual being assessed. There are also concerns regarding item sensitivity and item breadth, especially prevalent in the low IQ range.

Kaufman Battery

The KABC-II (Kaufman & Kaufman, 2004) was a response to the problems that plagued intelligence testing throughout much of the twentieth century, including translating IQ scores into contextualized learning settings. The KABC was originally developed as an assessment tool thoroughly grounded in theory. Its main goal was not merely to assess children for the sake of determining a single intelligence score, but rather to gain information about a child's learning potential so as to apply that knowledge to children's learning in the classroom (Lichtenberger et al., 2000). The KABC-II, designed for children between the ages of 3 and 18, consists of five scales: simultaneous processing, sequential processing, planning, learning, and knowledge. There is also a nonverbal scale that can be both administered and completed using gestures. Another major goal of the KABC-II was to provide an assessment tool that would be sensitive to a wide range of children including ethnic minorities and children with disabilities. In particular, the Kauffman has found much less of a difference in intelligence scores between African American and Caucasian children than the WISC-III.

Bayley Scales of Infant Development

The Bayley scales of infant development (BSID; Bayley, 1969) have a tradition that is different from other traditional intellectual assessments. In particular, the BSID, as well as the current revision, the BSID-II, is rooted in theories of infant development rather than intelligence per se. For this reason, Bayley scores have been found to be only moderately predictive of later IQ scores (Black & Matula, 2000). However, because the Bayley is appropriate for use with a wide range of children and is one of the few tools that can assess infant development, it tends to be especially sensitive in identifying both developmental delay and developmental disability. This is a particularly useful instrument for the early identification of developmental problems in young children (Black & Matula).

The second edition of the Bayley (BSID-II; Bayley, 1993) was designed for infants and children between the ages of 1 and 42 months and consists of three scales: a mental scale, a motor scale, and a behavioral rating scale. The mental scale provides a score for overall cognitive development whereas the motor scale yields a similar score for overall motor development. Of interest in the behavioral rating scales is the fact that the child's caregiver is also asked questions concerning the typicality of the child's behavior during the assessment (Black & Matula, 2000).

Each of the major intelligence tests in use today has specific advantages and disadvantages. The Stanford–Binet and Wechsler scales have remained the most popular instruments, even in the twenty-first century, but are not without competition. The Kaufman scales, in particular the KABC-II, are innovative in that they are more theoretically driven than other tests and are process-oriented rather than outcome-oriented. Finally, the Bayley scales offer promise in identifying early signs of delay in infants and very young children.

In the next sections, we offer three critiques of traditional assessments of intelligence from the viewpoints of dynamic assessment, contemporary theories of intellectual assessment, and an integration of the assessment of self-regulation within a dynamic assessment framework. The aim is to help bridge the gap between definitional assessment and the achievement of human potential through integrating assessment and learning.

STATIC VERSUS DYNAMIC ASSESSMENT

In the intelligence testing literature there has been a growing awareness of alternative forms of assessment due to the static, time-bound nature of the more traditional testing methods (Freeman & Miller, 2001). This section elucidates the ways in which traditional measures of intelligence are sometimes inadequate when measuring ID or learning disabilities and highlights how the dynamic assessment approach provides a richer understanding of each individual's potential for cognitive growth and development.

Shortcomings of Traditional Approaches to Assessment

Traditional intellectual assessments, based on the assertion that prior learning adequately predicts future performance, fail to address and measure the responsiveness of an individual to instructions and practice (Bransford, Delclos, Vye, Burns, & Hasselbring, 1987). Hence, the claim is made that traditional intelligence tests sometimes underestimate what a child or adult can learn and achieve. Traditional or static approaches are seen as lacking because they tend to represent a one-instance sampling of behavior, assume common preparatory backgrounds of examinees, focus on end products, use a standardized administration format that restricts the assessment of individual potential (Lidz, 1997), and hides or fails to identify nonintellectual factors that can affect performance (Tzuriel, 1992). It is not surprising that Fletcher, Francis, Rourke, Shaywitz, and Shaywitz (1992) argue that intelligence measures have been used to place children into special education settings based on assessments that underestimate their learning ability or reflect "nonstable" discrepancies between their potential and achievement.

Lastly, traditional assessment does not provide information for designing potentially effective instruction (Bransford et al., 1987; Haywood & Brown, 1990; Utley, Haywood, & Masters, 1992). Static assessments, in which children are expected to answer questions and solve problems without help, contain little information about performance in typical situations in which teaching and learning occur (Haywood & Brown). Thus, traditional assessment does not recognize the learner's potential to succeed when given adequate environmental supports (Jitendra & Kameenui, 1993).

The Nature and Purpose of Dynamic Assessment

Dynamic assessment differs from standardized assessment in a number of ways. The major goal of standardized assessment is to classify and group students for differential instruction (Lidz, 1997). In contrast, dynamic assessment is characterized by a pretest-intervene-posttest administration format that focuses directly on learning processes (Lidz & Pena, 1996; Missiuna & Samuels, 1989; Swanson, 1996). Swanson contends that any procedure that attempts to modify performance via examiner assistance, in an effort to understand learning potential, represents dynamic assessment. If the goal is to understand how a child learns, it is best to engage the child in a real-life learning process; this is the principle component of dynamic assessment (Lidz, 1997).

The theoretical grounding for dynamic assessment is Vygotsky's notion of the "zone of proximal development" (Vygotsky, 1986). Vygotsky suggested that development of higher mental functioning requires social interactions within zones of development at increasingly complex levels. In accord with Vygotsky, Feuerstein, Rand, and Hoffman (1979) suggested that a dynamic assessment process has the potential to assess the modifiability of basic cognitive structures. The intent is to provide information that can serve as the basis for enhancement of the cognitive functioning of the learner, regardless (but not independent) of his or her current level of performance (Freeman & Miller, 2001; Lidz, 1997).

Dynamic assessment identifies children's developmental abilities and limitations in relation to their learning context (Missiuna & Samuels, 1989) and encourages enthusiastic participation by both the clinician and the child (Nigram, 2001). The assessor actively engages the child in a true learning interaction and tries to promote changes in a positive direction (Freeman & Miller, 2001). Dynamic assessment yields three kinds of information: (1) "baseline" performance, i.e., learning without assistance; (2) amount and type of help required to reach a higher level of performance; and (3) the individual's response to that help. That is, to what extent has a person learned principles and strategies and then applied them to new problems that have the same cognitive requirements (Haywood & Brown, 1990; Lidz, 1997).

In sum, dynamic assessment sheds light upon children-as-learners, offers insight into the modifiability of cognitive skills (especially the extent to which children are capable of change in response to intervention), assists teachers and clinicians in generating hypotheses about children's learning potential, and based on these formulated hypotheses determines intervention strategies that might improve their performance (Lidz & Pena, 1996).

Implications for Assessment and Classification of MR or LD

Nigram (2001) suggested that because traditional assessment procedures using standardized tests do not provide information about children's learning potential, the concept of dynamic assessment is becoming more common in the field of communication disorders, special education, and other behavioral sciences. The utility of the dynamic assessment approach as a "nondiscriminatory" assessment is highlighted when assessing the learning potential of children who are culturally different, handicapped, or language-impaired (Haywood & Brown, 1990). As such, results from various studies have suggested that mediated learning helps "special" children to perform in zones of proximal development in which they formerly showed no competence (Gutierrez-Cellen & Pena, 2001; Pena, Iglesias, & Lidz, 2001).

Dynamic assessment is a valuable addition to traditional psychometric approaches, due to the fact that motivational and instructional factors are considered in the analysis of intellectual–cognitive performance (Jitendra & Kameenui, 1993). As such, the addition of dynamic assessment serves to compensate for the shortcomings of traditional assessments by approaching issues that otherwise are not considered, such as improving the understanding of the learner's knowledge of task features as well as discerning the learner's ability to maintain and transfer what was learned.

CONTEMPORARY PERSPECTIVES ON INTELLECTUAL ASSESSMENTS AND ID

Although there is a growing recognition of the need for dynamic assessment of intellectual abilities, the most commonly used intelligence tests still fail to take this into account. In fact, one of the major shortcomings of traditional measures of intellectual assessment is that these tools are generally not thoroughly grounded in underlying theories of intelligence. In fact, theory and measurement of intelligence have become separate areas of investigation, such that theories of intelligence are not always consistent with existing measures (Anderson, 1999; Deary, Austin, & Caryl, 2000; Harrison, Flanagan, & Genshaft, 1997; Styles, 1999). Nowhere is this more evident than in the models of intelligence provided by Gardner, Sternberg, and Borkowski.

Multiple Intelligences

Howard Gardner's model asserts that people have multiple intelligences (MI) rather than a single, general intelligence (Chen & Gardner, 1997; Gardner, 1983, 1993; Torff & Gardner, 1999). This approach posits that intelligence consists of vertical (i.e., separate, specialized) faculties, in contrast to the traditional horizontal view which accepts the notion of a single set of centralized processes that underlie intelligence (Torff & Gardner, 1999). Gardner has postulated that it is important to consider not only abstract thinking skills and problem-solving abilities in the definition of intelligence, but also the function of those skills and abilities when applied to real-world problems. Research has focused on atypical populations who display uneven cognitive profiles, survivors of brain damage who have lost some abilities yet maintained others, and cross-cultural studies that investigate culturally valued knowledge and abilities (Chen & Gardner, 1997). MI considers an intelligent person to be the one who can solve problems or create products that are valued by individuals of their culture (Gardner, 1983). Gardner emphasizes that the definition of intelligence is culture-laden; that what is considered intelligent in one culture may be different from what is considered intelligent in other cultures.

According to MI theory, humans possess at least eight distinct intelligences: linguistic, logical/mathematical, spatial, musical, bodily/kinesthetic, interpersonal, intrapersonal, and naturalist (Torff & Gardner, 1999). Each of these is thought to function as an autonomous faculty, yet they do not work in isolation from one another. The theory rests on the assumption that raw propensities in each domain are shaped and defined by cultural and educational experiences (Chen & Gardner, 1997). Furthermore, everyone is thought to possess the same ensemble of MI, but not everyone exhibits equal strengths or similar profiles (Gardner, 1997). Thus, MI theory suggests assessing individuals' patterns of aptitude rather than obtaining discrete scores in separate domains. No particular intelligence is assigned priority (Chen & Gardner). Rather, each is seen as equally important.

Implications of Gardner's Multiple Intelligences Approach

According to the MI approach to education, students should be able to carry out specific analyses, interpretations, comparisons, and critiques not only in a classroom setting, but also in a real-world setting. To attain this goal, Gardner (1991, 1993, 1997) has suggested that teachers should use a variety of instructional strategies. He argues that this multifaceted method of teaching would maximize students' abilities to learn in a way that is consistent with their own intellectual strengths to the extent that different strategies are effective in enhancing specific intelligences. Moreover, Gardner (1993, 1997) urges educators to employ multiple assessment techniques, rather than a single formal test, in order to better understand each student's abilities and performance. In this regard, Gardner's suggestions are conducive to the use of dynamic assessment rather than of traditional, static assessment.

Triarchic Theory of Intelligence

Like Gardner's MI theory, Sternberg's triarchic theory posits that the fundamental nature of intelligence consists of more than a single general factor (Sternberg, 1988). Sternberg has adopted a systems approach in which several aspects of intelligence are examined together in order to explain how intelligence operates as a system (Sternberg, 1997). This theory posits that there are three distinct, yet interrelated, types of intelligence: analytical, creative, and practical (Sternberg, 1988; Sternberg, Castejón, Prieto, Hautamaki, & Grigorenko, 2001). Although the three aspects of intelligence are theoretically distinct from one another, all make use of the same underlying set of information-processing abilities (Sternberg et al., 2001).

The first component of the triarchic theory, analytical intelligence, consists of executive processes, knowledge, and performance (Sternberg et al., 2001). Creative intelligence is represented in behaviors and strategies employed when a person is faced with an unfamiliar task or situation. Practical intelligence is demonstrated by positive adaptation to real-world environments. According to the theory, individuals may possess strengths in one or more aspects of intelligence. Like Gardner's MI approach, the triarchic theory assumes that the definition of intelligence may vary from culture to culture, based on the values of the particular culture (Cooper, 1999; Sternberg, 1999). Sternberg's triarchic theory indicates that intelligent behavior is demonstrated through the application of information-processing skills and abilities to coping with relatively novel tasks and situations. The Sternberg Triarchic Abilities Test (STAT), based on Sternberg's theory (Sternberg et al., 2001), uses verbal, quantitative, and figural items to assess analytical, practical, and creative intelligence. Because the goal of the STAT is to assess abilities that are not measured by traditional intelligence tests (Sternberg), there is little information available regarding correlations between the STAT and these other measures. Thus, it remains unclear whether the STAT may predict academic achievement more accurately than traditional measures of intelligence.

Implications of Sternberg's Triarchic Theory of Intelligence

The implications of the triarchic theory of intelligence are related to the notion that the goal of education should be to recognize and enhance talents that are important to pursuing a career and succeeding in later life. Sternberg asserts that intelligence is malleable, and as such he posits that psychologists and educators can, to some extent, remediate deficits in cognitive skills and abilities (Sternberg & Grigorenko, 2000). He emphasizes that school practices should be altered in several ways in order to make educational practices more consistent with research findings (Sternberg & Grigorenko, 2000). For example, he recommends that IQ scores should not be the sole determinant of assignment to educational tracks because traditional intellectual assessment procedures, in contrast to dynamic assessment procedures, do not provide information on a sufficiently broad range of abilities. Another recommended change is that instruction and assessment should be diversified to reflect analytical, practical, and creative abilities. Finally, Sternberg recommends that teachers should consider students' values and strive to encourage them to understand why it is important for them to learn to their full potential, thereby inducing students to enjoy learning more fully and ultimately to experience personal and career success.

A Process-Oriented Model of Metacognition

A third contemporary approach to intellectual assessment, Borkowski's process-oriented model of metacognition, attempts to explain strategy use and information processing in terms of links between motivation and executive functioning (Borkowski, Chan, & Muthukrishna, 2000). Borkowski's process-oriented model of metacognition describes the way in which people regulate their cognitive processes (Puustinen & Pulkkinen, 2001). This model takes the focus off of traditional views of intelligence and instead emphasizes the value of strategy selection and strategy-based learning (Borkowski et al., 2000). Metacognitive theory attempts to explain successes and failures in strategy generalization through providing an understanding of the ways in which strategies develop and explaining how their use becomes generalized over time and in various settings (Borkowski, Milstead, & Hale, 1988). According to this theory, which is essentially a model of self-regulated learning, strategy-based learning begins as a deliberate, effortful process for novice learners (Borkowski et al., 2000). In time, previously learned skills and knowledge are generalized to new situations and tasks through the use of regulatory processes and motivational beliefs (Borkowski & Muthukrishna, 1995). The successful integration of cognitive, motivational, personal, and situational characteristics—the main components of the metacognitive system—is at the heart of human intelligence and adaptation (Borkowski et al., Pressley, Borkowski, & Schneider, 1990).

Implications of Borkowski's Process-Oriented Model of Metacognition

The educational implications of Borkowski's model are rather straightforward: educational environments should teach students that they can gain personal control over their own academic outcomes through the use of self-regulatory strategies (Borkowski et al., 2000). Essentially, this recommendation centers around the development of self-regulation skills. In order to teach the type of self-regulation necessary for metacognitive success, educators should continually encourage students to appraise their problem solving and provide basic instruction, or frameworks, for students to effectively self-monitor their problem solving. This process will eventually aid students in developing a sense of control over their own learning. In turn, these perceptions of control are likely to have a positive impact on motivation, regulation, achievement processes, and academic outcomes. Moreover, these perceptions will influence students' judgments about their ability, their willingness to apply effortful strategies, and their feelings of satisfaction.

SELF-REGULATION, DYNAMIC ASSESSMENT, AND ID

Cognition and Social–Emotional Regulation as Intellectual Behaviors

In the metacognitive model of Borkowski et al. (2000), self-regulation plays a key role in an individual's understanding of the importance of task analysis, strategy selection, and monitoring. This specific type of cognitive regulation is at the root of most of the learning problems of individuals with ID, who often do not use strategies efficiently or fail to generalize newly acquired strategies appropriately. The latter problem is often due to immature forms of self-regulation. This higher order skill is also important for everyday learning. For instance, mental planning and monitoring are involved in practical skills such as preparing meals and keeping and re-membering appointments as well as relating to others and deciding who to trust (e.g., police officers, teachers) and whose advice is disputable (e.g., people who might attempt to manipulate them).

The "ideal" self-regulated student is unusually active during complex learning situations, especially through their utilization of strategies and the setting of realistic goals. In addition, self-regulated students actively monitor their learning progress and adapt strategies to fit the context and the goals at hand (Martinez-Pons, 1996; Pintrich, 2000). Unfortunately, many individuals with ID often experience problems in developing these high-order regulation skills. In fact, Whitman (1990) has proposed that self-regulation is the central problem in defining a variety of intellectual impairments.

The appropriate context and proper choice of tasks used in special ed-ucation classrooms may be important ways to increase the self-regulatory functioning of individuals with ID. For instance, Stright and Supplee (2002) compared small-group seat work to teacher-directed instruction, and found that students' monitoring of their progress varied considerably across settings, with small-group seat work being more conducive to active monitoring. Moreover, the type of task utilized by teachers for instruction has been shown to influence students' motivation (Turner, 1995). Open tasks requiring higher order thinking exert a stronger influence on stu-dents' motivation than do closed tasks involving memory skills. In addi-tion, role-playing, peer tutoring, and the practice of new strategic-based skills on a variety of tasks may allow mentally retarded individuals to be more likely to transfer and apply these strategies more efficiently and to a wide variety of learning settings.

Language and Regulation

Another related concern, particularly relevant when discussing self-regulation, is that of language abilities. Research has shown that language plays a central role in guiding all domains of self-regulation. In brief, language allows for self-reflection and response inhibition through the utilization of internal verbalizations (Abbeduto & Hesketh, 1997; Vygotsky, 1987). In fact, children with language problems tend to display significantly lower ratings on teacher's reports of emotional regulation than do their more "typical" counterparts (Fujiki, Brinton, & Clarke, 2002). Additionally, research has demonstrated that mature adolescents, and most adults, utilize private speech when attempting difficult tasks as their preferred means of problem solving (Duncan & Cheyne, 2002). In this sense, language abilities and skills set the stage for the emergence of mature forms of emotional and cognitive self-regulation and sequential reasoning.

Social–Emotional Regulation and Intellectual Disability

There is a strong link between emotional regulation and the quality of social relationships, with more adept emotional regulators exhibiting more successful social interactions. Gottman (1997) has shown that the same metacognitive skills needed for intellectual success are also crucial in managing one's emotional states. These include the abilities to recognize emotional states and to move from state-to-state in order to restore emotional equilibrium—essentially a form of emotional self-regulation. Some mentally retarded individuals are likely to experience difficulty in forming and developing social relationships—a defining characteristic of their disability—in large part because of deficiencies in basic skills related to emotional regulation (e.g., Geschwind, Boone, Miller, & Swerdloff, 2000).

Dynamic Assessment, Regulation, and ID

ID is not a static entity; instead, each individual manifests varying behaviors and differential ranges of salient behavioral characteristics. For this reason, it is essential that an accurate diagnosis of ID be made through assessment of each individual's range of task-related competencies, particularly in the domain of self-regulation, from emotional, cognitive, and social perspectives. In addition, creating goals, a treatment plan, and instructions based on the principles of dynamic assessment are efficient ways to ensure optimal assessment and development in many domains that encompass the definition of ID.

There are a number of ways to include self-regulation within a dynamic approach to assessment. Several tasks are available dependent upon which aspect of self-regulation and age of the child are the foci. In infancy, the *Still-Face* paradigm addresses regulatory abilities (Moore, Cohn, & Campbell, 2001). Early childhood tasks such as *Toy Cleanup* assess compliance, whereas the *Mother-in-Teaching Context* task measures motivational aspects of regulation (Kochanska, Tjebkes, & Forman, 1998). During adolescence, motivation and strategy use can be assessed with the *Motivational Strategies for Learning Questionnaire* (Pintrich, Smith, Garcia, & McKeachie, 1993).

Interventions aimed at self-regulation should always occur in multiple contexts. For instance, delays in behavioral regulation could be practiced and modeled both with parents at home as well as with teachers at school. Also, new strategies should be modeled and demonstrated; for example, using words to ask for another student's possession rather than simply grabbing the object. Moreover, games like *red-light, green-light* foster effortful control, placing children in touch with their body movements as governed by verbal instruction. In short, pre- and postassessment of emotional, social, and cognitive regulatory skills set the stage for discovering how well children and adolescents respond to appropriate instructions in the home and in the classroom.

INTELLECTUAL ASSESSMENTS: FUTURE PERSPECTIVES

Although new theories of intelligence, new approaches to assessments, and new definitional concerns with existing measures of IQ have all gained momentum during the past decade, the field of ID has not "budged" in terms of its reliance on traditional, static, and noncontextualized measures of intelligence. This lack of change in definitional direction seems attributable to several factors: (1) the "need" for a cutoff point (e.g., 70–75) that distinguishes individuals who meet, from those who do not meet, the major criterion (i.e., intelligence) associated with ID. This "need" is often more related to practical issues, such as securing additional school funding, establishing eligibility for other entitlements, or influencing judicial consequences for those convicted of serious crimes than to educationally relevant rationale (Reschly, Myers, & Hartel, 2002); (2) the psychometrically strong foundation upon which traditional IQ tests rest and their long histories of success in diagnosis; (3) the failure of the "new wave of theories" to find their way, as yet, into the arena of mainstream assessment; (4) a gap between the tools or instruments that might define and assess new constructs (such as self-regulation) and basic educational practices; and (5) the lack of a "clear-cut winner" among new theories and new constructs that reflect that multiple—sometimes interactive—components of intelligence.

From another perspective, it might be unreasonable to expect the old approach to be supplanted by the new, at least overnight. What might realistically occur is a phased-in approach wherein traditional assessments (appropriate for diagnoses) are augmented with contextually based tests (more useful for remedial education). Out of this dual approach to intellectual assessment could emerge renewed interests in creating an IQ test that is theoretically, diagnostically, and educationally relevant, although separate tests that evidence predictive validity for each of these purposes might also suffice for clinician use. Construction of a single test, or related tests, would satisfy the needs of many of the current stakeholders associated with intellectual assessments: testing corporations, researchers, educators, psychometricians, parents, the public at large, and all the children who will be assessed for ID in the future.

ACKNOWLEDGMENTS. This paper was supported, in part, by NIH grant HD-26456. Authors Carothers, Howard, and Farris were supported by NIH training grant HD-07184.

REFERENCES

Abbeduto, L., & Hesketh, L. J. (1997). Pragmatic development in individuals with mental retardation: Learning to use language in social interactions. *Mental Retardation and Developmental Disabilities Research Reviews, 3*, 323–333.

Anderson, M. (1999). Project development—Taking stock. In M. Anderson (Ed.), *The development of intelligence* (pp. 311–332). East Sussex, UK: Psychology Press.

Bayley, N. (1969). *Manual for the Bayley Scales of Infant Development*. San Antonio, TX: Psychological Corporation.

Bayley, N. (1993). *Manual for the Bayley Scales of Infant Development* (2nd ed.). San Antonio, TX: Psychological Corporation.

Black, M. M., & Matula, K. (2000). *Essentials of Bayley Scales of Infant Development—II Assessment*. New York: Wiley.

Borkowski, J. G., Chan, L. K. S., & Muthukrishna, N. (2000). A process-oriented model of metacognition: Links between motivation and executive functioning. In G. Schraw & J. C. Impara (Eds.), *Issues in the measurement of metacognition* (pp. 1–41). Lincoln, NE: Buros Institute of Mental Measurements.

Borkowski, J. G., Milstead, M., & Hale, C. (1988). Components of children's metamemory: Implications for strategy generalization. In F. E. Weinert & M. Perlmutter (Eds.), *Memory development: Universal changes and individual differences* (pp. 73–100). Hillsdale, NJ: Erlbaum.

Borkowski, J. G., & Muthukrishna, N. (1995). Learning environments and skill generalization: How contexts facilitate regulatory processes and efficacy beliefs. In F. E. Weinert & W. Schneider (Eds.), *Memory performance and competencies: Issues in growth and development* (pp. 283–300). Mahwah, NJ: Erlbaum.

Bransford, J. D., Delclos, V. R., Vye, N. J., Burns, M. S., & Hasselbring, T. S. (1987). Approaches to dynamic assessment: Issues, data, and future directions. In C. S. Lidz (Ed.), *Dynamic assessment: An interactional approach to evaluating learning potential* (pp. 479–496). New York: Guilford Press.

Chen, J. Q., & Gardner, H. (1997). Alternative assessment from a multiple intelligences theoretical perspective. In D. P. Flanagan, J. L. Genshaft, & P. L. Harrison (Eds.), *Contemporary intellectual assessment: Theories, tests, and issues* (pp. 105–121). New York: Guilford Press.

Cooper, C. (1999). *Intelligence and abilities* (pp. 39–65). New York: Routledge.

Deary, I. J., Austin, E. J., & Caryl, P.G. (2000). Testing versus understanding human intelligence. *Psychology, Public Policy, and Law, 6*, 180–190.

Duncan, R. M., & Cheyne, J. A. (2002). Private speech in young adults: Task difficulty, self-regulation, and psychological predication. *Cognitive Development, 16*, 889–906.

Feuerstein, R., Rand, Y., & Hoffman, M. B. (1979). *The dynamic assessment of retarded performers*. Baltimore, MD: University Park Press.

Flanagan, D. P., McGrew, K. S., & Ortiz, S. O. (2000). *The Wechsler Intelligence Scales and Gf–Gc Theory: A contemporary approach to interpretation*. Needham Heights, MA: Allyn & Bacon.

Fletcher, J. M., Francis, D. J., Rourke, B. P., Shaywitz, S. E., & Shaywitz, B. A. (1992). The validity of discrepancy-based definitions of reading disabilities. *Journal of Learning Disabilities, 25*, 555–561.

Freeman, L., & Miller, A. (2001). Norm-referenced, criterion-referenced, and dynamic assessment: What exactly is the point? *Educational Psychology in Practice, 17,* 3–16.

Fujiki, M., Brinton, B., & Clarke, D. (2002). Emotion regulation in children with specific language impairment. *Language, Speech, and Hearing Services in Schools, 33,* 102–111.

Gardner, H. (1983). *Frames of mind: The theory of multiple intelligences.* New York: Basic Books.

Gardner, H. (1991). *The unschooled mind: How children think and how schools should teach.* New York: Basic Books.

Gardner, H. (1993). *Multiple intelligences: The theory in practice.* New York: Basic Books.

Gardner, H. (1997). Multiple approaches to understanding. In C. M. Reigeluth (Ed.), *Instructional-design theories and models: Vol. II. A new paradigm of instructional theory* (pp. 69–89). Mahwah, NJ: Erlbaum.

Geschwind, D. H., Boone, K. B., Miller, B. L., & Swerdloff, R. S. (2000). Neurobehavioral phenotype of Klinefelter syndrome. *Mental Retardation and Developmental Disabilities Research Reviews, 6,* 107–116.

Gottman, J. (1997). *The heart of parenting.* New York: Simon and Schuster.

Grossman, H. (Ed.). (1983). *Classification in mental retardation.* Washington, DC: American Association on Mental Deficiency.

Gutierrez-Cellen, V. F., & Pena, E. (2001). Dynamic assessment of diverse children: A tutorial. *Language, Speech, and Hearing Services in Schools, 32,* 212–224.

Harrison, P. L., Flanagan, D. P., & Genshaft, J. L. (1997). An integration and synthesis of contemporary theories, tests, and issues in the field of intellectual assessment. In D. P. Flanagan, J. L. Genshaft, & P. L. Harrison (Eds.), *Contemporary intellectual assessment: Theories, tests, and issues* (pp. 533–561). New York: Guilford Press.

Haywood, H. C., & Brown, A. L. (1990). Dynamic approaches to psychoeducational assessment. *School Psychology Review, 19,* 411–422.

Hunt, M. (1993). *The story of psychology.* New York: Doubleday.

Jitendra, A. K., & Kameenui, E. J. (1993). Dynamic assessment as a compensatory assessment approach: A description and analysis. *Remedial and Special Education, 14,* 6–17.

Kamphaus, R. W., Petoskey, M. D., & Morgan, A. W. (1997). A history of intelligence test interpretation. In D. P. Flanagan, J. L. Genshaft, & P. L. Harrison (Eds.), *Contemporary intellectual assessment: Theories, tests, and issues* (pp. 3–16). London: Guilford Press.

Kaufman, A. S., & Kaufman, N. L. (2004). *KABC-II administration and scoring manual.* Circle Pines, MN: American Guidance Service.

Kaufman, A. S., & Lichtenberger, E. O. (2000). *Essentials of WISC-III and WPPSI-R assessment.* New York: Wiley.

Kochanska, G., Tjebkes, T. L., & Forman, D. R. (1998). Children's emerging regulation of conduct: Restraint, compliance, and internalization from infancy to the second year. *Child Development, 69,* 1378–1389.

Lichtenberger, E. O., Broadbooks, D. Y., & Kaufman, A. S. (2000). *Essentials of cognitive assessment with KAIT and other Kaufman measures.* New York: Wiley.

Lidz, C. S. (1997). Dynamic assessment approaches. In D. P. Flanagan, J. L. Genshaft, & P. L. Harrison (Eds.), *Contemporary intellectual assessment: Theories, tests, and issues* (pp. 281–296). New York: Guildford Press.

Lidz, C. S., & Pena, E. D. (1996). Dynamic assessment: The model, its relevance as a nonbiased approach, and its application to Latino American preschool children. *Language, Speech, and Hearing Services in Schools, 27,* 367–372.

Luckasson, R., Borthwick-Duffy, S., Buntinx, W. H. E., Coulter, D. L., Craig, E. M., Reeve, A., et al. (2002). *Mental retardation: Definition, classification, and systems of supports* (10th ed.). Washington, DC: American Association on Mental Retardation.

Luckasson, R., Coulter, D. L., Polloway, E. A., Reiss, S., Schalock, R. L., Snell, M. E., et al. (1992). *Mental retardation: Definition, classification, and systems of supports* (9th ed.). Washington, DC: American Association on Mental Retardation.

Martinez-Pons, M. (1996). Test of a model of parental inducement of academic self-regulation. *Journal of Experimental Education, 64,* 213–227.

Missiuna, C., & Samuels, M. (1989). Dynamic assessment of preschool children with special needs: Comparison of mediation and instruction. *Remedial and Special Education, 10*, 53–62.

Moore, G. A., Cohn, J. F., & Campbell, S. B. (2001). Infant affective responses to mother's still face at 6 months differentially predict externalizing and internalizing behaviors at 18 months. *Developmental Psychology, 37*, 706–714.

Nigram, R. (2001). Dynamic assessment of graphic symbol combinations by children with autism. *Focus on Autism and Other Developmental Disabilities, 16*, 190–197.

Pena, E., Iglesias, A., & Lidz, C.S. (2001). Reducing test bias through dynamic assessment of children's word learning ability. *American Journal of Speech–Language Pathology, 10*, 138–152.

Pintrich, P. R. (2000). The role of goal orientation in self-regulated learning. In M. Boekaerts, P. R. Pintrich, & M. Zeider (Eds.), *Handbook of self-regulation* (pp. 452–502). New York: Academic Press.

Pintrich, P. R., Smith, D. A. F., Garcia, T., & McKeachie, W. (1993). Reliability and predictive validity of the motivated strategies for learning questionnaire (MSLQ). *Educational and Psychological Measurement, 53*, 801–813.

Pressley, M., Borkowski, J. G., & Schneider, W. (1990). Good information processing: What it is and how education can promote it. *International Journal of Educational Research, 2*, 857–867.

Puustinen, M., & Pulkkinen, L. (2001). Models of self-regulated learning: A review. *Scandinavian Journal of Educational Research, 45*, 269–286.

Reschly, D. J., Myers, T. G., & Hartel, C. R. (Eds.). (2002). *Mental retardation: Determining eligibility for social security benefits*. Washington, DC: National Academy Press.

Riverside Publishing Company. (2002). *Stanford–Binet Intelligence Scales, Fifth edition features*. Retrieved November 14, 2002, from http://www.riverpub.com/products/clinical/sbis5/features.html

Roid, G. H. (2003). *Stanford-Binet Intelligence Scales, Fifth Edition, Technical Manual*. Itasca, IL: Riverside.

Saylor, C. F., Boyce, G. C., Peagler, S. M., & Callahan, S. A. (2000). Brief report: Cautions against using the Stanford–Binet-IV to classify high-risk preschoolers. *Journal of Pediatric Psychology, 25*, 179–183.

Sternberg, R. J. (1988). *The triarchic mind: A new theory of human intelligence*. New York: Viking.

Sternberg, R. J. (1997). The triarchic theory of intelligence. In D. P. Flanagan, J. L. Genshaft, & P. L. Harrison (Eds.), *Contemporary intellectual assessment: Theories, tests, and issues* (pp. 92–104). New York: Guilford Press.

Sternberg, R. J. (1999). A triarchic approach to the understanding and assessment of intelligence in multicultural populations. *Journal of School Psychology, 37*, 145–159.

Sternberg, R. J. (2000). Group and individual differences in intelligence: What can and should we do about them? In A. Kozulin & Y. Rand (Eds.), *Experience of mediated learning: An impact of Feuerstein's theory in education and psychology* (pp. 55–82). New York: Pergamon.

Sternberg, R. J., Castejón, J. L., Prieto, M. D., Hautamaki, J., & Grigorenko, E. L. (2001). Confirmatory factor analysis of the Sternberg Triarchic Abilities Test in three international samples. *European Journal of Psychological Assessment, 17*, 1–16.

Sternberg, R. J., & Grigorenko, E. L. (2000). Theme-park psychology: A case study regarding human intelligence and its implications for education. *Educational Psychology Review, 12*, 247–268.

Stright, A. D., & Supplee, L. H. (2002). Children's self-regulatory behaviors during teacher-directed, seat-work, and small-group instructional contexts. *Journal of Education Research, 95*, 235–245.

Styles, I. (1999). The study of intelligence—The interplay between theory and measurement. In M. Anderson (Ed.), *The development of intelligence* (pp. 311–332). Hove, East Sussex, UK: Psychology Press.

Swanson, H. L. (1996). Classification and dynamic assessment of children with learning disabilities. *Focus of Exceptional Children, 28*, 1–20.

Thorndike, R. L., Hagan, E. P., & Sattler, J. M. (1986). *Stanford–Binet Intelligence Scale* (4th ed.). Chicago: Riverside.

Thorndike, R. M. (1997). The early history of intelligence testing. In D. P. Flanagan, J. L. Genshaft, & P. L. Harrison (Eds.), *Contemporary intellectual assessment: Theories, tests, and issues* (pp. 3–16). London: Guilford Press.

Torff, B., & Gardner, H. (1999). The vertical mind—The case for multiple intelligences. In M. Anderson (Ed.), *The development of intelligence* (pp. 139–159). Hove, East Sussex, UK: Psychology Press.

Turner, J. C. (1995). The influence of classroom contexts on young children's motivation for literacy. *Reading Research Quarterly, 30,* 410–441.

Tzuriel, D. (1992). The dynamic assessment approach: A reply to Frisby and Braden. *Journal of Special Education, 26,* 302–324.

Utley, C. A., Haywood, H. C., & Masters, J. C. (1992). Policy implications of psychological assessment of minority children. In H. C. Haywood & D. Tzuriel (Eds.), *Interactive assessment* (pp. 445–469). New York: Springer-Verlag.

Vygotsky, L. S. (1986). *Thought and language.* Cambridge, MA: MIT Press.

Vygotsky, L. S. (1987). Thinking and speech. In R. Rieber & A. Carton (Eds.), *The collected works of L. S. Vygotsky: Vol. 1. Problems of general psychology* (pp. 39–285). New York: Plenum.

Wechsler, D. (1939). *The measurement of adult intelligence.* Baltimore: Williams & Wilkins.

Wechsler, D. (1967). *Manual for the Wechsler Preschool and Primary Scale of Intelligence (WPPSI).* San Antonio, TX: Psychological Corporation.

Wechsler, D. (1997). *Manual for the Wechsler Adult Intelligence Scale—third edition (WAIS-III).* San Antonio, TX: Psychological Corporation.

Wechsler, D. (2002). *Wechsler Preschool and Primary Scales of Intelligence* (3rd ed.). San Antonio, TX: Psychological Corporation.

Wechsler, D. (2003). *WISC-IV technical and interpretive manual.* San Antonio, TX: Psychological Corporation.

Whitman, T. L. (1990). Self-regulation and mental retardation. *American Journal on Mental Retardation, 94,* 347–362.

15

Adaptive Behavior

SHARON A. BORTHWICK-DUFFY

ADAPTIVE BEHAVIOR AND MENTAL RETARDATION

The early descriptions of persons with mental retardation emphasized their inability to adapt to the demands of everyday life (Biasini, Grupe, Huffman, & Bray, 1999; Greenspan & Driscoll, 1997; Scheerenberger, 1983). In 1850, Seguin argued that "sensibility, of intelligence, and will" could help to identify mental retardation in instances when, "to a casual observation, the question may arise whether any default in these particulars exists at all" (Wilbur, 1877, p. 31). In the early twentieth century Tredgold described mental retardation as incomplete mental development "of such a kind and degree that the individual is incapable of adapting himself to the normal environment of his fellows in such a way as to maintain existence independently of supervision, control, or external support" (Luckasson et al., 2002, p. 20). Thus, dating back to the original perceptions, limits in the ability adapt to the demands of everyday life, i.e., adaptive behavior, have been a central and distinguishing feature of mental retardation.

Current definitions of adaptive behavior are consistent with the early conceptualizations of mental retardation. The American Psychological Association describes adaptive behavior, for example, in terms of individual performance in relation to person–environment interactions and includes it with social skills and peer acceptance as a component of social competence (Jacobson & Mulick, 1996a). Similarly, the American Association on Mental Retardation (AAMR) refers to adaptive behavior as the collection of skills that people learn in order to function in everyday life (Luckasson et al., 2002). Although adaptive behavior is just one criterion in diagnosis, and may not be the criterion carrying the most weight in diagnostic decisions, it is clear that it is closely aligned with descriptors of mental retardation.

SHARON A. BORTHWICK-DUFFY • Graduate School of Education, University of California Riverside, Riverside, California 92521.

ADAPTIVE BEHAVIOR AND INTELLIGENCE

To understand adaptive behavior, it is important to consider its relationship to intelligence and the ways in which these two constructs fit in a model of overall personal competence. Most definitions of mental retardation imply that intelligence and adaptive behavior, or adaptive functioning, are distinct and nonoverlapping constructs, as diagnostic criteria include evidence of significant limitations in both intelligence and adaptive behavior. Accordingly, a person with low intelligence who does not have significant limitations in adaptive behavior should not receive a diagnosis of mental retardation and a person with significant limitations in adaptive behavior who does not have low intelligence also does not have mental retardation. The unique contributions and meaning of intelligence estimates (as measured by intelligence tests) and adaptive functioning or adaptive behavior (measured by adaptive behavior scales) to the assessment of a person's overall personal competence and what Greenspan, Switzky, and Granfield (1996) referred to as "the essence of mental retardation," however, are not as clear as the definitions imply. In Greenspan's (1979) widely cited theoretical model of personal competence, conceptual intelligence, practical intelligence, and social intelligence each contribute to a person's overall functioning. Greenspan suggested that practical and social intelligence are what people use in real-world settings and problems and that intelligence tests measure conceptual or academic intelligence. In its 2002 definition of mental retardation (Luckasson et al., 2002), AAMR refers to three dimensions of adaptive behavior that are reflected in conceptual, practical, and social skills. This is consistent in some respects with Greenspan's tripartite model. However, the AAMR model does not fully reflect the proposal that low social intelligence, rather than low conceptual intelligence (measured by IQ), is the most salient characteristic of mental retardation or that practical and social adaptive behavior or skills actually represent practical and social intelligence (Greenspan, 1979, in press; Greenspan & Driscoll, 1997). Thus, whether adaptive behavior is one of two defining characteristics of mental retardation, or is simply the "outward manifestation of intelligence," is a topic of continuing discussion (Leffert & Siperstein, 2002).

STRUCTURE OF ADAPTIVE BEHAVIOR

A growing consensus about the dimensionality and meaning of adaptive behavior is evident in the scientific literature and recent publications of professional organizations (Thompson, McGrew, & Bruininks, 1999). The American Association on Mental Retardation, the American Psychological Association, and the National Research Council Committee on Disability Determination for Mental Retardation have reached similar conclusions about the multidimensional structure of adaptive behavior and there is general agreement about the broad, or higher-order, dimensions that reflect adaptive functioning in persons with mental retardation.

Dimensions of Adaptive Behavior

Three dimensions of adaptive behavior are identified in the 2002 AAMR definition of mental retardation, expressed by observable, practical, conceptual, and social skills (Luckasson et al., 2002). The practical dimension refers to personal independence and is reflected in the demonstration of the practical skills needed for daily living. The social dimension refers to personal responsibility, such as meeting the social expectations of others and getting along in social contexts. Conceptual adaptive behavior is observed in cognitive and academic skills, including communication. As noted above, these AAMR dimensions emerged from a synthesis of factor analytic studies of psychometrically adequate measures of adaptive behavior, although none of the scales uses this exact set of terms to identify its higher order dimensions. Depending on the measure, for example, social skills might be represented by a subscale called "Personal–social responsibility," "Socialization," "Social Interaction," or "Social Skills." The National Research Council Committee on Disability Determination for Mental Retardation (National Research Council [NRC], 2002) identified domains generally similar to those in the AAMR definition (see Table 15.1). Slight variations in emphases within the broad areas are noted by the NRC Committee for different developmental periods (infancy/early childhood, childhood, and adolescence/adulthood), which suggests that different items within the domains are likely to discriminate persons with and without mental retardation at different ages or that different measures should be used at different ages.

The NRC committee included motor/mobility as a fourth dimension of adaptive behavior for all ages. Work skills and work-related behavior

Table 15.1. Dimensions of Adaptive Behavior Identified by AAMR and NRC

	Conceptual	Practical	Social	Motor	Work
AAMR[a]					
	Cognitive/ academic	Independence	Personal responsibility		
	Communication	Daily living skills	Meet social expectations		
NRC[b]					
0–4 years	Communication	Daily living skills Self-help skills	Social	Motor/ mobility	
5–17 years	Communication/ functional academic	Daily living skills	Social	Motor/ mobility	
>18 years	Communication	Daily living skills	Social	Motor/ mobility	Work skills/ related behavior
	Practical/cognitive				

[a] American Association on Mental Retardation.
[b] National Research Council Committee on Disability Determination for Mental Retardation.

appear as a separate construct only in adolescence and adulthood. AAMR instead considers motor skills and other indicators of health status to influence individual functioning and very important to consider in the evaluation of adaptive behavior (e.g., physical disability may affect a person's ability to perform certain skills), but not to be a separate dimension of adaptive behavior in the diagnostic criteria.

Indicators of Social Competence Not Found on Adaptive Behavior Scales

Current measures of adaptive behavior omit the sometimes subtle, and possibly even immeasurable, characteristics that differentiate persons with and without mental retardation and reflect the person–environment interaction that is understood to be adaptive behavior. One of the most distinguishing features of mental retardation is a limitation in the ability to understand people and social processes (Greenspan, 2004). Concerns that adaptive behavior scales are best at measuring nonsocial behavior and do not adequately address social adaptation have been noted in recent years (Greenspan, 2004; Gresham & Elliott, 1987; Leffert & Siperstein, 2002; MacMillan, Gresham, & Siperstein, 1993). Adaptive behavior scales gather information on socially relevant, discrete behaviors, but the items contained in the social domains most of these scales typically do not provide sensitive measures of social processes, such as picking up social cues or anticipating the reactions of others. Leffert and Siperstein (2002) argue that the construct of adaptive behavior should be expanded to highlight the role that social cognition plays in adaptive functioning, particularly for persons with mild forms of mental retardation. This social–cognitive perspective emphasizes the identification and measurement of cognitive processes that are associated with observed adaptive behavior in the social domain.

The importance of assessing gullibility and credulity in relation to a diagnosis of mental retardation, particularly with regard to victimization and exploitation, has also been emphasized in recent years (Greenspan, 1999). These indicators of low social competence do not appear on adaptive behavior measures but are now considered important indicators of limitations in adaptive behavior (Luckasson et al., 2002; NRC, 2002).

Reliable measurement of social processes and behaviors required to negotiate new or unusual circumstances present numerous challenges, but preliminary work provides optimism that relevant information can be collected for diagnosis and the development of a person's profile of adaptive behavior. We do not know whether the assessment of social processes and additional social behaviors will identify different individuals than with current adaptive behavior scales, but it will be important to address this question. If these are the behaviors that can distinguish between persons with and without mental retardation, they need to be examined. Until adequate measures are available, consideration of relevant characteristics that are not on adaptive behavior scales will require clinical judgment that is rooted in a high level of clinical expertise and experience with relevant groups (Luckasson et al., 2002).

RELATIONSHIP OF ADAPTIVE AND MALADAPTIVE BEHAVIOR

Many adaptive behavior scales address both adaptive behavior and problem, or maladaptive behavior. Although these constructs have functional and conceptual connections, it is generally agreed that maladaptive behavior is neither the absence of adaptive behavior nor the low end of a continuum of adaptive behavior (Greenspan, in press; Jacobson & Mulick, 1996a; NRC, 2002). This view is supported by empirical studies that have found relatively low correlations between adaptive and maladaptive behavior scores (Harrison, 1987). Greenspan (1999) suggested that the presence of maladaptive behavior items on many adaptive behavior scales has also contributed to misunderstandings about presumed relationships between mental retardation and mental illness, and between maladaptive behavior and social incompetence.

FACTORS TO CONSIDER IN THE ASSESSMENT OF ADAPTIVE BEHAVIOR

Availability of Measures

Precise and objective measures of adaptive behavior with adequate norms for all age groups were unfortunately not available when impairment in adaptive behavior was included in the criteria of the first AAMR definition of mental retardation (Heber, 1961). Thus, claims that adaptive behavior was an ill-defined and poorly measured construct and one that did not belong in the definition of mental retardation were common until the mid-1980s (Clausen, 1972; Zigler, Balla, & Hodapp, 1984).

The development in the past 20 years of psychometrically adequate, norm-referenced measures of adaptive behavior has led to a greater recognition of the value of the construct in diagnosis and planning supports. It has been estimated that at least 200 measures of adaptive behavior have been developed and marketed (Biasini et al., 1999; Spreat, 1999), not including measures developed for local use. Of these, a small number have excellent psychometric properties, i.e., reliabilities of about .90, evidence of strong validity (NRC, 2002), and data on appropriate norming samples. Not all tests need to be subjected to these criteria; however, if their primary purpose is to facilitate needs assessment and treatment planning and they are not used to determine eligibility or diagnose mental retardation. The APA *Manual of Diagnosis and Professional Practice in Mental Retardation* (Jacobson & Mulick, 1996b) and the AAMR *Mental Retardation: Definition, Classification, and Systems of Supports* (Luckasson et al., 2002) provide detailed guidelines for determining the psychometric adequacy of adaptive behavior measures. Adaptive behavior scales with strong psychometric properties and norms on nonhandicapped groups include the *Vineland Adaptive Behavior Scales: Second Edition, Vineland II* (Sparrow, Cicchetti, & Balla, 2005), the *ABAS: Adaptive Behavior Assessment System*

(Harrison & Oakland, 2000), the *AAMR Adaptive Behavior Scale—School and Community* (Lambert, Nihira, & Leland, 1993), the *Comprehensive Test of Adaptive Behavior* (Adams, 2000), and the *Scales of Independent Behavior* (Bruininks, Woodcock, Weatherman, & Hill, 1996). Before selecting an adaptive behavior scale users should determine whether updated versions of the scales listed here have become available with more recent norms and content and whether there are other scales not listed that have good psychometric properties.

Contextual Considerations

Context refers to the interrelated conditions within which people live their everyday lives, including the immediate social setting, community settings, and the overarching patterns of culture and sociopolitical influences that determine normative behavior (Luckasson et al., 2002). It is generally agreed that a person's adaptive behavior can vary across settings and time, as a function of different demands and environmental supports. Context should therefore be a consideration in the selection of measures, to the extent alternatives are available, and in clinical judgment if they are not.

Culture

Most definitions of adaptive behavior stress its relationship to cultural expectations. In fact, adaptive behavior is usually defined in terms of cultural or societal expectations. Unlike IQ tests that should be culture and context-free, some items on adaptive behavior measures purposely reflect the individual's behavior with reference to cultural norms. It would be impossible to obtain standardization samples to represent all cultural variations. Tassé and Craig (1999) noted the need for culturally sensitive or culturally specific adaptive behavior measures. Without these, test consumers must be made aware of problems involved in comparing test performance across cultural groups. Thus, the selection of a culturally appropriate measure of adaptive behavior and the interpretation of scores from a measure that is not a perfect fit to the individual's culture will require good clinical judgment. It is also important to recognize that cultural demands are likely to change over time (Demchak & Drinkwater, 1998).

Environment

In addition to broader cultural factors, an evaluation of adaptive behavior depends on the specific environments where people spend their time. Most definitions of mental retardation assume that a person's adaptive behavior will be considered in relation to behavior expectations in integrated settings. This means that for diagnosis, if the individual's actual environments are segregated from nonhandicapped age peers, i.e., in congregate living designated for persons with cognitive or emotional/behavioral disabilities or special day classes in schools, adaptive behavior should be assessed in terms of behaviors that would be expected in integrated contexts.

In some cases, people will adapt better to one environment (e.g., school) than another (e.g., home), depending on the demands and provision of supports in each setting. When there are differences in levels of performance in different settings, it may be that for a diagnosis, additional weight should be given to the context that has the strongest relationship to eligibility (Reschly, 1990).

Age

Age is a key factor in the selection of measures and interpretation of adaptive behavior scores because environmental demands and expectations change and become increasingly more complex as children move toward adulthood. Therefore, whether or not a behavior is considered adaptive will depend on the person's age and most definitions specify that adaptive behavior should be considered in relation to the individual's age peers. Although this implies that precise expectations of adaptive skills have been identified for different ages, we know that the expected age of skill acquisition varies widely, even among persons without mental retardation.

Physical Limitations

An important point made by the American Psychological Association (Jacobson & Mulick, 1996a) is that physical limitations are more likely to affect adaptive behavior scores than IQ scores, and that their effect on adaptive behavior is related to whether accommodations and environmental supports have been provided. Because the theoretical basis of adaptive behavior is based on performance, rather than on ability, adaptive behavior scales are usually scored according to levels of mastery in the norming group without consideration of physical conditions. Physical limitations should therefore be considered in the interpretation of scores on adaptive behavior measures because an individual may not be able to perform certain skills due to physical conditions or disability that is unrelated to the presence of mental retardation (Luckasson et al., 2002).

Skill Acquisition Versus Skill Performance

Intelligence tests measure maximum performance, or what individuals "can do," whereas typical performance, or what the individual actually "does do," is reported on most adaptive behavior scales. A second difference between IQ and adaptive behavior measures is that IQ scores are generally considered stable, whereas adaptive behavior scores are expected to fluctuate for a variety of reasons at different points of the individual's life.

A person with mental retardation is limited in the ability to negotiate successfully the demands of daily living. In the case of adaptive behavior, ability includes both skill acquisition and an understanding of the importance and appropriateness of using particular skills in different environments and at different times. If a person scores low on an IQ test but is able to compensate for his intellectual ability with various coping behaviors, this reflects an aspect of personal competence that is not captured by standardized IQ tests.

Adaptation to environmental demands (skill performance) can be influenced by many nonintellective factors (Widaman, Borthwick-Duffy, & Little, 1991). For example, motivation and personality have been identified as important determinants of whether individuals use the skills they have learned to benefit them in different situations (Greenspan, 2004; Switzky, 1997; Zigler & Hodapp, 1986). Behavior problems can also stand in the way of the appropriate use of acquired adaptive skills.

Leland (1991) distinguished between the "training" provided to persons with mental retardation that helps them acquire adaptive skills, and the "treatment" that follows skill acquisition, to promote the use of acquired skills. Leland noted that although there are obvious overlaps between training and treatment needs, the distinction could be useful in the determination of priorities for specific individuals and the understanding of potential barriers to success.

Sources of Information

Typical performance cannot be assessed in a testing or observation situation. This means that people who are familiar with the usual behavior of the person being rated must provide information for ratings. Those who know the person being rated, such as parents, teachers, residential caregivers, employers, and peers complete some rating scales that are in a checklist format. Other measures require that professionals rely on "third party" informants to provide information that will be recorded on adaptive behavior scales. An advantage of the informant method is that the interviewer is likely to learn more about the individual being rated than will be recorded on the rating scale. A number of cautions have been raised with regard to the selection of informants. The extent to which the informant can reliably determine typical performance depends on several factors, including how long and how well he or she knows the individual, the range of contexts in which performance has been observed, frequency of contact, knowledge of the individual's specific cultural and environmental demands, consequences of high or low scores to the rater and individual being rated, and whether the relationship between the two people is positive or negative (Harrison & Robinson, 1995; Reschly, 1990).

Harrison and Robinson (1995) stressed the importance of using multiple raters to provide adaptive behavior information relative to different settings, rater perspectives, etc. One has to be careful, though, about how multiple informants are used. Information from more than one informant should not be averaged. In some cases (e.g., Vineland Adaptive Behavior Scales Second Edition: Teacher Rating Form [TRF-II]; Sparrow, Cicchetti, & Balla, in press) raters are asked to estimate a person's ability in areas that they have not directly observed (and indicate the estimation made). Too much estimation raises a red flag with regard to the validity of summary scores.

Other Methods of Assessment

Harrison and Robinson (1995) argued strongly that ratings of people's *perceptions* of adaptive behavior should be considered one piece of information in the comprehensive assessment of adaptive behavior and that alternate methods (observation, informal interviews with different sources), should be used to supplement rating scale data. Alternate methods of assessment, such as interviews (other than for completion of a rating scale) or observations, can provide useful data regarding a person's adaptive behavior. Because other data can present serious problems of reliability, alternative methods should be used to supplement norm-referenced tests and should never be the only form of assessment used to document limitations in adaptive behavior.

ADAPTIVE BEHAVIOR IN PRACTICE

Multiple Purposes of Adaptive Behavior Measures

The first adaptive behavior scales were developed to identify behavior deficits needing treatment or remediation in persons who were already known to have mental retardation. Subsequent work focused on the assessment of adaptive behavior for the purpose of diagnosis and eligibility for special services. Most current scales are reported to be useful for these and other uses, including identifying strengths and weaknesses for individual program planning, diagnosis, documenting change, and providing information for administrative needs. Spreat (1999) discussed the problems of breadth and depth that come from using a single measure for multiple purposes. Measures that provide enough detail to assist with programming can be either too long to be useful for diagnostic testing, or are developed for persons with disabilities too severe to be useful for diagnosis of individuals at higher levels of functioning.

Relative Contributions of IQ and Adaptive Behavior in Diagnosis

IQ was the predominant and sometimes only criterion considered in the diagnosis of mental retardation for many years (Adams, 1973; Harrison & Robinson, 1995; Roszkowski, Spreat, & Isett, 1983; Smith & Polloway, 1979; Zigler & Hodapp, 1986). Resistance to the inclusion of adaptive behavior as a criterion was primarily due to a perceived inability of existing measures to identify reliably significant adaptive behavior deficits (Clausen, 1972). Measurement problems were attributed to the lack of an accepted definition of adaptive behavior. When used, adaptive behavior tended to be a secondary criterion and was primarily viewed as a mechanism for declassification, i.e., a person who was considered to have mental retardation on the basis of IQ could be subsequently declassified on the basis of adequate levels of adaptive behavior (Harrison & Robinson, 1995). An alternate explanation is that adaptive behavior was ignored in diagnostic practices because it was not clearly enough connected to intelligence and the historical meaning of mental retardation (Greenspan, in press). Zigler et al. (1984) argued that adaptive behavior was not intrinsic to mental retardation and should be dropped from the definition. They contended that adaptive behavior was a correlate but not a defining characteristic of mental retardation and should be used for classification purposes. They proposed that mental retardation "should be defined solely by subaverage performance on measures of intellectual abilities (p. 66)." This proposal generated much discussion and some support but subsequent definitions offered by AAMR, APA, and other organizations retained the adaptive behavior criterion.

The current availability of psychometrically sound adaptive behavior scales that have been normed on nonhandicapped samples and increased efforts to raise the profile of adaptive behavior have contributed to increased attention to adaptive behavior in theory and practice in recent years. Most professionals agree that intelligence tests and adaptive behavior scales are not substitutes for each other but that they provide complementary information (Prasher, 1999).

Cutoff Scores and Significant Limitations

The American Association on Mental Retardation (AAMR), the American Psychological Association (APA), and the National Research Council (NRC) Committee on Disability Determination for Mental Retardation concur that for the diagnosis of mental retardation adaptive behavior should be considered in relation to appropriate normative data on nonhandicapped people. Professional organizations differ in the specific cutoffs they recommend to establish significant limitations in adaptive behavior and these differences can influence who is identified as having mental retardation. As noted above, cutoffs must be based on instruments normed on nonhandicapped groups.

AAMR (Luckasson et al., 2002) requires a score of *two standard deviations below the mean on one of the three domains* or *two standard deviations below the mean on a total score* of a measure that examines all three domains of practical, social, and cognitive skills. The criterion of significant limitations in adaptive behavior, according to APA (Jacobson & Mulick, 1996a), is a score of *two standard deviations below the mean on a summary index score of a comprehensive measure of adaptive behavior or two standard deviations below the mean on two or more scores of a multidimensional scale that provides factor or summary scores.* The NRC committee (National Research Council, 2002) expressed concern that cutoff scores of two standard deviations for both IQ and adaptive behavior would result in under-identification of mental retardation in the population. On the basis of the results of Monte Carlo simulations, the NRC committee recommended a cutoff of *one standard deviation below the mean in*

*two adaptive behavior areas or 1.5 standard deviations below the mean
in one adaptive behavior area.* Given that the availability of adaptive behavior measures normed on nonhandicapped people is relatively recent,
it is not surprising that slight variations exist across the first definitions
to designate adaptive behavior limitations in terms of standard deviation
units.

Norms for Planning

After diagnosis, norms based on standardization samples of persons
with mental retardation may be more appropriate for identifying priorities for education and training, and evaluating relative rates of progress
and program effectiveness than are norms on nonhandicapped groups.
The most widely used adaptive behavior measures include both types of
norms. Norms based on age alone are not sufficient to determine an individual's true relative standing among peers, particularly on measures
of adaptive behavior, because age groups are not homogeneous with regard to developmental expectations. Ideally, individuals would be perfectly
matched on several other characteristics, such as physical limitations and
cultural group. Because it would be impractical to develop norms for all
possible subgroups within age categories, other factors that can influence
adaptive behavior performance must be taken into account when clinicians
interpret scores.

Measures for Planning and Evaluation

Criterion-referenced tests are particularly useful for needs assessment in the individual programming process and for evaluating program effectiveness for individuals or groups. Spreat (1999) suggested that
adaptive behavior scales represent a type of criterion-referenced measurement, because "mastery is indicated when an individual achieves
all possible points in a given area of adaptive behavior" (p. 114). The
achievement of a designated criterion that is useful in the individual's
environment, but not necessarily for everyone in a standardization sample
may also constitute an important goal related to programming and support
provision.

The recently published AAMR *Supports Intensity Scale* (SIS; Thompson
et al., 2004) is similar to adaptive behavior scales in that it is concerned
with typical performance of persons with mental retardation in their
everyday activities. These measures are also different in important ways.
The stems in adaptive behavior scales are skills and the purpose is to assess the individual's level of mastery of these skills. In contrast, SIS stems
are activities that are encountered in everyday life and item responses indicate the extent of support that the person needs to participate in or perform
the activity. The SIS also considers more than an individual's present level
of personal competence, such as medical and behavioral factors and the
complexity of the settings and life activities in which he or she participates.

CURRENT ISSUES AND FUTURE DIRECTIONS

Measurement advances in recent years have improved the ability to study researchable questions related to the development and decline of adaptive behavior in different subgroups of people with mental retardation. Relationships between general aging, dementia, and Alzheimer disease, for example, have been the focus of many studies that have utilized measures of adaptive behavior, particularly in relation to Down syndrome (Prasher, 1999). The growing body of research on behavioral phenotypes that are associated with different genetic disorders has also contributed in important ways to what we know about adaptive behavior (e.g., Hodapp & Dykens, 2001). The recent decision of the Supreme Court in Atkins v. Virginia (2002), that executions of persons with mental retardation are cruel and unusual punishments and prohibited by the Constitution, has generated new questions that are relevant to the assessment of adaptive behavior, the first-time diagnosis of mental retardation in adults, and the affects of incarceration on adaptive skills. Adaptive behavior issues related to deception, gullibility, vulnerability, malingering, and manipulation are especially relevant to this court decision and highlight the importance of continued study.

Conceptualization and measurement issues in adaptive behavior continue to be a focus of current research in mental retardation. The field has come a long way with regard to the psychometric adequacy and consistency of the dimensional structure of available instruments for research and practice. It is now possible to use reliable measures of adaptive behavior to identify significant limitations in adaptive skills. At the same time, there seems to be a consensus that, just as we know intelligence is not fully explained by an IQ score, adaptive behavior is also more than what even the best adaptive behavior scales measure. Although this should not diminish the value of current adaptive behavior assessments for diagnosis and planning, it is becoming increasingly evident that attention to cultural, environmental, motivational, personality, and other influences on behavior must be integrated into the assessment process. It is also apparent that the measurement challenges of the subtle indicators of mental retardation in the social domain that are not on current adaptive behavior scales need further study.

Related to these issues is the recent encouragement by AAMR (Luckasson et al., 2002) and the NRC committee (Reschly et al., 2002) to add to the information that is provided on standardized adaptive behavior scales. Observation, interviews, and other data can contribute contextual information and information on skills not on adaptive behavior scales. Obtaining separate adaptive behavior scale ratings from more than one informant or in relation to one or more environment can also add to the overall behavior profile. The field has not addressed how all this information should contribute to the overall decisions for diagnosis regarding significant limitations in adaptive behavior. In other words, the standardized adaptive behavior scale will provide a score in standard deviation units that determines whether a significant limitation is present. How will clinical judgment that utilizes a wide array of data contribute to decisions that include discrepancies found from different data sources? Guidelines for good clinical judgment should be developed for adaptive behavior assessment to assure that all pertinent data can contribute to reliable decisions.

Theoretical relationships between adaptive behavior, intelligence, and personal competence continue to be explored. Whether the conceptual, practical, and social skills that are measured by adaptive behavior scales represent a separate dimension of personal competence (i.e., adaptive behavior) or whether they are indicators of conceptual, practical, and social intelligence is a theoretical question. Regardless of the answer to this question, it is clear that information relevant to these dimensions, obtained from adaptive behavior scales and other sources, is directly relevant to what we understand to be the "essence" of mental retardation.

REFERENCES

Adams, G. (2000). *CTAB-R and NABC-R technical manual*. Seattle, WA: Educational Achievement Systems.

Adams, J. (1973). Adaptive behavior and measured intelligence in the classification of mental retardation. *American Journal of Mental Deficiency, 78*, 77–81.

Atkins v. Virginia, 536 U.S. 304 (2002).

Biasini, F., Grupe, L., Huffman, L., & Bray, N. W. (1999). Mental retardation: A symptom and a syndrome. In S. Netherton, D. Holmes, & C. E. Walker (Eds.), *Comprehensive textbook of child and adolescent disorders* (pp. 6–23). New York: Oxford University Press.

Bruininks, R. H., Woodcock, R. W., Weatherman, R. F., & Hill, B. K. (1996). *Scales of Independent Behavior—Revised*. Itasca, IL: Riverside.

Clausen, J. (1972). Quo vadis, AAMD? *Journal of Special Education, 6*, 51–60.

Demchak, M., & Drinkwater, S. (1998). Assessing adaptive behavior. In V. H. Booney (Ed.), *Psychological assessment of children: Best practices for school and clinical settings* (2nd ed., pp. 297–322). New York: Wiley.

Greenspan, S. (1979). Social intelligence in the retarded. In N. R. Ellis (Ed.), *Handbook of mental deficiency, psychological theory and research* (pp. 483–531).

Greenspan, S. (1999). A contextualist perspective on adaptive behavior. In R. L. Schalock (Ed.), *Adaptive behavior and its measurement: Implications for the field of mental retardation* (pp. 61–80). Washington, DC: American Association on Mental Retardation.

Greenspan, S. (2004). Why Pinocchio was victimized: Factors contributing to social failure in people with mental retardation. In L. Glidden (Ed.), *International review of research in mental retardation* (pp. 121–144). San Diego, CA: Academic Press/Elsevier.

Greenspan, S. (2006). Mental retardation in the real world: Why the AAMR definition is not there yet. In H. N. Switzky & S. Greenspan (Eds.), *What is mental retardation? Ideas for evolving disability* (Revised and updated Ed.) (pp. 165–184). Washington, DC: American Association on Mental Retardation.

Greenspan, S., & Driscoll, J. (1997). The role of intelligence in a broad model of personal competence. In D. P. Flanagan, J. L. Genshaft, & P. L. Harrison (Eds.), *Contemporary intellectual assessment: Theories, tests, and issues* (pp. 131–150). New York: Guilford Press.

Greenspan, S., Switzky, H., & Granfield, J. (1996). Everyday intelligence and adaptive behavior: A theoretical framework. In J. Jacobson & J. Mulick (Eds.), *Manual on diagnosis and professional practice in mental retardation* (pp. 127–135). Washington, DC: American Psychological Association.

Gresham, F. M., & Elliott, S. N. (1987). The relationship between adaptive behavior and social skills: Issues in definition and assessment. *Journal of Special Education, 21*, 167–181.

Harrison, P. L. (1987). Research with adaptive behavior scales. *Journal of Special Education,* *21,* 37–68.

Harrison, P. L., & Oakland, T. (2000). *ABAS: Adaptive behavior assessment system.* San Antonio, TX: Psychological Corporation.

Harrison, P. L., & Robinson, B. (1995). Best practices in the assessment of adaptive behavior. In A. Thomas & J. Grimes (Eds.), *Best practices in school psychology—III* (pp. 753–762). Washington DC: National Association of School Psychologists.

Heber, R. (Ed.). (1961). *A manual on terminology and classification in mental retardation.* Washington, DC: American Association on Mental Deficiency.

Hodapp, R. M., & Dykens, E. M. (2001). Strengthening behavioral research on genetic mental retardation syndromes. *American Journal of Mental Retardation, 106,* 4–15.

Jacobson, J. W., & Mulick, J. A. (1996a). *Manual of diagnosis and professional practice in mental retardation.* Washington, DC: American Psychological Association.

Jacobson, J. W., & Mulick, J. A. (1996b). Psychometrics. In J. W. Jacobson & J. A. Mulick (Eds.), *Manual of diagnosis and professional practice in mental retardation* (pp. 75–84). Washington, DC: American Psychological Association.

Lambert, N., Nihira, K., & Leland, H. (1993). *AAMR Adaptive Behavior scale—School and Community.* Austin, TX: Pro-Ed.

Leffert, J. S., & Siperstein, G. N. (2002). Social cognition: A key to understanding adaptive behavior in individuals with mild mental retardation. In L. Glidden (Ed.), *International review of research in mental retardation* (pp. 135–181). San Diego, CA: Academic Press/Elsevier.

Leland, H. (1991). Adaptive behavior scales. In J. L. Matson & J. A. Mulick (Eds.), *Handbook of mental retardation* (pp. 211–221). New York: Pergamon Press.

Luckasson, R., Borthwick-Duffy, S., Buntix, W. H. E., Coulter, D. L., Craig, E. M., Reeve, A., et al. (2002). *Mental retardation: Definition, classification, and systems of supports* (10th ed). Washington, DC: American Association on Mental Retardation.

MacMillan, D. L., Gresham, F. M., & Siperstein, G. N. (1993). Conceptual and psychometric concerns about the 1992 AAMR definition of mental retardation. *American Journal of Mental Retardation, 98,* 325–335.

National Research Council. (2002). *Mental retardation: Determining eligibility for social security benefits.* Committee on Disability Determination for Mental Retardation, Division of Behavioral and Social Sciences and Education, D. J. Reschly, T. G. Meyers, and C. R. Hartel editors. Washington, DC: National Academy Press.

Prasher, V. P. (1999). Adaptive behavior. In M. P. Janicki & A. J. Dalton (Eds.), *Dementia, aging, and intellectual disabilities: A handbook* (pp. 157–178), Philadelphia: Brunner/Mazel.

Reschly, D. J. (1990). Best practices in adaptive behavior. In A. Thomas & J. Grimes (Eds.), *Best practices in school psychology* (pp. 29–42). Washington, DC: National Association of School Psychology.

Roszkowski, M., Spreat, S., & Isett, R. (1983). Adaptive behavior. In S. Bruening, J. Matson, & R. Barrett (Eds.), *Advances in mental retardation and developmental disabilities* (Vol. 1). Greenwich, CT: JAI Press.

Scheerenberger, R. C. (1983). *A history of mental retardation.* Baltimore: Brookes.

Smith, J., & Polloway, E. (1979). The dimension of adaptive behavior in mental retardation research: An analysis of recent practices. *American Journal of Mental Deficiency, 84,* 203–206.

Sparrow, S. S., Cicchetti, D. V., & Balla, D. A. (2005). *Vineland Adaptive Behavior scales: Second edition (Vineland II), Survey interview form/caregiver rating form.* Bloomington, MN: Pearson Assessments.

Sparrow, S. S., Cicchetti, D. V., & Balla, D. A. (2006). *Vineland Adaptive Behavior scales: Second edition: Teacher rating form, second edition (Vineland II TRF).* Bloomington, MN: Pearson Assessments.

Spreat, S. (1999). Psychometric standards for adaptive behavior assessment. In R. L. Schalock (Ed.), *Adaptive behavior and its measurement: Implications for the field of mental retardation* (pp. 103–108). Washington, DC: American Association on Mental Retardation.

Switzky, H. N. (1997). Mental retardation and the neglected construct of motivation. *Education and Training in Mental Retardation and Developmental Disabilities, 32,* 194–200.

Tassé, M. J., & Craig, E. M. (1999). Critical issues in the cross-cultural assessment of adaptive behavior. In R. L. Schalock (Ed.), *Adaptive behavior and its measurement: Implications for the field of mental retardation* (pp. 161–184). Washington, DC: American Association on Mental Retardation.

Thompson, J. R., McGrew, K. S., & Bruininks, R. H. (1999). Adaptive and maladaptive behavior: Functional and structural characteristics. In R. L. Schalock (Ed.), *Adaptive behavior and its measurement: Implications for the field of mental retardation* (pp. 15–42). Washington, DC: American Association on Mental Retardation.

Thompson, J. R., Bryant, B., Campbell, E. M., Craig, E. M., Hughes, C., Rotholz, D. A., et al. (2004). *Supports Intensity scale.* Washington DC: American Association on Mental Retardation.

Widaman, K. F., Borthwick-Duffy, S. A., & Little, T. D. (1991). The structure and development of adaptive behaviors. In N. W. Bray (Ed.), *International review of research in mental retardation* (Vol. 17, pp. 1–54). San Diego, CA: Academic Press.

Wilbur, H. B. (1877). The classifications of idiocy. In *Proceedings of the Association of Medical Officers of American Institutions for Idiotic and Feeble-Minded Persons* (pp. 29–35). Philadelphia: Lippincott.

Zigler, E., Balla, D., & Hodapp, R. M. (1984). On the definition and classification of mental retardation. *American Journal of Mental Retardation, 89,* 215–230.

Zigler, E., & Hodapp, R. M. (1986). *Understanding mental retardation.* New York: Cambridge University Press.

16

Psychosocial and Mental Status Assessment

PETER STURMEY

Clinicians assess a client's psychosocial and mental status in a variety of contexts. Clients may be screened at intake to a service and at annual staffings, often to determine eligibility for professional services or supportive interventions. In this type of referral the important question is whether or not there is a clinically significant problem that requires attention. This can also take place during ongoing evaluation of response to various interventions such as psychotropic medications, behavioral interventions, other forms of therapy. In this context the key question is whether or not there has been a change in functioning in response to interventions. Assessment of psychosocial and mental status may also take place in response to a referral following a decline in functioning. On these occasions relevant questions often relate to determination of the causes in the change in functioning, requests for modifications and refinements to existing treatment plans, and development of new interventions or movement to new service settings, such as a residence. Recently a variety of practice guidelines and professional resources for assessment of individuals with intellectual disabilities (ID) or related conditions have become available (American Academy of Child and Adolescent Psychiatry [AACAP], 1999; Deb, Matthews, Holt, & Bouras, 2001; Fletcher & Greene, 2002; Poindexter, 2002; Royal College of Psychiatrists, 2001).

Assessment of psychosocial functioning and mental status in people with ID now has a long history, and often takes place within multidisciplinary teams of professionals and other concerned people. Yet, no unified view of this assessment process has evolved. Moss (1999) noted that there are fairly clear differences in how psychiatrists and psychologists formulate cases. Psychiatrists (and some psychologists with

---

PETER STURMEY • Department of Psychology, Queens College/CUNY, New York 10016.

a primary mental health background) search for patterns of symptoms and take a detailed history of the development of a problem in order to diagnose the underlying illness. For example, the AACAP (1999, p. 16S) guidelines clearly state, "The history is the cornerstone of the diagnostic process" (see also Levitas & Van Silka, 2001). According to the AACAP guidelines a history should include presenting symptoms [sic] and their evolution over time, management strategies and results, previous assessments, including medical assessments, premorbid and current personality, adaptive skills, past psychiatric diagnoses, therapies, drugs, behavioral interventions and their effectiveness, present and past environmental supports and stressors, and family variables (AACAP, 1999). Thus, a psychiatric history encompasses a broad aspect of assessment.

These psychiatric illnesses, which are just like other physical illnesses, have been discovered and described. They are described in authoritative, professional diagnostic manuals, such as *Diagnostic and statistical manual of mental disorders*, 4th ed., Text revision (American Psychiatric Association [APA], 1994), the *International classification of diseases*—10th ed. (ICD-10; World Health Organization, 1992a, 1992b) or the *Diagnostic criteria for psychiatric disorders for use with adults with learning disabilities/mental retardation* (DC-LD; Royal College of Psychiatrists, 2001). Most information used to diagnose comes from interviews with the patient or informants, usually conducted in clinics (see Hurley, 2001; Levitas, Hurley, & Pary, 2001). In contrast, behaviorally oriented psychologists develop functional explanations for observed and operationally defined behavior in terms of its establishing operations, antecedents, and consequences (Hanley, Iwata, & McCord, 2003; Iwata, Dorsey, Slifer, Bauman, & Richman, 1982/1994; Skinner, 1953; Sturmey, 1996; Sturmey & Bernstein, 2004; Sturmey, Reyer, Lee, & Robek, in press). The greatest weight is places on observational data from the natural environment acquired through analytical manipulation of environmental variables. History and information from the client and third parties are given less weight. This is because client verbal behavior is greatly influenced by extraneous environmental events. Thus, clients may be unable to accurately describe their own behavior and environment because they have not learned to describe their own behavior and the environment accurately or sufficiently. Verbal behavior may also be inaccurate because of present or past contingencies to speak inaccurately (e.g., to acquiesce or minimize problems). Thus, because of the potential inaccuracy of verbal report, emphasis is placed on observation in the current environment. In summary, psychiatric approaches emphasize the *form* of the presenting problem, whereas behavioral approaches emphasize the *function of the presenting, or related, problem(s)*. Moreover, psychological observations and interviews may differ on the basis of the primary therapeutic orientation of the observer or interviewer (e.g., behavior analytic, behavior therapeutic, cognitive–behavior therapeutic), or a blend of such orientations.

ASSESSMENT OF PSYCHIATRIC SYMPTOMS
AND DIAGNOSES

Rating Scales and Self-Report Measures

There are now a large number of instruments to assess psychopathology in people with ID. Reviews published in the early 1990s (Aman, 1991a, 1991b; Sturmey, Reed, & Corbett, 1991) are now outdated and incomplete. Deb et al. (2001) provide a very useful guide, but even this is not comprehensive; new instruments continue to develop and old ones refined.

There are several important general features of rating scales and self-report measures. Many are screening instruments that identify people who are at risk for a psychiatric diagnosis and require further evaluation. Cutoff scores on most of these measures merely indicate the need for further evaluation: they are not diagnostic. There has been little research on validity, sensitivity, and specificity of many of these measures. Therefore, the best use of these measures is to screen and identify people who may have a psychiatric disorder, and who may need to be referred on for a more comprehensive assessment. For example, the *Psychopathology Instrument for Mentally Retarded Adults* (Matson, Kazdin, & Senatore, 1984) and the *Reiss Screen* (Reiss, 1988) are useful screening instruments for people with mild and moderate ID. The *Diagnostic Assessment for the Severely Handicapped*, 2nd ed. (Matson, 1995; Sturmey, Matson, & Lott, 2004) is a useful screen for adults with severe or profound ID. Some authors have evaluated the use of scales to assess psychopathology with people with ID that were developed for people of average intelligence. For example, Lindsay, Michie, Baty, Smith, and Miller (1994) found that measures such as the Zung Self-Rating Anxiety Scale, the Zung Depression Inventory, the General Health Questionnaire, and the Eysenck–Withers Personality Test were acceptably reliable in use with people with mild and moderate ID. Measures for specific diagnoses are reviewed in Deb et al. (2001).

It is also important to distinguish scales used to assess psychopathology that are assembled rationally versus those assembled empirically. Scales that are assembled rationally adopt existing diagnostic criteria, such as those in *DSM-IV-TR*, and use these criteria as the basis for items on the checklist. Others take an empirical approach in which a large pool of items is assembled and scales are then derived using factor analysis and other psychometric data reduction methods. The rational approach has the advantage of producing scales that are easily translated into the diagnoses that clinicians must make. Additionally, these scales have considerable face validity. However, it is an empirical question as to whether or not this approach produces scales that are reliable and internally consistent. In the empirical approach scales are very likely to be reliable, internally consistent, and robust, because the items are selected on the basis of these criteria. However, the issue of validity remains problematic: the complex question of the construct validity always must be answered.

There are many scales that are used to assess the presence, frequency, and severity of maladaptive behaviors, such as aggression, self-injury behavior (SIB), and noncompliance. Commonly used measures include the *Aberrant Behavior Checklist* (Aman & Singh, 1986; Newton & Sturmey, 1988), the *Behavior Problem Inventory* (Rojahn, Matson, Lott, Esbensen, & Smalls, 2001; Rojahn, Tasse, & Sturmey, 1997), and the *Developmental Behavior Checklist* (Einfeld & Tonge, 1995). Such scales are usually developed empirically and can be a useful way to screen for maladaptive behaviors that may require further evaluation and intervention. Their role in diagnosis is unclear, because the relationship between maladaptive behaviors and psychiatric diagnosis is still debated (see below).

Both psychiatric and behavioral checklists are commonly used with informants, such as family members, direct care staff, and parents. People with mild and moderate ID can be reliable informants (Lindsay et al., 1994), but they may show biases such as response acquiescence, tendency to use the first or last of two alternatives, or simply be unable to answer questions that are open-ended or grammatically complex (Finlay & Lyons, 2001 2002). There are a number of solutions to this problem. Screening clients for response acquiescence may be desirable (Senatore, Matson, & Kazdin, 1985). People with ID have been successfully taught interview skills for job interviews (Mozingo, Ackley, & Bailey, 1994) and to participate in selecting preferred residences (Foxx, Faw, Taylor, Davis, & Fulia, 1993). It may be possible to prepare clients to participate in diagnostic interviews. Likewise, psychiatrists vary in the quality of their assessment interviews (Duckworth, Radhakrishnan, Nolan, & Fraser, 1993). Thus, another option would be to identify specific skills that differentiated skilled from unskilled interviewers and to train clinicians in these desirable skills (see Levitas et al., 2001).

Mental Status

Mental status refers to "appearance, mood, anxiety, disorders, perceptions (e.g., delusions, hallucinations), and all aspects of cognition (e.g., attention, orientation, memory)" (Folstein & Folstein, 2003). Assessment of mental status usually takes place as a quick screen to consider indications of serious mental disorders, such as psychotic disorders, delirium, or dementia, to track decline during a dementia, or to distinguish organic from functional psychiatric disorders. Assessment of mental status in people with ID poses special challenges for the diagnostician because it is not possible to make broad assumptions about premorbid functioning in the absence of good psychometric and historical data. Existing impairment in selected or broad areas of functioning due to ID means that baseline functioning is low prior to assessment.

A variety of assessments of mental status have been developed for use with people with ID, including generic screens and assessments to track change during old age. Myers (1987) evaluated the *Mini-Mental Status Exam* with people with ID and found that it was sufficiently sensitive for use with people with mild ID, although with greater impairment suggestive scores were common in the absence of any psychiatric disorder. The *Test for Severe Impairment* has also been shown to have good reliability and validity for adults with Down syndrome (Cosgrave et al., 1998). More recently, tests for mental status specific to people with ID, such as the *Dementia Scale for Down Syndrome* (Simon, Rappaport, Papka, & Woodruff-Pak, 1995) and the *Multi-Dimensional Observational Scale for Elderly Subjects* (Dalton & Fedor, 1997; Sturmey, Tsouris, & Patti, 2003) have been developed. There is some preliminary evidence that they are superior to generic measures of mental status in that they avoid floor effects, and sensitivity and specificity problems (Deb & Braganza, 1999). Given the high risk of dementia in older adults with Down syndrome, use of these measures as annual screens seems worthwhile.

Diagnostic Interviews

Structured diagnostic interviews were developed as a response to the unreliability of unstructured interviews. Unconstrained interviewers collect different information, combine information differently, and use different implicit criteria for diagnosis. In response, researchers have developed structured diagnostic interviews (Lord et al., 1997; Steinberg & Stein, 1994), clinical decision-making algorithms (Gilbert et al., 1998), and consensus guidelines (Rush & Frances, 2000) that constrain the collection and combination of information in a variety of ways.

Early work on structured psychiatric interviews with people with ID produced less than satisfactory results. Ballinger, Armstrong, Presly, and Reid (1975) evaluated the *Structured Psychiatric Interview* with 27 people with ID. Of the 31 items, 19 had adequate reliability, but the remainder were unreliable or could not be evaluated because of low frequency. Further, the reliability of actual diagnoses, as opposed to the presence or absence of individual symptoms was not reported. However, Meadows et al. (1991) used the *Schedule for Affective Disorders and Schizophrenia—Lifetime* to diagnose schizophrenia in adults with ID and Richards et al. (2001) used the *Present State Examination*. Both proved satisfactory.

Over the last 10 years considerable research effort has gone into developing the *Psychiatric Assessment Schedule for Adults with Developmental Disabilities* (PAS-ADD; Costello, Moss, Prosser, & Hatton, 1997; Moss et al., 1993, 1997; Moss, Prosser, Ibbotson, & Goldberg, 1996; Patel, Goldberg, & Moss, 1993). The PAS-ADD is a semi-structured clinical interview that probes for the presence of psychiatric symptoms using an algorithm for combining the information in order to make diagnoses of the more common ICD-10 psychiatric disorders. It is based on earlier research on semi-structured interviews used in the general population. Careful attention was given to the question format, use of simple words and simple grammar, splitting multiple questions, use of anchor events to enhance recall, and simplification of the questions and interview format. The PAS-ADD encompasses the ICD diagnoses of schizophrenia, unspecified nonorganic psychosis, hypomania, depressive episode, phobic anxiety disorders, panic and generalized anxiety disorders, and nonorganic hypersomnia. In addition to the PAS-ADD interview there is a screening checklist known as the *mini PAD-ADD*. This can be used to screen for the presence of depression, anxiety, expansive mood, obsessive compulsive disorder (OCD), psychosis, unspecified disorder (including dementia), and autism. The *mini PAS-ADD* is not used to make a diagnosis, rather is a screening tool to be completed by family members and direct care staff who know the client well. It can be completed with a moderate amount of training.

There is a considerable evidence base on the use of these two instruments. It should be noted that there is moderate-to-good evidence of reliability of both symptom recognition and diagnosis. Unusually, there is also some evidence of validity, and they have been used with a variety of populations, including seniors with ID and Spanish-speakers (Gonzalez-Gordon, Salvador-Carulla, Romero, Gonzalez-Saiz, & Romero, 2002). The PAS-ADD is probably the most carefully designed and extensively researched clinical interview for people with ID. Nevertheless, a number of limitations should be noted. First, it is based on ICD-10 rather than on *DSM-IV-TR* criteria. This limits its use in the United States. Future research should develop a structured interview based on *DSM-IV-TR* taking note of the methods used to develop the PAS-ADD. Although there is good evidence of reliability, the perplexing question of validity remains only partially answered (Gonzalez-Gordon et al., 2002; Moss et al., 1996, 1997). Finally, although the PAS-ADD has been used with adults with moderate and severe ID, the precise lower limit of the applicability, either in terms of degree of ID or prerequisite skills has yet to be determined.

Standardized psychiatric interviews only address some of the problems that clinicians face when conducting an assessment. Although professionals may agree on the kind of problem that is presented, they may not agree as to the cause of the problem. Behavioral and psychiatric symptoms can present for a number of reasons. A very wide range of undiagnosed medical problems may first be noticed because of changes in behavior. Although textbook examples, such as hypothyroidism presenting as depression should be considered, a wide range of medical problems might present as psychiatric or behavior disorders. Headaches, allergies, constipation, infections, menstrual discomfort, dental problems, pain, arthritis, undiagnosed cancer, and other illnesses can all be present as withdrawal, noncompliance, SIB, or other maladaptive behaviors. Careful screening for these problems and a thorough history can sometimes be helpful. However, often no clear cause to a presenting behavioral or psychiatric problem can be found and no medical diagnosis can be made. This situation can be hard to interpret because there may be an undiagnosed illness or no illness at all. Likewise, a wide variety of negative side effects of psychotropic and other medication can cause discomfort or more serious medical problems and careful screening for these problems is important (Kalachnik & Sprague, 1993). In both these examples, excluding these explanations for presenting symptoms can be difficult, especially in clients who have limited or no speech.

Behavioral Equivalents

A cursory glance at *DSM* or ICD diagnostic criteria reveals significant problems for their use in people with ID (Sturmey, 1993, 1995a, 1999). Most standardized diagnostic criteria require sufficient language to be able to report a wide range of internal states such as mood, cognition, and so on. Yet, people with mild or moderate ID have considerable impairment related to these functions (Baroff & Oliver, 1999) and often have problems in describing emotional states. Most people with severe or profound ID have very limited or no expressive language. Hence, strict application of standardized criteria would often mean that a diagnosis could not be made because many of the criteria could not be used. Empirical studies have lent some support to different presentation of psychiatric disorders in this population. For example, Meadows et al. (1991) compared symptoms in 25 people with mild ID and schizophrenia and 25 people with no intellectual impairment and schizophrenia using a standardized psychiatric interview. Although they found that the standardized diagnostic criteria for schizophrenia could be readily applied to people with ID they did find some simplification in presentation of symptoms in this group. Linaker and Heller (1994) found that people with ID were less likely to show delusions, but did show more incoherence and flat affect than a matched group of people with schizophrenia.

In response to this problem authors have often modified diagnostic criteria for use with people with ID. Sturmey's (1993) review of empirical studies using ICD or *DSM* diagnostic criteria with people with ID revealed that *all* published empirical studies at that time had modified standardized diagnostic criteria. This trend has continued. Many published papers have proposed a variety of modifications. AACAP (1999), Clarke and Gomez (1999), Jawed, Krishnan, Prasher, and Corbett (1993), Marston, Perry, and Roy (1997), and Pary, Levitas, and Hurley (1999) have all proposed a broad range of behavioral equivalents for mood disorders including aggression, SIB, pica, and so on. SIB has been conceptualized as a form of OCD, at least when accompanied by self-restraint (AACAP, 1999) or compulsive features (Bodfish, Powell, Golden, & Lewis, 1995). The DC-LD project (Royal College of Psychiatrists, 2001) used extensive literature reviews and a consensus panel approach to develop behavioral equivalents for a wide range of ICD-10 psychiatric disorders for people with moderate through profound ID.

There have been a number of empirical studies that have evaluated the relationship between maladaptive behaviors and psychiatric diagnoses. Bodfish, Crawford, et al. (1995) used questionnaire measures of compulsions, stereotypy, and SIB and found positive correlations between compulsions and stereotypy and SIB within this group of participants. Bodfish, Powell, et al. (1995) reported convergent validity data for the OCD hypothesis of stereotypy and SIB. They found that blink rate, a putative measure of low dopamine, was higher in people with stereotypies and SIB. Although people with compulsions did not have an elevated blink rate, those that also had stereotypies and SIB did have higher blink rates. Lewis, Bodfish, Powell, and Golden (1995) and Lewis, Bodfish, Powell, Parker, and Golden

(1996) provided yet further convergent validity data in two double-blind trials of clomipramine for repetitive behaviors. They found that clomipramine was associated with decreases in repetitive behaviors as well as increases in engagement, and decreases staff interventions for maladaptive behaviors. These studies provide good convergent validity data for the OCD hypothesis of stereotypies and SIB.

Practitioners should recall that these studies only report statistical associations between scores in a group of participants. These studies do not support a one-to-one correspondence between stereotypies or SIB and OCD in every case. Further, it should be noted that compulsive features were systematically assessed using a psychometric checklist, rather than interview data or clinical impressions. Thus, clinicians should be cautious in interpreting these data to justify the use of clomipramine for SIB in the absence of similar systematic diagnostic procedures. Further, independent replications of these results have yet to be published.

Data on behavioral equivalents and depression have been less clear. Although some surveys have found an increased risk of depression associated with aggressive behavior (Reiss & Rojahn, 1993), other studies have failed to find such a relationship (Rojahn, Borthwick-Duffy, & Jacobson, 1993). Marston et al. (1997) proposed a checklist of symptoms of depression and proposed behavioral equivalents; however, this checklist was developed rationally rather than empirically. Subsequent studies using this checklist by Tsiouris, Mann, Patti, and Sturmey (2004) and a similar empirical study by Ross and Oliver (2003a) found no relationship between measures of mood and maladaptive behaviors. Clarke, Reed, and Sturmey (1991) found that staff had considerable difficulty identifying when people with ID were sad, which might explain why no relationship was observed in these studies. Ross and Oliver's (2003b) subsequent review suggested that the literature on identification of mood symptoms in people with severe and profound ID is marked by problems with reliability and validity, as well as conceptual problems in identifying when a maladaptive behavior may be a behavioral equivalent of depression. At this time there is little evidence to support the use of behavioral equivalents for depression in people with severe or profound ID.

FUNCTIONAL ANALYSIS AND DUAL DIAGNOSIS

The second major approach to psychosocial assessment is based on applied behavior analysis (ABA) and is known as functional analysis. In *Science and human behavior*, Skinner (1953) defined functional analysis as "The external variables of which behavior is a function provide for what may be caused a causal or functional analysis. We undertake to predict and control the behavior of the individual organism" (p. 35). Baer, Wolf, and Risley (1968) defined functional analysis as: "...the analysis of a behavior...(that) requires a believable demonstration of the events that can be responsible for the occurrence or nonoccurrence of a behavior...an ability of an experimenter to turn the behavior on and off..." (pp. 93–94). Noting that practitioners were only interested in independent variables that have a large affect on the behavior of interest and only those independent variables that they can control, Haynes and O'Brien (1990) went on to define functional analysis as "...the identification of important, controllable, causal, functional relationships applicable to a specified set of target behaviors for an individual client..." (p. 654).

Early work in ABA included many studies and interventions with people with mental illness (Kazdin, 1977), including direct functional analysis of psychiatric symptoms (Haughton & Ayllon, 1965). Since the beginning of ABA many functional analyses have been conducted extensively with SIB (Hanley et al., 2003), as well as a very wide range of maladaptive behaviors in people with ID, including aggression disruption, vocalization, property destruction, stereotypy, noncompliance, tantrums, elopement, pica, and other problem behaviors (Hanley et al., 2003; Sturmey & Bernstein, 2004). ABA has also been used within clinical psychology to address a wide range of child, adolescent, and adult disorders (Sturmey, 1996) as well as other applications including autism, psychotherapy, staff training and organizational interventions, industry, business, sports, and college teaching (Austin & Carr, 2000).

Harris (*this volume*) provides a detailed review of the methods of functional assessment and analysis. Briefly, functional analysis identifies relationships between environmental variables, such as consequences, antecedents, and establishing operations and publicly observable behavior. Descriptive methods, also known as functional assessment, such as interviews, questionnaires, and naturalistic observation may be used to describe the relationship between specific environmental variables and behavior. These methods do not manipulate independent variables and thus produce correlational data only. Experimental functional analyses directly manipulate independent variables—for example, by analyzing the effects of contingent versus noncontingent attention on a target behavior. Hence, conclusions about causes of behavior are possible. Common hypotheses about causes include positive reinforcement, by access to attention or objects, negative reinforcement, or perhaps, by removal of academic or work demands or other aversive environmental conditions, or perhaps by automatic reinforcement. Other idiosyncratic causes, multiple causes, and the impact of variables more distant in time, such as deprivation and satiation, are also possible. Maladaptive behaviors often occur in chains. In response chains, earlier responses reliably lead to some terminal response. For example, Fisher, Lindauer, Alterson, and Thompson (1998) analyzed the relationship between property destruction and stereotypy. They found that property destruction was reinforced by access to presumably reinforcing stereotypic manipulation of pieces of broken objects. When access to unbroken objects was blocked and toys providing apparently equivalent stimulation were available both property destruction and stereotypy were greatly reduced. Thus, analysis of response chains is another method of assessing the functions of maladaptive behaviors.

Clinicians use the results of a functional assessment or analysis in order to develop an intervention based on the hypotheses that this assessment generates. It may be used to identify replacement behaviors, rearrange the environment to remove or modify antecedents, remove reinforcers maintaining the target behavior, or develop reinforcement schedules for the absence of the target behavior using the reinforcers maintaining the target behavior. Most interventions are complex packages of several components such as these (O'Neill et al., 1999; Sturmey, 1996). Several meta-analyses have made similar conclusions (Carr et al., 1999; Didden, Duker, & Korzilius, 1997) and have found that interventions based on pre-assessment of behavioral function are associated with larger effect sizes (Didden et al., 1997).

ABA has been used to analyze and intervene with a wide range of mental health issues in people with ID (Sturmey, Lee, Reyer, & Robek, 2006). One problem that has been addressed is bizarre and psychotic speech and psychotic disorders in people with ID. Mace, Browder, and Lin (1987) conducted a functional analysis of bizarre speech in a 29-year-old woman with mild ID. Bizarre speech included references to things that were not present, sexual speech, etc. Initial functional assessment suggested two possible hypotheses. The first hypothesis was that that the speech was maintained by escape from requests to participate in activities and the second hypothesis was that it was maintained through attention as positive reinforcement for that bizarre speech. In the functional analysis, bizarre speech was more likely when the woman was allowed to escape from demands. Therefore, guided compliance was provided and this procedure was effective in reducing bizarre speech. Burgio, Brown, and Tice (1985), Dixon, Benedict, and Larson (2001), Durand and Crimmins (1987), Fisher, Piazza, and Page (1989), and Stephens, Matson, Westmoreland, and Kulpa (1981) have reported similar results in both children and adults with ID and psychoses. Similar results have been reported in behavioral treatment of psychotic symptoms in adults of average intelligence (Fichter, Wallace, Liberman, & Davis, 1976; Foxx, McMorrow, Davis, & Bittle, 1988; Mace & Lalli, 1991; Matson, Zeiss, Zeiss, & Bowman, 1980; Wilder, Masuda, O'Conner, & Baham, 2001). ABA has also been used extensively to address the motivational aspects of psychotic disorders and to establish and reestablish the skills necessary for everyday life (Liberman et al., 1998).

Depression has been conceptualized from a behavioral perspective. Behavioral models of depression have defined it in terms of deficits, such as poor social skills, slow motor movements, long latencies to respond to questions, and behavioral excesses, such as excessive complaining, crying, and agitation. The behavioral changes associated with the onset of depression might reflect a paucity of reinforcers in the person's life, inappropriate contingencies, or a history of punishment (e.g., Ferster, 1973; Lejuez, Hopko, & Hopko, 2001, 2003; Lewinsohn, Hoberman, Teri, & Hantsinger 1988). Matson (1983) noted these behavioral features also characterize depression in people with ID (Helsel & Matson, 1988). Although other correlational studies have confirmed the association between poor social skills and other factors related to depression in people with ID, no experimental analyses of depressed behavior in people with ID have been published. However, there are a few intervention studies indicating that the behavioral characteristics of depression, such as poor eye contact, lack of speech (Matson, 1982), psychosomatic complaints (Matson, 1984), and suicidal threats (Sturmey, 1995a, 1995b) can be effectively reduced through various combinations of reinforcement of appropriate speech and prosocial behaviors, and through role-play, modeling, feedback, and contingency management. There is also some evidence that cognitive behavior therapy may be effective for people with mild ID and depression (Lindsay, Howells, & Pitcaithly, 1993; Sturmey, 2004).

As with depression, relatively little attention has been paid to functional analysis of anxiety disorders (also see Jones and Friman, 1999). Obviously, avoidance of feared objects is a powerful consequence maintaining phobic behavior, although comfort from others is another candidate consequence that should be considered. Functional assessment of school refusal (Burke & Silverman, 1987; Kearney & Silverman, 1990) has indicated that avoidance of school demands, avoidance of fear, avoidance of social anxiety, gaining attention from others, and access to positive reinforcers at home are all potential reinforcers maintaining school refusal. Kearney and Silverman (1990) developed a questionnaire to assess these possible functions and found that treatments based on appropriate hypotheses were highly successful. A wide range of fears and phobias in people with ID have been successfully treated using a variety of exposure, shaping, and relaxation training procedures (Sturmey et al., 2006).

Obsessional features, such as problems with transitions from activity to activity, have been studied. McCord, Thompson, and Iwata (2001) demonstrated that termination of the pretransition activity, initiation of the posttransition activity, and the transition itself, were consequences that might be avoided through maladaptive behaviors such as self-injury. They found that giving warnings of transitions and reinforcement alone without extinction were ineffective treatments. Only reinforcement combined with extinction and response blocking was an effective treatment. Rincover, Newsom, and Carr (1979) analyzed the sensory consequences that characterize some ritualistic behaviors seen in children with autism. They found that sensory extinction was an effective intervention if the form of extinction matched the reinforcer maintaining the behavior (Rincover et al., 1979).

Methods based on ABA, such as self-regulation (e.g., self-management) training, have also been used to address impulsive behaviors related to Attention Deficit Hyperactivity Disorder such as impulsive responding (Finch, Wilkinson, Nelson, & Montgomery, 1975). Other impulse control disorders that have been addressed include pyromania (Kolko, 1983), and problematic behaviors of sexual offenders with ID, such as stalking, exhibitionism, and pedophilia (Lindsay, 2002). Substance abuse disorders in people with ID have also been addressed through education, social support, training, and education of family members and professional staff, social skills training, and refusal training (Annand, 2002; Sturmey et al., 2006).

INTEGRATING ASSESSMENT FORMULATIONS

Relationship Between Psychiatric and Behavioral Formulations

Given the disparity between these two approaches is some kind of rapprochement possible? Emerson, Moss, and Kiernan (1999) speculated about four possible relationships between psychiatric diagnosis and maladaptive behaviors. First, there may be common developmental pathways of both psychiatric disorders and maladaptive behaviors in people with ID. They speculated that family histories characterized by disruption, poor quality care, discord, instability and disorganization, poor parental adjustment and poor parent–child relationships, and poverty were risk factors for both groups of conditions. They also note that for people with severe and profound ID that these factors might have a less powerful influence than for those people with mild or moderate ID. A second potential relationship is that maladaptive behavior could be an atypical symptom of a psychiatric disorder (e.g., as behavioral equivalents). They cite SIB as a possible example of an atypical presentation of an underlying OCD. A third relationship is that maladaptive behaviors may be a secondary feature of psychiatric disorder. Finally, a psychiatric disorder might be an establishing operation for the maladaptive behavior. For example, depression might be an establishing operation that potentiates escape from tasks as negative reinforcers. Baker, Blumberg, Freeman, and Wieseler (2002) present a model case that can be used as a method to integrate psychiatric diagnosis with functional assessment using the notion of establishing operations.

These potential relationships as well as others exist. The AACAP (1999) guidelines boldly state that "In virtually every mental disorder there might be behavioral manifestations that are learned, conditioned by environmental factors, and under voluntary control. *In addition, every behavioral presentation that is serious enough to cause significant discomfort or dysfunction can be characterized by a DSM-IV designation, even if a relatively nonspecific one or a V code is used*" (italics added, p. 15S). The essence of this latter claim seems to be that all severe forms of maladaptive behaviors represent some form of mental illness, or possibly susceptible to mental health treatment methods.

A final possibility is that there is no relationship between a maladaptive behavior and a psychiatric disorder. Classic studies suggest that SIB and other severe and dangerous and even life-threatening behaviors can be shaped in primates and rats that presumably did not have a mental illness. Schaefer (1970) was able to shape SIB using attention and food in Rhesus monkeys and bring SIB under the stimulus control of the presence of the experimenter. Similar phenomena have been known for many years in humans. Haughton and Ayllon (1965) reported that they shaped walking around holding a broom using cigarettes in a psychiatric inpatient with schizophrenia. When mental health professionals were then asked to explain this behavior they supposed that it was a symptom of various kinds of unobserved mental illnesses, or a symbol of a conflict such as a Queens scepter or the inevitable phallic symbol. (These explanations are of course dated. The study was conducted in the 1960s when psychoanalysis was still in vogue. Presumably today it would be explained as due to an imbalance in neurotransmitters, perhaps as an atypical presentation of an OCD that should be treated by clomipramine.) Thus, mental health professionals may be prone to interpret bizarre human behavior that is known to be learned, as a sign of an underlying illness when that is not the cause of the observed behavior.

Some large-scale epidemiological studies based on case registers have found no relationship between psychiatric diagnosis and the presence of maladaptive behaviors (Rojahn et al., 1993). However, these results might simply reflect the poor quality of psychiatric diagnoses of record, problems with the integrity of databases, and unreliability in assessing the target behaviors (Emerson et al., 1999). Some studies have found moderate associations between aggression and depression (e.g., Reiss & Rojahn, 1993). In contrast, Deb, Thomas, and Bright (2001a) used standardized measures of behavior problems and the mini PAS-ADD with a representative sample of adults using community services. They found that although some 60% (Deb, Thomas, & Bright, 2001b) showed significant behavior problems, only 14% showed a psychiatric disorder. The overall point prevalence of psychiatric disorders was similar to that in the general population and the majority of participants with a behavior problem had no psychiatric disorder. If the latter finding is generalizable, then one would expect to find low correlations between specific behavior problems and presence of psychiatric diagnosis.

Integration of Psychiatric and Behavioral Formulations in Treatment Plans

In educational settings a student's education is coordinated through an Individual Education Plan that is periodically reviewed. Most adult services in the United States are coordinated in a similar fashion through an annual staffing. In the United Kingdom a similar process takes places for adult services and results in a plan of care. A similar process occurs at admission to services, major transitions (e.g., admission to residential care), and perhaps in response to emergencies. More recently such plans have been recast in terms of person-centered planning. Whichever way these plans are put together they are based on contributions from varied sources including client, family members, and an array of professionals: psychiatric and behavioral assessments and treatment plans are only some of the elements in the plan.

Recommendations from behavioral and psychiatric plans might enhance or contradict other recommendations in the proposed plan. For example, a dietician might recommend weight reduction and no high-calorie foods, whereas a behavioral assessment might indicate use of preferred edibles as part of a reinforcement-based intervention. Another example, of such a potential conflict, might be that every time a client makes a suicide threat a psychiatrist might insist on conducting an assessment of suicide risk. During this assessment the psychiatrist might attempt to persuade the client not to kill himself or herself, and then place them on one-to-one staffing for at least 24 h. In contrast, a behavioral assessment might indicate that suicide threats are maintained by attention from medical and nursing staff (Sturmey, 1995a, 1995b). Good team functioning and careful case management skills are needed to integrate conflicting recommendations. These include setting priorities and resolving conflicting recommendations. In these two examples, weight management might be explicitly not addressed because the team might consider it to be of a lower priority than a behavioral or psychiatric emergency or it might be addressed through an exercise program, instead of changing diet. Likewise, behavioral interventions to manage suicidal threats could be devised that both ensure client safety, address professional liability issues, and reduce the problem (Sturmey, 1995a, 1995b).

FUTURE DIRECTIONS

The last 20 years has seen considerable expansion of assessment procedures for psychiatric diagnosis in people with ID. In the past there were relatively few measures, often of unknown psychometric properties (Aman, 1991a, 1991b; Sturmey et al., 1991). However, there are now so many instruments, many for specific diagnoses or subpopulations (Deb et al., 2001) that practitioners may be confused by the relative merits of different instruments designed to be used for similar purposes. Similarly, there are now a number of structured psychiatric interviews that could be used, at least with people with mild and moderate ID. Although there are instruments such as the DASH-II for screening people with severe and profound ID (Sturmey et al., 2006), there is a relative dearth of tools for this population and empirical research on behavioral equivalents has only just begun (Ross & Oliver, 2003b). Therefore, future research should address the conceptual basis and assessment procedures for people with severe and profound ID in a rigorous fashion.

Staff training and dissemination of existing information on dual diagnosis is inadequate to support high quality services. Although resources are becoming available (Fletcher & Greene, 2002; Poindexter, 2002), such resources are not as widely disseminated as they should be and the vexing question of if and how staff, including professional staff, should change their behavior to better address the assessment and treatment of people with dual diagnosis has yet to be addressed (see Singh et al., 2002, for an example of consulting to professional teams about such concerns). Many psychologists still need practice models, continuing support and training in integrating functional assessment when working with persons with dual diagnosis. Future research should address this issue. Finally, although a number of decision-making algorithms are available for clinicians, none have yet been evaluated with this population.

REFERENCES

Aman, M. G. (1991a). *Assessing psychopathology and behavior problems in persons with mental retardation: A review of available instruments* (DHSS Publication No. ADM 91-1712). Rockville, MD: US Department of Health and Human Services.

Aman, M. G. (1991b). Review and evaluation of instruments for assessing emotional and behavioral disorders. *Australia and New Zealand Journal of Developmental Disabilities, 17*, 127–145.

Aman, M. G., & Singh, N. N. (1986). *Aberrant Behavior Checklist manual.* East Aurora, NY: Slosson Educational Publications.

American Academy of Child and Adolescent Psychiatry. (1999). Summary of the practice parameters for the assessment and treatment of children, adolescents, and adults with mental retardation and comorbid mental disorders. *Journal of the American Academy of Child and Adolescent Psychiatry, 38*(Suppl.), 5S–31S.

American Psychiatric Association. (1994). *Diagnostic and statistical manual of mental disorder* (4th ed., *DSM-IV-TR*). Washington, DC: Author.

Annand, J. (2002). *More than accommodation: Overcoming barriers to effective treatment of persons with both cognitive disabilities and chemical dependency.* Beaverton, OR: Nightwind.

Austin, J., & Carr, J. E. (Eds.). (2000). *Handbook of applied behavior analysis.* Reno, NV: Context Press.

Baer, D. M., Wolf, M. M., & Risley, T. R. (1968). Some current dimensions of applied behavior analysis. *Journal of Applied Behavior Analysis, 1*, 91–97.

Baker, D. J., Blumberg, R., Freeman, R., & Wieseler, N. A. (2002). Can psychiatric disorders be seen as establishing operations? Integrating applied behavior analysis and psychiatry. *Mental Health Aspects of Developmental Disabilities, 5*, 118–124.

Ballinger, B. R., Armstrong, J., Presly, A. S., & Reid, A. H. (1975). Use of a standardized psychiatric interview in mentally handicapped patients. *British Journal of Psychiatry, 127*, 540–544.

Baroff, G. S., & Oliver, J. G. (1999). *Mental retardation. Nature, cause and management* (3rd ed.). Ann Arbor, MI: Taylor and Francis.

Bodfish, J. W., Crawford, T. W., Powell, S. B., Parker, D. E., Golden, R. N., & Lewis, M. H. (1995a). Compulsions in adults with mental retardation: Prevalence, phenomenology, and comorbidity with stereotypy and self-injury. *American Journal on Mental Retardation, 100*, 183–192.

Bodfish, J. W., Powell, S. B., Golden, R. N., & Lewis, M. H. (1995b). Blink rate as an index of dopamine function in adults with mental retardation and repetitive behavior disorders. *American Journal on Mental Retardation, 99*, 335–344.

Burgio, L., Brown, K., & Tice, L. (1985). Behavioral covariation in the treatment of delusional verbalization with contingency management. *Journal of Behavior Therapy and Experimental Psychiatry, 16*, 173–182.

Burke, A. E., & Silverman, W. K. (1987). The prescriptive treatment of school refusal. *Clinical Psychology Review, 7*, 353–362.

Carr, E. G., Horner, R. H., Turnbull, A. P., Marquis, J. G., McLaughlin, D. M., et al. (1999). *Positive support for people with developmental disabilities. A research synthesis.* Washington, DC: AAMR.

Clarke, A., Reed, J., & Sturmey, P. (1991). Staff perceptions of sadness among people with mental handicaps. *Journal of Mental Deficiency Research, 35*, 147–153.

Clarke, D. J., & Gomez, G. A. (1999). Utility of modified DCR-10 criteria in the diagnosis of depression associated with intellectual disabilities. *Journal of Intellectual Disability Research, 43*, 413–420.

Cosgrave, M. P., McCarron, M., Anderson, M., Tyrell, J., Gill, M., & Laws, B.A. (1998). Cognitive decline in Down syndrome: A validity/reliability study of the test for severe impairment. *American Journal on Mental Retardation, 103*, 193–197.

Costello, H., Moss, S., Prosser, H., & Hatton, C. (1997). Reliability of the ICD 10 version of the Psychiatric Assessment Schedule for Adults with Developmental Disabilities (PAS-ADD). *Social Psychiatry, and Psychiatric Epidemiology, 32*, 339–343.

Dalton, A. J., & Fedor, B. L. (1997). The Multi-Dimensional Observation Scale for Elderly Subjects applied for persons with Down syndrome. In *Proceedings of the International Congress III on the Dually Diagnosed* (pp. 173–178). Washington, DC: National Association for the Dually Diagnosed.

Deb, S., & Braganza, J. (1999). Comparison of rating scales for the diagnosis of dementia in adults with Down syndrome. *Journal of Intellectual Disabilities Research, 43,* 400–407.

Deb, S., Matthews, T., Holt, G., & Bouras, N. (2001). *Practice guidelines for the assessment and diagnosis of mental health problems in adults with intellectual disability.* Brighton, UK: Pavillion.

Deb, S., Thomas, M., & Bright, C. (2001a). Mental disorders in adults with intellectual disability. 1: Prevalence of functional psychiatric illness among community-based population aged between 16 and 64 years. *Journal of Intellectual Disability Research, 45,* 506–514.

Deb, S., Thomas, M., & Bright, C. (2001b). Mental disorders in adults with intellectual disability. 2: The rate of behaviour disorders among community-based population aged between 16 and 64 years. *Journal of Intellectual Disability Research, 45,* 506–514.

Didden, R., Duker, P. C., & Korzilius, H. (1997). Meta-analytic study on treatment effectiveness for problem behaviors with individuals who have mental retardation. *American Journal on Mental Retardation, 30,* 387–399.

Dixon, M. R., Benedict, H., & Larson, T. (2001). Functional analysis and treatment of inappropriate verbal behavior. *Journal of Applied Behavior Analysis, 34,* 361–363.

Duckworth, M. S., Radhakrishnan, G., Nolan, M. E., & Fraser, W. I. (1993). Initial encounters between people with a mild mental handicap and psychiatrists: An investigation of a method of evaluating interview skills. *Journal of Intellectual Disability Research, 37,* 263–276.

Durand, V. M., & Crimmins, D. B. (1987). Assessment and treatment of psychotic speech in an autistic child. *Journal of Autism and Developmental Disorders, 17,* 17–28.

Einfeld, S. L., & Tonge, B. J. (1995). The Developmental Behavior Checklist: The development and validation of an instrument to assess behavioral and emotional disturbance in children and adolescents with mental retardation. *Journal of Autism and Developmental Disorders, 25,* 81–104.

Emerson, E., Moss, S., & Kiernan, C. (1999). The relationship between challenging behaviour and psychiatric disorders in people with severe developmental disabilities. In N. Bouras (Ed.), *Psychiatric and behavioural disorders in developmental disabilities and mental retardation* (pp. 38–48). Cambridge, UK: Cambridge University Press.

Ferster, C. B. (1973). A functional analysis of depression. *American Psychologist, 28,* 857–870.

Fichter, M. M., Wallace, C. J., Liberman, R. P., & Davis, J. R. (1976). Improving social interaction in chronic psychotic using discriminated avoidance ("nagging"): Experimental analysis and generalization. *Journal of Applied Behavior Analysis, 9,* 377–386.

Finch, A. J., Wilkinson, M. D., Nelson, W. M., III, & Montgomery, L. E. (1975). Modification of an impulsive cognitive tempo in emotionally disturbed boys. *Journal of Abnormal Child Psychology, 3,* 49–52.

Finlay, W. M., & Lyons, E. (2001). Methodological issues in interviewing and using self-report questionnaires with people with mental retardation. *Psychological Assessment, 13,* 319–335.

Finlay, W. M., & Lyons, E. (2002). Acquiescence in interviews with people who have mental retardation. *Mental Retardation, 40,* 14–29.

*Fisher, W., Piazza, C. C., & Page, T. J. (1989). Assessing the independent and interactive effects of behavioral and pharmacological interventions for a client with dual diagnosis. *Journal of Behavior Therapy and Experimental Psychiatry, 20,* 241–250.

Fisher, W. W., Lindauer, S. E., Alterson, C. J., & Thompson, R. H. (1998). Assessment and treatment of destructive behavior maintained by stereotypic object manipulation. Journal of Applied Behavior Analysis, 3, 513–527.

Fletcher, R. J., & Greene, E. (Eds.). (2002). *Dual diagnosis: Mental health /mental retardation. A reference guide for training.* Kingston, NY: NADD Press.

Folstein, M. F., & Folstein, S. E. (2003). Mental status examination. In M. H. Beers & R. Berkow (Eds.), *The Merck manual of geriatrics* (Chapter 38). Retrieved July 18, 2003, from http://www.merck.com/pubs/mm_geriatrics/sec5/ch38.htm

Foxx, R. M., Faw, G. D., Taylor, S., Davis, P. K., & Fulia, R. (1993). "Would I be able to..."? Teaching clients to assess the availability of their community living life style preferences. *American Journal on Mental Retardation, 98*, 235–248.

Foxx, R. M., McMorrow, M. J., Davis, L. A., & Bittle, R. G. (1988). Replacing a chronic schizophrenic man's delusional speech with stimulus appropriate responses. *Journal of Behavior Therapy and Experimental Psychiatry, 19*, 43–50.

Gilbert, D. A., Altshuler, K. Z., Rago, W. V., Shon, S. P., Crismon, M. L., & Toprac, M.G. (1998). Texas Medication Algorithm Project: Definitions, rationale, and methods to develop medication algorithms. *Journal of Clinical Psychiatry, 59*, 345–351.

Gonzalez-Gordon, R. G., Salvador-Carulla, L., Romero, C., Gonzalez-Saiz, F., & Romero, D. (2002). Feasibility, reliability and validity of the Spanish version of Psychiatric Assessment Schedule for Adults with Developmental Disability: A structured psychiatric interview for intellectual disability. *Journal of Intellectual Disability Research, 46*, 209–217.

Hanley, G. P., Iwata, B. A., & McCord, B. E. (2003). Functional analysis of problem behavior: A review. *Journal of Applied Behavior Analysis, 36*, 147–185.

Haughton, E., & Ayllon, T. (1965). Production and elimination of symptomatic behavior. In L. P. Ullner & L. Krazner (Eds.), *Case studies in behavior modification* (pp. 94–98). New York: Holt, Reinhart & Winston.

Haynes, S. N., & O'Brien, W. H. (1990). Functional analysis in behavior therapy. *Clinical Psychology Review, 10*, 649–668.

Helsel, W. J., & Matson, J. L. (1988). The relationship of depression to social skills and intellectual functioning in mental retarded adults. *Journal of Mental Deficiency Research, 32*, 411–418.

Hurley, A. D. (2001). Psychiatric diagnostic interview evaluation. *Mental Health Aspects of Developmental Disabilities, 4*, 21–30.

Iwata, B. A., Dorsey, M. F., Slifer, K. J., Bauman, K., & Richman, G. S. (1982/1994). Toward a functional analysis of self-injurious behavior. *Journal of Applied Behavior Analysis, 27*, 197–209. (Reprinted from *Analysis in Developmental Disabilities*, 1982, 2, 3–20).

Jawed, S. H., Krishnan, V. H., Prasher, V. P., & Corbett J. A. (1993). Worsening of pica as a symptom of depressive illness in a person with severe mental handicap. *British Journal of Psychiatry, 162*, 835–837.

Jones, K. M., & Friman, P. C. (1999). A case study of behavioral assessment and treatment of insect phobia. *Journal of Applied Behavior Analysis, 32*, 95–98.

Kalachnik, J. E., & Sprague, R. L. (1993). The Dyskinesia Identification System Condensed User Scale (DISCUS): Reliability, validity, and a total score cut-off for mentally ill and mentally retarded populations. *Journal of Clinical Psychology, 49*, 177–189.

Kazdin, A. E. (1977). *The token economy: An evaluative review.* Baltimore: Brookes.

Kearney, C. A., & Silverman, W. K. (1990). A preliminary analysis of a functional analysis model of assessment and treatment for school refusal behavior. *Behavior Modification, 14*, 340–366.

Kolko, D. J. (1983). Multicomponent parental treatment of firesetting in a six year old boy. *Journal of Behavior Therapy and Experimental Psychiatry, 14*, 349–353.

LeJuez, C. W., Hopko, C. W., & Hopko, S. D. (2001). A brief behavioral activation treatment for depression. Treatment manual. *Behavior Modification, 25*, 255–286.

LeJuez, C. W., Hopko, C. W., & Hopko, S. D. (2003). *The brief behavioral activation treatment for depression (BATD). A comprehensive patient guide.* Boston: Pearson.

Levitas, A., Hurley, A. D., & Pary, R. (2001). The mental status examination in patients with mental retardation and developmental disabilities. *Mental Health Aspects of Developmental Disabilities, 4*, 2–16.

Levitas, A. S., & Van Silka, R. (2001). Mental health clinical assessment of persons with mental retardation and developmental disabilities: History. *Mental Health Aspects of Developmental Disabilities, 4*, 31–42.

*Lewinsohn, P. M., Hoberman, H. M., Teri, L., & Hantsinger, M. (1988). An integrated theory of depression. In S. Reiss & R. R. Bootsin (Eds.), *Theoretical issues in behavior therapy* (pp. 331–359). New York: Academic Press.

Lewis, M. H., Bodfish, J. W., Powell, S. B., & Golden, R. N. (1995). Clomipramine treatment for stereotype and related repetitive movement disorders with mental retardation: A double-blind comparison with placebo. *American Journal on Mental Retardation, 100,* 299–312.

Lewis, M. H., Bodfish, J. W., Powell, S. B., Parker, D. E., & Golden, R. N. (1996). Clomipramine treatment for self-injurious behavior of individuals with mental retardation: A double-blind comparison with placebo. *American Journal on Mental Retardation, 100,* 654–665.

Lewis, M. H., Bodfish, J. W., Powell, S. B., Parker, D. E., Golden, R. N., & Mintz, J. (1995). Compulsions in adults with mental retardation: Prevalence, phenomenology, and comorbidity with stereotypy and self-injurious behavior. *American Journal on Mental Retardation, 100,* 183–192.

Liberman, R. P., Wallace, C. J., Blackwell, G., Kopelowicz, A., Vaccaro, J. V., et al. (1998). Skills training versus psychosocial occupational therapy for persons with persistent schizophrenia. *American Journal of Psychiatry, 155,* 1087–1091.

Linaker, O. M., & Heller, J. (1994). Validity of the schizophrenia diagnosis of the psychopathology instrument for mentally retarded adults (PIMRA): A comparison of schizophrenic patients with and without mental retardation. *Research in Developmental Disabilities, 15,* 473–486.

Lindsay, W. R. (2002). Research literature on sex offenders with intellectual and developmental disabilities. *Journal of Intellectual Disability Research, 46,* 74–85.

Lindsay, W. R., Howells, L., & Pitcaithly, D. (1993). Cognitive therapy for depression with individuals with intellectual disabilities. *British Journal of Medical Psychology, 66,* 135–141.

Lindsay, W. R., Michie, A. M., Baty, F. J., Smith, A. H., & Miller, S. (1994). The consistency of reports about feelings and emotions from people with intellectual disability. *Journal of Intellect Disability Research, 38,* 61–66.

Lindsay, W. R., Taylor, J., & Sturmey, P. (2004). *Offenders with developmental disabilities.* New York: Wiley.

Lord, C., Pickles, A., McLennan, J., Rutter, M., Bregman, J., Folstein, S., et al. (1997). Diagnosing autism: Analyses of data from the Autism Diagnostic Interview. *Journal of Autism and Developmental Disorders, 27,* 501–517.

Mace, F. C., Browder, D. M., & Lin, Y. (1987). Analysis of demand conditions associated with stereotypy. *Journal of Behavior Therapy and Experimental Psychiatry, 18,* 25–31.

Mace, F. C., & Lalli, J. S. (1991). Linking descriptive and experimental analyses in the treatment of bizarre speech. *Journal of Applied Behavior Analysis, 24,* 553–562.

Marston, G. M., Perry, D. W., & Roy, A. (1997). Manifestations of depression in people with intellectual disabilities. *Journal of Intellectual Disability Research, 41,* 476–480.

Matson, J. L. (1982). The treatment of behavioral characteristics of depression in the mentally retarded. *Behavior Therapy, 13,* 209–218.

Matson, J. L. (1983). Depression in the mentally retarded: Toward a conceptual analysis of diagnosis. *Progress in Behavior Modification, 15,* 57–79.

Matson, J. L. (1984). Behavioral treatment of psychosomatic complaints of mental retarded adults. *American Journal of Mental Deficiency, 88,* 638–648.

Matson, J. L. (1995). *The Diagnostic Assessment for the Severely Handicapped revised (DASH-II).* Baton Rouge, LA: Disability Consultants, LLC.

Matson, J. L., Kazdin, A. E., & Senatore, V. (1984). Psychometric properties of the psychopathology instrument for mentally retarded adults. *Applied Research in Mental Retardation, 5,* 81–89.

Matson, J. L., Zeiss, A. M., Zeiss, R. A., & Bowman, W. (1980). A comparison of social skills training and contingent attention to improve behavioural deficits of chronic psychiatric patients. *British Journal of Social and Clinical Psychology, 19,* 57–64.

McCord, B. E., Thomson, T., & Iwata, B. A. (2001). Functional analysis and treatment of self-injury association with transitions. *Journal of Applied Behavior Analysis, 34,* 195–210.

Meadows, G., Turner, T., Campbell, L., Lewis, S. W., Reveley, M. A., & Murray, R. M. (1991). Assessing schizophrenia in adults with mental retardation. A comparative study. *British Journal of Psychiatry, 158,* 103–105.

Moss, S. (1999). Assessment: Conceptual issues. In N. Bouras (Ed.), *Psychiatric and behavioural disorders in developmental disabilities and mental retardation* (pp. 18–37). Cambridge, UK: Cambridge University Press.

Moss, S., Ibbotson, B., Prosser, H., Goldberg, D., Patel, P., & Simpson, N. (1997). Validity of the PAS-ADD for detecting psychiatric symptoms in adults with learning disability (mental retardation). *Social Psychiatry, and Psychiatric Epidemiology, 32,* 344–354.

Moss, S., Patel, P., Prosser, H., Goldberg, D., Simpson, N., Rowe, N., et al. (1993). Psychiatric morbidity in older people with moderate and severe learning disability: I. Development and reliability of the patient interview (PAS-ADD). *British Journal of Psychiatry, 163,* 471–480.

Moss, S., Prosser, H., Ibbotson, B., & Goldberg, D. (1996). Respondent and informant accounts of psychiatric symptoms in a sample of patients with learning disability. *Journal of Intellectual Disability Research, 40,* 457–465.

Mozingo, D., Ackley, G. B., & Bailey, J. S. (1994). Training quality job interviews with adults with developmental disabilities. *Research in Developmental Disabilities, 15,* 389–410.

Myers, B. A. (1987). The Mini Mental State in those with developmental disabilities. *Journal of Nervous and Mental Diseases, 175,* 85–89.

Newton, T., & Sturmey, P. (1988). The factor structure of the Aberrant Behaviour Checklist: A British replication. *Journal of Mental Deficiency Research, 32,* 87–92.

O'Neill, R. E., Horner, R. H., Albin, R. W., Sprague, J. R., Storey, K., & Newton, J. S. (1999). *Functional assessment and program development for problem behavior. A practical handbook.* Albany, NY: Brooks/Cole.

Pary, R. J., Levitas, A. S., & Hurley, A. (1999). Bipolar disorder in persons with developmental disabilities. *Mental Health Aspects of Developmental Disabilities, 2,* 37–49.

Patel, P., Goldberg, D., & Moss, S. (1993). Psychiatric morbidity in older people with moderate and severe learning disability: II. The prevalence study. *British Journal of Psychiatry, 163,* 481–491.

Poindexter, A. (2002). *Facilitating behavioral/psychiatric assessment for persons with mental retardation.* Kingston, NY: NADD Press.

Reiss, S. (1988). *The Reiss screen for maladaptive behavior test manual.* Worthington, OH: IDS.

Reiss, S., & Rojahn, J. (1993). Joint occurrence of depression and aggression in children and adults with mental retardation. *Journal of Intellectual Disability Research, 37,* 287–294.

Richards, M., Maugham, B., Hardy, R., Hall, I., Strydon, A., & Wadsworth, M. (2001). Long-term affective disorder in people with mild learning disability. *British Journal of Psychiatry, 179,* 523–527.

Rincover, A., Newsom, C. D., & Carr, E. G. (1979). Using sensory extinction procedures in the treatment of compulsive like behavior of developmentally disabled children. *Journal of Consulting and Clinical Psychology, 47,* 695–701.

Rojahn, J., Borthwick-Duffy, S. A., & Jacobson, J. W. (1993). The association between psychiatric diagnoses and severe behavior problems in mental retardation. *Annals of Clinical Psychiatry, 5,* 163–170.

Rojahn, J., Matson, J. L., Lott, D., Esbensen, A. J., & Smalls, Y. (2001). The Behavior Problems Inventory: An instrument for the assessment of self-injury, stereotyped behavior, and aggression/destruction in individuals with developmental disabilities. *Journal of Autism and Developmental Disorders, 31,* 577–588.

Rojahn, J., Tasse, M., & Sturmey, P. (1997). The Stereotyped Behavior Scale for adolescents and adults with mental retardation. *American Journal on Mental Retardation, 102,* 137–146.

Ross, E., & Oliver, C. (2003a). The relationship between levels of mood, interest and pleasure and 'challenging behaviour' in adults with severe and profound intellectual disability. *Journal of Intellectual Disability Research, 46,* 191–197.

Ross, E., & Oliver, C. (2003b). The assessment of mood in adult who have severe or profound mental retardation. *Clinical Psychology Review, 23,* 225–245.

Royal College of Psychiatrists. (2001). *DC-LD (Diagnostic criteria used with adults with learning disabilities/mental retardation).* Occasional paper OP 48. London, UK: Gaskell.

Rush, A. J., & Frances, A. (2000). Expert consensus guidelines series. Treatment of psychiatric and behavioral problems in mental retardation. *American Journal on Mental Retardation, 105,* 159–228.

Schaefer, H. H. (1970). Self-injurious behavior: Shaping "head-banging" in monkeys. *Journal of Applied Behavior Analysis, 3,* 111–116.

Senatore, V., Matson, J. L., & Kazdin, A. E. (1985). An inventory to assess psychopathology of mentally retarded adults. *American Journal of Mental Deficiency, 89,* 459–466.

*Simon, E. W., Rappaport, D. A., Papka, M., & Woodruff-Pak, D. S. (1995). Fragile-X and Down syndrome: Are there syndrome-specific cognitive profiles at low IQ levels? *Journal of Intellectual Disability Research, 39,* 326–330.

Singh, N. N., Wahler, R. G., Sabaawi, M., Goza, A. B., Singh, S. D., & Molina, E. J. (2002). Mentoring treatment teams to integrate behavioral and psychopharmacological treatments in developmental disabilities. *Research in Developmental Disabilities, 23,* 379–389.

Skinner, B. F. (1953). *Science and human behavior.* New York: MacMillan.

Steinberg, M., & Stein, M. (1994). *Interviewer's guide to the Structured Clinical Interview for DSM-IV Dissociative Disorders (SCID-D).* Arlington, VA: American Psychiatric Press.

Stephens, R. N., Matson, J. L., Westmoreland, T., & Kulpa, J. (1981). Modification of psychotic speech with mentally retarded patients. *Journal of Mental deficiency research, 25,* 187–197.

Sturmey, P. (1993). The use of ICD and DSM criteria in people with mental retardation: A review. *Journal of Nervous and Mental Disease, 181,* 39–42.

Sturmey, P. (1995a). DSM-III-R and persons with dual diagnoses: Conceptual issues and strategies for research. *Journal of Intellectual Disability Research, 39,* 357–364.

Sturmey, P. (1995b). Suicidal threats and behavior in a person with developmental disabilities: Effective psychiatric monitoring based on functional assessment. *Behavioral Interventions: Theory and Practice in Residential and Community-Based Clinical Programs, 9,* 235–245.

Sturmey, P. (1996). *Functional analysis in clinical psychology.* London: Wiley.

Sturmey, P. (1999). Assessment of psychiatric disorders in adults with dual diagnosis. *Journal of Developmental and Physical Disabilities, 11,* 317–330.

Sturmey, P. (2004). Cognitive therapy with people with intellectual disabilities: A selective review and critique. *Clinical Psychology and Psychotherapy, 11,* 222–232.

Sturmey, P., & Bernstein, H. (2004). Functional analysis of maladaptive behaviors: Current status and future directions. In J. L. Matson, R. B. Laud & M. L. Matson (Eds.), *Behavior modification for persons with developmental disabilities.* Kingston, NY: National Association for the Dually Diagnosed.

Sturmey, P., Lee, R., Reyer, H., & Robek, A. (2006). Applied behavior analysis and dual diagnosis: Behavioral approaches to dual diagnosis. In N. Cain & P. Davidson (Eds.), *Training handbook of mental disorders in individuals with intellectual disability.* Kinigsten, NY: NADD Press.

Sturmey, P., Matson, J. L., & Lott, J. D. (2004). The factor structure of the DASH-II. *Journal of Developmental and Physical Disabilities, 16,* 247–255.

Sturmey, P., Reed, J., & Corbett, J. (1991). Psychiatric disorders in people with learning difficulties: A psychometric review of available measures. *Psychological Medicine, 21,* 143–155.

Sturmey, P., Reyer, H., Lee, R., & Robek, A. (in press). *Substance-related disorders in persons with mental retardation.* Kingston, NY: NADD Press.

Sturmey, P., Tsouris, J. A., & Patti, P. (2003). The psychometric properties of the Multi-Dimensional Observational Scale for Elderly Subjects (MOSES) in middle age and older populations with mental retardation. *International Journal of Geriatric Psychiatry, 18,* 131–134.

Tsiouris, J. A., Mann, R., Patti, P. J., & Sturmey, P. (2004). Symptoms of depression and challenging behaviors in people with intellectual disabilities: A Bayesian analysis. *Journal of Intellectual and Developmental Disabilities, 29,* 65–69.

Wilder, D. A., Masuda, A., O'Conner, C., & Baham, M. (2001). Brief functional analysis and treatment of bizarre vocalizations in an adult with schizophrenia. *Journal of Applied Behavior Analysis, 34,* 65–68.

World Health Organization. (1992a). *The ICD-10. International classification of diseases and behavioral disorders. Clinical descriptions and diagnostic guidelines.* Geneva, Switzerland: Author.

World Health Organization. (1992b). *The ICD-10. International classification of diseases and behavioral disorders. Diagnostic criteria for research.* Geneva, Switzerland: Author.

17

Functional Behavioral Assessment in Practice: Concepts and Applications

SANDRA L. HARRIS and BETH A. GLASBERG

The technology of functional assessment is among the most important developments in several decades for the education and treatment of people with mental retardation, autism, and other developmental disabilities. These powerful methods for understanding maladaptive behavior and linking intervention closely to assessment have made a difference in the lives of countless people with developmental disabilities and should be part of the repertoire of every service provider who works with these clients and students. In this chapter, we first review the research documenting the benefits of functional assessment and then illustrate the application with a case report highlighting the transfer of functional assessment research into clinical practice.

Harmful aggression, self-injurious behavior (SIB), and stereotypic behavior are among the behaviors that most challenge practitioners serving people with developmental disabilities. Sometimes these behaviors pose a danger to the client and others in the environment. In other cases the behaviors, although not immediately dangerous, interfere with learning and are stigmatizing in the community. In brief, these behavioral excesses intrude on the quality of life for the client, the family, and others who form that person's community.

Functional assessment has enabled applied behavior analysis to shift from a mixed reinforcement and punishment consequences based approach to severe aberrant behavior to one that is mainly reliant on positive reinforcement and environmental changes (e.g., interventions emphasizing

SANDRA L. HARRIS and BETH A. GLASBERG • Douglass Developmental Disabilities Center, Rutgers, The State University of New Jersey, New Brunswick, New Jersey 08901.

stimulus control; Pelios, Morren, Tesch, & Axelrod, 1999). Throughout the 1970s and continuing into much of the 1980s most efforts to control maladaptive behavior often included punishment contingencies. Without a technology for assessment, the tools in the behavior analyst's repertoire were relatively crude when compared the more elegant methods available today. In 1977, Carr suggested that a greater understanding of the variables that influenced maladaptive behavior such as SIB (self-injury) could produce more effective and precise interventions (Carr, 1977). Iwata, Dorsey, Slifer, Bauman, and Richman (1982) described functional analysis techniques for better understanding SIB. This seminal article was reprinted in the *Journal of Applied Behavior Analysis* in 1994 (Iwata, Dorsey, Slifer, Bauman, & Richman, 1994) to signify its importance in initiating the body of research that forms the heart of the functional assessment literature. Their report described the use of analog (contrived) assessment situations to expose nine children and adolescents with developmental problems and SIB to a range of situations that might evoke SIB. The analog settings involved manipulating the presence or absence of play materials, high or low adult demands, and social attention as absent, noncontingent or contingent. Importantly, Iwata et al. found considerable variability both within individual clients and across clients with respect to motivating factors for SIB. For example, one child showed a high level of SIB while alone in a room whereas another showed very little. This variation in responding, documenting that no single set of conditions evoked SIB in all the children, highlighted the urgency of doing an assessment with every client.

In another much-cited paper, Carr and Durand (1985) described an assessment method for identifying variables influencing the appearance of behavior problems and for developing interventions based on these assessments. In that study, they found that low levels of adult attention and high levels of task difficulty were most likely to evoke behavior problems in their participants. On the basis of their initial assessments, Carr and Durand (1985) developed an appropriate alternative communicative behavior for each youngster. For example, a child might be taught to say, "I don't understand," when faced with a hard task. This early demonstration of the power of functional communication training following a functional analysis led to scores of studies examining the link between functional assessment and skill training to remediate communication deficits (e.g., Kahng, Hendrickson, & Vu, 2000; Winborn, Wacker, Richman, Asmus, & Geier, 2002).

FUNCTIONAL ASSESSMENT

O'Neill et al. (1997) described three components of a functional assessment: (1) interviews with key informants to generate hypotheses about the variables that may be linked to the behavior, (2) direct observation of the client in a naturalistic context to collect data about the behavior as it occurs in real time (sometimes called a descriptive analysis), and (3) for some clients a functional analysis in which variables are systematically manipulated to identify factors that may evoke the problem behavior. Consistent with that description, we will use the term functional assessment as the broad category within which fall a range of assessment techniques including the analog (contrived) methods of a functional analysis.

Interviews

Almost every behavioral assessment begins with an interview with parents, teachers, and when possible, the client. That information allows the formulation of preliminary hypotheses to be supported or refuted by systematic observations. O'Neill et al. (1997) described in detail one model for gathering interview data and using these data to organize one's observations. As long as the hypotheses generated from interviews are "held lightly" and not assumed to be necessarily accurate reflections of a client's behavior, these preliminary guesses can be valuable in guiding initial observations, and may contribute structure to subsequent interviews or suggest an initial focus of descriptive observations. The same is true of paper and pencil scales such as the *Motivation Assessment Scale* (Durand and Crimmins, 1988) that must be used with caution as one's bias can influence the outcome, and the scale's and reliability and construct validity are linked in part to the frequency and the topography of specific behaviors (Duker, Sigafoos, Barron, & Coleman, 1998). The *Motivation Assessment Scale* should not be used in isolation for a functional assessment, although it is useful for generating hypotheses.

Descriptive Analyses

One approach to the systematic assessment of problem behavior in the client's natural environment was described by Anderson and Long (2002). They first developed definitions of the children's problem behaviors through parent interviews and direct observation. For purposes of the research an analog functional analysis was done for each child to form a basis of comparison for the more naturalistic observations that followed. In these structured descriptive assessments, the sessions were conducted at the time of day when the events associated with the behaviors would normally occur and with a teacher or parent presenting the activity. In this respect the assessment resembled a naturalistic assessment. However, these adults were asked to create specific antecedent conditions related to attention, task, tangible items, and play, and to respond to any problem behaviors as they normally would, and this creation of artificial demands more closely parallels an analog analysis. For three of the four children the naturalistic observations yielded results similar to those from tightly controlled analog assessments. The authors conclude that for some clients this less contrived form of assessment done in the natural context provides sufficient data to generate a useful intervention, but for others with more complex or subtle patterns of behavior an analog assessment is essential.

An assessment in the natural environment is sometimes key to identifying subtle events related to aberrant behavior. For example, the noise of another child crying may evoke stereotypical ear covering (Tang, Kennedy, Koppekin, & Caruso, 2002), level of food deprivation (meal schedule) has been linked to SIB (Wacker et al., 1996), aggression may vary with sleep deprivation (O'Reilly, 1995), and curriculum content can evoke inappropriate behavior (Dunlap, Kern-Dunlap, Clarke, & Robbins, 1991). A contextual variable can influence the potency of an intervention. For example, Haring and Kennedy (1990) noted that during a work task, a Differential Reinforcement of Other behavior (DRO) procedure reduced aberrant behavior while time-out was not effective; however, during a leisure activity time-out was effective and DRO was not. This might reflect a higher level of access to reinforcement for clients during recreational tasks as contrasted with work. For another child, a variation in the route to school influenced problem behavior in school (Kennedy & Itkonen, 1993). When a city street with a number of stops and delays was taken she engaged in more problematic behavior at school than when a highway was taken. This kind of relatively subtle setting event can often only be detected through careful observation of a client's entire routine. Stimuli that have such effects are known as either setting events, establishing operations (Michael, 1993) or most recently as motivating operation (Laraway, Snycerski, Michael, & Poling, 2003). Once identified it is often possible to alter such setting events as the route taken or the amount of sleep a client had the night before.

Although functional assessment requires a complex set of skills, motivated staff can learn the fundamentals fairly quickly and do this work under the supervision of a senior behavior analyst. In a recent study, Iwata et al. (2000) trained naive undergraduates to use the technology of functional analysis and found that they were able to quickly master the basic skills required to employ these methods. Wallace, Doney, Mintz-Resudek, and Tarbox (2004) used a 3-h group format to teach three educators to implement functional analyses. The workshop used videotapes and role-play as well as questions and answers. For two of the three, the group format was sufficient and for one some additional brief individual feedback was used.

Direct observation of clients using a descriptive analysis and the use of analog assessments in a functional analysis may both have a role to play in the same assessment process. Sasso et al. (1992) compared descriptive analyses done by experts and by classroom teachers with a functional analysis in the classroom and found that both procedures identified negative reinforcement (i.e., escape or avoidance) as the maintaining variable for two children. In another comparison of descriptive analysis and functional analyses of SIB by six adults with profound mental retardation, Lerman and Iwata (1993) found that the naturalistic observations were helpful in determining how SIB was linked to social versus nonsocial behavior, but was less helpful in distinguishing conditions linked to attention (positive reinforcement) or escape (negative reinforcement).

Functional Analysis

The potentially dangerous nature of SIB makes it the target of many studies of functional analysis. These have included identifying a variety of

stimulus conditions linked to SIB and development of techniques for precisely targeting these variables to decrease SIB. For example, Iwata, Pace,
Kalsher, Cowdery, and Cataldo (1990) used a series of analog conditions
to identify variables maintaining SIB in seven children and adolescents.
For six of them a demand condition in which they had to respond to learning tasks increased the probability of SIB. Based on that analysis an extinction procedure, tailored to the needs of each child, was put in place
so that SIB no longer resulted in the termination of academic demands.
That intervention resulted in a significant decrease in, or elimination of,
SIB and an increase in task compliance. For one participant whose SIB
occurred during an analog of a medical examination, the extinction procedure required tolerance of the examination process. A number of other
studies have found escape or avoidance to be the maintaining variables
for SIB (e.g., Mazaleski, Iwata, Vollmer, Zarcone, & Smith, 1993; Vollmer,
Marcus, & Ringdahl, 1995).

Not all SIB is escape-motivated. For example, Moore, Fisher, and
Pennington (2004) found automatic reinforcement was a factor in a
12-year-old girl's SIB. Vollmer and Vorndran (1998) illustrate the importance of a functional assessment/analysis to identify the relevant variables
for every client. These authors did such an analysis with a young woman
with severe mental retardation and a history of aggression and SIB. She
employed a form of self-restraint in which she wrapped herself tightly in a
leather jacket and she would engage in high rates of SIB when not allowed
to do so. However, she did not demonstrate SIB when alone, even if not
given access to the jacket for self-restraint. On the basis of their assessment, and the identification of the jacket as a positive reinforcement for
SIB, she was first taught to ask for the jacket, and then that request was
shifted to a cardigan sweater that was viewed as more appropriate to wear
indoors than the heavy leather jacket. With this functional communication
skill in place the client regularly asked for her sweater, and engaged in low
rates of SIB.

In another illustration of nonescape related SIB, Kuhn, DeLeon, Fisher,
and Wilke (1999) found in a preliminary functional analysis that the SIB
of a man with autism and mental retardation was maintained by escape,
by sensory reinforcement, or by both. Given this ambiguity in the data
they examined two different treatments, one involving sensory extinction,
another escape extinction, and the combination of these two. This assess-
ment/intervention phase revealed that sensory extinction was sufficient
to extinguish the behavior and thus indicated that escape motivation was
not a potent factor, demonstrated that initial interventions often serve as
a valuable source of assessment information, and underscored the importance of accurate data collection to enable continuing assessment of the
impacts of an intervention.

The subtlety of functional analysis is illustrated in a report by Moore,
Mueller, Dubard, Roberts, and Sterling-Turner (2002) in a case of SIB in a
6-year-old girl. Initially they found that her SIB was maintained by adult
attention and tangible reinforcement. However, when the tangible reinforcement condition was examined more closely by comparing a tangible
condition that included verbal attention and another tangible condition

that did not, they found that when verbal attention was removed from the tangible condition, SIB declined. Thus, verbal attention alone was the key factor in her SIB and tangible reinforcement was not important. This study highlights the importance of looking closely at the events occurring in any functional assessment or analysis. In another study examining the details of the analog context, Fisher, Piazza, and Chiang (1996) noted how the duration of the interval of access to reinforcement can influence the rate of aberrant behavior.

Another category of behavior that has received the attention of applied behavior analysts is the occurrence of stereotypic behavior such as rocking, hand flapping, and light gazing. Although these behaviors are sometimes called self-stimulatory in reference to their inherently reinforcing quality for some people (automatic reinforcement), in other cases different variables may maintain the stereotypic behavior and a functional assessment is important. For example, Kennedy, Meyer, Knowles, and Shukla (2000) describe the multiple functions of stereotypic behavior in youths with autism. They measured the frequency of stereotypic behavior in analog conditions of attention, demand, no attention, and recreation and found that the occurrence of the stereotypic behavior was associated with a range of conditions for the children and that in many cases these functions were not linked to the topography (form) of the stereotyped behavior. For example, for two of the children stereotyped behavior was maintained by escape or avoidance of teaching situations. This highlights the importance of not assuming that the function of stereotyped behavior is automatic reinforcement.

The variables influencing aberrant behavior may be idiosyncratic and require close attention to identify. Van Camp et al. (2000) describe items such as a particular toy or social interaction that was linked to increases in problem behavior on the part of two boys with mental retardation. Similarly, Ringdahl and Sellers (2000) found that whether a child's caretaker or an inpatient staff member was present during an analog condition influenced the rate of problem behaviors.

As illustrated by the studies cited above, even after doing a functional analysis and implementing a related intervention plan, the occurrence of behavior may remain variable. Wacker, Berg, Asmus, Harding, and Cooper (1998) suggest that this variability may be related to unidentified influential antecedent stimuli. They point out that functional analysis examines the response–reinforcer relationship. To complement this, they offer models for conducting experimental analyses of antecedent variables. These authors recommend that the behavior analyst begin by completing a descriptive assessment including antecedent–behavior–consequence (A-B-C) observations and interviews to develop hypotheses about antecedent stimuli that may be influencing the target behavior. Next, the analyst can choose between two basic approaches to assessment. First, antecedents may be systematically manipulated while all responses are consequated with extinction. Alternatively, antecedents may be systematically manipulated while all responses are reinforced. The analyst can then evaluate changes in behavior that occur with changes in the antecedents. For example, a behavior analyst may compare compliance to task demands as it varies according to which staff member delivers the demands, the context in which the demands occur, or the materials utilized. Similarly, antecedent assessment may focus on the systematic manipulation of establishing operations (e.g., which route is taken by the school bus, as in the earlier example) in order to determine their impact on the target response.

Brief Assessment

Functional analyses need not always be long to be useful. Derby et al. (1992) report data from 79 functional assessments collected over 3 years at the University of Iowa. Initial hypotheses for functional analyses were based on interviews with the client's caregiver and scores on the *Motivation Assessment Scale*, a paper-and-pencil measure of factors that may motivate aberrant behavior (Durand & Crimmins, 1988). On the basis of this initial information, targeted functional analyses of 90-min duration were done to pinpoint the contingences of aberrant behavior. For clients with relatively high frequency behaviors these brief assessments were often sufficient to allow a useful assessment. However, for behaviors of low frequency, brief sessions did not always yield data about the behavior. Vollmer, Marcus, Ringdahl, and Roane (1995) did relatively brief assessments of 60–120 min and then carried out more extended assessments with 20 clients seen for severe behavior problems. For about 30% of clients the brief period was sufficient to identify the factors involved in the behavior whereas for others as much as 12 h were needed to determine the functions that were involved; there were a few individuals for whom function could not be identified even after extended assessments. Kahng and Iwata (1999) found that in approximately two-thirds of cases of SIB, a brief assessment yielded results consistent with a longer assessment. Indeed, Wallace and Iwata (1999) examined session duration and found that shorter assessment sessions may be nearly as effective as longer ones.

Assessment of Choice and Preference

Giving people with developmental disabilities choices of clothing, foods, daily routines, work activities, and recreational events treats them with respect and allows them control over important aspects of their lives. The positive impact of respecting preferences on client behavior was illustrated by Foster-Johnson, Ferro, and Dunlap (1994), who assessed the activity preferences of three students with moderate to severe mental retardation and behavior problems and found that when these youngsters engaged in preferred curricular activities their behavior problems decreased and appropriate behavior increased. However, many clients with severe mental retardation or autism may have little experience making choices and may lack the verbal ability to name their preferences, and unfortunately caregiver guesses about client preferences are not always accurate (Newton, Ard, & Horner, 1993). In a study of hypothesized preferences identified by staff as part of "person-centered planning" to design supports for clients with profound disabilities it was found that although some of the items were indeed preferred, others were not (Reid, Everson, & Green, 1999). Staff opinions should be regarded as hypotheses, and not as proven facts. In addition, client preferences shift over time (Zhou, Iwata, Goff, & Shore, 2001). As a result, it is important to do ongoing assessments (e.g., Parsons & Reid, 1990). Fortunately there is a body of research to guide the practitioner in doing these assessments. The feasibility of using preference assessments in clinical settings was documented by Lavie and Sturmey (2002), who found that using brief instruction, a videotape, and feedback on a rehearsal were sufficient to train staff in about 80 min per person.

Pace, Ivancic, Edwards, Iwata, and Page (1985) described a preference-assessment procedure for clients with profound mental retardation in which the client is systemically presented with 16 different stimuli to assess the extent to which he or she approaches each item. Green, Reid, Canipe, and Gardner (1991), using the Pace et al. (1985) technique, found that caregiver opinions were not consistent with the results of client choice, and that highly preferred stimuli were effective reinforcements in a learning context whereas stimuli that were less highly preferred were less effective.

Fisher et al. (1992) noted that a limitation of the Pace et al. model is that some clients approach all the items and it may be difficult to determine a hierarchy of preferences. They developed a forced choice model in which the client chooses between two items. This technique was more effective for identifying items with potentially greater reinforcement value than was a method that did not require forced choice. Similar findings by Piazza, Fisher, Hagopian, Bowman, and Toole (1996) indicated that high-preference items were more consistently reinforcing than were middle- and low-preference items. These preferred items can be used to address both skill acquisition and reduction of behavior problems (e.g., Lalli & Kates, 1998). In a preference assessment designed to identify alternative stimuli to decrease SIB, Ringdahl, Vollmer, Marcus, and Roane (1997) found that providing clients with preferred items to manipulate, and reinforcing this object use, reduced the frequency of SIB.

Although some preference assessments rely on actual objects such as food, toys, or clothing, other potential choices must be presented in a symbolic form such as a line drawing or a photograph. For some clients without much choice making experience and with limited verbal abilities it may be necessary to teach the link between a picture and an event. Hanley, Iwata, and Lindberg (1999) documented that when the connection between pictures and activities was made concrete by, for example, giving the person brief access to a bike after showing a picture of the bike, people with profound mental retardation learned to select a picture representing a preferred future activity.

In doing preference assessments it is important to consider the effects of establishing operations (motivational level). An individual who has been deprived of an activity for a period of time may find access to that item more reinforcing than does someone who has had free access to that stimulus. Gottschalk, Libby, and Graff (2000) showed that periods of deprivation increased item preference whereas having extensive exposure to an item just before the assessment decreased preference. There are at least two implications of this finding. One is that in doing a formal preference assessment it is important to consider the client's level of deprivation. The second is that in identifying an item as potentially reinforcing for a specific teaching session one must consider the student's current level of deprivation. For this reason doing an extensive one-time assessment of a client's stimulus preferences and then relying on staff choices from that list to select potential reinforcements is not sufficient to maximize the motivating value of the items being offered to the client. Consistent with this, Carr, Nicolson, and Higbe (2000) described a brief, preteaching session preference assessment in which the items chosen by the children were effective reinforcements. Establishing operations shift and change in a continuous fashion. For this reason moving the preference assessment to within the session may be even more potent than doing it just before the session. Graff and Libby (1999) found that when people with developmental disabilities selected their reinforcements throughout a session they made selections that differed from their choices presession and the opportunity for making choices improved performance. One advantage of this procedure is that it adds little complexity to intervention sessions, while demonstrating potential for increased responsiveness of the client.

FUNCTIONAL ASSESSMENT IN PRACTICE: A CASE STUDY

The first section of this chapter provided ideal models for assessing behavior problems. In practice, special challenges may arise that require specific modifications to these models and careful evaluation of data regarding behavior change. The following case study illustrates the principles of functional assessment as implemented within an applied setting.

As a behavior analyst who consults to a private school for elementary school students with disabilities, Kristen's services were requested by Josie, a special education teacher, who sought help in decreasing tantrum behavior being exhibited by her student, Kyle. Kyle is a 4-year-old boy with autism who had been described as "untestable" during cognitive assessments. Kyle was one of the six students in Josie's classroom, which was staffed by six paraprofessional instructors under her supervision. Instructor assignments were rotated so that students worked with different staff each day. Josie's classroom was rooted in the principles of behavior analysis. Within this framework, she incorporated a variety of specific teaching practices centering on interspersed discrete trials. Curriculum was based on developmental guidelines as well as Skinner's (1957) analysis of verbal behavior.

Kyle's tantrums involved a variety of behaviors including throwing himself to the floor, screaming "No!," and sometimes hitting his head on the floor, kicking the floor, and hitting his instructor. Tantrums occurred primarily at school and very rarely in the home. Because the behavior was primarily a problem in the classroom setting, Kristen began her assessment by interviewing teaching staff. Her questions focused primarily on gaining a thorough description of the behavior and identifying influential variables including the conditions under which the behavior was most likely to occur, the conditions under which the behavior was least likely to occur, staff reactions to the behavior, other changes in the environment pursuant to the behavior, factors that exacerbated the behavior, and factors that seemed to terminate the behavior. Additionally, patterns regarding the relationship of the behavior to certain staff, tasks, settings, or activities were evaluated. Finally, Kristen asked staff members for their impressions regarding the possible function of the behavior on the environment.

On the basis of these interviews, Kristen learned that Kyle was most likely to exhibit tantrum behavior during work sessions. Some staff believed that Kyle was trying to "get a rise" out of them, whereas others described him as "oppositional." Other staff thought that he was simply trying to get out of work. Typically, staff responded to Kyle by attempting to prompt him back to the work area or by bringing his work to the floor with him. Attempts to ignore Kyle escalated the behavior, whereas prompts back to the table ended the behavior fairly quickly. However, after being prompted back to work, the latency until the next tantrum began was brief. Staff interviews also led to the identification of precursor behaviors for the tantrum including laying on the instructor's lap, and jumping out of his seat then quickly sitting back down. There was no apparent relationship between Kyle's tantrums and staff, specific tasks, activities, or settings, other than that they occurred during work periods rather than lunch, recess, or breaks.

Kristen also reviewed ABC (antecedent–behavior–consequence) data collected by staff over a 5-day period as part of her assessment. These data revealed that tantrum behavior and its precursors typically occurred immediately after an instruction was given. Consequences for the behavior varied but always involved either a delay in or escape from the task at hand. Tantrums were intermittently consequated by physical attention in the form of prompts to return to his desk or his chair. Taken together with interview data, it seemed likely that Kyle's behavior was maintained by negative reinforcement in the form of task removal. However, the possibility remained that tantrums might also be maintained by attentional variables because social attention also occurred as a part of the typical consequences.

Although the staff had been collecting their ABC data, Kristen spent time observing Kyle at different times of the day in his classroom. She was able to articulate some qualitative variables that clarified some of the impressions reported by teachers. Although it was clear that the occurrence of tantrums was linked to task demands, Kyle seemed to enjoy the intense interactions with staff that followed. After jumping out of his seat or falling to the ground, Kyle would look at his instructor expectantly. He would sometimes smile or giggle when being physically prompted. In contrast, during the periods when Kyle was on-task, instructors were fairly muted in their style. Although praise was offered as a reward, it was often not very animated and was infrequently paired with physical attention (e.g., high fives). Taken together with the interview and ABC data, Kristen was confused as to whether the behavior was maintained by escape, attention, or some combination of the two. She decided to implement a series of systematic manipulations in order to complete her assessment.

Kristen worked with Josie and her staff to count the frequency of both precursor behaviors and tantrums under three conditions: (1) *Control*: Kyle was given a high level of attention from his instructor, preferred materials, and no demands; (2) *Low attention*: Kyle was given preferred activities and no demands, but the teacher turned away from him and pretended to be busily engaged in another task; and (3) *Task*: Kyle was given difficult programs on which to work with his teacher, who offered high-intensity verbal praise and physical attention. Each condition lasted 5 min and was replicated on a second day. Target behaviors were ignored.

Results indicated that tantrums did not occur in any condition, and only one precursor behavior occurred during the escape condition on the first day. No precursor behaviors occurred on the second day.

At first, the failure of the analog conditions to elicit the behavior puzzled Kristen. However, she soon noted that the analog task condition assessing whether or not the behavior might be occurring as a means of escaping tasks differed from naturalistic task situations in the quality of attention. During the assessment, in order to insure that only one motivation (escape from task demand) was evaluated at a time, instructors had been told to deliver high-intensity attention during tasks. The high-intensity attention presented during the task condition in the analog assessment sharply contrasted with the quiet praise offered during everyday work periods. This led Kristen to a new hypothesis. Perhaps tantrums resulted from Kyle's motivation to obtain high-intensity attention, and task demands acted as a cue for him that this quality of attention was available.

To asses this possibility, Kristen created an additional assessment condition for low attention, which she juxtaposed with a replicated control condition. In this new condition, Kyle was again given free access to preferred activities and no demands with the teacher turned away from him pretending to be busily engaged in another task. However, every 30 s, Josie delivered an instruction requiring no behavior change. For example, she might say "Keep playing with your toys." In this way, it was hoped that deprivation of high-intensity attention could be examined without the confound of an actual demand. However, if her thinking was correct, it would seem to Kyle that reinforcement in the form of physical attention might now be available for tantrums. The hypothesis was confirmed when this condition led to an increased rate of the behavior. There were six precursor behaviors on the first day of this condition and four precursors and a tantrum on the second day of this assessment. Recall that only one precursor behavior was seen across two sessions in the escape condition and no target behaviors were seen in the original low attention condition. This sharp contrast, especially when considered in light of his daily frequency and the length of the assessment interval, highlights the impact of a subtle environmental manipulation.

On the basis of the assessment results, a behavior plan was written for Kyle addressing his pursuit of high-intensity attention. The plan was organized to provide a great deal of high-intensity noncontingent attention as an antecedent intervention to reduce Kyle's motivation to seek additional attention of this quality, to identify replacement skills through which Kyle could obtain high-intensity attention appropriately if motivated, and to shift the consequences of his behavior in such a way that staying on task resulted in high-intensity attention whereas off-task behavior resulted in decreased attention. Specifically, this plan included the following components:

1. Staff was trained to provide high-intensity attention throughout work periods including tickles, hugs, high fives, and animated praise.
2. All curricular programs were modified to make them more compatible with teaching using an interactive format.
3. A number of social initiation skills were added to his curriculum.
4. Attention was withdrawn during tantrums. If prompting was necessary to preserve Kyle's safety, this was done without eye contact or any vocal interaction.
5. Signs of quieting during tantrums were reinforced with attention (e.g., "I'm glad you're calm now, let's finish up this work.")

Staff used the number of minutes spent off-task engaged in tantrums or precursors as the measure of the effectiveness of this intervention. The plan had an immediate impact on this behavior, as the number of minutes off-task dropped from 64 per day to 3 per day during the first month. Unfortunately, during the second month, time spent engaging in off-task behavior began to increase. Additionally, Kyle's behavioral data became quite variable. Minutes spent off-task ranged from 0 to 18 on different days with no clear pattern. Frustrated, Josie again called for Kristen's assessment services.

This time, Kristen began her assessment with a review of the data. She decided to begin by trying to identify the sources of variability in the behavior. As was the case during baseline, tantrums did not vary by task, activity, or context. However, at this time, the behavior did not occur at all with some staff members and occurred at high rates with other staff members. Kristen shared this feedback with Josie and together they observed each staff member working with Kyle. Although some staff members were adhering very strictly to the teaching strategies dictated by Kyle's intervention plan, others fell victim to procedural drift: they were not implementing the designated procedures. Not surprisingly, those instructors delivering instruction with a high degree of procedural fidelity saw the least tantrum behavior from Kyle. In contrast, those instructors who failed to offer high-intensity attention or practice social initiation programs lost the most time on task.

To address these issues and again decrease Kyle's tantrum behaviors, Kristen and Josie agreed upon a two-pronged approach. First, all staff members were retrained on the various components of the behavior intervention plan. As part of this training, Josie videotaped herself working with Kyle, which she viewed with staff as a model of high-intensity attention. She also videotaped staff members working with Kyle. Each staff member was given her/his video and asked to complete a self-evaluation regarding the level of intensity of attention. Secondly, Kristen created a treatment integrity checklist for Josie to use to complete staff evaluations and for staff to use for self-evaluations. This checklist operationally defined each component of the plan so that adherence to this plan could be quantified. Josie used completed treatment integrity checks as a jumping off point for feedback in supervision with her staff.

Finally, with these follow-up structures in place, the plan was effective in eliminating Kyle's tantrums. This had such a profound impact on Kyle's educational performance that he progressed to a less restrictive classroom the following academic year. Decreasing the tantrums both allowed more time for skill acquisition and increased the possibility for exposure to higher functioning peers without the threat of stigmatization.

CONCLUSIONS

In this case example, many of the general principles of functional assessment described in the first part of this chapter are exemplified. First, we see the powerful impact that an effective assessment and intervention plan can have on the lives of individuals with developmental disabilities. Kyle was able to move to a less restrictive setting partially as a result of benefiting from an effective behavioral intervention plan. Next, we see the importance of linking intervention to careful, individualized assessment. Because the plan described above involved withdrawal of attention during a tantrum, which necessarily involves the withdrawal of demands, this intervention would likely have strengthened the tantrums had they been motivated by escape. In fact, the consequences utilized within Kyle's plan could only have been successful in the event that the behavior was maintained by attention. Finally, we see that multiple sources of information are often necessary to identify a behavior's communicative function. Kristen needed interview, ABC data, naturalistic observation, and systematic manipulations in order to finally recognize the pattern of variables leading to Kyle's tantrums.

This case study also highlights the challenges of completing a functional assessment and developing an effective intervention plan in an applied setting. Kristen's interviews revealed conflicting ideas about the tantrums from different staff members. Her initial functional analysis did not lead to clear results (i.e., unambiguous hypotheses about maintaining factors) and Kyle's routine had to be disrupted for two additional days whereas a second round of manipulations were run. In many settings, Kyle's teacher or parents might have refused this approach. Finally, a plan viewed to be effective initially was rendered ineffective by poor treatment integrity. Luckily, Josie had access to a skilled behavior analyst as a consultant. However, without these services in place, she might have dropped what would have been an otherwise effective intervention.

In summary, functional assessment is an invaluable methodology for identifying the motivations for challenging behaviors and their maintaining variables. Although obstacles may arise in implementing these approaches in an applied setting, with creativity and persistence, these barriers can be surmounted and a successful intervention can be devised. As a result, the lives of individuals with developmental disabilities can be significantly improved.

REFERENCES

Anderson, C. M., & Long, E. S. (2002). Use of a structured descriptive assessment methodology to identify variables affecting problem behaviors. *Journal of Applied Behavior Analysis, 35*, 137–154.

Carr, E. G. (1977). The motivation of self-injurious behavior: A review of some hypotheses. *Psychological Bulletin, 84*, 800–816.

Carr, E. G., & Durand, V. M. (1985). Reducing behavior problems through functional communication training. *Journal of Applied Behavior Analysis, 18*, 111–126.

Carr, J. E., Nicolson, A. C., & Higbe, T. S. (2000). Evaluation of a brief multiple-stimulus preference assessment in a naturalistic context. *Journal of Applied Behavior Analysis, 33*, 353–357.

Derby, K. M., Wacker, D. P., Sasso, G., Steege, M., Northup, J., Cigrand, K., et al. (1992). Brief functional assessment techniques to evaluate aberrant behavior in an outpatient setting: A summary of 79 cases. *Journal of Applied Behavior Analysis, 25*, 713–721.

Duker, P. C., Sigafoos, J., Barron, J., & Coleman, F. (1998). The Motivation Assessment Scale: Reliability and construct validity across three topographies of behavior. *Research in Developmental Disabilities, 19*, 131–141.

Dunlap, G., Kern-Dunlap, L., Clarke, S., & Robbins, F. R. (1991). Functional assessment, curricular revision, and severe behavior problems. *Journal of Applied Behavior Analysis, 24*, 387–397.

Durand, V. M., & Crimmins, D. B. (1988). Identifying the variables maintaining self-injurious behavior. *Journal of Applied Behavior Analysis, 18*, 99–117.

Fisher, W. W., Piazza, C. C., Bowman, L. G., Hagopian, L. P., Owens, J. C., & Slevin, I. (1992). A comparison of two approaches for identifying reinforcers for persons with severe and profound disabilities. *Journal of Applied Behavior Analysis, 25*, 491–498.

Fisher, W. W., Piazza, C. C., & Chiang, C. L. (1996). Effects of equal and unequal reinforcer duration during functional analysis. *Journal of Applied Behavior Analysis, 29*, 117–120.

Foster-Johnson, L., Ferro, J., & Dunlap, G. (1994). Preferred curricular activities and reduced problem behaviors in students with intellectual disabilities. *Journal of Applied Behavior Analysis, 27*, 493–504.

Gottschalk, J. M., Libby, M. E., & Graff, R. B. (2000). The effects of establishing operations on preference assessment outcomes. *Journal of Applied Behavior Analysis, 33*, 85–88.

Graff, R. B., & Libby, M. E. (1999). A comparison of presession and within-session reinforcement choice. *Journal of Applied Behavior Analysis, 32*, 161–173.

Green, C. W., Reid, D. H., Canipe, V. S., & Gardner, S. M. (1991). A comprehensive evaluation of reinforcer identification processes for persons with profound multiple handicaps. *Journal of Applied Behavior Analysis, 24*, 537–552.

Hanley, G. P., Iwata, B. A., & Lindberg, J. S. (1999). Analysis of activity preferences as a function of differential consequences. *Journal of Applied Behavior Analysis, 32*, 419–435.

Haring, T. G., & Kennedy, C. H. (1990). Contextual control of problem behavior in students with severe disabilities. *Journal of Applied Behavior Analysis, 23*, 235–243.

Iwata, B. A., Dorsey, M. F., Slifer, K. J., Bauman, K. E., & Richman, G. S. (1982). Toward a functional analysis of self-injury. *Analysis and Intervention in Developmental Disabilities, 2,* 3–20.

Iwata, B. A., Dorsey, M. F., Slifer, K. J., Bauman, K. E., & Richman, G. S. (1994). Toward a functional analysis of self-injury. *Journal of Applied Behavior Analysis, 27,* 197–209.

Iwata, B. A., Pace, G. M., Kalsher, M. J., Cowdery, G. E., & Cataldo, M. F. (1990). Experimental analysis and extinction of self-injurious escape behavior. *Journal of Applied Behavior Analysis, 23,* 11–27.

Iwata, B. A., Wallace, M. D., Kahng, S. W., Lindberg, J. S., Roscoe, E. M., Conners, J., et al. (2000). Skill acquisition in the implementation of functional analysis methodology. *Journal of Applied Behavior Analysis, 33,* 181–194.

Kahng, S. W., Hendrickson, D. J., & Vu, C. P. (2000). Comparison of single and multiple functional communication training responses for the treatment of problem behavior. *Journal of Applied behavior Analysis, 33,* 321–324.

Kahng, S. W., & Iwata, B. A. (1999). Correspondence between outcomes of brief and extended functional analyses. *Journal of Applied Behavior Analysis, 32,* 149–159.

Kennedy, C. H., & Itkonen, T. (1993). Effects of setting events on the problem behavior of students with severe disabilities. *Journal of Applied Behavior Analysis, 26,* 321–327.

Kennedy, C. H., Meyer, K. A., Knowles, T., & Shukla, S. (2000). Analyzing the multiple functions of stereotyped behavior for students with autism: Implications for assessment and treatment. *Journal of Applied Behavior Analysis, 33,* 559–571.

Kuhn, D. E., DeLeon, I. G., Fisher, W. W., & Wilke, A. E. (1999). Clarifying an ambiguous functional analysis with matched and mismatched extinction procedures. *Journal of Applied Behavior Analysis, 32,* 99–102.

Lalli, J. S., & Kates, K. (1998). The effects of reinforcer preference on functional analysis outcomes. *Journal of Applied Behavior Analysis, 31,* 79–90.

Laraway, S., Snycerski, S., Michael, J., & Poling, A. (2003). Motivating operations and terms to describe them: Some further refinements. *Journal of Applied Behavior Analysis, 36,* 407–414.

Lavie, T., & Sturmey, P. (2002). Training staff to conduct a paired-stimulus preference assessment. *Journal of Applied Behavior Analysis, 35,* 209–211.

Lerman, D. C., & Iwata, B. A. (1993). Descriptive and experimental analyses of variables maintaining self-injurious behavior. *Journal of Applied Behavior Analysis, 26,* 293–319.

Mazaleski, J. L., Iwata, B. A., Vollmer, T. R., Zarcone, J. R., & Smith, R. G. (1993). Analysis of the reinforcement and extinction components in DRO contingencies with self-injury. *Journal of Applied Behavior Analysis, 26,* 143–156.

Michael, J. (1993) Establishing operations. *The Behavior Analyst, 16,* 191–206.

Moore, J. W., Fisher, W. W., & Pennington, A. (2004). Systematic application and removal of protective equipment in the assessment of multiple topographies of self-injury. *Journal of Applied Behavior Analysis, 37,* 73–77.

Moore, J. W., Mueller, M. M., Dubard, M., Roberts, D. S., & Sterling-Turner, H. E. (2002). The influence of therapist attention on self-injury during a tangible condition. *Journal of Applied Behavior Analysis, 35,* 283–286.

Newton, J. S., Ard, W. R., & Horner, R. H. (1993). Validating predicted activity preferences of individuals with severe disabilities. *Journal of Applied Behavior Analysis, 26,* 239–245.

O'Neill, R. E., Horner, R. H., Albin, R. W., Sprague, J. R., Storey, K., & Newton, J. S. (1997). *Functional assessment and program development for problem behavior* (2nd ed.). Pacific Grove, CA: Brooks/Cole.

O'Reilly, M. F. (1995). Functional analysis and treatment of escape maintained aggression correlated with sleep deprivation. *Journal of Applied Behavior Analysis, 28,* 225–226.

Pace, G. M., Ivancic, M. T., Edwards, G. L., Iwata, B. A., & Page, T. J. (1985). Assessment of stimulus preference and reinforcer value with profoundly retarded individuals. *Journal of Applied Behavior Analysis, 18,* 249–255.

Parsons, M. B., & Reid, D. H. (1990). Assessing food preferences among persons with profound mental retardation: Providing opportunities to make choices. *Journal of Applied Behavior Analysis, 23,* 183–195.

Pelios, L., Morren, J., Tesch, D., & Axelrod, S. (1999). The impact of functional analysis methodology on treatment choices for self-injurious and aggressive behavior. *Journal of Applied Behavior Analysis, 32,* 185–195.

Piazza, C. C., Fisher, W. W., Hagopian, L. P., Bowman, L. G., & Toole, L. (1996). Using a choice assessment to predict reinforcer effectiveness. *Journal of Applied Behavior Analysis, 29,* 1–9.

Reid, D. H., Everson, J. M., & Green, C. W. (1999). A systematic evaluation of preferences identified through person-centered planning for people with profound multiple disabilities. *Journal of Applied Behavior Analysis, 32,* 467–477.

Ringdahl, J. E., & Sellers, J. A. (2000). The effects of different adults as therapists during functional analyses. *Journal of Applied Behavior Analysis, 33,* 247–250.

Ringdahl, J. E., Vollmer, T. R., Marcus, B. A., & Roane, H. S. (1997). An analogue evaluation of environmental enrichment: The role of stimulus preference. *Journal of Applied Behavior Analysis, 30,* 203–216.

Sasso, G. M., Reimers, T. M., Cooper, L. J., Wacker, D. P., Berg, W., Steege, M., et al. (1992). Use of descriptive and experimental analyses to identify the functional properties of aberrant behavior in school settings. *Journal of Applied Behavior Analysis, 25,* 809–821.

Skinner, B. F. (1957). *Verbal behavior.* New York: Appleton-Century-Crofts.

Tang, J. C., Kennedy, C. H., Koppekin, A., & Caruso, M. (2002). Functional analysis of stereotypical ear covering in a child with autism. *Journal of Applied Behavior Analysis, 35,* 95–98.

Van Camp, C. M., Lerman, D. C., Kelley, M. E., Roane, H. S., Contrucci, S. A., & Vorndran, C. M. (2000). Further analysis of idiosyncratic antecedent influences during the assessment and treatment of problem behaviors. *Journal of Applied Behavior Analysis, 33,* 207–221.

Vollmer, T. R., Marcus, B. A., & Ringdahl, J. E. (1995). Noncontingent escape as treatment for self-injurious behavior maintained by negative reinforcement. *Journal of Applied Behavior Analysis, 28,* 15–26.

Vollmer, T. R., Marcus, B. A., Ringdahl, J. E., & Roane, H. S. (1995). Progressing from brief assessment to extended experimental analyses in the evaluation of aberrant behavior. *Journal of Applied Behavior Analysis, 28,* 561–576.

Vollmer, T. R., & Vorndran, C. M. (1998). Assessment of self-injurious behavior maintained by access to self-restraint material. *Journal of Applied Behavior Analysis, 31,* 647–650.

Wacker, D. P., Berg, W. K., Asmus, J. M., Harding, J. W., & Cooper, J. L. (1998). Experimental analysis of antecedent influence on challenging behaviors. In J. K. Luiselli & M. J. Camerson (Eds.), *Antecedent control* (pp. 67–86). Baltimore, MD: Brookes.

Wacker, D. P., Harding, J., Cooper, L. J., Derby, K. M., Peck, S., Asmus, J., et al. (1996). The effects of meal schedule and quantity on problematic behavior. *Journal of Applied Behavior Analysis, 29,* 79–87.

Wallace, M. D., Doney, J. K., Mintz-Resudek, C. M., & Tarbox, R. S. F. (2004). Training educators to implement functional analyses. *Journal of Applied Behavior Analysis, 37,* 89–92.

Wallace, M. D., & Iwata, B. A. (1999). Effects of session duration on functional analysis outcomes. *Journal of Applied Behavior Analysis, 32,* 175–183.

Winborn, L., Wacker, D. P., Richman, D. M., Asmus, J., & Geier, D. (2002). Assessment of mand selection for functional communication packages. *Journal of Applied Behavior Analysis, 35,* 295–298.

Zhou, L., Iwata, B. A., Goff, G. A., & Shore, B. A. (2001). Longitudinal analysis of leisure-item preferences. *Journal of Applied Behavior Analysis, 34,* 179–184.

18

Psychoeducational Assessment

CAROLINE I. MAGYAR, VINCENT PANDOLFI, and CHRISTINE R. PETERSON

Students with developmental disabilities (DD) display characteristics that present unique challenges to practitioners conducting psychoeducational assessments. Developmental characteristics can vary widely across disorders and among individuals with the same disorder. Evaluators must be prepared to respond appropriately to unique needs so that assessments validly inform educational decision-making for identified students. This requires a thorough understanding of how various psychoeducational assessment practices contribute to the decision-making process for students with disabilities. This chapter reviews the process and issues affecting the psychoeducational assessment of students with DD and the importance of linking assessment outcomes to intervention.

School psychologists often do not receive sufficient training in DD, making the identification of an appropriate assessment protocol difficult (e.g., Drotar & Sturm, 1996). Given the paucity of research in best assessment practices with students with DD, a pragmatic approach needs to be articulated for selecting an appropriate assessment protocol. Although many assessment procedures discussed in this chapter likely represent best practices for any student, they are critical for students with DD. The assessment protocol selected depends on the referral question and type of information needed for decision-making. The following discussion presents an overview of assessment considerations relevant to DD, preservice

CAROLINE I. MAGYAR • Strong Center for Developmental Disabilities and STAART Center, School of Medicine and Dentistry, University of Rochester, Rochester, New York 14642. **VINCENT PANDOLFI** • School Psychology Program, College of Liberal Arts, Rochester Institute of Technology, Rochester, New York 14623-5604.   **CHRISTINE R. PETERSON** • Strong Center for Developmental Disabilities, School of Medicine and Dentistry, University of Rochester, Rochester, New York 14642.

training issues relevant to school psychologists, and the contributions and limitations of various assessment practices to educational decision-making.

DEVELOPMENTAL DISABILITY

General Characteristics

DD constitute a heterogeneous group of disorders (Developmental Disabilities Assistance and Bill of Rights Act of 2000) and this book focuses on five broad types of DD including pervasive developmental disorder, cerebral palsy, epilepsy, intellectual disability (ID), and developmental and traumatic neurological impairment. Although these disorders have different etiologies and behavioral phenotypes, most if not all students with DD will demonstrate difficulty in one or more areas of language and communication, cognition, motor skills, sensory processing, and behavior. Deficits in these areas can impact the individual's ability to attend, concentrate, and sustain performance on tasks. Many students with DD also present with comorbid disorders such as anxiety, depression, and visual or auditory impairments. The presence of a comorbid condition can extend the range of difficulties the individual might have as a result of the primary disorder. These difficulties often interfere with academic achievement, the development of adaptive skills, and social relationships. Like many individuals, students with DD also experience ongoing personal and social challenges related to aging and development that require systematic assessment over time.

Best Assessment Practices

Best practices in psychoeducational assessment for all students suggest that assessment be comprehensive and include more than one set of valid evaluation measures. The measures must be selected and administered in a nondiscriminatory manner that considers the student's individual communication abilities. Before evaluating a student with special needs, the evaluator should assess the student for the presence of specific communication difficulties and preferred mode of communication (e.g., vocal speech, sign, and communication device). The evaluator should also identify the student's specific disorder(s) and ensure that his or her physical condition and health status have been examined. This information guides the evaluator in the selection of tests, the process of assessment, and any special accommodations used to make the assessment results more meaningful and useful for developing interventions. An idiographic assessment is indicated to profile both the relative strengths and needs of the student and to generate information used for designing appropriate intervention programs. A strength-based approach, rather than a strict deficit model approach to assessing students with DD is preferred. Identifying strengths helps determine starting points for intervention and the preferred modalities through which instruction is delivered (e.g., visually based methodologies for learners with significant communication deficits).

General Considerations in Assessing Students with DD

The following is a list of suggestions to assist the practitioner in assessing students with developmental disorders (Shontz, 1977; Wright, 1983):

- Become familiar with the identified student's specific disorder(s).
- Be prepared to work at establishing rapport.
- Plan on many, brief testing sessions, if required. Monitor the student for fatigue, frustration, and attention.
- Ensure that the student uses any adaptive equipment that is routinely used, including alternative or augmentative communication devices.
- Ensure that the student understands your questions, directions, and instructions.
- Listen carefully to the student, especially when assessing students with significant expressive or articulation deficits.
- Be sensitive to the lighting in the room, ambient temperature, the positioning of the student with regard to his or her physical limitations to maximize physical comfort and provide appropriate access to testing materials.
- Incorporate visual aids for additional support, especially for students with an autism spectrum disorder or a traumatic brain injury. Visual aids include picture symbols, photographs, written words, and gestures. They can inform the student about the sequence of events in the testing situation, signal a change in activity, and prompt the student for attending skills (e.g., "look and listen").
- Incorporate positive reinforcement into the testing situation. Determine student preferences in advance, through interview and/or observation, and attempt to use the preferred stimuli to maximize motivation and task engagement. Implement the student's existing behavior support strategies where applicable to maximize test performance.

PSYCHOEDUCATIONAL ASSESSMENT

Definition and Conceptualization

Psychoeducational assessment refers to a process of collecting information on a student's skills, performance, learning history, and instructional context, in order to make decisions about what supports and interventions might be needed for that student (Salvia & Ysseldyke, 1978). It can be broadly conceptualized as the process of effective problem solving: (a) determining the referral question, "What information do we need to know?"; (b) deciding on the most efficient and effective methods of assessment, "How can we get the necessary information?"; and (c) using the results to develop an effective academic and/or behavioral intervention plan, "How do we use the information?". There are at least five specific reasons for conducting a psychoeducational assessment: screening, placement, intervention planning, intervention evaluation, and measurement of student progress.

When evaluating students with DD, a traditional "discrepancy-focused" model of assessment (e.g., IQ vs. academic scores) may be inadequate. Rather, a functional, competency-based assessment should be used to gather information on self-help skills, social skills, independence, and community living skills, in addition to information on academic performance. The assessment should include direct measurement of the student's behavior (e.g., behavioral observations, standardized testing, curriculum-based assessment) and indirect measurement (e.g., interviews and rating scales completed by the student or key informants). This multi-method assessment process is necessary to obtain information across developmental domains to facilitate valid educational decision-making and strength-based intervention planning.

Personnel Preparation

The unique characteristics of students with DD require the evaluator to be specifically trained in assessment of this population and to be familiar with the potential contributions and limitations of each test or assessment method used in educational decision-making for a particular student. Although child clinical psychologists and pediatric psychologists conduct psychological assessments of children with DD (Drotar & Strum, 1996), school psychologists are often the primary providers of psychoeducational assessments for school-aged children. Unfortunately, little published literature supports consistency among school psychology graduate programs in their training of students in the assessment and treatment of specific populations of disabled students. According to the graduate training guidelines set forth by the National Association of School Psychologists (NASP) in their *Standards for Training and Field Placement in School Psychology* (NASP, 2000), educational programs will produce professionals trained in a broad range of assessment, consultation, intervention, and professional skills described as "building blocks for effective practice" (p. 6). Although these domain driven guidelines provide educational training programs with a general "blueprint" or outline for broad-based skill development for professional competency, they do not provide specific skill-based competencies or address the application of such skills to individuals with DD.

Training programs, therefore, are generally challenged to prepare qualified professionals to conduct well-planned and executed psychoeducational assessments with lower incidence populations including learners from culturally and linguistically diverse backgrounds, individuals with traumatic brain injury, and individuals with DD (e.g., Walker, Boling, & Cobb, 1999). Surveys of school psychology practitioners and faculty over the last decade reveal a rather static pattern of training and practice that emphasizes the use of more traditional assessment measures (e.g., standardized intelligence tests), apparently without regard to the specific referral questions or unique characteristics of the student to be evaluated (Haney & Evans, 1999; Wilson & Reschly, 1996). Less traditional assessment measures are not likely to be used either in place of or in addition to norm-referenced measures, with some exceptions noted at the preschool level (Riccio, Houston, & Harrison, 1998). Particularly amid ever-evolving federal mandates such as the Individuals with Disabilities Education Act Amendments of 1997 (IDEA) and Individuals with Disabilities Education Improvement Act of 2004 (IDEA), which call for more accountability in making the link from assessment to intervention for diverse learners there is growing criticism within the professional community that there has been a slow reaction on the part of university-based training programs in incorporating less traditional methods of assessment (e.g., curriculum-based assessment, dynamic assessment, functional behavior assessment [FBA]) into school psychology curriculums and field experience requirements. Such "alternative" methods have been found particularly beneficial for use in developing effective intervention plans, as well as in enriching information gathered in evaluations that utilize more traditional methods. Although research indicates that these less traditional methods of assessment have gained slightly more prominence in training programs and in use with practitioners over the last two decades, changes have been very slow to occur (Wilson & Reschly, 1996). And, with the emphasis on performance-based assessments in the Reauthorization of IDEA (2004) school psychologists may require continuing education to acquire competencies in alternative assessment methods in order to meet new assessment mandates.

ASSESSMENT METHODS

The review below discusses the strengths and limitations of norm- and criterion-referenced testing, curriculum-based assessment, and FBA in educational decision-making for students with DD. The type of tests used in a particular assessment protocol depends on the referral question. Some tests address multiple purposes, whereas others might be used for a specific purpose (Salvia & Ysseldyke, 1978).

Norm-Referenced Testing

Norm-referenced testing is one of the most commonly used methods of evaluating students. Its uses include identifying learning or behavioral disabilities, determining eligibility for special services, and for making placement decisions. Norm-referenced tests feature standardized test instructions and scoring procedures used with every examinee regardless of ability or handicapping condition. They provide information about the student's performance in relation to a representative sample of same age or same grade peers, rather than mastery of a particular content area. Conclusions regarding relative standing are valid to the extent that standardized procedures are followed. Many times, the unique characteristics of students with DD require modifications to test administration procedures. This limits the validity of obtained test scores because of departures from standardized procedures for test administration.

Samples of the more commonly used norm-referenced tests for assessing intelligence, academic achievement, and adaptive behavior are presented below. The review is not meant to be exhaustive and is presented to identify characteristics of tests that pertain to specific purposes of psychoeducational assessment of students with DD. Our review suggests that norm-referenced tests have utility in screening, diagnosis, and classification, but they provide less information on how students learn or what types of interventions are useful in the remediation of specific learning or behavior problems.

Intelligence Tests

Traditional norm-referenced intelligence tests have not been substantially influenced by theory, and some argue that they offer an incomplete account of intelligence (e.g., Das & Naglieri, 1996). Reschly and Wilson (1990) indicated that empirical data are needed to substantiate the treatment validity of these traditional tests as well as newer tests such as the Cognitive Assessment System (CAS; Naglieri & Das, 1997) that are based on theories of cognitive processing. As a new measure of cognitive processing, the CAS has apparently not gained widespread acceptance and more research is needed to evaluate its clinical utility (Sattler, 2001).

Comprehensive reviews of the psychometric properties of norm-referenced intelligence tests exist elsewhere (e.g., Salvia & Ysseldyke, 2001; Sattler, 2001) and this section discusses characteristics of commonly used tests that should be considered by practitioners when preparing to test an individual with a developmental disability. Table 18.1 presents the targeted age range of commonly used instruments, the skills, and abilities they purport to assess, and their role in educational decision-making.

The intelligence tests in Table 18.1 appear adequately suited to screen cognitive functioning; however, the instruments vary in their usefulness for placement and instructional planning decisions, and have limited utility for student outcome evaluations. For preschool age children, the relatively high floors of the Differential Ability Scales (DAS; Elliot, 1990a, 1990b) might not permit adequate discrimination between students functioning below the upper moderate/mild range of deficiency on the Verbal Ability scale and for school age children on the Verbal, Nonverbal, and Spatial scales. Out of level testing allows for an extrapolation downward into estimates of severe ID (see DAS manual for specifics across age ranges). Concerns for high floors also exist for individuals functioning below the moderate range of ID tested with the Mullen Scales of Early Learning (Mullen, 1995), WISC-III (Wechsler, 1991), WISC-IV (Wechsler, 2003), WPPSI-R (Wechsler, 1989), WPPSI-III (Wechsler, 2002), WAIS-III (Wechsler, 1997), and Stanford–Binet Fifth Edition (Roid, 2003). Insufficient floors for subtest or composite scores require additional data collection from

Table 18.1. Norm-referenced Tests Used in Educational Decision-Making for Students with Developmental Disabilities

Tests	Age range	Skills/abilities assessed	Role in educational decision-making
Intelligence			
CAS	5 years 0 months to 17 years 0 months	Planning, attention, simultaneous processing, successive processing	These tests are generally well suited for screening and placement decisions for persons at or above the moderate range of intellectual disability. They are useful for identifying general targets for instruction, but have more limited utility for comprehensive instructional planning and outcome evaluation
DAS	2 years 6 months to 17 years 11 months	General ability, verbal, nonverbal, spatial	
Mullen scales	0 to 69 months	General ability, expressive and receptive language, visual reasoning, motor skills	
WPPSI-III	2 years 6 months to 7 years 3 months	General ability, verbal, performance, processing speed, general language composite	
WISC-IV	6 years 0 months to 16 years 11 months	General ability, verbal comprehension, perceptual reasoning, working memory, processing speed	
WAIS-III	16 years 0 months to 89 years	General ability, verbal comprehension, perceptual organization, working memory, processing speed	
Stanford–Binet, 5th ed.	2 years 0 months to >90 years	Verbal/nonverbal fluid reasoning, knowledge, quantitative reasoning, visual–spatial processing, working memory	
Academic achievement			
PIAT-R	Kindergarten to 12th grade	Information, math, reading comprehension/recognition, spelling, writing	These tests have limited utility for students with intellectual disabilities
WIAT-II	4 years 0 months to 85 years	Reading, math, written, and oral language	
Adaptive behavior			
Vineland	0 years to 18 years 11 months	Communication, daily living skills, socialization, motor, maladaptive behavior (birth to 5:11)	These tests are adequate for screening. Can assist in beginning instructional planning. More limited utility for placement and outcome evaluation

(cont.)

Table 18.1. (*Continued*)

Tests	Age range	Skills/abilities assessed	Role in educational decision-making
SIB-R	0 to >80 years	Motor, social interaction and communication, personal living, problems behaviors	
AAMR ABS-S:2	3 years 0 months to 18 years 11 months	Scales personal self-sufficiency, community self-sufficiency, personal-social responsibility, social adjustment, personal adjustment	
ABS-RC:2	18 years 0 months to 79 years	Same as ABS-S:2	
ABAS-II	0 to 89 years	Conceptual, social, and practical	

curriculum-based assessment devices (discussed below) or adaptive be-havior inventories to accurately estimate the present level of a student's cognitive functioning and to help determine the most appropriate educa-tional placement and subsequent intervention planning.

Several abbreviated measures of intelligence are available (e.g., Kaufman Brief Intelligence Test—K-BIT, Kaufman & Kaufman, 1990; Wechsler Abbreviated Scale of Intelligence—WASI, The Psychological Corporation, 1999). These tests sample a narrow range of intellectual abili-ties, often two or four ability areas, but allow the examiner to estimate over-all intelligence of an examinee in a short amount of time. Given their narrow focus however, abbreviated measures are not considered appropriate for initial diagnostic and educational classification decisions for any student.

Referencing test composites and subscales supports decision-making regarding the targeting of skills for instruction and intervention. A test's composites and subscales indicate the constructs the test purports to mea-sure; however, empirical data are required to support the construct valid-ity of the scales. Except for the Mullen Early Learning Composite and DAS one-factor model at ages 2–6 to 3–5, Sattler (2001) reported that multifactor models for the CAS, DAS, WPPSI-R, WISC-III, and WAIS-III have empirical support. Technical manuals for the WPPSI-III, WISC-IV, and Stanford–Binet Fifth Edition present data supporting multifactor models but the field awaits convergent data from independent samples. Measuring differ-entiated abilities (e.g., verbal and nonverbal abilities) not only provides for broad-based assessment but is also important in the assessment of students with DD that prevent them from participating adequately in one or more intellectual tasks (e.g., verbal expression or reception). Consult-ing each test's technical manual, and empirically based reviews, such as Sattler (2001) and Salvia and Ysseldyke (2001), assists in determining the appropriateness of identifying specific intervention targets based on composite scaled scores or subtest scaled scores purporting to measure specific abilities within the broader composites (e.g., consulting subtest specificity data).

Although the norm-referenced intelligence tests appear adequately suited for identifying cognitive profiles and general intervention targets, they are limited in their usefulness for further instructional planning and assessing student outcome. These tests might guide the selection of curricular content, but they will not specify instructional scope or sequence. Results from a norm-referenced intelligence test do not provide sufficient information about effective teaching methods for a particular student. Retesting a student, on an annual or triennial basis, might not reveal significant changes in scores, in part because scaled scores are age or grade normed (however, changes in raw scores might be of interest on some measures). These tests will not reveal information regarding response to instructional approaches, advancement in a curriculum, degree of independence in learning activities, and required environmental and behavioral support. In addition, the range of scores available on composites and subscales might not be equivalent across the age range, making year-to-year comparisons difficult to interpret. Thus, educators should not rely exclusively on changes in intelligence test scores as an outcome index.

Achievement Tests

Norm-referenced achievement tests are often used in conjunction with intelligence tests to identify learning disabilities. Test content samples a cross section of various curricula used in schools throughout the United States but might not adequately sample the curriculum to which the student has been exposed. Moreover, these tests provide little direct information as to which instructional and behavioral supports need to be in place for the student to both acquire and display knowledge. Two commonly used tests include the Wechsler Individual Achievement Test—2nd Edition (WIAT-II, Psychological Corporation, 2001) and the Peabody Individual Achievement Test—Revised/Normative Update (PIAT-R/NU, Markwardt, 1997). The WIAT-II appears to sample a wider range of academic content and may be useful as a broad screen of academic achievement, whereas the multiple choice response format for the majority of the subtests on the PIAT-R makes it useful for assessing students with poor expressive language ability (Sattler, 2001). However, as norm-referenced tests, they can pose limitations for educational decision-making similar to those for the norm-referenced intelligence tests (e.g., high subtest floors, nonuniformity of scores across the age range).

Adaptive Behavior Scales

Sattler (2002) and Salvia and Ysseldyke (2001) reviewed commonly used measures of adaptive behavior and their psychometric properties. Most scales reviewed were developed prior to the American Association on Mental Retardation (AAMR, 2002) revised definition of mental re-tardation. Aside from intellectual impairment, adaptive behavior deficits across one or more areas of conceptual skills (e.g., language skills, money concepts, time), social skills (e.g., interpersonal skills, rule-following), and practical skills (e.g., activities of daily living, occupational skills) must exist for a diagnosis of intellectual disability. The more commonly used norm-referenced adaptive behavior measures include the Vineland Adaptive Behavior Scales (Sparrow, Balla, & Cicchetti, 1984), the AAMR Adaptive Behavior Scales (School, 2nd edition; Lambert, Nihira, & Leland, 1993; Residential and Community, 2nd edition; Nihira, Leland, & Lambert, 1993), the Scales of Independent Behavior—Revised (Bruininks, Woodcock, Weatherman, & Hill, 1996), and the Adaptive Behavior Assessment System, 2nd edition (ABAS-II; Harrison & Oakland, 2003). Each test samples behaviors from the AAMR categories; however, only the ABAS-II is organized under AAMR's conceptual, social, and practical framework.

Aside from general concerns with norm-referenced testing, additional caveats regarding adaptive behavior assessment are offered. Adaptive be-havior is conceptualized differently across diagnostic and classification systems (see Reschly, Myers, & Hartel, 2002, and Simeonsson & Short, 1996, for excellent reviews). The assessor should select an assessment in-strument appropriate to the age, functioning level, and context in which the examinee functions as the breadth of adaptive domains and specific behav-iors sampled will likely vary as a function of these variables (Reschly et al., 2002). In addition, research indicates low correlations between teacher and parent ratings of adaptive behavior (Sattler, 2002); therefore, data should be collected from the home and school environments to capture differential performance that might be a function of the setting or informant bias. Data collected by these instruments represent the frequency at which an individ-ual typically performs specific behaviors, or in some instances the quality of that performance (e.g., fluency); however, information is often not provided to help the evaluator distinguish between skill-based and motivation-based performance deficits across settings. Thus, there is a need for the func-tional assessment of adaptive repertoires. For skill-based deficits, adaptive behavior samples indicated on the record forms are broad-based and offer a useful starting place to develop performance-based goals, akin to curricu-lum objectives. The data, however, will not inform the assessor as to how the student will best learn new skills; thus task analyses of instructional targets and a teaching methodology must be developed and directly applied to determine baseline performance of any given student. With respect to motivational deficits, functional assessment of interfering behaviors and identification of potential reinforcers (i.e., motivation) via preference as-sessments become essential elements of the evaluation process in order to determine the appropriate behavioral supports that will maximize student learning.

Criterion-Referenced Testing

Criterion-referenced tests measure a student's skill development in terms of mastery of particular skills or concepts. Comparisons are made against an absolute standard reflecting skill acquisition, rather than against a normative group of peers as in norm-referenced assessment (Shapiro, 1996). Scores are interpreted by determining whether the obtained score meets a preestablished standard (criterion) reflecting mastery of a targeted skill. Criterion-referenced instruments may be used for screening for potential learning problems, and for identifying target areas for subsequent educational intervention. They can also be used to identify the specific strengths and weaknesses of a student's academic profile (Shapiro, 1996). Criterion-referenced tests can be either commercially available (e.g., Brigance Inventories; Brigance, 1977, 1978, 1981) or teacher made (often referred to as 'informal tests'). Although criterion-referenced tests are widely used to monitor student progress, they are generally limited in their usefulness in educational classification and in developing specific intervention strategies.

Curriculum-Based Assessment

Curriculum-based assessment (CBA; Gickling, Shane, & Croskery, 1989) is a method of assessment of student knowledge, skills, and abilities that links assessment results to instruction. It can be used for the ongoing monitoring of student performance relative to self and peers receiving the same instruction (Deno, 1985). CBA's ecological perspective focuses on assessing the student's performance within the local curriculum, the quality of the instruction received, and the instructional methods used by the teacher. CBA also assesses the student's skill and motivation for learning tasks, as well as the learning environment in order to determine its relationship to identified learning difficulties (Lentz & Shapiro, 1986).

The strengths of CBA are clearly in linking assessment to instruction, and providing a method for monitoring student performance. Although limited in its usefulness for eligibility determination and making placement decisions, this method of assessment may provide the most comprehensive method for assessing the ongoing performance of students with DD. It provides the most direct measurement of a student's academic progress and assists in identifying the functional relationships among the student's skill, the learning environment, and motivation to learn. The information gathered from a CBA can be used to adjust instruction, modify curriculum, and develop behavior support plans that increase the student's motivation to learn.

Functional Behavior Assessment

The unique cognitive, behavioral, and physical characteristics of individuals with DD make accurate diagnosis of behavioral disorders more challenging. Further, there has been concern as to whether topographically based assessment systems (e.g., *DSM-IV*, American Psychiatric Association, 1994) and functional assessment clearly demonstrate treatment utility (e.g., Kratochwill & Plunge, 1992). The Carr et al. (1999) research synthesis on positive behavior support for individuals with DD provided empirical evidence for enhanced treatment utility when behavioral interventions are based on an FBA. FBA is a type of ecological inventory designed to identify behavior–environment relationships. For students with DD, the FBA is an important part of the psychoeducational assessment process and has direct relevance to his or her educational programming. Thus, the following discussion focuses on FBA and the reader is referred elsewhere for information on norm-referenced behavioral (i.e., behavior rating scales) and diagnostic assessment for students with DD (e.g., Reschly et al., 2002).

O'Neill et al. (1997) specified five important outcomes of the FBA: (a) an objective description of the problem behavior; (b) the identification of variables predicting the occurrence and nonoccurrence of problem behavior; (c) the identification of consequences maintaining the behavior; (d) the development of hypotheses regarding behavioral function (e.g., attention, tangible-seeking, avoidance/escape, sensory stimulation); and (e) data supporting the hypotheses. Best practice calls for FBAs to be comprising a combination of both direct and indirect (e.g., interviews, rating scales) observations. This approach directly ties student needs with precise dictates for evaluation, behavioral support, and instructional planning.

Evaluative procedures include the analysis of medical conditions related to problem behaviors, behavioral excesses, and behavioral deficits (Kanfer & Saslow, 1969), as well as problems with stimulus control. *Behavioral excesses* are behaviors that occur too often, with too much intensity or duration, or are not considered socially appropriate (e.g., self-injury, aggression, self-stimulation). *Behavioral deficits* are behaviors that occur with insufficient frequency, intensity, or duration, or with inadequate topography (e.g., social withdrawal, poor coping skills, and underdeveloped play skills). Problems with *stimulus control* refer to behaviors that occur at the wrong time or place (e.g., talking during teacher-directed instruction, wandering about the classroom during lessons). These problems can interfere with a student's ability to learn from the educational intervention or participate in the least restrictive educational setting; therefore, these behaviors need to be evaluated for intervention.

Assessment-based behavior support and intervention plans (BSIPs) are generated from the FBA and should be a part of the student's IEP. BSIPs identify (a) targeted behaviors for reduction or elimination; (b) proactive skills instruction procedures (e.g., social skills, coping skills, self-management instruction) for replacement or alternative skill development; (c) antecedent or environmental alterations (e.g., modifying task demands, instituting predictable daily schedules); (d) consequence strategies to strengthen functionally equivalent alternative skills that support appropriate academic and social engagement; and (e) methods for data collection and performance evaluation. Findings from an FBA may also indicate useful modifications of general classroom management practices (e.g., frequency and method for displaying and reviewing classroom rules, frequency of teacher-delivered reinforcement) or changes in instructional methods (e.g., providing a visual model of the task to be completed, modifying teaching materials to contain fewer math problems per page) that may have broad impact on a student's learning.

At this writing, in early 2004, IDEA mandates schools to conduct an FBA when a student's behavior results in his or her removal from the current educational placement for more than 10 school days in an academic year or when the school commences a removal that constitutes a change in placement (Turnbull, Wilcox, Stowe, & Turnbull, 2001). However, the 2004 Reauthorization of IDEA has modified language regarding discipline and manifest determination, but final federal regulation is necessary to determine what specific changes may be required with regard to FBA in the school.

LINKING ASSESSMENT TO INTERVENTION

Process and Practice

Assessment should include the selection of instruments that will adequately measure the behavior(s) of interest, the instructional setting, instructional methods, and curriculum. A comprehensive support plan can then be developed that will assist the student in learning and performing more effectively in the least restrictive environment. Students with a DD are likely to require multiple objectives in many developmental areas.

But, how do you translate assessment results to intervention? Translation of assessment results into instructional planning requires multidisciplinary input. Educational teams often consist of the primary educator, related service providers, and family members. Together, evaluators translate results into targeted interventions to meet student needs and valued family outcomes. Intervention begins by summarizing the assessment results into goal statements and then translating those goal statements into measurable objectives. Once objectives have been identified, instructional methods and curricula are identified. The methods and curricula chosen should be directly related to the acquisition of the skill(s) stated in the objective. Thus, the method chosen for the establishment of one skill may not be the method chosen for the development of another. For example, an instructor may choose task analysis with graduated guidance to teach a student with ID how to wash his hands, but may use direct instruction with scripting to teach the same student some basic social skills (see Davis & Rehfeldt, this volume). The educational team is ultimately responsible for the ongoing assessment of the student's response to the intervention plan and any needed modifications, such as changes in instructional strategies.

Below is a case example of a psychoeducational assessment of a student with autism that demonstrates the use of assessment for educational planning. A list of the instruments used in the assessment protocol and a rationale for choosing each instrument is provided. Following that, a description of the recommended intervention plan is provided that demonstrates the linking of assessment results into specific educational planning for the student.

CASE EXAMPLE

"Mark," a 5-year and 1-month-old student with autism, is preparing to transition from home-based special education and speech services into a school placement. He is a verbal child who shows interest in others, but is described as having great difficulty around other children with joining in, sharing and taking turns, and maintaining conversations. There are also questions as to how well he uses language. His parents describe him as using "a lot of language" at home; however special educators working with Mark in the home report that he most often repeats phrases from his favorite television shows and movies, both in a repetitive fashion and to communicate wants and needs. An evaluation was requested to help determine the most appropriate school-based supports for Mark. The following question was of primary interest to the educational team, "Where is Mark functioning developmentally?"

Given the nature of the referral question as well as Mark's age, the Mullen Scales of Early Learning was used to assess language, motor, and basic preacademic skills. The MacArthur Communicative Developmental Inventory (Fenson et al., 1993) was completed by Mark's parents to assess his use of language. The Vineland Adaptive Behavior Scales—Interview Form was administered to the parents to assess Mark's independence and adaptive functioning across daily living, socialization, communication, and motor-skill domains. As young children with autism generally display better developed nonverbal reasoning skills than language processing skills, a more detailed analysis of Mark's nonverbal skills was to be assessed using the Leiter International Performance Scale—Revised (Roid & Miller, 1997) at a later date. Parent semi-structured interview and observation of Mark in the home setting were also completed.

Assessment results identified areas for intervention across all developmental domains. Results of the Mullen yielded an Early Learning Composite standard score of 64, indicating that Mark was functioning within the mild range of intellectual disability. Results indicated visual reception skills at an age-equivalent of 3 years, 2 months. For example, he was able to match by shape alone, but not by size and color combined, and he was not able to match most letters and words presented. Mark displayed a relative strength in his expressive language skills, which were assessed at the 3-year, 7-month age equivalent, compared to his receptive understanding, which was assessed at the 2-year, 11-month age equivalent. Findings of the McArthur were consistent with results of the Mullen's language subscales, as his parents reported a rather extensive labeling vocabulary (e.g., nouns, adjectives, and verbs) but poor ability to comprehend simple two or more step direction. Pragmatic language skills and ability to communicate wants and needs effectively were reportedly even less well developed than were basic language skills. Results on the Communication and Socialization domains of the Vineland indicated skill deficits in both areas. Further evidence of Mark's reported difficulty with pragmatics was noted during the assessment as evidenced by his attempt to engage the evaluator socially by using verbal scripts that were repeated several times during the assessment (e.g., "Hey, you see that?" to draw attention; "You want more?" to make a request), but were not consistent with the social context.

With regard to daily living skills, results from the Vineland's Daily Living Skills domain indicated that Mark required parental assistance to complete grooming and hygiene activities. Moreover, a general lack of compliance with completing these activities often resulted in a "power struggle" between him and his parents. Progress with toilet training has reportedly been very slow, with behavioral difficulties recently emerging (e.g., flopping to the ground when asked to go to the bathroom; crying when sitting on the toilet). A recommendation was made for an FBA to be completed to determine the motivational issues interfering with successful grooming and hygiene behaviors.

Results of the psychoeducational assessment helped identify the most appropriate educational supports, which included a recommendation for an educational setting, initial instructional targets, and corresponding teaching methods. On the basis of these results, the team concluded that Mark would benefit from a self-contained special education kindergarten with a low teacher-to-student ratio. Given the level of assistance required with such tasks as toileting, dressing, and eating, as described by the Vineland, Mark would likely need significant adult support in the school setting that might include a 1:1 aide, to assist him in acquiring and applying the necessary skills to be successful in the classroom setting. Given Mark's significant receptive language difficulties, instruction should occur in a highly structured fashion, with opportunities for 1:1 direct instruction and discrimination training for new and difficult concepts (e.g., attributes, functions, classes of objects). Newly acquired concepts should be generalized to small group settings.

To assist with the development of independent daily living and classroom readiness skills, specific skills should be prioritized on the basis of assessment results and taught sequentially, using direct instruction methods and prompt and reinforce procedures. For example, a visual system could be developed that includes visual cues for prompting discrete classroom skills (e.g., waiting in line, raising hand in group) and behavior chains (e.g., common classroom routines such as arriving to school, lining up and preparing for lunch) and a token system for reinforcing correct skills application. Additionally, a picture schedule of his daily activities could enhance Mark's independence in following the daily classroom routine (i.e., transitioning from one activity to the next). A data collection system should be developed to track progress with regard to skill acquisition and application in targeted and generalized settings.

To assist Mark with developing social communication skills (i.e., social skills and pragmatic language skills), social skills training using a direct instruction method with script fading should be implemented in a systematic manner. Direct instruction would be useful in developing specific social behaviors (e.g., joining in) and scripts would be useful in assisting Mark to acquire the necessary language associated with the social skill. In addition, social stories could be incorporated into the training sessions to increase Mark's understanding of the social context in which the social skills will be applied. Peer-mediated strategies should be included as part of the intervention plan for teaching and generalizing peer social interaction across settings, as these strategies will enhance the likelihood that acquired skills will transfer across settings and be maintained within the generalized setting(s). Finally, opportunities for inclusion with typically developing peers in the general education kindergarten should be planned for and initiated when appropriate, with the assistance of a 1:1 aide for support in targeted skill application (e.g., group participation skills, social skills). Additional assessment using curriculum-based checklists, rating scales, and direct observation of initiations, responses, and turn-taking in conversation may be necessary to assist in prioritizing targets for social skills training.

In sum, all the aforementioned interventions will require ongoing assessment to ascertain their effectiveness. Therefore, direct observation methods should be used to continually assess discrete skill acquisition and performance (e.g., new language concepts, social skills, daily living skills). Data collected should be analyzed and used to make modifications to skills training programs. In addition, criterion-referenced testing and curriculum-based assessment methods should be used to assess academic progress and to inform revision or modification to curriculum or instructional methods.

CONCLUSION

Students with DD present unique challenges to the psychoeducational assessment process. Psychoeducational assessment can be conceptualized as effective and efficient problem solving for student needs, to provide them with educational benefit in the least restrictive setting, as mandated by IDEA. Achieving this end requires familiarity with the unique needs of students with low incidence disabilities and understanding the contributions of different assessment methods to various educational decision-making priorities.

A functional, competency-based assessment is indicated for students with DD and must include both direct and indirect measurement of relevant behaviors. Assessment results not only contain information regarding a student's standing on skills in relation to age- or grade-level peers, but must also be translated into measurable goals and objectives with effective individualized instructional methods and curricular selection.

Although NASP training guidelines for school psychologists represent a general "blueprint" for training, they fall short of specific competencies required for professionals working with students with DD. Preservice training programs and applied researchers are challenged to keep pace with shifts in professional practice and federal policy favoring inclusive education, as well as proactive approaches to instruction and behavior support. With increasing numbers of students with disabilities participating in general education classrooms, the capacity-building efforts of schools need to be directed at (a) identifying the knowledge, skills, and abilities of their personnel to implement effective instruction and behavior support for students with disabilities; and (b) developing or refining organizational resources and processes to support multidisciplinary assessment practices directly linked to intervention. Preservice programs can assist this effort by preparing trainees to apply research-validated behavior intervention practices and best practices in assessment for students with DD. Finally, more research is needed on the effects that testing accommodations have on the validity of norm-referenced assessment and on the differential utility of various assessment procedures in developing effective educational programs.

REFERENCES

American Association on Mental Retardation. (2002). *Mental retardation: Definition, classification, and systems of support* (10th ed.). Washington, DC: Author.

American Psychiatric Association. (1994). *Diagnostic and statistical manual of mental disorders* (4th ed.). Washington, DC: Author.

Brigance, A. (1977). *Brigance Diagnostic Inventory of Basic Skills.* North Billerica, MA: Curriculum Associates.

Brigance, A. (1978). *Brigance Inventory of Early Skills.* North Billerica, MA: Curriculum Associates.

Brigance, A. (1981). *Brigance Diagnostic Inventory of Essential Skills.* North Billerica, MA: Curriculum Associates.

Bruininks, R. H., Woodcock, R., Weatherman, R., & Hill, B. (1996). *Scales of Independent Behavior—Revised.* Chicago, IL: Riverside.

Carr, E. G., Horner, R. H., Turnbull, A. P., Marquis, J. G., McLaughlin, D. M., & McAtee, M. L. (1999). *Positive behavior support for people with developmental disabilities: A research synthesis.* Washington, DC: American Association on Mental Retardation.

Das, J. P., & Naglieri, J. A. (1996). Mental retardation and assessment of cognitive processes. In J. W. Jacobson & J. A. Mulick (Eds.), *Manual of diagnosis and professional practice in mental retardation* (pp. 115–126). Washington, DC: American Psychological Association.

Davis, P. K., & Rehfeldt, R. A. (2006). Functional skills training for people with intellectual and developmental disabilities. In J. W. Jacobson, J. A. Mulick, & J. Rojahn (Eds.), *Handbook of intellectual and developmental disabilities* (pp. xxx). New York: Springer.

Deno, S. L. (1985). Curriculum-based measurement: The emerging alternative. *Exceptional Children, 52,* 219–232.

Drotar, D. D., & Sturm, L. A. (1996). Interdisciplinary collaboration in the practice of mental retardation. In J. W. Jacobson & J. A. Mulick (Eds.), *Manual of diagnosis and professional practice in mental retardation* (pp. 393–401). Washington, DC: American Psychological Association.

Elliot, C. D. (1990a). *DAS administration and scoring manual.* San Antonio, TX: The Psychological Corporation.

Elliot, C. D. (1990b). *DAS introductory and technical handbook.* San Antonio, TX: The Psychological Corporation.

Fenson, L., Dale, P. S., Reznick, J. S., Thal, D., Bates, E., & Hartung, J. P. (1993). *MacArthur Communicative Development Inventories: Users guide and technical manual.* San Diego, CA: Singular Publishing.

Gickling, E. E., Shane, R. L., & Croskery, K. M. (1989). Developing mathematics skills in low achieving high school students through curriculum-based assessment. *School Psychology Review, 18,* 344–355.

Haney, M. R., & Evans, J. G. (1999). National survey of school psychologists regarding use of dynamic assessment and other nontraditional assessment techniques. *Psychology in the Schools, 36,* 295–304.

Harrison, P., & Oakland, T. (2003). *Adaptive behavior assessment system* (2nd ed.). San Antonio, TX: The Psychological Corporation.

Individuals with Disabilities Education Act Amendments of 1997, P.L. 105-17, 20 U.S.C. §1400 *et seq.*

Individuals with Disabilities Education Improvement Act of 2004 (H.R. 1350).

Kanfer, F. H., & Saslow, G. (1969). Behavioral diagnosis. In C. M. Franks (Ed.), *Behavior therapy: Appraisal and status* (pp. 417–444). New York: McGraw-Hill.

Kaufman, A. S., & Kaufman, N. L. (1990). *Kaufman Brief Intelligence Test.* Circle Pines, MN: American Guidance Service.

Kratochwill, T. R., & Plunge, M. (1992). DSM-III-R, treatment validity, and functional analysis: Further considerations for school psychologists. *School Psychology Quarterly, 7,* 227–232.

Lambert, N., Nihira, K., & Leland, H. (1993). *AAMR Adaptive Behavior Scale—School* (2nd ed.). Austin, TX: Pro-Ed.

Lentz, F. E., Jr., & Shapiro, E. S. (1986). Functional assessment of the academic environment. *School Psychology Review, 15,* 346–357.

Markwardt, F. C. (1997). *Peabody Individual Achievement Test—Revised/Normative Update.* Circle Pines, MN: American Guidance Service.

Mullen, E. M. (1995). *Mullen Scales of Early Learning.* Circle Pines, MN: American Guidance Service.

Naglieri, J. A., & Das, J. P. (1997). *Cognitive assessment system.* Itasca, IL: Riverside.

National Association of School Psychologists. (2000). *Standards for training and field placement programs in school psychology.* Bethesda, MD: Author.

Nihira, K., Leland, H., & Lambert, N. (1993). *AAMR Adaptive Behavior Scale—Residential and Community* (2nd ed.). Austin, TX: Pro-Ed.

O'Neill, R. E., Horner, R. H., Albin, R. W., Sprague, J. R., Storey, K., & Newton, J. S. (1997). *Functional assessment and program development for problem behavior: A practical handbook.* Pacific Grove, CA: Brooks/Cole.

Reschly, D. J., Myers, T. J., & Hartel, C. (Eds.). (2002). *Mental retardation: Determining eligibility for social security benefits.* Washington, DC: National Academy Press.

Reschly, D. J., & Wilson, M. S. (1990). Cognitive processing versus traditional intelligence: Diagnostic utility, intervention implications, and treatment validity. *School Psychology Review, 19,* 443–458.

Riccio, C. A., Houston, F., & Harrison, P. L. (1998). Assessment practices for children with severe mental retardation. *Journal of Psychoeducational Assessment, 16,* 292–301.

Roid, G. H. (2003). *Stanford–Binet Intelligence Scales* (5th ed.). Itasca, IL: Riverside.

Roid, G. H., & Miller, L. J. (1997). *Leiter International Performance Scale (Revised).* Wood Dale, IL: Stoelting.

Salvia, J., & Ysseldyke, J. E. (1978). *Assessment in special and remedial education.* Boston: Houghton Mifflin.

Salvia, J., & Ysseldyke, J. E. (2001). *Assessment* (8th ed.). Boston: Houghton Mifflin.

Sattler, J. M. (2001). *Assessment of children: Cognitive applications* (4th ed.). San Diego, CA: Author.

Sattler, J. M. (2002). *Assessment of children: Behavioral and clinical applications* (4th ed.). La Mesa, CA: Author.

Shapiro, E. S. (1996). *Academic skill problems: Direct assessment and intervention* (2nd ed.). New York: Guildford Press.

Shontz, F. C. (1977). Six principles relating disability and psychological adjustment. *Rehabilitation Psychology, 24,* 207–210.

Simeonsson, R. J., & Short, R. J. (1996). Adaptive development, survival roles, and quality of life. In J. W. Jacobson & J. A. Mulick (Eds.), *Manual of diagnosis and professional practice in mental retardation* (pp. 137–146). Washington, DC: American Psychological Association.

Sparrow, S. S., Balla, D. A., & Cicchetti, D. V. (1984). *Vineland Adaptive Behavior Scales.* Circle Pines, MN: American Guidance Service.

The Developmental Disabilities Assistance and Bill of Rights Act of 2000, 42 U.S.C. §15001, Pub. L. No. 106-402 (2000).

The Psychological Corporation. (1999). *Wechsler Abbreviated Scale of Intelligence.* San Antonio, TX: Author.

The Psychological Corporation. (2001). *Wechsler Individual Achievement Test: Examiner's manual* (2nd ed.). San Antonio, TX: Author.

Turnbull, H. R., Wilcox, B. L., Stowe, M., & Turnbull, A. P. (2001). IDEA requirements for use of PBS: Guidelines for responsible agencies. *Journal of Positive Behavioral Interventions, 3,* 11–18.

Walker, N. W., Boling, M. S., & Cobb, H. (1999). Training of school psychologists in neuropsychology and brain injury: Results of a national survey of training programs. *Child Neuropsychology, 5,* 137–142.

Wechsler, D. (1989). *Wechsler Preschool and Primary Scale of Intelligence* (rev. ed.). San Antonio, TX: The Psychological Corporation.

Wechsler, D. (1991). *Wechsler Intelligence Scale for Children* (3rd ed.). San Antonio, TX: The Psychological Corporation.

Wechsler, D. (1997). *Wechsler Adult Intelligence Scale* (3rd ed.). San Antonio, TX: The Psychological Corporation.

Wechsler, D. (2002). *Wechsler Preschool and Primary Scale of Intelligence* (3rd ed.). San Antonio, TX: The Psychological Corporation.

Wechsler, D. (2003). *Wechsler Intelligence Scale for Children* (4th ed.). San Antonio, TX: The Psychological Corporation.

Wilson, M. S., & Reschly, D. J. (1996). Assessment in school psychology training and practice. *School Psychology Review, 25,* 9–23.

Wright, B. A. P. (1983). *Physical disability: A psychosocial approach* (2nd ed.). New York: Harper & Row.

19

Developmental and Behavioral Screening

FRANCES PAGE GLASCOE

Early intervention for children with disabilities and those at psychosocial risk is facilitated by screening—a brief method for sorting those who probably have difficulties from those who probably do not (Frankenburg, 1974). Most screening tests do not make discrete identification among types of conditions but are instead designed to detect a range of common disabilities, i.e., intellectual disability (ID), learning disabilities, and language impairment. Such tools are referred to as broadband measures. Narrow-band screens (e.g., those for ADHD or autism) are typically developed on and used with referred samples and are beyond the scope of this chapter.

Screening tests are typically administered by paraprofessionals via screening fairs, by educators and psychologists at school entrance, and through child-find programs funded by the Individuals with Disabilities Education Act (IDEA). Even more common is the use of screens in public health departments and pediatric clinics. Professionals in such settings have contact with almost all children prior to kindergarten and are exhorted by their professional societies to deploy screens during routine health supervision visits (American Academy of Pediatrics [AAP], 2001; National Association of Pediatric Nurse Practitioners, 2000). Indeed, Medicaid recipients and those receiving services under the State Children's Health Insurance Programs are entitled by law to comprehensive health, developmental, and mental health screening (Centers for Medicare & Medicaid Services, 1989).

Such policies recognize that development (1) is malleable and easily influenced by the transactions of caretakers and environments (Aylward, 1996; Sameroff, Seifer, Barocas, Zax, & Greenspan, 1987). Children with psychosocial risk factors (e.g., those whose parents have less than a high

FRANCES PAGE GLASCOE • Vanderbilt University, Nashville, Tennessee 37205.

school education, mental health problems, frequent stressful life events, do not provide mediated learning experiences for their children), often exhibit delays, below average performance, or disabilities. Thus developmental status occurs on a continuum making a single effort to discrimination of those with and without probable disabilities challenging, although not impossible, and (2) has age-related manifestations, meaning that skills as well as problems often manifest with age. Children without any early signs of developmental problems may exhibit deficits as they grow older (Bell, 1986). Thus most professional groups suggest repeated, routine developmental screening including some effort to identify those at-risk as well as those with true disabilities. In health care, this generally involves efforts at detection during each of the 12 well-child visits recommended for children between 0 and 5 years of age. In nonmedical settings, routine screening is somewhat less common because repeated contact with children may be limited. Even so, more than 60% of all children under age 5 attend day care, preschool, or Head Start and so are available for multiple screenings.

The varied settings and skills of those using screening measures has resulted in a proliferation of tools—some of good quality—some not. The publication of screening instruments is a largely unregulated industry, at least in the United States. Other countries, notably Canada, require evidence of test accuracy and thus provide consumers and purchasers more guidance in selection of measures (Canadian Psychological Association, 1996). To aid readers in critically examining tools, a summary of standards for screening test construction follows (AAP, 2001; American Educational Research Association, American Psychological Association, & National Council on Measurement in Education, 1999).

STANDARDS FOR SCREENING TEST CONSTRUCTION

Screening test construction involves both traditional and unique psychometry. Nevertheless, screens should adhere to standards for any other educational and psychologist test including evidence of:

(a) *Standardization.* This should include a large nationally representative population (rather than a referred population). Ideally, the sample should be a naturalistic one and not a concatenation of groups known to be either normal or abnormal (because this generally eliminates gradations in functioning that characterize children to whom screening tests are applied (e.g., those with below average but not disabled performance).

(b) *Reliability.* Information should be included on internal consistency, interrater reliability, and test–retest reliability. Stability (longer-term test–retest reliability) is sometimes included although given the rapid changes in developmental performance set against a small set of items; stability indicators are not likely to be strong or meaningful.

(c) *Validity* including concurrent validity (a comparison of screening measures to diagnostic measures). Ideally concurrent validation should involve a test battery that samples the same range of developmental tasks measured by the screening test (e.g., if motor, language, and academic skills are measured, the diagnostic battery should include motor, language, and academic tasks). Discriminant validity studies are also desirable because they show how well a screening test detects the specific kinds of problems. In the case of broadband developmental screens, discriminant validity studies should illustrate the extent to which the more common disabling conditions such as language impairment, ID, learning disabilities, autism, and cerebral palsy are detected, and for mental health screens, how well internalizing and externalizing disorders are detected. Predictive validity studies are not common but are desirable because they reflect how well screening test items and overall screening test performance measure enduring and meaningful dimensions of child development.

(d) *Criterion-related validity.* This is the "acid test" of screening instrumentation and takes a unique form in screening test construction. Generally referred to as accuracy indices, criterion-related validity for screening tests is expressed as follows:

Sensitivity. In a random sample of children, if all were administered a diagnostic battery and categorized into the presence or absence of disabilities (e.g., by viewing eligibility for services under IDEA), some would be found to have disabilities. If screening tests were then given to the same group, ideally, all children with disabilities would score below cutoffs on the screen and thus be identified as needing referrals for diagnostic workups and special services. In reality, detection of disabilities is imperfect due to behavioral noncompliance, psychosocial malleability, and age-related manifestations, and the brevity of screens. Thus, sensitivity, sometimes called copositivity, is percentage of children with true problems correctly identified by a screening test (e.g., by failing, abnormal, or positive results). Ideally, 70–80% of those with difficulties should be identified. While this figure may seem low, many tests fail to attain this level of accuracy and none attain sensitivity that is substantially higher. More importantly, repeated screening is thought to improve detection rates over time.

Specificity. To continue the above example, most children in a random sample who are given diagnostic tests would be found to have normal development. Screening tests given to the same group would ideally identify all the children with typical development as normal (e.g., above cutoffs, passing, or negative scores). Reality differs of course, and so specificity (or conegativity) indicates the percentage of children without disabilities correctly identified, usually by passing or above cutoff scores on the screen. At least 70–80% of those with normal development should be correctly identified. Still, because there are many more children developing normally than not, specificity closer to 80% or higher is desirable.

Other Accuracy Indicators. Screening test research sometimes includes information on other accuracy indicators. Positive predictive value answers the question, to what extent does a suboptimal screening test score, reflect a true problem? If all children performing poorly on a screening test are pooled and administered diagnostic tests, at least a few will perform in the broad range of normal (because of the limits of specificity) and the rest will have disabilities. For example, if 9 out of 10 children with failing scores on screening tests are later found to have developmental diagnoses, the test's positive predictive value is 9/10 or 90% meaning that for any screening test failure, there would be an 90% chance of a true developmental problem. In reality, positive predictive value is rarely 90% with values ranging from 30 to 50% being far more common (i.e., one of every two or three referrals will render a diagnosis. While this may seem troublingly inaccurate, the costs of overreferral (approximately $1000 for a comprehensive diagnostic evaluation) are substantially less than the cost of undertreatment, (a lifetime loss to the child and society of more than $100,000 if needed early intervention is not offered—Barnett & Escobar, 1990; Glascoe, Foster, & Wolraich, 1997). Also reassuring are results from a recent study showing that approximately 70% of children overreferred on developmental screening tests have numerous psychosocial risk factors and score on diagnostic measures of intelligence, language, and academic achievement well below the 25th percentile (the point below which regular classroom instruction is less than optimally effective—Glascoe, 2001a, 2001b). This suggests that almost all children performing poorly on screening tests need at least some additional scrutiny and intervention and that a range of responses is desirable (e.g., Head Start, Title I services, parent training, as well as special education and related services).

Negative predictive value is somewhat less commonly presented but involves determining the degree to which an optimal (above cutoff, passing, or not-at-risk) score reflects typical or nondelayed development. For example, if 95 out of 100 children with passing scores on screening tests are later found on diagnostic testing to have typical development, the test's negative predictive value is 95/100 or 95% meaning that for any passing score, there would be an 95% chance of a no developmental problem.

Some measures also report over and underreferral rates. This reflects the proportion of the entire sample who should have been referred but were not correctly identified (underreferral rates) or should not have been referred (overreferral rates).

Figure 19.1 provides an example and illustrates how the various statistics are computed: Hit rates are occasionally reported and are simply the total number of children for whom a screening test gave accurate information i.e., copositives and conegatives are added together and then divided by the entire sample (copositives + conegatives + false positives + false negatives). Hit rates are an extremely misleading statistic and should not be used as an indicator of test accuracy. In the example shown in Figure 19.1, the hit rate is (70 + 16)/100 = 86%. Because there are far more conegatives, specificity carries excessive weight in the computation of hit rates and as can be seen, the hit-rate is closer to the specificity index than to

Diagnosis

		No	Yes	
Diagnosis	Pass	70 conegatives/ true negatives	4 false negatives	47
	Fail	10 false positives	16 copositives/ true positives	26
		80	20	

Sensitivity (true positives divided by true positives + false negatives) = 16/20 = 75%
Specifiity (true negatives divided by true negatives + false positives) = 70/80 = 88%
Positive Predictive Value (true positives divided by true positives + false positives) = 16/26 = 62%
Negative Predictive Value (true negatives divided by true negatives + false negatives = 70/74 = 94
Over-referral rate (false positives divided by total sample) = 10/100 = 10%
Under-referral rate (false negatives divided by total sample) = 4/100 = 4%

Figure 19.1. Computation of accuracy indices for screening tests.

the sensitivity index. If in the above example, sensitivity were only 50% (10 children with disabilities correctly identified and 10 underdetected), the hit-rate would still remain deceptively attractive [(70 + 10)/100 = 80%] and mask serious flaws in accuracy.

Utility. Less of a psychometric construct and more a function of practical attributes, screens should be studied for their usefulness to diverse professionals in varied settings. Such studies often address length of administration and scoring, acceptability to parents and children, readability, amount of training required, cost of administration in terms of professional time to deliver the measure, score and interpret it, and descriptions of other amenities helpful to specific applications (e.g., ability to aggregate results for program evaluation, availability of growth indicators for use in plotting progress over time).

Prescreening. In an effort to conserve educational and health care dollars, it is obviously desirable to select measures with a high degree of positive predictive value. Given the subtlety and gradations of developmental outcomes, high positive predictive value remains elusive. Nevertheless, positive predictive value can be improved by administering a second screening test or by using part of a screen (e.g., a subtest) as a *prescreen.* Prescreening tests are extremely brief measures with a high degree of sensitivity but limited specificity. Prescreens are administered routinely and are followed by screening tests only when children fail the prescreen. Although prescreening can simply compound error and lead to underreferrals, accurate prescreening improves detection rates, and saves considerable time, since prescreens reduce, often by one-half to two-thirds, the numbers of children requiring complete screening.

SPECIFIC DEVELOPMENTAL AND BEHAVIORAL/ EMOTIONAL SCREENING INSTRUMENTS

What follows is a description of several tests, selected for discussion because they: (a) cover most or all developmental domains (although some emotional/behavioral/mental health screens are discussed separately since few developmental screens also measure this domain); (b) cover wide age ranges; and (c) meet or approach standards for screening test accuracy, i.e., have sensitivity and specificity of at least 70–80%.

Not included are measures that fail to comply with basic psychometric values. Excluded tests were the Denver-II and its prescreening derivative, the PDQ-R, because they were standardized only in Colorado, lack any validity research by the authors, and as a consequence provide no information on specificity and specificity. Studies by researchers other than the test authors showed that the Denver-II consistently overrefers or underdetects depending on how the questionable score is handled (Glascoe et al., 1992). Also excluded were the Early Screening Profile, the DIALIII, and the Gesell which while nationally standardized and validated, have poor sensitivity or specificity; the CAT-CLAMS which, although heavily language oriented was validated only against measures of intelligence on referred rather than general pediatric samples (rendering its sensitivity and specificity likely inflated), the Early Screening Inventory, because it was validated against an antiquated measure of intelligence (and so does not contain proof that it measures language and academic skills) and deploys draconian cutoffs that enable identification of only the lowest scoring 6% (problematic given that the prevalence of disabilities approaches 18%— Newacheck et al., 1998).

Measures are divided into those relying on information from parents and those relying on direct elicitation of children's skills. The former are particularly useful for statewide or regional screening initiatives because they can be mailed to families, used in telephone surveys, completed by interview, or via self-administration in waiting rooms. Measures involving information from parents are increasingly popular in pediatrics and public health in which early detection is one of many competing activities and where the volume of patients or clients is high. In contrast, screens relying on direct elicitation typically take longer to administer but provide more in-depth information. As such, they can be considered secondstage screens in primary care (meaning that they would be administered only to a subset of patients identified by briefer measures as at higher risk) but are useful in settings where there is time (and often greater skill in child management) to work individually with children (e.g., outreach screening clinics, child-find programs, behavioral practices, neonatal intensive care follow-up programs, school system prekindergarten screening initiatives).

For each of the measures below, information is provided about the publisher, price for a complete set of materials, age range, administration time, scores produced, descriptions of item content, supporting research, and other relevant details.

DEVELOPMENTAL SCREENS RELYING ON INFORMATION FROM PARENTS

Parents' Evaluation of Development Status (PEDS—Ellsworth & Vandermeer Press, Ltd., 1013 Austin Caurt, Nolensville, TN 37136 Phone: 615-776-4121; fax: 615-776-4119; $30.00; http://www.pedstest.com)
PEDS is a 10-item tool for children 0–8 years of age and takes 2–5 min to administer and score. PEDS elicits parents' concerns, which makes it helpful in initiatives with an interest in family-centeredness, collaboration, and cultural competence. Two of the questions are open-ended and the remaining ones probe various developmental domains. Readability is 4th to 5th grade. A longitudinal score form with columns for each age range (tied to the American Academy of Pediatrics well-visit schedule) shows which concerns are predictive of developmental and behavioral problems and sorts children into low, moderate, versus high-risk levels for various developmental as well as behavioral or mental health problems. The score form leads users to a longitudinal interpretation form that guides a range of evidence-based decisions: when to refer and what kinds of referrals are needed, when to screen further (or in the case of primary care, refer for screening), when to offer parents advice and counseling on developmental and behavioral issues, when to monitor development vigilantly, and when to provide reassurance that development appears on target. Because PEDS identifies a subset in need of additional screening it can be considered, at least in part, a prescreening tool. Available in Spanish, English, Vietnamese, and other languages, the test was validated and cross-validated on national samples with sensitivity between 74 and 84% and specificity between 70 and 80% (Glascoe, 1991, 1994, 1999; Glascoe et al., 1997; Glascoe, Altemeier, & MacLean, 1989). These studies consistently show that although parents with limited education and other risk factors are less likely to raise concerns independently, that once asked, they are as able as educated parents to report concerns reflective of developmental status. Overly concerned parents can be identified by unique patterns of nonpredictive concerns for which optimal responses include offering advice or parent training rather than referrals for diagnostic services.Recent

research illustrated a high level of predictive validity over a 2-year period with parents who held predictive concerns at age five, and had children at age seven who tended to perform below average in academic and language skills (Wake & Gerner, 2002). A nonclinical survey version is widely used in evaluating the quality of developmental services within health care plans (Bethell, Peck, & Schor, 2001). Another study compared PEDS to a range of other developmental screens and found it to be the least expensive of the measures studied (Dobrez et al., 2001).

PEDS- Developmental Milestones (PEDS-DM) Ellsworth & Vandermeer Press, Ltd.

1013 Austin Court, Nolensville, TN 37136 Phone: 615-776-4121; fax: 615-776-4119 http://www.pedstest.com, in press (October, 2006) and to be online at www.forepath.org PEDS-DM is a validated checklist of milestones for children 0–8 years of age. It consists of 6–8 items at each age level (spanning the well visit schedule). Each item taps a different domain (fine/gross motor, self-help, academics, expressive/receptive language, social-emotional). The PEDS-DM can be used to complement PEDS or stand-alone. It can be administered either by parent report or directly to children. Each version at each age is produced on forms that are laminated and scannable. Items are tied to cutoffs tied to performance above and below the 16th percentile for each item and its domain which is the point at which children experience failure with typical curricula. The PEDS-DM is 75% to 87% sensitive and 71$ to 88% specific to performance above and below the 16th percentile. Across age ranges, the measure is 70% to 94% sensitive and 77% to 93% specific. It takes about 1 minute to score, and about 5 to administer. About 3 minutes (October, 2006, in press)

Ages and Stages Questionnaire—Paul H. Brookes, Publishers, PO Box 10624, Baltimore, MD 21285 (1-800-638-3775); http://www.pbrookes.com. ($199)

For children 4 months—to 6 years of age, the Ages and Stages Questionnaire (ASQ) uses parental report (descriptions of children's skills to which parents endorse "not yet, sometimes, or yes") and provides simple drawings and directions for eliciting careful responses. Separate forms tied to a well-child visit schedule each have 30–35 items. Overall reading level is approximately 5th grade although some individual questions are more challenging and reach the 12th-grade level. Modifications are available for screening children between specified intervals. The measure takes 10–15 min to complete and score. Well-standardized, the ASQ is validated on national samples against a range of criterion measures. It provides an overall pass–fail score but optional scoring enables a view of strengths and weakness in developmental domains. Sensitivity ranged 70–90% at all ages except the 4-month level. Specificity ranged from 76 to 91%. A related publication, the ASQ-SE, works in much the same way but focuses on social and emotional development in children 0–9 years of age. Both measures are available in English, Spanish, and French. The test(s) are purchased and photocopying of forms is then permitted, although the numbers of pages required (4–5 per age level per test) elevate the cost substantially (Dobrez et al., 2001).

DEVELOPMENTAL SCREENS USING DIRECT ELICITATION OF CHILDREN'S SKILLS

Brigance Screens—Curriculum Associates, Inc. (2004), 153 Rangeway Road, N. Billerica, MA 01862 (1-800-225-0248 ($501.00); http://www. curriculumassociates.com/

For children 0–90 months, the test has nine separate forms, approximately one for each 12- month age range. Originally developed as a criterion-referenced measure, many of the items are a part of complete skill sequences (e.g., naming of *all* colors, *all* letters, *all* body parts). Items tap speech-language, motor, readiness, and general knowledge at younger ages and also reading and math at older ages. Only the 0–2-year version includes a measure of social–emotional development but research on the Screens with older children shows that problematic performance is associated with psychiatric issues as well as developmental problems (Murphy et al., 2000). Measurement is accomplished via direct elicitation and observation except in the 0–2-year age range, where items can also be administered by parent interview. The measure takes 10–15 min to complete and produces quotients, percentiles, and cutoff and age-equivalent scores for various domains. Sensitivity and specificity range from 73 to 86% in detecting delays and academic problems. Although there are some studies critical of the measures, these failed to use the empirically derived cutoffs or age restrictions on selection among forms (Mantzicopoulos, 1999, 2000). The Brigance Screens are one of the few measures that also detect advanced or gifted development. Additional features include a growth indicator score for monitoring progress over time, and separate psychosocial risk cutoff scores for careful allocation of diagnostic services for children recently enrolled in programs like Head Start (where the majority of new enrollees are screened, tend to perform poorly, but often make rapid progress). Instructional videos, scoring software, and recently an online-web-based scoring application facilitate data aggregation useful in program evaluation. The focus of abundant research, a range of predictive validity studies provide support for the quality of items. The test is published in numerous languages including English, Spanish, Vietnamese, Cambodian, and Tagalog.

Bayley Infant Neurodevelomental Screen (BINS). San Antonio, Texas: The Psychological Corporation, 1995. 555 Academic Court, San Antonio, TX 78204 (1-800-228-0752) ($265); http://www.psychcorp.com

For children 3–24 months, the BINS has 10–13 directly elicited items per 3–6-month age range. The tool assesses neurological processes (reflexes and tone); neurodevelopmental skills (movement, and symmetry); and developmental accomplishments (object permanence, imitation, and language). Test results categorize performance into low, moderate, or high risk via cut scores for each of the three domains. Specificity and sensitivity are 75–86%. Examiner skill is essential (especially for items requiring judgment of motor tone and object permanence) which may explain why the tool is largely used in neonatal follow-up clinics (Leonard, Piecuch, & Cooper, 2001). A video illustrating item administration is a helpful adjunct to using the tool. The BINS takes 10–15 min to administer.

First Step Screening Test for Evaluating Preschoolers. San Antonio, Texas: The Psychological Corporation, 1995. 555 Academic Court, San Antonio, TX 78204 (1-800-228-0752) ($195); http://www.psychcorp.com

For children 2 years, 9 months to 6 years, 2 months, the FirstStep relies largely on direct elicitation of skills from children although parent report is used to obtain adaptive behavior information. The measure has 14 subtests that coalesce into five optional domains: Cognition, Communication, Motor with a Social–Emotional Scale and Adaptive Behavior Checklist. Scaled scores and a risk status indicator (acceptable, caution, at-risk) are produced. The test takes about 15 min to complete. FirstStep was standardized on a large sample stratified on a number of variables. However, higher SES groups were oversampled and disabled children were excluded, resulting in potential inflation of normative performance. The measure has excellent sensitivity and specificity although these indices were computed by adding into the standardization sample a disproportionately large group of children with known disabilities (30% of the total sample). As a consequence overreferrals are likely and evident as reported by one school system (Dr. Judith Lombana, Director, Research and Development, Hillsborough County Schools, personal communication, April 1995).

BEHAVIORAL AND MENTAL HEALTH SCREENING MEASURES

Eyberg Child Behavior Inventory/Sutter-Eyberg Student Behavior Inventory—Revised (SESBI).Psychological Assessment Resources, P.O. Box 998 Odessa Florida: 33556 (1-800-331-8378) ($120.00); http://www. parinc.com/

For children 2–16 years of age, the Eyberg Child Behavior Inventory (ECBI) consists of 36 short statements of common behavior problems written at about the 6th-grade level to which parents respond, while the SESBI consists of 38 statements that teachers rate. Both measures tap externalizing disorder (e.g., attention, conduct, aggression). Each item includes a severity rating (essentially frequency of occurrence) and an indicator of whether the behavior is perceived as a problem. The measure is available in English only. Scoring takes about 5 min. Sensitivity is 80% to disruptive behavior problems and specificity is 86% to their absence. Several studies showed that the ECBI is responsive to the effects of behavioral training for a range of populations (Brestan, Jacobs, Rayfield, & Eyberg, 1999; McNeil, Capage, Bahl, & Blanc, 1999).

Pediatric Symptom Checklist and Youth-Pediatric Symptom Checklist Jellinek MS, Murphy JM, Robinson J, et al. Pediatric Symptom Checklist: Screening school-age children for psychosocial dysfunction. Journal of Pediatrics, 1988;112:201–209 and Psychology in the Schools, 2000; 37: 91–106 (and downloadable without charge at www.pedstest.com)

For children 4–16 years, this screener is comprised of 35 short statements of problem behaviors (including those which are internalizing versus externalizing). Parents (or youth ages nine and older) rate items, written at approximately the 6th-grade level) as never/sometimes/often. A value of 0–2 is assigned and a total of 28 requires a referral, except at younger ages for which some items are eliminated and scoring criteria change slightly. All but one study showed high sensitivity (80–95%) but somewhat scattered specificity (68–100%), and much applicability to a variety of pediatric settings including inpatient and ambulatory services (Jellinek, Bishop, Murphy, Biederman, & Rosenbaum, 1991; Murphy, Arnett, Bishop, Jellinek, & Reede, 1992; Murphy, Reede, Jellinek, & Bishop, 1992; Rauch et al., 1991). Recent research identified factor scores that accurately detect internalizing disorders (depression and anxiety), externalizing disorders (e.g., oppositional defiance, conduct), and attentional deficits (Gardner et al., 1999). The measure is available in Spanish, English, and Chinese. A pictorial version, the PPSC, is useful for Latino families, improves sensitivity and specificity in this population, and can be downloaded at www.dbpeds.org.

SCREENING HOME ENVIRONMENTS

The close relationship between the psychosocial well-being of parents and that of children suggests that comprehensive screening programs should address environmental contributors to children's developmental and behavioral status. Use of the following screens can help identify families in need of referrals for substance abuse, depression, domestic violence, parenting skills, and mental health services. Some pediatric clinics use family screens as routine intake questionnaires required from families when obtaining medical and developmental histories on new patients. Although identification of family risk factors do not substitute for a developmental screen (because resilience is common), identification of psychosocial risk factors can help focus referrals to a range of social and mental health services.

Family Psychosocial Screen. Kemper, KJ & Kelleher KJ. Family psychosocial screening: Instruments and techniques. Ambulatory Child Health. 1996;4:325–339. (and downloadable at www.pedstest.com)

This questionnaire is a series of validated items drawn from several studies conducted by Dr. Kathi Kemper and colleagues. The items, along with other questions about psychosocial risk factors comprise the clinic intake form at the University of Washington. The validated questions include: (1) a four-item measure of parental history of physical abuse as a child (Kemper, Carlin, & Buntain-Ricklefs, 1994); (2) a six-item measure of parental substance abuse (Kemper, Greteman, Bennett, & Babonis, 1993); and (3) a three-item measure of maternal depression (Kemper & Babonis, 1992). All are written at approximately the 6th-grade level. Each of these measures was validated against larger inventories and had sensitivity and specificity of 80–90%. Guidelines for administering, scoring are included with the screen.

Home Screening Questionnaire (HSQ). Denver Developmental Materials, Inc., PO Box 6919, Denver, Colorado 80206 (303-355-4729). ($18.00)

Designed for children 0–6 years of age, the HSQ uses parental report to identify children at risk for delays due to negative environmental influences. Items were selected to be predictive of the HOME Inventory (which requires a home visit). The HSQ was standardized only on low income families. Subsequent studies found it to correlate highly with developmental status and social competence after the age of 15 months. The test meets standards for sensitivity but specificity is below acceptable levels which suggest administration should be restricted to referral populations and it should be deployed largely to refine treatment plans. Fortunately, the HSQ is known to be responsive to intervention as shown in the National Evaluation of The Even Start Family Literacy Program (1998 (http://www.ed.gov/pubs/evenstart_final/chap7pt2.html).

SCREENING SCHOOL-AGED CHILDREN FOR ACADEMIC DYSFUNCTION

Despite the plethora of academic testing to which school-age children are exposed, few group (or subsets of diagnostic) achievement tests are studied for their sensitivity and specificity (a notable exception being Maryland's school performance assessment program—Morgan, 1999). Children experiencing difficulties with curricula, as well as those with symptoms of attention deficit disorder, acting out behavior, school avoidance, and other troubling behaviors, should be scrutinized for the potential contribution of academic deficits. Although the Brigance Screens, Battelle Developmental Inventory Screening Test, and Parents' Evaluation of Developmental Status screen children up to age 8, for older children, the following measures can also be considered.

Comprehensive Inventory of Basic Skills – Revised Screener (CIBS-R Screener), Curriculum Associates, Inc. (1985), 153 Rangeway Road, N. Billerica, MA 01862 (1-800-225-0248 ($224.00); http:// www. curriculumassociates.com/

For children 6–14 years age, the CIBS-R Screener deploys three of the 10 scales that comprise the complete CIBS-R. The three scales measure reading comprehension, computational skills, and sentence writing and produce quotients, raw score cutoffs, age-equivalents, and percentiles. All three can also be timed to produce an indicator of information processing. The remaining subtests can then be administered if a complete educational diagnostic battery is required and include word recognition, word analysis, reading vocabulary comprehension, math problem-solving, spelling, and listening vocabulary. A survival sight word vocabulary measure is optional but has been validated as a brief primary care screen for academic problems called the Safety Word Inventory and Literacy Screen (SWILS; Glascoe, 2002). Although one review was critical of the CIBS-R for failing to determine performance stability, (i.e., long-term test–retest reliability—Bradley-Johnson, 1999), sensitivity and specificity were appropriate and ranged from 73 to 78%. The CIBS-R Screener takes 15–20 min to administer and is available in English only.

Einstein Assessment of School-Related Skills. Slossen Educational Publications, 538 Buffalo Road, East Aurora, NY 14052, Phone: 716 652-0930; http://www.slosson.com, $75.00

For children from K through grade 5, this instrument measures reading, arithmetic, auditory memory, language cognition, and visual-motor abilities. The measure takes 7–10 min to administer and uses separate forms for each grade level. Standardization is somewhat limited (to the Northeast U.S.) and information on parents' level of education is not available. Other limitations include use of the WRAT-R, a limited measure of achievement, as the criterion and computations of sensitivity and specificity conducted on a preidentified sample of children with restricted disabilities (i.e., learning disabilities). Strengths include predictive validity and cross-validation studies (Bennett, Gottesman, Cerullo, & Rock, 1991; Gottesman, Cerullo, Bennett, & Rock, 1991) and sensitivity and specificity produced at each grade level and at different points during the school year ranging from 70 to 91%. The measure is available in English only.

Glascoe, F. P. The Safety Word Inventory and Literacy Screener (SWILS). Free download at www.pedstest.com

The SWILS presents children between 6 and 14 years of age, 29 common safety words, most in the context of their typical logos (e.g., the poison label on household products). Administration time is about 7 min. The measure correlates highly with academic performance in all subjects but most closely with reading skills. Its sensitivity and specificity ranged from 78 to 84% across age levels. The content of the measure makes it a helpful springboard to safety and injury-prevention counseling.

ISSUES IN APPLICATION OF SCREENS IN PRIMARY CARE MEDICINE

The opinions of psychologists and educators are often solicited when primary care clinicians debate the virtues of various approaches to screening. In such cases, it is helpful to recognize the following:

(a) In primary care, screening typically occurs at well-child visits. Time frames for these visits range from 11 to 18 min on the average and include a physical exam, anticipatory guidance, developmental promotion, safety counseling, hearing, dentition, nutrition, and vision screening. The time available for psychosocial screening is extremely limited. Thus measures relying on information from parents, because these can be completed in waiting or medical exam rooms, are advisable.

(b) Because of the time constraints of primary care, most primary care providers rely on clinical judgment, informal checklists, and assessment of (often motor) milestones (Bierman, Connor, Vaage, & Honzik, 1964; Scott, Lingaraju, Kilgo, Kregel, & Lazzari, 1993; Shonkoff, Dworkin, Leviton, & Levine, 1979; Smith, 1978). Research suggests these techniques are inadequate and identify only

20–30% of children with developmental or mental health problems (Halfon et al., 2001; Lavigne et al., 1993; Pavluri, Luk, Clarkson, & McGee, 1995). Dissuading clinicians of this practice and encouraging use of validated measures is often necessary.

(c) Primary care providers tend not to refer when faced with poor performance on screening tests and prefer a "wait and see approach" sometimes coupled with in-office counseling and medication management (Rushton, Bruckman, & Kelleher, 2002). Decision support (i.e., specific guidelines for optimal responses to screening test performance) is often needed. Some tools (i.e., PEDS) include decision support as part of the measure's protocols. When other tests are used, it may be helpful to generate a flow chart for encouraging prompt referrals to various kinds of services.

(d) Primary care providers are often unfamiliar with local nonmedical services and this reduces the likelihood of referrals (Forrest, Nutting, Starfield, & von Schrader, 2002). Creating opportunities for practitioners to learn about available early intervention programs, psychological services, speech-language clinics, and other resources can help. Also invaluable is offering a list of phone numbers and brochures about local programs. Ultimately, providing routine and prompt feedback (e.g., a follow-up letter or phone call) is critical, and should include treatment suggestions, history, diagnosis, and other pertinent information (Forrest et al., 2000).

ISSUES IN THE APPLICATION OF SCREENING MEASURES BY EDUCATORS, PSYCHOLOGISTS, AND OTHER PROFESSIONALS

In addition to their explicit value in case-finding, screening tools are deployed for a variety of other purposes. Some applications stretch the viability of interpretation given the restricted range of items inherent in screening tests. Nevertheless, alternative applications reflect the limitations of time, dollars, and personnel that preclude administration of in-depth measures. Understandably, screening tests offer an attractive method for obtaining information inexpensively while still ensuring at least some evidence in support of established indicators and benchmarks:

Prioritizing Referrals and Parsimonious Allocation of Diagnostic Resources

In settings such as Head Start, it is not uncommon for 70–80% of children to perform suboptimally upon enrollment (Campbell & Ramey, 1994). Offering diagnostic testing for such a large group is neither feasible nor desirable, especially in light of the rapid gains many children with psychosocial risk factors make when first placed in highly enriching environments. Nevertheless, psychosocial risk factors remain closely associated with disabilities so the task at hand is to make efficacious decisions about referral priorities. The Brigance Screens contain a separate cutoff for children (kindergarten age and younger) at psychosocial risk who have been recently enrolled in programs. The cutoff is applied to the factor most predictive of disabilities according to children's ages and enables program personnel to meet diagnostic services carefully and with reasonable wisdom. Rescreening later in the year is recommended for the remaining children who scored below overall cutoffs but above psychosocial risk factors. Other measures, such as PEDS, Battelle, and FirstStep sort children into varying levels of risk or by performance departures at varying distances from the mean. Risk sorting also provides an opportunity to identify children at high risk and in prompt need of further testing while offering watchful waiting to those at moderate risk levels.

Determining Entry Points Into Curricula

In programs offering individualized instruction, screening tests are sometimes used for instructional planning. The dangers of teaching directly to a screening test are imminent and the limited range of items would make for dull and restricted curricula. Recognizing this, screens linked to more complete assessments provide teachers more substantive direction. The Battelle Developmental Inventory Screening Test is one such tool and is linked item for item with the diagnostic measure, the diagnostic-level Battelle Developmental Inventory. Similarly, the Brigance Screens are part of the Brigance Inventory of Early Development and the Brigance Screens technical manual offers specific guidance about prerequisite and postrequisite skill. Substantially more is written on the topic of linking assessment with intervention, most notably, Bagnato, Neisworth, and Munson's text *Linking Assessment and Early Intervention: An Authentic Curriculum-Based Approach (1997)*.

Monitoring Progress

Screening measures are occasionally used as an interim step in program evaluation and as brief way to determine whether children are making progress with curricular goals. To the extent that items on the screen are part of curricula, it makes some sense to repeat the measures during the school year (although with insufficient frequency that test validity is not violated due to excessive retesting). The Brigance Screens provide growth indicators derived from normative data on expected changes in performance if testing is conducted at multiple points during the school year. Information is given on the average changes in raw scores over time banded by standard deviations in order to show when progress is exceptionally slow or rapid. Because the Screens are also criterion-referenced, growth indicator data can be interpreted as rate of skill gains (e.g., percent or number of skills mastered) as well as by departures from expected changes in raw scores, quotients, percentiles, or age-equivalent changes.

Program Evaluation and Outcomes Assessment

Aggregating results of screening at the beginning and again at the end of the year is a typical method for evaluating programs and viewing child outcomes. Ideally, unenrolled children or those attending programs with a different kind of curriculum would also be tested in order to offer generalizable information on how children fare under a range of conditions as well as a comparison point for benchmarking outcomes. The availability of scoring software (e.g., Battelle, Brigance) and online data entry (i.e., Brigance Screens) facilitate data aggregation. Such software also generates domain or factor scores that are easily produced and thus enables a more nuanced view of the developmental areas in which interventions are more or less effective. An excellent example of program evaluation using screening tools is seen in the Fayette County Schools (Lexington, Kentucky, at http://www.fcps.net/sa/eval/default.htm) in which administrators reviewed the effects of full versus half-day kindergarten, large versus small-class size, and other issues of interest, in order to make evidence-based decisions about program improvements and resource allocation.

Teacher Accountability

Program evaluation when conducted across sites often prompts an interest in comparing teacher performance. This is a serious task and probably one that should not be conducted with screening tests—given that they sample only a few developmental tasks and have a larger margin of error than lengthier measures. Even so, screening tests are put to this task and so cautions are in order. First and most importantly is the question of whether children within classrooms are comparable. Children with greater numbers of psychosocial risk factors may make fewer gains than those with fewer risk factors. It is essential to ensure that comparisons are fair, in essence by matching children on critical environmental indicators, before considering teacher performance. It is also helpful to view differences in teacher experience, training, and curricula and to consider whether substantiated differences in performance are an indicator that additional training or alternative curricula are needed.

CONCLUSION

Although most screening tests are used as brief methods for generating an index of suspicion about the probability of developmental or mental health problems, resource constraints and accountability initiatives have expanded the range of issues that screening tests are expected to address. As a consequence, the selection among screens becomes even more critical and should be based on strong psychometric support. Of the many standards for test construction, substantial attention should be paid to sensitivity and specificity. Tests reaching standards for screening test accuracy are presented above together with measures that appear promising but in need of additional research.

REFERENCES

American Academy of Pediatrics, Committee on Children with Disabilities. (2001). Developmental surveillance and screening of infants and young children. *Pediatrics, 108,* 192–196. Retrieved on 24 May 2006 http://aappolicy.aappublications.org/cgi/content/abstract/pediatrics;108/1/192

American Educational Research Association, American Psychological Association, & National Council on Measurement in Education. (1999). *Standards for educational and psychological testing.* Washington, DC: Authors.

Aylward, G. P. (1996). Environmental risk, intervention and developmental outcome. *Ambulatory Child Health, 2,* 161–170.

Barnett, W. S., & Escobar, C. M. (1990). Economic costs and benefits of early intervention. In S. J. Meisels & J. P. Shonkoff (Eds.), *Handbook of early childhood intervention* (pp. 560–582). Cambridge, UK: Cambridge University Press.

Bell, R. Q. (1986). Age-specific manifestations in changing psychosocial risk. In D. C. Farran & J. C. McKinney (Eds.), *Risk in intellectual and psychosocial development* (pp. 169–185). Orlando, FL: Academic.

Bennett, R. E., Gottesman, R. L., Cerullo, F. M., & Rock, D. A. (1991). The validity of Einstein assessment subtest scores as predictors of early school achievement. *Journal of Psychoeducational Assessment, 9,* 67–79.

Bethell, C., Peck, C., & Schor, E. (2001). Assessing health system provision of well-child care: The Promoting Healthy Development Survey. *Pediatrics. 107*(5), 1084–1094.

Bierman, J. M., Connor, A., Vaage, M., & Honzik, M. P. (1964). Pediatricians' assessment of the intelligence of two-year olds and their mental test scores. *Pediatrics, 43,* 680–690.

Bradley-Johnson, S. (1999). Test review: Brigance Diagnostic Comprehensive Inventory of basic skills—revised. *Psychology in the Schools, 36,* 523–528.

Brestan, E. V., Jacobs, J. R., Rayfield, A. D., & Eyberg, S. M. (1999). A consumer satisfaction measure for parent child treatments and its relation to measures of child behavior change. *Behavior Therapy, 30,* 17–30.

Campbell, F. A., & Ramey, C. T. (1994). Effects of early intervention on intellectual and academic achievement: A Follow-Up Study of Children from Low-Income Families. *Child Development, 65,* 684–698.

Canadian Psychological Association. (1996). *Guidelines for advertising preschool screening tests.* Ottawa, Ontario, Canada: Canadian Psychological Association. Retrieved 24 May 2006 http://www.cpa.ca/documents/PsyTest.htm

Centers for Medicare & Medicaid Services. (1989). *MEDICAID and EPSDT.* Retrieved October 2005 from http://www.cms.hhs.gov/medicaid/epsdt/default.asp.

Dobrez, D., Lo Sasso, A., Holl, J., Shalowitz, M., Leon, S., & Budetti, P. (2001). Estimating the cost of developmental and behavioral screening of preschool children in general pediatric practice. *Pediatrics, 108,* 913–922.

Forrest, C. B., Glade, G. B., Baker, A. E., Bocian, A., von Schrader, S., & Starfield, B. (2000). Coordination of specialty referrals and physician satisfaction with referral care. *Archives of Pediatrics and Adolescent Medicine, 154,* 499–506.

Forrest, C. B., Nutting, P. A., Starfield, B., & von Schrader, S. (2002). Family physicians' referral decisions: Results from the ASPN referral study. *Journal of Family Practice, 51,* 215–222.

Frankenburg, W. K. (1974). Selection of diseases and tests in pediatric screening. *Pediatrics, 54,* 1–5.

Gardner, W., Murphy, J. M., Childs, G., Kelleher, K., Pagano, M., Jellinek, M., McInerny, T. K., Wasserman, R. C., Nutting, P., & Chiapetta, L. (1999). The PSC-17: A brief pediatric symptom checklist psychosocial problem subscales: A report from PROS and ASPN. *Ambulatory Child Health, 5,* 225–236.

Glascoe, F. P. (1991). Can clinical judgement detect children with speech–language problems? *Pediatrics, 87,* 317–322.

Glascoe, F. P. (1994). It's not what it seems: The relationship between parents' concerns and children's global delays. *Clinical Pediatrics, 33,* 292–298.

Glascoe, F. P. (1999). Toward a model for an evidence-based approach to developmental/behavioral surveillance, promotion and patient education. *Ambulatory Child Health, 5,* 197–208.

Glascoe, F. P. (2001a). Are over-referrals on developmental screening tests really a problem? *Archives of Pediatrics and Adolescent Medicine, 155,* 54–59.

Glascoe, F. P. (2001b). Teacher's global ratings and students' academic achievement. *Journal of Developmental and Behavioral Pediatrics, 22,* 163–168.

Glascoe, F. P. (2002). The Safety Word Inventory and Literacy Screener. *Clinical Pediatrics, 41,* 697–704.

Glascoe, F. P., Altemeier, W. K., & MacLean, W. E. (1989). The importance of parents' concerns about their child's development. *American Journal of Diseases of Children, 143,* 855–958.

Glascoe, F. P., & Byrne, K. E. (1993). The accuracy of three developmental screening tests. *Journal of Early Intervention, 17,* 368–379.

Glascoe, F. P., Byrne, K. E., Chang, B., Strickland, B., Ashford, L. G., & Johnson, K. L. (1992). Accuracy of the Denver-II in developmental screening. *Pediatrics, 89*(6), 1221–1224.

Glascoe, F. P., Foster, F. M., & Wolraich, M. L. (1997). An economic evaluation of four methods for detecting developmental problems. *Pediatrics, 99,* 830–837.

Gottesman, R. L., Cerullo, F. M., Bennett, R. E., & Rock, D. (1991). A predictive validity of a screening test for mild school learning difficulties. *Journal of School Psychology, 29,* 191–205.

Halfon, N., Hochstein, M., Sareen, H., O'Connor, K., Inkelas, M., & Olson, L. (2001). Barriers to the provision of developmental assessments during pediatric health supervision visits. *Pediatric Research, 49,* 26A.3.

Jellinek, M. S., Bishop, S. J., Murphy, J. M., Biederman, J., & Rosenbaum, J. F. (1991). Screening for dysfunction in the children of outpatients at a psychopharmacology clinic. *American Journal of Psychiatry, 148,* 1031–1036.

Kemper, K. J., & Babonis, T. R. (1992). Screening for maternal depression in pediatric clinics. *American Journal of Diseases of Children, 146,* 876–878.

Kemper, K. J., Carlin, A. S., & Buntain-Ricklefs, J. (1994). Screening for maternal experiences of physical abuse during childhood. *Clinical Pediatrics, 33,* 333–339.

Kemper, K. J, Greteman, A., Bennett, E., & Babonis, T. R. (1993). Screening mothers of young children for substance abuse. *Journal of Developmental and Behavioral Pediatrics, 14,* 308–312.

Lavigne, J. V., Binns, J. H., Christoffel, K. K., Rosenbaum, D., Arend, R., Smith, K., Hayford, J. R., McGuire, P. A., and the Pediatric Practice Research Group. (1993). Behavioral and emotional problems among preschool children in pediatric primary care: Prevalence and pediatricians' recognition. *Pediatrics, 91,* 649–655.

Leonard, C. H., Piecuch, R. E., & Cooper, B. A. (2001). Use of the Bayley Infant Neurodevelopmental Screener with low birth weight infants. *Journal of Pediatric Psychology, 26,* 33–40.

Mantzicopoulos, P. Y. (1999). Risk assessment of head start children with the Brigance K&1 Screen: Differential performance by sex, age, and predictive accuracy for early school achievement and special education placement. *Early-Childhood-Research-Quarterly, 14,* 383–408.

Mantzicopoulos, P. Y. (2000). Can the Brigance K&1 Screen detect cognitive/academic giftedness when used with preschoolers from economically disadvantaged backgrounds? *Roeper-Review, 22,* 185–191.

McNeil, C. B., Capage, L. C., Bahl, A., & Blanc, H. (1999). Importance of early intervention for disruptive behavior problems: Comparison of treatment and waitlist control groups. *Early Education and Development, 10,* 445–454.

Morgan, K. R. D. (1999). Validation of performance assessments: Maximizing their utility and positive impact (Maryland school performance assessment program). *Dissertation Abstracts International Section A: Humanities and Social Sciences, 59*(11-A), 4057.

Murphy, J. M., Arnett, H. L., Bishop, S. J., Jellinek, M. S., & Reede, J. Y. (1992). Screening for psychosocial dysfunction in pediatric practice. A naturalistic study of the Pediatric Symptom Checklist. *Clinical Pediatrics, 31*, 660–667.

Murphy, J. M., Pagano, M. E., Smith, D., Nowlin, C., Ramirez, Y., Dickinson, L., et al. (2000). Enhanced mental health services and the educational impact of psychosocial problems in Head Start: A model program in Ventura County. *Early Education and Development* [Special Issue on Project Head Start and Mental Health], 11(3), 247–385.

Murphy, J. M., Reede, J., Jellinek, M. S., & Bishop, S. J. (1992). Screening for psychosocial dysfunction in inner-city children: Further validation of the Pediatric Symptom Checklist. *Journal of the American Academy of Child and Adolescent Psychiatry, 31*, 1105–1111.

National Association of Pediatric Nurse Practitioners (NAPNAP). (2000). *Standards of practice for PNPs.* Retrieved from http://www.napnap.org/practice/pnpstandards/

Newacheck, P. W., Strickland, B., Shonkoff, J. P., Perrin, J. M., McPherson, M., McManus, M., Lauver, G., Fox, H., & Arango, P. (1998). An epidemiologic profile of children with special health care needs. *Pediatrics, 102*, 117–123.

Pavluri, M. N., Luk, S. L., Clarkson, J., & McGee, R. A. (1995). Community study of preschool behavior disorder in New Zealand. *Australian and New Zealand Journal of Psychiatry, 29*, 454–462.

Rauch, P. K., Jellinek, M. S., Murphy, J. M., Schachner, L., Hansen, R., Esterly, N. B., Prendiville, J. S., Bishop, S. J., & Goshko, M. (1991). Screening for psychosocial dysfunction in pediatric dermatology practice. *Clinical Pediatrics, 30*, 493–497.

Rushton, J., Bruckman, D., & Kelleher, K. (2002). Primary care referral of children with psychosocial problems. *Archives of Pediatrics and Adolescent Medicine, 156*, 592–598.

Sameroff, A. J., Seifer, R., Barocas, R., Zax, M., & Greenspan, S. (1987). Intelligence quotient scores of 4-year-old children: Social–environmental risk factors. *Pediatrics, 79*, 343–350.

Scott, F. G., Lingaraju, S., Kilgo, J., Kregel, J., & Lazzari, A. (1993). A survey of pediatricians on early identification and early intervention services. *Journal of Early Intervention, 17*, 129–138.

Shonkoff, J. P, Dworkin, P. H., Leviton, A., & Levine, M. D. (1979). Primary care approaches to developmental disabilities. *Pediatrics, 64*, 506–514.

Smith, R. D. (1978). The use of developmental screening tests by primary care pediatricians. *Journal of Pediatrics, 93*, 524–527.

Wake, M., & Gerner, B. (2002, May). *Parent and teacher developmental concerns at school entry: What happens to academic outcomes two years later?* Presentation to the Pediatric Academic Societies, Baltimore, MD.

20

Forensic and Psychosexual Assessment

MARC GOLDMAN

Most individuals with developmental disabilities are law-abiding citizens. In some cases, where individuals with developmental delay have clearly engaged in dangerous criminal activity, support providers, police, and prosecutors are reluctant to initiate legal proceedings. Those prosecuted are vulnerable to disproportionate incarceration, susceptible to abuse in correctional settings, and likely to experience cessation of significant treatment.

Webster's New Universal Unabridged Dictionary (1989) defines forensics as an adjective "pertaining to, connected with, or used in courts of law or public discussion and debate." Forensic psychology, it follows, entails the interchange between psychology and the law. This intersection is the application of the science of psychology to a variety of legal issues involving victims, offenders, and suspected offenders. Forensic psychology is clinical in nature and provides the criminal justice system with relevant expert opinion. Forensic psychologists and psychiatrists advise the court on a variety of matters including an individual's competence for criminal proceedings, criminal culpability, and the probability of reoffence.

The reports of mental health professionals are used by the criminal justice system to consider a wide range of issues. Assessment of criminal behavior can vary in focus but frequently includes determination of risk for dangerousness and violence. Even though the decision in any matter remains that of the judge or administrator, the foundation for the decision is often that provided by the mental health professional.

Assessment of sexual offenders is often referred to as sex-offence-specific evaluation. They rely on specialized techniques developed to predict risk of sexual reoffence. The mental health professional makes

MARC GOLDMAN • Consultant, Private Practice, Durham, North Carolina 27707.

recommendations concerning safety, treatment, and supervision requirements of the sexual offender.

This chapter will focus on a relatively few issues pertaining to individuals having developmental disabilities and the criminal justice system and
is relevant to care, treatment, or support for individuals at risk of criminal behavior, regardless of whether or not they have been charged with
criminal activity. It is important to note that the majority of research on
the topic concerns adult males generally functioning within the mild range
of mental retardation, for several reasons that will become evident in the
sections of this chapter that follow.

PREVALENCE OF CRIMINAL BEHAVIOR

Social concern and clinical activity reflecting the relationship between
crime and developmental disabilities can be traced back to a century and
remains of considerable, and perhaps growing, significance today (Gardner,
Graeber, & Machkovitz, 1998; Lindsay, 2002). In particular, there has been
an increase in research on forensic issues and services for people with
developmental disabilities during the last 10 years (Lindsay, 2002).

Goddard (1914) speculated that one-half of the inmates of reformato-
ries and prisons were intellectually impaired. He concluded that "feeble-
mindedness" was responsible for "social sores" that included "paupers,
criminals, prostitutes, drunkards, and examples of all forms of social pest
with which modern society is burdened" (p. 116). Goddard proposed "segregation through colonization" and argued that people with intellectual
deficits be sterilized, "because the conditions have become so intolerable"
(p. 117). Goddard's statements reflect perspectives that appear to have
gained acceptance among some leaders, but not all, in the field of mental
retardation in the United States from the late 1890s to the 1920s; emphasizing that people with mental retardation and other disabilities were
vulnerable to engaging in a wide range of immoral behaviors. Goddard, and
others who sympathized with this perspective, later repudiated such generalizations and assertions, but lingering effects of these broadly promulgated viewpoints have since lingered as undercurrents of popular culture,
in the sense that people with mild mental retardation may be thought to be
vulnerable to immoral conduct, a generalization not supported by research
or evaluation through the past decades.

Although research indicates that people having developmental disabilities can be identified within the criminal justice system, prevalence
estimates of the proportion of inmates with mental retardation or other developmental disabilities have varied widely, and often do not include those
on probation or parole, or diverted to other programs (Goldman, 1997;
Hawk, Rosenfeld, & Warren, 1993; Mason & Murphy, 2002). State correctional agency data that have been reported suggest prevalence rates among
U.S. states within inmate populations ranging from 0.5 to 19.1% (Noble &
Conley, 1992). Although it is possible that prisoners with developmental
disabilities are unequally distributed throughout the United States, it is

more likely that the disparities in state-specific prevalences are the result of different screening or assessment method used to identify people with developmental disabilities among state correctional agencies (Gardner et al., 1998; Noble & Conley, 1992; Petrella, 1992). In addition to those arrested and incarcerated, it appears that a significant number of individuals with developmental disabilities who are never prosecuted despite evidence that they have engaged in serious criminal acts (Mikkelsen & Stelk, 1999). Police and prosecutors may be reluctant to proceed for a variety of reasons (Coleman & Haaven, 2001; Kearns, 2001). Unfortunately, in many instances when criminal proceedings could occur, but do not, this may prevent service systems from implementing interventions that reflect significant consequences and court-sanctioned conditions that may motivate the offender to change his or her behavior and comply with treatment and community restrictions related to the nature of the criminal acts.

Although estimates of the percentage of persons having developmental delay within the population of sexual offenders are also wide in range, they do suggest a higher than expected rate. Hawk et al. (1993) argued that estimates of prevalence of sex offenders having developmental disabilities might significantly underestimate true prevalence because they are based on data obtained from prisons and do not include those charged but diverted to alternative settings. They investigated the specific charges against individuals who underwent forensic assessment in Virginia over a 6-year period and found that the rate of sex offense charges was almost twice as high among developmentally disabled individuals than among other defendants. Day (1997) reported that people with developmental disabilities are overrepresented in all studies of sex offences. Griffiths (2002) reported percentages of persons with developmental disabilities among the population of sexual offenders ranging from 3–4% to 15–33%.

Noble and Conley (1992) concluded that there was "little point" in attempting to determine the exact percentage of people with developmental delay in the prison system. They assert that the numbers are "significant" and many people with developmental disabilities are not receiving appropriate services while in prison. Their contention that prisons often fall short in providing adequate services for offenders with disabilities seems intuitively applicable to such offenders residing in the community as well.

SUSCEPTIBILITY TO THE CRIMINAL JUSTICE SYSTEM

Upon his or her first interaction with police, a person with mental retardation is likely to speak and behave in ways that increase possibility of arrest and punishment (Perske, 1991). Fear or lack of comprehension might result in behaviors interpreted by the criminal justice system as cavalier, arrogant, or defiant. Poor comprehension of the serious nature of their situation, lack of support, and lack of adequate counsel results in the individual being vulnerable to more assertive booking, interrogation, incarceration, and retention by the criminal justice system than is experienced by nondisabled peers (Lindsay, 2002). It is doubtful that many individuals with developmental disabilities, unless they have had specific training, understand that police are entitled to employ devious methods in order to obtain confessions or that everyone has a constitutional right to an attorney when charged with a crime. Ericson and Perlman (2001) reported that individuals with developmental disabilities demonstrated poor comprehension of a variety of legal terms that were believed to "undoubtedly arise in typical legal situations." For example, many of the participants in this study (45%) did not understand the concept of "guilty" and some reversed the meaning of "guilty" and "innocent."

Motivation to hide one's disability as well as motivation to please others can lead to false confessions (Perske, 1991). A person with a disability generally lacks the capacity to understand that a confession might lead to serious consequences.

Adjustment to prison by individuals with developmental disabilities has been observed to be poor. Smith, Algozzine, Schmid, and Hennly (1990) found that prisoners with developmental disabilities were two to three times more likely to receive disciplinary reports "than were matched convicts who were not disabled." Poor disciplinary records as well as assignment of longer sentences because of inadequate representation in court may explain why prisoners with developmental disabilities are likely to be somewhat older than the general prison population and have greater difficulty obtaining parole (Noble & Conley, 1992).

RESEARCH ON ABERRANT SEXUAL EXPRESSION

The majority of significant developments in the treatment of sexual offenders have occurred over the past 30 years (Marshall & Serran, 2000). Early treatment during this era primarily consisted of behavioral techniques designed to suppress sexual expression (Griffiths, Quinsey, & Hingsburger, 1989). Individuals with developmental delays who had engaged in sexual expression that others considered "inappropriate" have historically been vulnerable to institutional placement and behavioral suppression techniques targeting sexual expression. In the 1970s aversive procedures were readily accepted as the treatment of choice for sexual offenders without evident developmental delays, principally for classical deconditioning of sexual arousal to inappropriate cues. Despite the popularity of such methods, there remains a lack of evidence that such techniques resulted in long-term change in sexual expression (Marshall, Anderson, & Fernandez, 1999). Griffiths et al. (1989) have noted that despite an understanding that the reduction of undesirable behaviors is best achieved through the learning of desirable behaviors, such teaching has rarely occurred when addressing aberrant sexual expression.

There are few studies of sexual offenders with developmental delay (Day, 1997; Timms & Goreczny, 2002). The majority of research is descriptive and provides information that has implications for prevention as well as treatment. One survey and literature review reported that sexual offenders who have developmental disabilities exhibited more social skill deficits and were sexually naive than their peers (Tudiver, Brockstra, Josselyn, & Barbaree, 1997). Day (1997) reported that poor interpersonal skills and lack of sexual knowledge and experience were prevalent among sex offenders with intellectual impairment.

Day (1997) reported that "true sexual deviance is rare" (p. 88). It seems evident that therapeutic interventions for individuals who are not aroused by deviant stimuli will vary in at least some respects from those diagnosed with paraphilias. Hingsburger, Griffiths, and Quinsey (1991) suggested that some individuals with developmental disabilities who do engage in aberrant sexual expression are influenced by variables such as lack of appropriate interpersonal skills or sexual knowledge. Such "counterfeit deviance" may also be influenced by agency-created environments and rules, which may lead to lack of opportunity for sexual expression, and absence of agency policy that involve rights or grounds for restriction of rights to sexual expression. Coleman and Haaven (2001) have cautioned that sex-offence-specific evaluation referrals for individuals with developmental disabilities must be screened to determine if the problem is the result of the referring agency's policies, practices, or structure rather than individual factors. Lambrick and Glaser (2004) noted that the initial task in assessment of individuals with intellectual disability who had engaged in offensive sexual behavior is to determine if the behavior was due to knowledge or understanding deficits versus more serious processes such as deviant arousal or antisocial attitudes and beliefs.

Although there are clearly uncertainties about the prevalence of sex offense among people with mental retardation, the proportion of people who are at risk of being sexually abused appears greater than among the general population, albeit the reported percentage of increased risk varies as a result of experimental design used (Mansell & Sobsey, 2001; Ryan, 1994). Research has demonstrated that higher-than-expected percentages of sex offenders with developmental disabilities were themselves sexually victimized (Knight & Prentky, 1993). Although there is a well-established association between victimization and subsequent offensive behavior, research has not established that offending is the result of victimization (Menard, 2002). Victimization is not considered the exclusive reason for aberrant sexual expression nor a justification. Moreover, the great majority of members of the general population who have reported being sexually abused do not engage in sexually abusive behavior; thus, a history of being abused is not an effective predictor of the likelihood that a given individual will abuse others.

Current treatment approaches for sex offenders consider and treat multiple aspects of the individual and emphasize cognitive–behavioral techniques. Some argue that cognitive–behavioral treatment can require skills lacking in people with developmental disabilities (Barbaree & Marshall, 1998), but others report successful use of this approach when a variety of accommodations are implemented (Haaven, Little, & Petre-Miller, 1990; Rea, Dixon, Parker, & Martin, 2003; Ward & Bosek, 2002). Given the lacking solid research base for treatment and the absence of a clear consensus from the community of professionals supporting individuals having developmental disabilities, Fedoroff, Fedoroff, and Peever (2002) possibly understated that, "Few topics in clinical practice raise more controversy than the question of how to best manage sex offenders" (p. 355).

ASSESSMENT OF DANGEROUSNESS

Risk assessment has been described as the evaluation of the likelihood that a person will commit a new offense and the conditions that influence possible reoffense (McGrath, 1991, 1992, cited in Mussack & Carich, 2001). There are numerous points within the criminal justice system where the assessment of risk of future violent behavior is germane (Heilbrun & Griffin, 1998). Courts consider such predictions when making important decisions concerning sentencing and conditional release. Risk assessments are considered when determining if an individual can be safely supervised in the community. Under these circumstances, the court seeks an answer to the question, "Will the offender commit this or a similar crime again?" In addition to completion of risk assessments in order to inform the criminal justice system of recidivism risk, many providers of services for people having developmental disabilities seek such information for individuals believed to be dangerous despite limited or nil court involvement. Turner (2000) reported that service providers are under increasing pressure to measure and control risks despite conceptual and measurement problems pertaining to the concept of dangerousness. Such noncourt-related risk assessments are completed to determine appropriate safety, treatment or habilitation, and staff support needs. Although risk assessment instruments are becoming increasingly sophisticated and combine various sources of information, they are based on studies of populations that may present risks or risk factors that are directly generalizable to individuals with mental retardation. Currently, there is a lack of empirical evidence supporting the validity of forensic assessment tools when used in evaluation of people having developmental disabilities (Johnston, 2002; Turner, 2000). Griffiths (2002) has cautioned that some risk assessment instruments are being used with people with developmental disabilities despite lack of evidence that they are valid for the population.

Modern day risk assessments are based on actuarial models and focus on static or historical variables such as criminal history, childhood adjustment, and paraphilia. Those treating or supervising individuals at risk of criminal behavior must also consider dynamic or variable risk factors. Dynamic factors include those that might change rapidly, such as access to victims, and might result in destabilization such as mental status and mood, drug use, and social or environmental influences (e.g., changes in level of available supervision, association with other people who themselves present risk of criminal offence). Dynamic risk factors can be used in the community to assist in determining when the level of supervision should be changed to lower an individual's risk (Quinsey, 2004).

Mikkelsen and Stelk (1999) developed a model of assessment for people with developmental disabilities who may be at risk of criminal behavior.

Their approach considers static and dynamic variables. The model also considers system issues that might influence likelihood of reoffense. Although this model provides an organized framework that a community team supporting people with developmental delays will find useful in assessment of risk and development of treatment interventions, the authors of the approach caution that those unfamiliar with criminal offenders and risk assessment are vulnerable to errors of interpretation that may result in overestimation or underestimation of risk.

PREDICTORS OF SEXUAL RECIDIVISM

There are many published reports indicating that sex offenders show evidence of disordered patterns of sexual arousal (Barbaree & Marshall, 1998). Hanson and Bussiere's (1998) meta-analysis reported that the strongest predictors of sexual offense recidivism were variables related to sexual deviancy, prior sexual offenses, early age of onset of sexual offenses, and victims who are strangers. The strongest predictor was pronounced, phallometrically measured, sexual interest in children. These and additional variables reported by Hanson and Bussiere have been replicated in at least four studies and do indeed appear to be related to recidivism risk (Hanson, 2000), at least among known, identified offenders.

Phallometric techniques (typically referred to as plethysmography, penile plethysmography, or psychophysiological assessment) involve measuring penile circumference or volume during exposure to varied pictures or audiotapes of deviant and nondeviant sexual stimuli. Earlier studies utilizing plethymography tended to use pictures as (visual) stimuli, whereas more recent research protocols generally use audiotaped (auditory) stimuli. Langevin and Curnoe (2002) have noted that sex offenders in general might be unable to specify a sexual preference for children and that this may be "particularly difficult for individuals having developmental disabilities" (p. 394) They reported that phallometric assessment is "especially valuable" in evaluations of people with developmental delay who have engaged in sexual behavior with children. Phallometric results of individuals with developmental disabilities should be interpreted with caution. It has been reported that individuals with developmental delay tend to respond generally on phallometric tests with higher levels of sexual arousal than that of their peers (Association for the Treatment of Sexual Abusers, 2001; Haaven et al., 1990).

Haaven et al. (1990) reported that the use of plethysmograpy in their residential treatment program for sex offenders with developmental disabilities aided in the development of individualized treatment plans, facilitated lessening of denial, better measured the effectiveness of interventions, and provided a "sense of hope and accomplishment" to those making progress in treatment of deviant arousal. The program adapted the technique to include discussions of the process with staff and peers familiar with the assessment, preparatory visitations to the assessment area during which offenders became familiar with the equipment, and engagement in "trial runs." Assessment was not initiated until it was determined that the individual was "psychologically prepared." There is a lack of information concerning use, and predictive validity, of phallometric techniques with individuals with developmental disabilities. Even when accommodations are made, results of phallometric assessments of individuals with developmental delays should be interpreted with caution and should not be used without additional assessment information when making decisions concerning community safety and least restrictive residential settings.

Although current instruments predicting risk of reoffense generally rely on historical or static variables, changeable (dynamic) factors should also be considered when providing treatment (Hanson, 2000) and developing of safety plans. Gathering such information challenges the examiner. Sex offenders are generally believed to be unreliable historians who are well versed in deception. Coleman & Haaven (2001) caution that when working with sex offenders with developmental disabilities, one must distinguish denial from memory impairment. The examiner must refer to past records, including arrest reports and court records, and seek collateral interviews in an attempt to discern numerous variables that might have influenced the individual at the time of criminal behavior.

ASSESSMENT OF SEXUAL DANGEROUSNESS

Determination of the likelihood that an individual will engage in aberrant sexuality in the future and understanding the circumstances under which such behavior would most likely occur makes up the process of risk assessment of sexual offense. Although Doren (cited in Mussack & Carich, 2001) developed a list of 30 risk assessment instruments and Prentsky and Edmunds (1977) compiled over ninety instruments that are used by clinicians who work with sex offenders, there is no instrument that is adequately validated for assessment purposes with people with developmental disabilities.

Fedoroff, Smolewska, Selhi, Ng, and Bradford (2001) noted that the violence risk appraisal guide (VRAG) and the sex offender risk appraisal guide (SORAG) are gaining acceptance as the best predictors of risk for violence (VRAG) and sexual offences (SORAG). Research on these actuarial scales, developed by Quinsey, Harris, Rice, and Cormier (1998), is at the early stage (Seghorn & Ball, 2000). Fedoroff et al. (2001) reported that it appeared that both instruments falsely elevated scores of offenders who with developmental delays when matched with offenders of normal intellectual abilities who had the same number of known victims. Griffiths (2002) noted that people with developmental disabilities are more susceptible to over-rating on some of the items on these instruments, while being possibly favored by other items.

Given the minimal amount of actuarial, or descriptive, data available on risk and offenders with developmental delay, clinical models of assessment are often used (Johnston, 2002).

Bays and Freeman-Longo (1995) have considered 29 factors as a basis for estimating risk. These factors include static, or unchangeable variables such as history of offenses, anger associated with offenses, and the presence and number of paraphilias. Their instrument, the Bays & Freeman-Longo Evaluation of Dangerousness for Sexual Offenders, also considers numerous variables that can change over time (dynamic factors) such as motivation for treatment and willingness to discuss the offense. Use of this unvalidated approach serves as a useful guide for evaluation when used along with additional instruments and interview information.

RISK ASSESSMENT OF INDIVIDUALS HAVING DEVELOPMENTAL DISABILITIES

Along with determining risk, a comprehensive assessment provides information that guides treatment strategies (Mikkelsen, 2004). Given the lack of validated approaches to assessment of offenders and non-adjudicated people having developmental disabilities who are suspected of dangerous behavior, or known to have engaged in such behavior, care should be taken to gather as much information as possible from the individual, records, and collaterals, prior to estimating risk and developing treatment and intervention recommendations or plans. Assessment should remain ongoing; not only to obtain additional static information but to also consider changes in dynamic factors. Risk prediction, restrictions, and treatment interventions should be developed through a combination of assessment results, information concerning offenders without intellectual impairment, and information from the field of developmental disabilities. Relying solely on research concerning offenders without developmental disabilities may result in inaccurate predictions, inappropriate interventions, or lack of needed treatments. Relying on one or several static or dynamic factors may result in an underestimate or overestimate of risk and will limit the development of treatment interventions.

Evaluation of an individual with developmental disabilities at risk of criminal behavior should include comprehensive examination of individual, social, and system characteristics (Gardner et al., 1998; Griffiths, 2002; McGee & Menolascino, 1992). Seghorn and Ball (2000) and Ward and Bosek (2002) have described static and dynamic variables that should be considered in risk assessment of sex offenders having developmental disabilities. These include sex offense and other criminal behavior history, willingness to discuss the offense and cooperate with the assessment, acceptance of responsibility, remorse, deviant sexual interests, victim typology, mental illness, substance abuse, willingness for treatment, adaptive and emotional functioning, social skills, and sexual knowledge and attitudes.

Quinsey (2004) reported that the Short Dynamic Risk Scale was useful in predicting antisocial behavior in individuals with a history of criminal behavior. The scale includes ratings on dynamic factors including accountability for one's behavior, constructive coping skills, anxiety, anger, and

frustration, offensive, teasing and obnoxious verbal behavior, lack of consideration for others, poor housekeeping skills, and poor self-care skills.

Griffiths et al. (1989) stress that reasons why more appropriate or typical psychosexual development failed to occur should be pursued in order to
provide a partial basis for proactive and preventative treatment of aberrant
sexual expression. Griffiths (2002) suggested consideration of aberrant behavior, including abnormal sexual expression, through the "Multimodal
Contextual Model," which evaluates biomedical, psychological, and socioenvironmental variables, such as genetic factors, history of opportunities
to acquire culturally typical sexual behavior repertoires, and availability of
peers and family members with whom one might discuss issues surrounding sexuality.

Although these variables, and those outlined below, are extensive, it
must be emphasized that there is little empirical evidence of the importance
of these risk factors for people having developmental disabilities (Lindsay,
2002).

When evaluating individuals with developmental disabilities who are
at risk of criminal behavior, a combination of evaluation approaches is necessary. The established approaches to assessing the offender without intellectual impairment cannot be ignored. Haaven et al. (1990) and Coleman
and Haaven (2001) report that although there are differences between sex
offenders with and without developmental disabilities, there are meaningful clinical similarities. Variables known to be associated with risk should
indeed be evaluated, but these results should be interpreted with particular care. Evaluations must also consider the vulnerabilities to aberrant
sexual expression associated with individuals having developmental disabilities. The individual and guardian (if indicated) should be informed of
the nature and purpose of the evaluation. It is important to describe the
evaluation process and limited confidentiality of the report in a simple but
complete manner that the client understands, and to obtain either consent or assent for evaluation, depending upon relevant state regulations or
laws. Evaluations of individuals who have been charged but as yet not convicted of an offense should be avoided because a person who understands
that information obtained during the evaluation may be revealed during
the trial will be more likely to withhold or underreport salient information.
Generally, an assessment conducted with an unresponsive or uncooperative individual is likely to obtain sufficiently accurate information and
correspondingly likely to distort estimates of risk or reoffense.

The following should be considered a guide for forensic assessment,
including determining the risk of future criminal behavior. Static and dynamic information obtained from such an assessment should be used
to develop individualized treatment and intervention recommendations or
plans.

1. Review information from the systems that have been involved with
   the individual. Prior to interviewing the client, the examiner should
   be thoroughly familiar with the facts of the offense as well as the
   individual's history. Determine the context and facts of the criminal

behavior. This will require review of information from the criminal justice system, community providers of supports, the offender, and the offender's family. Detailed information concerning the individual's documented and undocumented criminal history should be gathered, including dates and age of the client at the time of the offense(s), description of the offense(s) and its context, the degree and method of violence, the type of victim (age, sex, relationship to the offender), and the client's attitudes and reasoning concerning the offences. Documentation of past criminal behavior is likely to be lacking due to the reluctance on the part of some support providers and criminal justice systems to pursue charges. The examiner must often aggressively seek information from a variety of sources. Past and present environmental responses to such behavior in the home, school, and community should be gathered. When assessing responses to previous treatment, the adequacy of the treatment should be considered. That is, did the treatment address variables of plausible salience, was its duration and nature sufficient to engender therapeutic effects, and were features of the treatment modified to take into account the individual's special needs?

2. Background information should include developmental history and an understanding of the environment that influenced the individual. Indicators that the individual was exposed to chaotic or traumatic settings or events are useful and may assist in determining if the individual was likely to have been taught culturally typical values and a sense of responsibility. The possibility of neglect and physical, emotional, and sexual abuse should be investigated. School history should be reviewed, as well as marital or other significant social or sexual relationships and substance use history. Information concerning psychiatric admissions, depression, and suicide attempts should be reviewed. The offender's use of leisure time, vocational history and current employment, and daily activities should be established.

3. A history of diagnoses should be gathered. Reliability of historical diagnoses should be estimated. Diagnoses of personality disorders should be carefully reviewed for substantiating information and confirmed rather than accepted as reliable. The role or influence of any mental disorder should be determined. That is, is the offender more or less likely to engage in criminal behavior when symptoms are florid or the person is noncompliant with medication?

4. Determine internal and external variables that influence the offensive behavior. Griffiths (2002) provides a thorough discussion of such influential variables as they pertain to aberrant sexual expression. They include biological, psychological, habilitative, social, and environmental influences. After establishing rapport, emotional characteristics, social skills, and psychosexual knowledge and attitudes (if the crime is of a sexual nature) should be assessed. The individual should be screened as a possible victim of abuse. The individual's willingness to discuss the offense and their willingness

to take responsibility for their behavior as opposed to denying or minimizing said behavior should be determined. The individual's amenability for treatment and willingness to abide by community restrictions should be evaluated. Assessment of remorse is challenging. The individual is aware that he or she is in trouble. The examiner is challenged to determine if the individual regrets his or her behavior due to the resulting predicament or is feeling regret for harming others.

5. If the assessment focus is aberrant sexual behavior, the interview should include assessment of deviant interest and fantasies, and planning of the behavior. A detailed sexual history should be completed that includes how the individual learned about sex and his or her deviant and nondeviant sexual experiences. Documented and nondocumented history of sexual assaults should be reviewed with the client and victim preferences should be determined. That is, the clinician should determine what type of individual is most at risk of victimization. The client's access to potential victims should be considered, both with respect to past incidents and intervention planning. The methods used to select victims should be investigated. Assessment of the individual's sexual knowledge and attitudes should be completed, including beliefs regarding sexual activity and interpretations of the responses of victims (e.g., the belief that victim resistance to sexual advances is not genuine). If the individual resides in a restrictive setting, agency policies or restrictions that may have influenced the client's behavior should be considered.

6. The attitudes of those supporting the individual should be assessed. Of particular interest is whether the individual's network denies or minimizes the individual's offensive behavior, inadvertently increases risk of reoffense (e.g., allows access to potential victims, provides insufficient oversight), or considers such behavior as serious and in need of intervention.

7. Throughout the evaluation of an individual at risk of sexual offenses, information concerning risk should be gathered. Mussack and Carich (2001) summarized the factors believed to increase the risk of sexual offending to include denial of offense, multiple victims, multiple victim types, multiple deviant sexual interests, history of nonsexual criminal behavior, younger victims, history of violence, history of substance abuse if it was involved in the aberrant sexual behavior, ritualistic offending, lack of remorse or empathy, presence of a significant personality disorder, previous probation/parole failure, history of the individual being subjected to extensive sexual abuse that is similar to the individual's own victimization pattern, failure to complete previous treatment or aftercare, and the presence of cognitive distortions and defensive coping techniques that are used to deny or minimize the aberrant sexual expression. As previously emphasized, care must be taken to view such factors in the context of the individual's disability. Coleman and Haaven (2001) have noted that individuals with developmental disabilities

are likely to use denial to defend against any perceived threat, thus, denial may be seen as an adaptive coping strategy rather than a self-defensive response in the context of accusation or discussion of criminal behavior.

8. Determine the resources required so those influential physiological, psychological, or social and environmental variables that increase risk can be eliminated, reduced, treated, or controlled.

9. The final session with the offender should include an explanation of findings and treatment recommendations. This provides an opportunity to discuss the serious nature of the problem and the person's situation, as well as instilling hope and motivating the individual to actively participate in treatment. It is often productive to inform the offender at the time of the initial interview and provide subsequent reminders that such feedback will be provided.

Care must be taken to gather sufficient risk assessment information prior to providing community support for an individual who has engaged in sexually aggressive behavior or other criminal behavior. When, where, and toward whom the individual is most likely to reoffend should be determined. The person's willingness to cooperate with supervision and comply with rules for community protection must be established through frank discussion with the individual. If community treatment is indicated, the residential provider and others in the offender's support network must take offense risk seriously and become willing participants in assuring safety of the individual and those around him or her (Cumming & Buell, 1997). Clear consequences for violations of conditions of treatment should be established and agreed upon by the offender, service providers, family or advocates as relevant, and if indicated, the court.

COMMUNITY SAFETY PLANNING

Regardless of involvement of the criminal justice system or whether the offensive behavior was of a sexual or nonsexual type, those supporting an individual having developmental disabilities in the community who is at risk of criminal behavior should develop and implement a safety plan designed to minimize risk of reoffence. The safety plan should be based on risk assessment information and include indicators of when the individual is at higher risk due to dynamic stressors. The plan should include the following:

1. *Control of social and environmental risk factors:* Access to potential victims must be restricted. This might include restrictions of housing location, visitors in the home, and community access, including intensity of supervision. Other influences established through assessment, such as use of pornography or drug and alcohol use that influence offending behavior should be restricted.

2. *Interventions designed to reduce dynamic internal factors:* Therapeutic interventions addressing psychological variables should be

ongoing and provided by qualified providers. These might include teaching and practice of specific skills often provided by developmental disability agencies such as anger management or social skills training. Other interventions may require involvement of specialized providers experienced in accommodated sex offence or felony-specific treatment.

3. *Emergency or crisis indicators:* The network of support providers should be aware of dynamic factors or indicators that the individual is at increased risk of offending. A process of notification of such indicators to a responsible party or treatment coordinator should be established. A change in management and supervision level should be considered when increased risk is observed.

4. *Emergency or crisis procedures:* Specific responses to crisis indicators that are designed to protect the individual and community from reoffence should be implemented when crisis indicators are recognized. Responses might include increased supervision or restrictions, additional treatment interventions, and notification to probation or parole officers depending upon the specifics of court orders or correctional history.

5. *Established consequences of aberrant behaviors or offending behaviors:* The individual and serving agencies and professionals should understand preestablished responses to offending behavior and provisions must be established to assure that agencies and professionals can immediately implement such responses to offending behavior. Minimizing criminal behavior or giving the individual a "second chance" merely makes such behavior more likely in the future (on an actuarial basis), placing potential victims at risk of harm and the offender at risk of increasingly restrictive community sanctions, incarceration, or reincarceration.

SUMMARY

Despite growing interest in recent years in forensic issues pertaining to people with developmental disabilities, considerable philosophical deliberation and empirical investigation is needed. There is no consensus in the developmental disabilities field concerning methods and alternatives to serve and support offenders or individuals at risk of criminal behavior. The disability community has developed assessment processes that identify areas of individual need for services or supports, but for the most part has been reluctant to expand the process to include criminal behavior. Functional Analysis, a traditional tool used in the developmental disabilities field, could be modified to evaluate the offender with intellectual disability (Lambrick & Glaser, 2004). On the one hand, some people with developmental disabilities engage in criminal behavior, and it seems that many can benefit from alternative sentencing or other special provisions, whereas on the other hand therapeutic offender services may be increasingly controversial in a context of changing social values in the larger culture that increasingly favor retribution and extended incarceration as responses to a range of offenses, but especially in response to sex offenses. Given the apparent general reluctance of the developmental disability field to consider many of these difficult issues and provide specialized services, providers of assessment and treatment services to offenders without developmental disabilities are often called upon to assess people with developmental disabilities without the advantage of understanding their special needs. Developmental disabilities professionals who are willing to provide services often find little research-based evidence to support the selection of assessment tools and their responsible interpretation.

Assessment of individuals having developmental disabilities at risk of criminal behavior requires the careful application of knowledge from two scientific fields. Both fields report a lack of information concerning offenders with developmental disabilities. Both fields advocate assessment of multiple influences on aberrant behavior. Both fields acknowledge the need for a clearer understanding of numerous variables. Those involved in the support of individuals with developmental disabilities at risk of criminal behavior must cautiously apply information from both fields as they question, evaluate, and modify their approaches to assessment and planning.

REFERENCES

Association for the Treatment of Sex Abusers. (2001). *Practice standards and guidelines for members of the association for the treatment of sexual abusers.* Beaverton, OR: Author.

Barbaree, H. E., & Marshall, W. L. (1998). Treatment of the sexual offender. In R. Wettstein (Ed.), *Treatment of offenders with mental disorders* (pp. 265–328). New York: Guilford Press.

Bays, L., & Freeman-Longo, R. (1995). Evaluation of dangerousness for sexual offenders. In M. S. Carich & D. Adkerson (Eds.), *Adult sexual offender assessment packet* (pp. 88–93). Brandon, VT: Safer Society Press.

Coleman, E. M., & Haaven, J. (2001). Assessment and treatment of intellectually disabled sexual abusers. In M. Carich & S. Mussack (Eds.), *Handbook for sexual abuser assessment and treatment* (pp. 193–209). Brandon, VT: Safer Society Press.

Cumming, G., & Buell, M. (1997). *Supervision of the sex offender.* Brandon, VT: Safer Society Press.

Day, K. (1997). Clinical features and offence behavior of mentally retarded sex offenders: A review of research. *The NADD Newsletter, 14*(6), 86–90.

Ericson, K. I., & Perlman, N. B. (2001). Knowledge of legal terminology and court proceedings in adults with developmental disabilities. *Law and Human Behavior, 25,* 529–545.

Fedoroff, J. P., Smolewska, K., Selhi, Z., Ng, E., & Bradford, J. (2001). Assesment of violence and sexual offense risk using the "VRAG" and "SORAG" in a sample of men with developmental delay and paraphilic disorders. A case-controlled study. *International Academy of Sex Research Twenty-Seventh Annual Meeting Abstracts,* p. 17.

Fedoroff, P., Fedoroff, B., & Peever, C. (2002). Consent to treatment issues in sex offenders with developmental delay. In D. Griffiths, D. Richards, P. Fedoroff, & S. Watson (Eds.), *Ethical dilemmas: Sexuality and developmental disability* (pp. 355–386). Kingston, NY: NADD Press.

Gardner, W. I., Graeber, J. L., & Machkovitz, S. J. (1998). Treatment of offenders with mental retardation. In R. Wettstein (Ed.), *Treatment of offenders with mental disorders* (pp. 329–364). New York: Guilford Press.

Goddard, H. H. (1914). *The Kallikak family.* New York: Macmillan.

Goldman, M. (1997). The criminal justice system vs. the criminal mentally retarded: Is justice being served? *The NADD Newsletter, 14*(6), 81–85.

Griffiths, D. M. (2002). Sexual aggression. In W. I. Gardner (Ed.), *Aggression and other disruptive behavioral challenges: Biomedical and psychosocial assessment and treatment* (pp. 328–398). Kingston, NY: NADD Press.

Griffiths, D. M., Quinsey, V. L., & Hingsburger, D. (1989). *Changing inappropriate sexual behavior: A community based approach for persons with developmental disabilities.* Baltimore: Brookes.

Haaven, J., Little, R., & Petre-Miller D. (1990). *Treating intellectually disabled sex offenders.* Brandon, VT: Safer Society Press.

Hanson, R. K. (2000). *Risk assessment: Prepared for the association for the treatment of sexual abusers.* Beaverton, OR: Association for the Treatment of Sexual Abusers.

Hanson, R. K., & Bussiere, M. T. (1998). Predicting relapse: A meta-analysis of sexual offender recidivism studies. *Journal of Consulting and Clinical Psychology, 66*, 348–362.

Hawk, G. L., Rosenfeld, B. D., & Warren, J. I. (1993). Prevalence of sexual offenses among mentally retarded criminal defendants. *Hospital and Community Psychiatry, 44*, 784–786.

Heilbrun, K., & Griffin, P. A. (1998). Community-based forensic treatment. In R. Wettstein (Ed.), *Treatment of offenders with mental disorders* (pp. 168–210). New York: Guilford Press.

Hingsburger, D., Griffiths, D., & Quinsey, V. (1991). Detecting counterfeit deviance: Differentiating sexual deviance from sexual inappropriateness. *The Habilitative Mental Healthcare Newsletter, 9*, 51–54.

Johnston, S. J. (2002). Risk assessment in offenders with intellectual disability: The evidence base. *Journal of Intellectual Disability Research, 46*(Suppl. 1), 47–56.

Kearns, A. (2001). Forensic services and people with learning disability: In the shadow of the Reed report. *Journal of Forensic Psychiatry, 12*, 8–12.

Knight, R. A., & Prentky, R. A. (1993). Exploring characteristics for juvenile sex offenders. In H. Barbaree, W. Marshall, & S. Hudson (Eds.), *The juvenile sex offender* (pp. 45–83). New York: Guilford Press.

Lambrick, F., & Glaser, W. (2004). Sex offenders with an intellectual disability. *Sexual Abuse: A Journal of Research and Treatment, 16*(4), 381–392.

Langevin, R., & Curnoe, S. (2002). Assessment and treatment of sex offenders who have a developmental disability. In D. Griffiths, D. Richards, P. Fedoroff, & S. Watson (Eds.), *Ethical dilemmas: Sexuality and developmental disability* (pp. 387–416). Kingston, NY: NADD Press.

Lindsay, W. R. (2002). Research and literature on sex offenders with intellectual and developmental disabilities. *Journal of Intellectual Disability Research, 46*(Suppl. 1), 74–85.

Mansell, S., & Sobsey, D. (2001). *The Aurora Project: Counseling people with developmental disabilities who have been sexually abused.* Kingston, NY: NADD Press.

Marshall, W. L., Anderson, D., & Fernandez, Y. (1999). *Cognitive behavioral treatment of sexual offenders.* New York: Wiley.

Marshall, W. L., & Serran, G. A. (2000). Improving the effectiveness of sexual offender treatment. *Trauma, Violence, and Abuse: A Review Journal, 1*, 203–222.

Mason, J., & Murphy, G. (2002). Intellectual disability amongst people on probation: Prevalence and outcome. *Journal of Intellectual Disability Research, 46*, 230–238.

McGee, J. J., & Menolascino, F. J. (1992). The evaluation of the defendants with mental retardation in the criminal justice system. In R. W. Conley, R. Luckasson, & G. N. Bouthilet (Eds.), *The criminal justice system and mental retardation: Defendants and victims* (pp. 55–77). Baltimore: Brookes.

McGrath, R. (1991). Sex offender risk assessment and disposition planning: A review of empirical and clinical findings. *International Journal of Offender Therapy and Comparative Criminology, 35*(4), 328–350.

Menard, S. (2002). *Youth violence research bulletin.* Washington, DC: Office of Juvenile Justice and Delinquency Prevention.

Mikkelsen, E. J. (2004). The assessment of individuals with developmental disabilities who commit criminal offenses. In W. R. Lindsay, J. R. Taylor, & P. Sturmey (Eds.), *Offenders with developmental disabilities* (pp. 111–129). West Sussex, England: Wiley.

Mikkelsen, E. J., & Stelk, W. J. (1999). *Criminal offenders with mental retardation: Risk assessment and the continuum of community based programs.* Kingston, NY: NADD Press.

Mussack, S. E., & Carich, M. S. (2001). Sexual abuser evaluation. In M. Carich & S. Mussack (Eds.), *Handbook for sexual abuser assessment and treatment* (pp. 11–36). Brandon, VT: Safer Society Press.

Noble, J. H., & Conley, R. W. (1992). Toward an epidemiology of attributes. In R. W. Conley, R. Lucckasson, & G. N. Bouthilet (Eds.), *The criminal justice system and mental retardation: Defendants and victims* (pp. 17–53). Baltimore: Brookes.

Perske, R. (1991). *Unequal justice.* Nashville, TN: Abingdon.

Petrella, R. C. (1992). Defendants with mental retardation in the forensic service system. In R. W. Conley, R. Lucckasson, & G. N. Bouthilet (Eds.), *The criminal justice system and mental retardation: Defendants and victims* (pp. 79–96). Baltimore: Brookes.

Prentsky, R., & Edmunds, S. B. (1977). *Addressing sexual abuse: A resource guide for practitioners.* Brandon, VT: Safer Society Press.

Quinsey, V. L. (2004). Risk assessment and management in community settings. In W. R Lindsay, J. R. Taylor, & P. Sturmey (Eds.), *Offenders with developmental disabilities* (pp. 132–141). West Sussex, England: Wiley.

Quinsey, V. L., Harris, G. T., Rice, M. E., & Cormier, C. A. (1998). *Violent offenders: Appraising and managing risk.* Washington DC: American Psychological Association.

Rea, J. A., Dixon, M., Parker, T., & Martin, C. (2003). A generalization analysis of relapse prevention skills of four sex offenders with mental retardation. *NADD Bulletin, 6,* 14.

Ryan, R. (1994). Posttraumatic stress syndrome: Assessing and treating the aftermath of sexual assault. *The NADD Newsletter, 11,* 51–53.

Seghorn, T. K., & Ball, C. J. (2000). Assessment of sexual deviance in adults with developmental disabilities. *Mental Health Aspects of Developmental Disabilities, 3,* 47–53.

Smith, C., Algozzine, B., Schmid, R., & Hennly, T. (1990). Prison adjustment of youthful inmates with mental retardation. *Mental Retardation, 28,* 177–181.

Timms, S., & Goreczny, A. J. (2002). Adolescent sex offenders with mental retardation: Literature review and assessment considerations. *Aggression and Violent Behavior, 7,* 1–19.

Tudiver, J., Brockstra, S., Josselyn, S., & Barbaree, H. (1997). *Addressing needs of the developmentally delayed sex offenders: A guide.* Toronto, Ont.: Clark Institute of Psychiatry.

Turner, S. (2000). Forensic risk assessment in intellectual disabilities: The evidence base and current practice in one English region. *Journal of Applied Research in Intellectual Disabilities, 13,* 239–255.

Ward, K. M., & Bosek, R. L. (2002). Behavioral risk management: Supporting individuals with developmental disabilities who exhibit inappropriate sexual behaviors. *Research and Practice for Persons with Severe Disabilities, 27,* 27–42.

Webster's New Universal Unabridged Dictionary. (1989). New York: Dilithium Press.

21

Family Assessment and Social Support

LARAINE MASTERS GLIDDEN and
SARAH A. SCHOOLCRAFT

An explosion of research on families and developmental disabilities occurred during the last two decades of the 20th century and is continuing
into the 21st century. The Mental Retardation/Developmental Disabilities
Branch of the National Institute of Child Health and Human Development
sponsored conferences, workshops, and requests for applications on many
aspects of family adjustment. The American Association on Mental Retardation published a special collection of journal articles (Blacher & Baker,
2002) and special issues of the *American Journal on Mental Retardation*
(1989) and the *Journal of Intellectual Disability Research* (2003) were devoted to the topic. Driven by the greater likelihood that persons with developmental disabilities (DD) would live longer and with their families, the
need for understanding the influence of the family assumed a high priority.
This influence was seen as transactional, with attention directed both to
understanding the effect of a person with DD on the family, as well as the
effect of the family on persons with DD.

In the 1998 *Handbook of Mental Retardation and Development* (Burack,
Hodapp, & Zigler, 1998), no fewer than five different chapters addressed, as
their primary content, issues related to family influences and adaptation.
Because of these chapters and a comprehensive review by Stoneman
in *Ellis' Handbook of Mental Deficiency, Psychological Theory and Research* (MacLean, 1997), we have adopted the following guidelines for this
chapter:

1. Focusing on material published from 1997 to the present, the last
   year cited in any of the six chapters mentioned above.

LARAINE MASTERS GLIDDEN and SARAH A. SCHOOLCRAFT • Department of Psychology,
St. Mary's College of Maryland, 18952 E. Fisher Road, St. Mary's City, Maryland 20686–3001.

2. Differentiating family assessment and social support research with a clinical rather than research purpose, and concentrating on the latter, while
3. Identifying research that has implications for practice, and
4. Emphasizing methodological considerations with an aim to developing recommendations for future research.

CHALLENGES TO FAMILY ASSESSMENT

Definitional Issues

Assessment is predicated on a shared consensus, an agreement regarding a definition of that which is being assessed. Families, however, are highly variable on many dimensions, making definition difficult. Even the seemingly simple issue of "what constitutes a family" introduces complexity. Thus, a family may be a collection of individuals that (says, believes) it is a family—in other words, family as attitude (Myerhoff & Tufte, 1979). If such a tack seems absurd, then consider what to call a 38-year-old never-married man fostering an 8-year-old boy with an intellectual disability (ID). If they are not a family, then what are they? They have geographic, legal, and psychological ties to each other just as "traditional" families do. Consider them 15 years later when the 8-year-old is 23 and lives in a supervised apartment, and the geographic and legal ties have disappeared, but the (former) foster father and his son still have regular contact, and the father acts as a guide and a mentor and a benefactor. Are they not still a family?

It is essential, therefore, to recognize that the variability in the composition of families poses special problems in family assessment. These problems are likely to be multiplied when the family contains a person with an intellectual or other developmental disability, a child who may never become an independent adult, or who as a child may not live in the parental home because of his or her special needs. Despite definitional and other obstacles, however, family assessment does take place, and most investigators and clinicians accept that individuals who assume parenting roles can be considered parents. For example, Hampson, Beavers, and Hulgus (1990) included families that were nuclear, multi-generational, single parent, foster/adoptive, or blended in their paper on interactional assessment of White, Black, and Mexican-American families.

Theoretical Mélange

In addition to the challenges posed by a broad definition of family, an even greater difficulty results from the lack of a widely accepted theory of family functioning. As Bray (1995) pointed out, consensus standards of healthy nor unhealthy family functioning do not exist nor does an evidence-based system for diagnosing dysfunction. Whereas most practitioners may agree on some symptoms of dysfunction as in neglectful and abusive families, healthy families undoubtedly have a remarkably varied topography. As well, because notions of function and dysfunction are largely culturally determined, they are not fixed in time and place; in the 1950's, the functional family with a child with severe mental retardation institutionalized that child. Indeed, hypotheses predicting family dysfunction if a child was not institutionalized were common (Farber, 1959). Fifty years later, the cultural norms have changed.

Instrumentation/Measurement Techniques

The *Handbook of Family Measurement Techniques* (Touliatos, Perlmutter, & Straus, 1990) lists and describes 976 instruments that have been used to measure facets of family functioning. Schumm (1990) notes that in the past, most measures were used only once and investigators frequently created and used new measures without conducting or reporting appropriate psychometric data. This problem exists also in the research on families with children with disabilities (Padula, 1995). Measures are applied that are newly created or modified substantially and adopted without critical scrutiny of reliability and validity, making it difficult to compare new and previous results. For example, we reviewed a sample of 25 articles measuring the demands, burden, or stresses of rearing children with DD published in *American Journal on Mental Retardation, Journal on Intellectual Disability Research* or *Mental Retardation* from 1997 to 2002. Nineteen different instruments were used to operationalize one or more of these constructs, and the most frequently used instrument was used only four times. Thus, when results are not consistent, it is often impossible to determine the reason, e.g., sampling differences, measurement differences, or differences due to independent variables of interest.

In part because of these definitional, theoretical, and instrumentation challenges, methodological considerations are particularly important in understanding the procedures and results of family assessment. Who and what is measured can be as revealing as the results of the measurement. Therefore, we focus on instrumentation and methodology as well as on findings in order to provide the details essential for evaluation of the strengths of the field and the challenges that face it.

WHO AND WHAT IS ASSESSED

Although families as systems are sometimes the focus of assessment, it is also likely that attention is directed toward one or more members of a family. Many investigators (e.g., Dakof, 1996; Hayden et al., 1998) emphasize that family assessment can be at the family, marital, or parent–child interaction level.

Individual Family Members: Parents

Overwhelmingly, early research on family members studied mothers (Minnes, 1998). Although mothers still more frequently serve as the primary respondent reporting on their perceptions, either for themselves or for other family members, increasingly, fathers are being included. In the 1997–2002 period, 51 articles including some aspect of family assessment were published in *American Journal on Mental Retardation. Journal of Intellectual Disability Research*, or *Mental Retardation*. We will use these 51 articles as the basis for drawing conclusions about current emphases and practices in the field of family assessment and social support, and will refer to them in this chapter as the *Recent Journal Sample*. Of these 51, 98% included at least one parent, and 74% of those included both parents. However, fathers are still underrepresented, because frequently their inclusion represents small numbers of fathers. For example, Baker and Blacher (2002) studied the impact of residential placement on 106 families, represented by 73 mothers, 24 fathers, and 9 other family members.

Moreover, fathers who do participate are not necessarily representative of all fathers. Costigan and Cox (2001) examined just how nonrepresentative they were in 661 families that were part of the NICHD Early Child Care Study. Of the eligible fathers, 64.6% agreed to participate. Nonparticipants differed from participants on a number of dimensions. They were less educated and more likely to be of an ethnic/racial minority and working-class; their marriages and current parenting environments were less positive. Their children were more likely to have difficult temperaments and to have more health problems. We do not have comparable information on fathers of children with disabilities, and until we do the assumption should be made that participating fathers are likely to be different from non-participating fathers.

Negative Outcomes: Depression

Depression and stress have been measured extensively in mothers, and, increasingly, in fathers. At this point, there is some consensus that depression, although elevated at the time of diagnosis of a child disability, declines substantially over time, and is elevated only slightly or not at all in comparison to mothers of children and adults without DD or to norms for the instrument (Chen, Ryan-Henry, Heller, & Chen, 2001; Glidden & Schoolcraft, 2003; Gowen, Johnson-Martin, Goldman & Appelbaum, 1989; Harris & McHale, 1989; Hoare, Harris, Jackson & Kerley, 1998; Orsmond, Seltzer, Krauss, & Hong, 2003; Seltzer, Greenberg, Floyd, Pettee, & Hong, 2001). However, not all investigators have obtained this finding. For example, Olsson and Hwang (2001, 2002) compared families with children with ID, autism, and typical development. Mothers of children with ID had depression that was significantly higher than mothers of typically developing children, but also significantly lower than mothers of children with autism. Of additional interest in this research is that fathers in each group reported lower depression than did mothers, and the differences in depression among fathers in the three groups were smaller than those for mothers. Somewhat different mean levels and patterns of responding for mothers and fathers are not unusual.

Stores, Stores, Fellows, and Buckley (1998) found higher scores on the Malaise Inventory for mothers of children with ID other than Down syndrome (DS) than for mothers of children with DS or of typically developing children, with the latter two groups not differing significantly from each other. The Malaise Inventory is more heterogeneous than most depression scales. In Stores et al., it was conceptualized as a measure of stress, and others have used it to assess anxiety (e.g., Gutman, Sameroff, & Cole, 2003).

The longitudinal research of Glidden and colleagues (Flaherty & Glidden, 2000; Glidden & Floyd, 1997; Glidden & Schoolcraft, 2003; Schoolcraft & Glidden, 2002, March) has studied multiple family members, including mothers, and utilizes a unique comparison group: families who have knowingly and voluntarily adopted children with DD, and whose adjustment, therefore, is expected to be positive. Their findings span a 17-year-period with the latest time of measurement taken when the children are entering adulthood. At the time of diagnosis, birth mothers were substantially more depressed than adoptive mothers as measured by the Beck Depression Inventory (Beck, Ward, Mendelson, & Erbaugh, 1961). However, at all time points after that depression was low and not significantly different for birth and adoptive mothers.

Research results have led us to believe that a variety of cultural or personal characteristics are risk factors for depression. For example, Blacher, Lopez, Shapiro and Fusco (1997) found that Latina mothers of children with ID reported elevated depression in comparison both to Latina mothers rearing children without ID and to non-Latina mothers rearing children with ID. Magaña (1999), also in a Latina sample, reported that maternal health, larger support networks, and more satisfaction with social support, as well as having additional young children at home, all were associated with lower depression. Olsson and Hwang (2002) demonstrated greater risk for depression among parents who have a low sense of coherence (Antonovsky, 1993). Relatedly, Glidden and Schoolcraft (2003) demonstrated that personality characteristics such as anxiety, hostility, impulsiveness and self-consciousness as measured by the Neuroticism factor of the NEO-FFI (Costa & McCrae, 1992) are risk factors for depression, as was earlier depression. Thus, both birth and adoptive mothers who reported higher depression at an earlier time were more likely also to report higher depression as long as 17 years later.

Negative Outcomes: Stress

More investigators have studied *stress* than any other negative outcome. In the *Recent Journal Sample*, 49% of the articles assessed some version of this construct, broadly defined as including perceived demands and burden, as well as psychological impact of that burden. The most frequently used instrument was some version or portion of a version of the Questionnaire on Resources and Stress (QRS—Holroyd, 1987). Other commonly used instruments such as the Parenting Stress Inventory (PSI—Abidin, 1982) have considerable overlap with the QRS (Sexton, Burrell,

Thompson & Sharpton, 1992). Although the results of these assessments have yielded a wide spectrum of findings (Guralnick, Neville, Connor, & Hammond, 2003; Honig & Winger, 1997; Hoare et al., 1998) many investigators have concluded that stress levels are higher among parents rearing children with DD than among parents of typically developing children (Baker et al., 2003; Emerson, 2003; Padeliadu, 1998; Roach, Orsmond, & Barratt, 1999; Sarimski, 1997; Stores et al., 1998). This conclusion is different from that of Shapiro, Blacher, and Lopez (1998) and Stoneman (1997) who, at the time they were writing, considered the results to be too contradictory to permit firm conclusions. Certainly it is still the case that not all studies find higher stress within families rearing children with DD. However, many do, and no studies report lower stress in comparison to families with typically developing children. Contradictions may result from sampling and instrument differences, from diagnosis and age differences and many other variables that may moderate the influence of disability on parental stress. A meta-analysis attending to these variables would help to determine the degree of and the process by which the stress is ameliorated or exacerbated. At this point, the only variable that has a reasonably certain claim on stress causation is child behavior problems.

Other qualifications are also essential to interpreting both older and more recent findings. First, the admonitions of a number of investigators (Beckman, 1991; Glidden, 1993; Shapiro, Blacher & Lopez, 1998) with regard to the mixing of demands, stresses, and strains have been largely ignored by most investigators. Glidden used the QRS as a case example, and demonstrated that its items often referred to the *demands* of parenting a child with disabilities (e.g., frequency of doctor visits, child irritability, child physical incapacitation), rather than to physical stress or psychological strain that these demands imposed. Equating demands with stresses and strains inevitably leads to an overestimation of what most investigators label *stress*. This qualification is pertinent to almost all the research published since 1997.

Data from Padeliadu (1998) provide confirmation of the need to be wary of these distinctions. In a study of 41 Greek mothers of children with DS and a comparison group of 41 mothers of typically developing children, she measured demands separately from stress. In addition to completing a Greek version of the QRS, mothers described the type and frequency of child demands on their time and how they felt about those demands. Mothers of children with DS reported higher QRS scores and more time demands than control mothers. However, they also perceived the time demands as more fun than did the control mothers, suggesting that at least some of these demands were not stressful. Indeed, correlations indicated that only demands seen as unpleasant by the mothers of the children with DS were correlated with the separately measured stress score.

Although some version of the QRS is used more than any other single measure, of the 25 articles reviewed in which stress was included as a construct, 19 different instruments (including variations of the QRS and the PSI) were used to operationalize stress. Yet, with the exception of Sexton et al. (1992) no good psychometric research provides data on how these instruments are related and it is difficult, therefore, to compare findings across investigators.

Negative Outcomes: Child Characteristics

In addition to the qualified finding of greater stress for parents caring for children with DD, some consensus is emerging with regard to diagnostic differences and how they relate to various family assessment measures. Although not a universal finding (see Cahill & Glidden, 1996 and Glidden & Cahill, 1998 for different results), many studies report fewer perceived negative outcomes for families rearing children with DS, and more perceived negative outcomes for families rearing children with autism (Hodapp, 1999; Holroyd & McArthur, 1976).

Recent work has also begun to address outcomes for families rearing children with other disabilities such as Cornelia-de-Lange, fragile-X, Prader-Willi, Smith-Magenis, 5p-, and Williams syndromes, among others (Dykens, 1999; Hodapp, Fidler, & Smith, 1998; Hodapp, Wijma, & Masino, 1997; Sarimski, 1997). As Dykens (1999) and Hodapp (1999) have pointed out, some effects on families may be direct consequences of characteristics of the children, whereas others may be more indirect as child characteristics result in changes in the environment which, in turn, influence the development of children. Interest in behavioral phenotypes and how they affect, and are affected by, the family will influence research and continue to intrigue researchers for some time. Indeed, as more specific syndromes are "discovered" and mapped behaviorally, the field will need to guard against fragmentation. Although it is essential to understand the unique characteristics of etiology-specific ID, it is also critical to recognize the similarities related to low general intellectual functioning and deficits in adaptive behavior, similarities that determine the life course of individuals and their families.

Many investigators have hypothesized that more severe disabilities may result in more negative outcomes for family members. Relevant findings, however, are inconsistent, especially when stress and strain are measured independently from demands. In reviews of the research through the mid-1990's, neither Shapiro, Blacher and Lopez (1998) nor Stoneman (1997) was able to draw firm conclusions about severity of disability and negative outcomes. In our *Recent Journal Sample*, although many articles described severity of disability, only five tested it as a variable that influenced outcomes for one or more family members. Only one of these studies presented an unequivocal result: Blacher et al. (1997) reported that mothers were more depressed when their children had more severe levels of ID. Shin (2002) found no significant correlations between adaptive behavior levels and maternal stress in either a Korean or an American sample. As well, Heller, Miller and Factor (1997) found that adaptive behavior was *negatively* correlated with care giving satisfaction, and adaptive behavior was unrelated to a separate measure of care giving burden.

In contrast to mixed findings with regard to severity of disability, there is consensus that regardless of severity of disability, parents report a variety of more negative outcomes when children exhibit behavior problems (Baker et al., 2003; Hastings, 2003; Hastings & Brown, 2002; Miltiades & Pruchno, 2001; Orsmond et al., 2003; Ricci & Hodapp, 2003). Floyd and Gallagher (1997) demonstrated this nicely in a study of mothers and fathers rearing children with or without behavior problems. Some of the children also had either ID or chronic illness. They found that child behavior problems, rather than type of disability, were associated with greater reported stress on various subscales of the QRS.

The realization that behavior problems contribute to negative outcomes has led to intervention programs to reduce maladaptive behavior and thereby the stress, depression, and other negative outcomes for family members. For example, Hudson, Matthews, and Gavidia-Payne (2003) reported on an intervention system called Signposts designed to help caretakers reduce or manage behavior problems in children with DD. Pre- and post-test data indicated success in improving behavior as well as reducing stress and hassles and increasing parental efficacy, adding to the general finding that parent training programs can be quite effective (Harris, Alessandri & Gill, 1991; Mulick, Hammer & Dura, 1991).

Negative Outcomes: Mother/Father Similarities and Differences

Minnes (1998) summarized mother and father differences by concluding that the limited research indicated (1) that mothers generally experienced higher levels of negative outcomes such as stress and depression; and (2) that the pattern of responding was also somewhat different. In our Recent Journal Sample, 10 articles directly compared mothers and fathers rearing children with DD. Hastings and Brown (2002) reported findings that indicate the importance of assessing both levels and patterns in these comparisons. In their study of mothers and fathers of children with autism, they measured self-efficacy as a mediating or moderating variable for the influence of level of child behavior problems on anxiety and depression outcomes. More than twice as many mothers as fathers reported anxiety and depression that was in the clinical or borderline range. Moreover, for mothers, the significant prediction of anxiety and depression by child behavior problems disappeared when maternal self-efficacy was included in the regression analysis, indicating that self-efficacy had a mediating effect for mothers. In contrast, fathers' anxiety and depression were not predicted by self-efficacy, but for fathers of children with high levels of behavior problems, anxiety was low if self-efficacy was high, indicating a different moderating effect of self-efficacy.

Positive Outcomes

In 1998, Helff and Glidden concluded that despite a trend toward a less pathology-oriented view of family adjustment between 1971 and 1993, most investigators still wrote about it in a predominantly negative tone. Although that conclusion may still be true, the trend toward a positive view of families has continued and been given impetus by the national move-ment toward a positive psychology (Diener, 2000; Seligman & Csikszent-mihalyi, 2000; Sheldon & King, 2001). A recent review article by Hastings and Taunt (2002) concluded that parents of children with disabilities re-port more stress, but not fewer positive outcomes than parents of children without disabilities. Moreover, positive and negative perceptions are not op-posite ends of the same dimension, but seem to be predicted by different variables. We believe that in the next decade family assessment research will continue a focus on positive outcomes (Gibson, 1995; Grant, Ramcha-ran & Goward, 2003; Grant, Ramcharan, McGrath, Nolan & Keady, 1998; Scorgie & Sobsey, 2000), reinforcing their co-existence and differentiation from negative outcomes. Seltzer and Heller (1997) stated it accurately and poignantly when they wrote the following in their introduction to a special issue of the journal *Family Relations*:

> "One point on which all studies agree is that there is great heterogeneity in the subjective experience of parent care-givers ... Some parents cope extremely well with this challenge and are able to maintain a sense of personal well-being. Other parents ... have a more difficult time coping and they feel bur-dened by their life circumstances, depleted by the physical and psychological demands of providing care, and pessimistic about the future. Many parents feel all of these emotions at different points in their lives" (p. 321).

Individual Family Members: Siblings

Although the predominant focus of family research has been on par-ents, siblings have not been ignored. Indeed, early work by Bernard Farber (Farber, 1959; Farber & Jenné, 1963) discovered that older sisters of chil-dren with ID exhibited more role tension than did brothers, and that com-plex differences in parent–child communication patterns existed, depend-ing upon whether the child with ID was institutionalized or living at home, the sex of the sibling, and the sex of the parent. Stoneman (1997, 1998) and others (Hannah & Midlarsky, 1999) have pointed out that hypotheses that siblings are prone to pathology and maladjustment have generally not been confirmed, although there are reports of negative impact (Cuskelly & Gunn, 1993; McHale & Gamble, 1989; McHale & Pawletko, 1992). In our Recent Journal Sample, only five articles, less than 10%, studied siblings. In a well-designed study, Hannah and Midlarsky (1999) compared siblings who had a brother or sister with ID and those who had a typically develop-ing brother or sister. In general, their findings indicated no differences in well-being or problems between the two groups. One significant difference for male siblings of a brother or sister with ID was lower-maternal ratings of sibling school performance. Teacher ratings of this variable, however, were comparable for female and male siblings.

Clearly, the impact of growing up with a brother or sister with DD still needs substantial research effort involving questions of processes, inter-actions, and mediating and moderating effects. Moreover, looking only for quantitative differences in the childhood period may not be the best approach. It is reasonable to expect that the characteristics of one's brother or sister will have an influence and that the influence is likely to be lifelong. An analogy with the attempt to identify effects of intensive early intervention is appropriate. Early efforts studied changes in IQ that were sometimes found, but typically faded once intervention ceased. However, the impact has been uncovered, still there years later, in the form of fewer special education placements, lower school drop-out, and a variety of other cognitive and social benefits (Lazar & Darlington, 1982; Ramey & Ramey, 1998).

Some research on siblings has also taken this broadened approach. Particularly noteworthy is the work of Seltzer, Krauss and colleagues in their longitudinal study of aging families caring for an adult with ID (Orsmond & Seltzer, 2000; Seltzer, Krauss, Hong, & Orsmond, 2001). They have found that in the normative life course some siblings remain involved both instrumentally and emotionally with their brother or sister with ID and that this involvement increases with the ailing health or death of their care taking parent. They have also noted continuation of the gendered nature of the sibling relationship, with sisters more involved than brothers.

Individual Family Members: Grandparents

Grandparent involvement in the care of children with DD has received little attention. As an understudied group, there is inadequate documentation as to their participation or the impact of their care giving on them, on their grandchildren, or on their adult sons or daughters who are the parents of the children for whom they are caring. Recently, however, evidence of increasing interest has been demonstrated by a review of the literature on grandparents of children with disabilities (Hastings, 1997); a thematic issue of the *Journal of Gerontological Social Work* (2000) that focused on grandparents as carers of children with disabilities; and a book on custodial grandparents that included a chapter on grandparent caregivers to children with DD (Kinney, McGrew, & Nelson, 2003). Grandparent primary care giving appears to be more common among low income families, disproportionately among African American or Latino families (Burnette, 2000). Typically, the parent of the child with DD is unable to fulfill the responsibilities of primary care taking, e.g., due to substance abuse or jail. These grandparent caregivers are frequently grandmothers (Janicki, McCallion, Grant-Griffin, & Kolomer, 2000), who seem to report many of the same consequences of care giving as do mothers. Of course, these older women are at greater risk for negative consequences because of their age and greater likelihood of poor health, as well as the context of their assuming primary care giving: inability of their own children to fulfill the parental role. Among grandparent caregivers, the child's DD status may not be a major determinant of outcome. For example, Force, Botsford, Pisano and Holbert (2000) compared grandparent care giving when a child did or did not have DD, and found the two groups to be remarkably similar. However, the grandparents of children with DD were more likely to need a variety of benefits and services, and thus were more vulnerable to changes in social and economic policy.

Family Systems

By far, most of the research in DD on family impact and functioning has focused on individual family members using a self-report methodology, with little or no attempt to describe the family as a whole. Convenient and easy to administer, and providing summary information about domains that may be impossible to observe, this methodology has dominated. Without a doubt, family assessment is far more complex and difficult than individual assessment, requiring multiple facets and multiple levels (Snyder, Cavell, Heffer, & Mangrum, 1995).

Self-report methodology also has been used extensively in the study of family systems, despite admonitions regarding its limitations (Sabatelli & Bartle, 1995). Although many whole-family oriented self-report instruments exist, consensus has developed that the three best-accepted self-report measures of family systems are the family environment scale (FES— Moos & Moos, 1986), the family assessment measure (FAM—Steinhauer, 1987; Skinner, Steinhauer & Sitarenios, 2000) and the family adaptability and cohesion scale (FACES—Olson, et al., 1985; Olson, Tiesel & Gorall, 1996). Psychometric information is readily available for them (Bloom & Naar, 1994) and Jacob and Windle (1999) have demonstrated that these instruments measure the same three dimensions—affect, activities, and control—regardless of which family system or sub-system is the focus and whether the reporter is a mother, a father or a child. These dimensions are clearly important in families who have children with DD, but the three instruments have been used to greatly differing degrees—the FES and the FACES far more than the FAM.

The FES

The FES is a 90-item true-false inventory with 10 subscales, characterizing the social climate dimensions of interpersonal relationships, personal growth, and maintenance of the family system. It has been used in hundreds of studies including ones with children with DD (Dyson, Edgar, & Crnic, 1989; Rousey, Wild, & Blacher, 2002; Skinner, 1987). Research in the 1980's by Mink and her colleagues (Mink, Meyers & Nihira, 1984; Mink & Nihira, 1987) identified different family types using dimensions of the FES as well as other variables. Although family types such as cohesive, control-oriented, and child-oriented were replicated by these investigators, other research has not adopted this model or extended it to determine long-term effects. Others have used the FES or one of its subscales to study differences between families with DS and other disabilities (Seltzer, Krauss & Tsunematsu, 1993); the prediction of unmet service need (Smith, 1997); cognitive ability in girls with fragile-X (Kuo, Reiss, Freund & Huffman, 2002); and how conflict and cohesion relates to depression in Latina mothers rearing children with or without DD (Blacher et al., 1997).

Because its use has been sporadic, it has related scores to different variables, and studies have not generally been replicated, it is impossible to draw generalizations about the effects of family social climate as the FES measures it upon other family or child outcomes.

The FACES

FACES is a self-report scale that exists in four different versions (Craddock, 2001; Olson et al., 1996). All versions use a Likert scale with individual respondents and measure degree of family adaptability and cohesion. According to Olson's circumplex model (Olson, Sprenkle & Russell, 1979), healthy families are characterized by moderate or balanced levels of adaptability and cohesion. High or low degrees can be problematic, leading to families that are rigid or chaotic, overly enmeshed, or disengaged. Research on families with children with DD has applied this model (Krauss, 1993; Martin & Cole, 1993), and it demonstrates that families with children with DD do not differ in any marked way on either adaptability or cohesion from other families (Hassiotis, 1997; Sgandurra, 2001).

Gottlieb (1998) reports on an especially vulnerable sample: low-income single mothers rearing school-age children with a variety of disabilities, including autism, ID, and cerebral palsy. She found that they were more likely to be rigid and separated on the FACES, rather than adaptable and cohesive. Nonetheless, mothers with a high sense of coherence (Antonovsky, 1993; Antonovsky & Sourani, 1988) were more adaptable and cohesive than mothers with lower sense of coherence. These high coherence mothers were also less depressed, and reported less parenting stress, fewer health problems, and greater well-being.

The FAM

Of these three self-report family system measures the FAM has been the least used in studies of families rearing children with DD. It consists of three levels of self-reporting: whole family, dyadic, and individual, and has been used both for research and clinical assessment (Skinner et al., 2000). Trute and his collaborators have used it in a number of studies. For example, Trute and Hauch (1988) reported data from parents with children with DD, finding that both mothers and fathers who had been judged by clinicians to have positive adjustment also demonstrated positive adjustment on the FAM. More recently, Trute and Hiebert-Murphy (2002) found that both mother and father scores on a short form of the FAM were correlated with a separate measure of marital adjustment and self-esteem, but not with a 15-item scale designed to measure both the positive and negative impacts of childhood disability on the family. Neither of these studies utilized comparison groups of families rearing children without disabilities.

An earlier study by Westhues and Cohen (1990) predicted disruption of special-needs adoptions based on FAM scores, demonstrating its potential utility in adoptive placement. However, no detailed description of the special-needs adoptive children was provided. Because a minority of special-needs children have DD, its relevance to family assessment in a DD sample remains unknown.

In sum, based on investigations of these three family system measures as well as others (e.g., Hampson, Hulgus, Beavers & Beavers, 1988) there is no substantial evidence that families rearing children with DD have systems characteristics that differ from those of other families. In large measure, necessary and carefully controlled studies have not yet been conducted.

Subsystems: Marital

Many of the earliest investigations of family functioning hypothesized that children with DD strained marital relationships, leading to dysfunction and divorce (Farber, 1959; Friedrich & Friedrich, 1981; Gath, 1977). Several decades later Stoneman (1997) concluded that relevant findings were inconsistent and Risdal and Singer (2004), using a meta-analytic technique, found a small effect size for greater marital strain and divorce in parents rearing children with DD. In our sample of 51 articles from 1997–2002, only two measured marital functioning. Baker and Blacher (2002) studied families after they had placed their children in a residential facility. Only 16% of the married respondents rated their marriage as less than happy, but parents of younger children tended to report lower marital adjustment scores than parents of older children. They also reported more stress and greater burden of care taking. Glidden and Floyd (1997) demonstrated that marital satisfaction was correlated negatively with depression in two different samples, for both mothers and fathers.

Research conducted with epidemiological methodologies using large samples such as the National Health Interview Survey or the Fragile Families Study suggest a somewhat different conclusion. Several studies have found that children's chronic poor health or disability is associated with higher risk of divorce (Corman & Kaestner, 1992; Joesch & Smith, 1997; Mauldon, 1992). Nonetheless, a variety of qualifications limit a strong conclusion. For example, Joesch and Smith found an effect for children with cerebral palsy, but not developmental delay and Corman and Kaestner found it for white women but not black women. Most recently, Urbano and Hodapp (2005) found a slightly lower divorce rate for parents of children with Down syndrome, in comparison to those of children without disabilities.

Reichman, Corman, and Noonan (2004) focused not on divorce only but on whether the parents were living together and were more or less involved in their relationship. Children's poor health, measured as birthweight less than 4 pounds, a physical or intellectual disability, or not achieving developmental milestones decreased the likelihood that parents would be married or cohabiting and increased the likelihood of lower involvement in the 12–18 months after the birth. They acknowledged, however, that although large, their sample was urban and not nationally representative, thus limiting the generalizability of the results.

In sum, based on current research, there is some evidence, although far from conclusive, that marital adjustment may be negatively influenced when a couple is rearing a child with DD rather than a child without DD. Undoubtedly, it is likely that rearing a child with disabilities interacts in complex ways with other variables just as other stressors do. Moreover, given normative changes that occur in family adaptation, it is essential to avoid drawing conclusions using studies that are decades old and with small or non-representative samples. For example, Amato, Johnson, Booth, and Rogers (2003) have documented substantial differences in marital quality, both declines and increases between 1980 and 2000. Finally, the methodology in the study of marital adjustment, even large sample studies, is almost exclusively self-report. Although there is some evidence that self-report and observational assessment are concordant for at least some measures of marital quality in families in general (Hahlweg, Kaiser, Christensen, Gehm-Wolfsdorf & Groth, 2000), this careful comparative work has not been done with families rearing children with DD.

Subsystems: Parent–child

Observational techniques have been used to study the parent–child subsystem of the family, frequently relying on some imposed structure for the interaction. For example, the work of Floyd and colleagues (Costigan, Floyd, Harter, & McClintock, 1997; Floyd & Phillippe, 1993; Floyd, Costigan, & Phillippe, 1997) allowed families to interact in a relatively free manner, following a few experimenter-imposed rules. Some investigators have obtained results that they have interpreted as problematically high levels of directiveness, and concomitant low levels of responsiveness for parents of children with DD (see reviews by Marfo, 1990; Marfo, Dedrick, & Barbour, 1998), although high directiveness is not always accompanied by low responsiveness (Tannock, 1988). Furthermore, reinterpretations have suggested that differences in parents of children with and without DD may be the result of child factors such as poor readability of cues (Hodapp, 1995). Floyd et al. (1997) provided some evidence for the child factor explanation. They conducted two family interaction assessments separated by approximately two years and found that mothers changed their levels of directiveness depending on their children's compliance or noncompliance. Further complicating conclusions is the recognition that children with DD may benefit from higher levels of directiveness, at least at certain developmental stages. The long-term effect of this interaction style is still unknown.

A quite different methodology was used by Keogh, Garnier, Bernheimer and Gallimore (2000). These investigators were interested in whether accommodations that were made by families rearing children with DD were in response to the child's characteristics and behaviors, or whether they were transactional, with child and care taking environment characteristics each influencing the other. Using a combination of standardized tests, self-reports, and detailed interview responses over an 8-year time period, their conclusion was that a child-driven model was the best fit to the data. Specifically, families with children who were less competent made more accommodations, but these accommodations did not alter the child's relative competence at a later time of measurement.

Perhaps not surprisingly, among the 51 articles in the *Recent Journal Sample*, only one, Floyd et al. (1997), used a traditional interactional observational methodology. Moreover, the May/June 2003 Special Issue on Family Research of the *Journal of Intellectual Disability Research* did not include any articles using this methodology. Because of the practical difficulties of conducting this type of research, including the expense and time commitment of coding, it will likely remain under-utilized. This situation is unfortunate because as the science of family relations develops it must be anchored in techniques that provide a perspective that broadens the information obtained from self-report. In order to interpret the data from any one method, we must understand its biases (e.g., social desirability) and how it compares with information collected from other methods.

In sum, positive and negative outcomes such as well-being, depression, and stress are rarely the result of single variables such as severity of disability or parental personality. Rather, they are likely mediated or moderated by other processes originating and operating within or outside the family. Because family assessment frequently embodies an applied focus with regard to interventions and services, one research emphasis has been the influence of social support. Social support is often included in models of parental adaptation to children with DD, and is frequently used to operationalize the Resources or "B" factor in McCubbin and Patterson's (1982) double ABCX model (Herman & Marcenko, 1997; Minnes, 1988).

SOCIAL SUPPORT

Definition

The definition of social support has evolved over time, gathering dimensions as the general understanding of families living with persons with DD has changed and broadened. Cohen and Willis (1985), as a result of an extensive literature review consisting of articles published through 1983, defined social support as a multidimensional construct consisting of instrumental support, informational support, esteem or emotional support, and social companionship. A similar multidimensional construct was described by Dunst, Trivette, and Cross (1986) who defined social support as physical and instrumental assistance, emotional support, and information and resource sharing.

Perhaps because of the multidimensional nature of social support, its measurement has been somewhat fragmented. Some investigators have focused only on one or two dimensions (Olstad, Sexton, & Sogaard, 2001), whereas others have used five or more types of support (Cutrona & Suhr, 1992). In addition to this troublesome segmentation, a multitude of ad hoc measurements have been used.

Support Schema

Despite these inconsistencies, certain patterns have emerged. Researchers distinguish among the different types of networks—formal versus informal; the sources of support found within each network; and the recipients of support. In addition to these dimensions, two other concepts are relevant to interpreting the effects of social support: (1) whether it acts directly or as a buffer, and (2) the distinction between perceived and received support.

Informal networks generally consist of those within the family unit, including extended family, or close friends, and sources of support within these networks are most likely to provide emotional support, social companionship, and care taking assistance. Sources of support found in formal networks consist of professionals such as doctors, psychologists, social workers, teachers, and others who may provide medical, psychological, informational, advocacy and other types of assistance. Although the focus of most research has been on the primary caregivers of persons with disabilities, the family member with DD has also been studied as a provider or recipient of support.

Buffer versus Direct Main Effects

Cohen and Willis (1985) noted two competing models of social support in the literature: the buffering model and the main effect model. Adherents of the buffering model claim that social resources are beneficial only when persons are experiencing stressful events. Thus, the buffering model predicts differences in adjustment between low and high social support in stressed, but not in unstressed, conditions. However, the main effect model posits that differences in adjustment in unstressed conditions differ with low and high social support, and that support is beneficial at all times, stressful or not.

Perceived Rather than Received

Perceived support measures the amount of support that individuals believe they receive, or that they believe would be available if needed, whereas received support refers to actual support behaviors (Norris & Kaniasty, 1996). Both theories and findings suggest that perceived support is correlated more highly with outcome variables than received support (Cohen & Willis, 1985; Lunsky & Benson, 2001). Norris and Kaniasty (1996) claim that perceived support has a direct effect on stress and well-being, whereas received support has an indirect effect, serving mainly to influence perception of support.

Measures of Support

Measures of social support abound. Touliatos et al. (1990) in the *Handbook of Family Measurement Techniques*, listed 24 measures of kinship support alone. These included measures of spousal support, support from the nuclear family, and support from the extended family. Our review of the most recent research found a myriad of social support assessments, many designed specifically for a single study, with questionable psycho-metric reliability and validity. As with other aspects of family assessment, findings are difficult to compare, threatening the accuracy of summary and generalization.

Despite the numerous assessment measures designed solely for indi-vidual studies, there has been some consistency of measurement in the field. Boyd (2002), reviewing 20 years of research on social support allevia-tion of stress in mothers of children with autism, found that one of the most commonly used measures of social support was the Family Support Scale (FSS—Dunst, Trivette & Cross, 1984). It has been used widely with families rearing children with DD, in both the United States and other countries (Crowley & Taylor, 1994; Kelley & Whitley, 2003; Pal, Chaudhury, Das & Sengupta, 2002; Rodgers, 1998; Schoolcraft & Glidden, 2003, March). The FSS is a self-report instrument for which respondents rate the usefulness of each of 18 possible sources of informal or formal support. Respondents are asked to rate the usefulness of each source of support.

Findings on Social Support

After a thorough review of prior research spanning several decades, Stoneman (1997), was able to conclude that social support does indeed buffer the effects of stress on individuals and families caring for individuals with DD. Although these parents generally report smaller support networks than comparison parents, they often find that social support to be more satisfying and beneficial. Stoneman concluded that higher levels of social support are correlated with less stress, less depression, happier marriages, more positive family functioning, greater parental self-efficacy, positive ad-justment to the parental role, reduced care giving burden, greater life sat-isfaction, and fewer parent/child problems. Stoneman also cited etiological differences, with families of individuals with DS reporting more satisfaction with social support than families of children with other forms of ID.

Similar results have been reported in studies conducted in 1997 and thereafter. Leung and Erich (2002) found that greater supports from both informal and formal sources were associated with better family function-ing. Boyd (2002) concluded that the strongest predictors of maternal de-pression and anxiety were low levels of social support, replicating the Horton and Wallander (2001) finding that higher social support was as-sociated with lower maternal distress. Manuel, Naughton, Balkrishnan, Smith, & Koman (2003) also found that mothers of children with cerebral palsy who reported low levels of perceived social support had more depres-sive symptoms than did mothers with high perceived social support.

The vitality of this domain of research is evident within our *Recent Journal Sample*, which yielded 12 articles pertaining to social support. This sample mirrored the field as a whole in terms of instrument selection, with the FSS being used in three of the articles and no other instrument used more than once. Despite variability in instrumentation, in general, the results supported earlier conclusions with regard to benefits of social support and problems when it was missing. For example, Magaña (1999) reported that greater maternal well-being for Puerto Rican mothers caring for adult children with DD was associated with larger social support networks and greater satisfaction with that support and Bruns (2000) found that lack of social support influenced parental decisions to place young children outside the home. Heller, Miller, and Factor (1997) demonstrated that care giving relationships can be reciprocally supportive. Greater instrumental, emotional, and informational support from the adult child with DD to his or her caretaker was associated with less care taking burden and increased satisfaction.

Two studies, both with minority families, stressed the use of family support. Bailey et al. (1999) found that Latino families of children with DD reported using more support from family than from friends or other informal sources. Chen and Tang (1997), in a study of Chinese mothers of children with DD, found that they were more likely to report receiving support from family members than any other source.

Studies that have compared mothers and fathers have sometimes, but not always, found differences. Crowley and Taylor (1994) administered the FSS to a large sample of 922 parents of children with varying disabilities. They compared mother and father scores on the family, spouse, social, and professional sub-scores and the total score. Mothers and fathers differed significantly on each of the subscales. An item-by-item analysis found that mothers received greater support from parents, relatives, friends, parent groups, physicians, professional helpers, and early intervention services. Fathers reported greater levels of support from their spouses than did mothers, a finding shared by Schoolcraft and Glidden (2003, March) in a study comparing 29 pairs of mothers and fathers on the FSS. Mothers reported receiving greater support than fathers from friends and social groups or clubs in the Schoolcraft and Glidden study. In contrast, Dyson (1997) found that mothers and fathers of children with DD did not differ from one another on perceived family support. In those studies where differences have been found, mothers generally express greater need than fathers for family and social support (Bailey, Blasco & Simeonsson, 1992), and fathers report more support from wives than wives do from husbands (Crowley & Taylor, 1994; Goldberg, Marcovitch, MacGregor & Lojkasek, 1986; Schoolcraft & Glidden, 2003).

Social support is also beneficial to family members other than parents, including siblings of children with DD both during childhood and when they age and may assume primary care taking. Fisman, Wolf, Ellison and Freeman (2000) found that perceived social support of siblings of children with DS predicted adjustment three years later. Wolf, Fisman, Ellison, and Freeman (1998) also examined sibling perception of differential parental treatment in sibling dyads with one child diagnosed with either a pervasive developmental disorder or DS. For both groups, social support had a positive effect on all families, more so over time. In a study of 39 adult siblings of Irish men and women with DD, Egan and Walsh (2001) concluded that perceived social support was significantly negatively correlated with the amount of stress reported by the siblings. Research on social support and grandparents has also found positive effects (Kelley, Whitley, Sipe, & Yorker, 2000; Kelley & Whitley, 2003).

Finally, some investigators have examined the effect of social support provided to the individual with DD. King et al. (2003) found that social support provided by family, friends, and others in the community served as a strong protective factor against stress. This positive effect may be offset by the generally smaller support networks that individuals with DD have in comparison to those without DD (Guralnick, 1997), networks consisting primarily of family members (Bigby, 1997).

Social Strain

Although most research does find that greater social support leads to more positive outcomes, there have been recent suggestions that support can actually be not only neutral, but negative in its effect. Lunsky and her colleagues (Lunsky & Benson, 2001; Lunsky & Havercamp, 1999) have studied social strain: If "supports" are unwanted by the recipient, they can lead to strain and distress rather than well-being, thereby confirming the importance of perceived rather than received support. In a study of adults with mild ID, Lunsky and Benson concluded that unwanted social supports added significantly to the prediction of depressive symptoms and somatic complaints in the future.

In sum, the social support research exhibits a number of problems, foremost of which is a plethora of measuring instruments. Additionally, many of the studies that measure social support do so incidentally as one of many variables rather than as the primary interest of the research. Frequently, social support itself is not manipulated as a variable, resulting in scanty knowledge with regard to the process by which it influences outcomes. Thus, although we are reasonably confident in the conclusion that social support is usually associated with benefits and its absence with difficulties, we are tentative with regard to the confirmation of other hypotheses. There is some, but limited evidence that (1) informal support is more effective as a buffer than formal support; and (2) that perceived support is more likely to lead to positive outcomes than is received support. There have not been enough well-designed studies of the direct versus buffering model to make even a tentative choice between them. With regard to cultural differences, although recent research has sampled groups with more cultural diversity than in older studies, no trends with regard to either main effects or interactions are yet apparent.

RECENT DEVELOPMENTS IN FAMILY ASSESSMENT AND SOCIAL SUPPORT

Multiculturalism

Disability diagnosis is not race or culture blind, and historically, individuals from minority cultures have been at greater risk for having a child diagnosed with DD. Since 1976, the first year following the passage of P.L.

94–142, a dramatic decline has occurred in the percentage of children, ages 0–21, diagnosed with ID, from 26% in the 1976–1977 school year to 9.7% in the 1999–2000 school year (U.S. Department of Education, 2001). Nonetheless, this smaller percentage is still disproportionately African American. In 1999–2000, the number of African. American children classified with ID or DD was 2.4 times greater than the number of Whites, although Whites outnumbered African Americans by almost 5:1 in the school population (Hallahan & Kauffman, 2003; U.S. Department of Education, 2000). This factor, accompanied by the increasing diversity of American society, has generated more research interest in the influence of different cultures, races, and ethnicities on family adjustment. Whereas some studies have found non-majority families to have more negative reactions (Blacher et al., 1997), others have reported the opposite finding (Flynt & Wood, 1989; Pruchno, Patrick, & Burant, 1999). Work by Rogers-Dulan and colleagues (Glidden, Rogers-Dulan, & Hill, 1999; Rogers-Dulan, 1998; Rogers-Dulan & Blacher, 1995) suggest that for African-American families, religiousness and spirituality may be a protective factor. Skinner, Rodriguez and Bailey (1999), using a qualitative methodology, have described several themes in the religious interpretations of their child's disability by Latino parents. Although the research is still too limited to draw any firm conclusions about the role of race, culture, and ethnicity in adjusting the rearing of children with disabilities, there is general agreement that it needs to be included in order to understand the process of adaptation (Lynch & Hanson, 1992; McCallion, Janicki, & Grant-Griffin, 1997; Tate & Pledger, 2003).

A multicultural orientation has influenced research on social support. Whereas some studies have confirmed culturally derived hypotheses (Bailey et al., 1999; Magaña, 1999) not all have done so. For example, Shin (2002) studied 38 American and 40 Korean mothers raising children with ID hypothesizing that, since Korean culture is collective and places its emphasis on the family, these mothers would be more apt to turn to family members than would American mothers, thus reporting higher levels of informal support. This hypothesis was not confirmed—American mothers reported greater informal and formal supports than did Korean mothers, in addition to reporting greater satisfaction with these supports. Korean mothers also reported more stress, perhaps due to lack of availability of and satisfaction with support.

Broader Conceptions of the Family

Interest has extended from a predominant focus on mothers to other family members such as fathers, siblings, and grandparents. This extension has encompassed families at different life stages. Whereas earlier research focused mostly on families with young children with DD, currently, families in later life stages are included in the research. Furthermore, longitudinal studies have provided valuable information about families making transitions across life stages (Blacher, Baker & Feinfield, 1999; Kraemer & Blacher, 2001; Menard, Schoolcraft, Glidden, & Lazarus, 2002, March; Schoolcraft & Glidden, 2002, March; Seltzer, Krauss et al., 2001).

One broader conception of the family that has flooded the research studying families with typically developing children is that of blended and step-families (Casper & Bianchi, 2002; Cherlin, 1992; Coleman, Ganong & Fine, 2000; DeFrain & Olson, 1999; Henderson, Hetherington, Mekos, & Reiss, 1996; Hetherington & Stanley-Hagan, 2002; Nelson & Levant, 1991). In research with families with children with DD, family structure has been studied in some of its variants such as foster, adoptive, and single versus married. Blended families, however, have not occupied investigators studying families of children with DD.

Emphasis on Different Diagnostic Groups

Although family research has historically included diagnostic and level of functioning information in descriptions of samples, with the exception of DS and autism, researchers had not usually focused on different diagnostic categories. Recently, however, the increasing sophistication of diagnostic techniques accompanying the advances in mapping and understanding the human genome, has led to more interest in diagnostic categories and behavioral phenotypes (Dykens, 1999; Hodapp, 1999). This emphasis is likely to lead to an increased understanding of both the direct and indirect effects of phenotypic characteristics on families. However, we must be careful that the emphasis on diagnostic differences does not obscure the similarities shared by families with children with DD.

CLINICAL IMPLICATIONS

With the advent of positive psychology (Seligman & Csikszentmihalyi, 2000) has come the widespread acceptance that a family with a disabled child is not automatically a disabled family. For many families, rearing a child with DD is only one of the many life events that will bring with it both sorrows and joys. Thus, assumptions about a need for clinical intervention must be examined. On the other hand, childrearing is challenging for all parents, and the demands on parents who have a child with DD are usually greater than for those who are rearing typically developing children. If the child exhibits high levels of maladaptive behavior, and if the family is at risk because of other stressors such as low income, family discord, low levels of informal social support, and vulnerable personality traits, then professional support may be useful.

Professional intervention may assume various forms. Sometimes it will be for the child, to reduce maladaptive and strengthen adaptive behavior. For example, intensive behavioral programs can reduce autistic behaviors and increase intellectual functioning (Lovass, 1987; Mulick, 2003, August). Because maladaptive behaviors have been linked to negative outcomes for families, reducing them should result in amelioration of negative family outcomes. Prevention may be an even better alternative. It is possible that effective programs to optimize child behavior should be delivered to all children with DD, and that, in the long run, this would be cost-effective, saving many dollars in treatment and avoiding psychological distress for the child and other family members.

Of course, it is not only the child, but also other family members and the family as a system that may be the target for clinical intervention. Given that there is little evidence that families with children with DD are systemically different from families, in general, implications for clinical intervention in this population are not unique. However, others have remarked that such research has brought little benefit to clinical practice (Coyne & Racioppo, 2000; Somerfield & McCrae, 2000), despite the exponential increase in publications. More optimistically, however, our review of research leads us to reiterate that, for the most part, if clinicians are treating families that include a child with DD they should assume neither function nor dysfunction. They should recognize that demands may be greater than for families with only typically developing children, but that personal growth and positive affect may also be the result, as individuals make meaning of life events (Folkman & Moskowitz, 2000).

ACKNOWLEDGMENTS. The writing of this chapter was supported, in part, by Grant No. 21993 from the National Institute of Child Health and Human Development awarded to Laraine M. Glidden and to faculty development grants from St. Mary's College of Maryland. Thanks go to Kevin Meyer and Brian Jobe for their assistance.

REFERENCES

Note: Articles included in the *Recent Research Sample* are marked with an asterisk.

Abidin, R. R. (1982). *Parenting Stress Index manual.* Charlottesville, VA: Pediatric Psychology Press.

Amato, P. R., Johnson, D. R., Booth, A., & Rogers, S. J. (2003). Continuity and change in marital quality between 1980 and 2000. *Journal of Marriage and the Family, 65,* 1–22.

Antonovsky, A. (1993). The implications of salutogenesis: An outsider's view. In A. P. Turnbull, J. M. Patterson, S. K. Behr, D. L. Murphy, J. G. Marquis, & M. J. Blue-Banning (Eds.), *Cognitive coping, families, and disability* (pp. 111–122). Baltimore, MD: Paul H. Brookes.

Antonovsky, A., & Sourani, T. (1988). Family sense of coherence and family adaptation. *Journal of Marriage and the Family, 50,* 79–92.

Bailey, D. B., Jr., Blasco, P. M., & Simeonsson, R. J. (1992). Needs expressed by mothers and fathers of young children with disabilities. *American Journal on Mental Retardation, 97,* 1–10.

*Bailey, D. B., Jr., Skinner, D., Correa, V., Arcia, E., Reyes-Blanes, M. E., Rodriguez, P., et al. (1999). Needs and supports reported by Latino families of young children with developmental disabilities. *American Journal on Mental Retardation, 104,* 437–451.

*Baker, B. L., & Blacher, J. (2002). For better or worse? Impact of residential placement on families. *Mental Retardation, 40,* 1–13.

Baker, B. L., McIntyre, L. L., Blacher, J., Crnic, K., Edelbrock, C., & Low, C. (2003). Pre-school children with and without developmental delay: Behavior problems and parenting stress over time. *Journal of Intellectual Disability Research, 47,* 217–230.

Beck, A. T., Ward, C. H., Mendelson, M., & Erbaugh, J. (1961). An inventory for measuring depression. *Archives of General Psychiatry, 4,* 561–571.

Beckman, P. J. (1991). Comparison of mothers' and fathers' perceptions of the effect of young children with and without disabilities. *American Journal on Mental Retardation, 95,* 585–595.

Bigby, C. (1997). Parental substitutes? The role of siblings in the lives of older people with intellectual disability. *Journal of Gerontological Social Work, 29*(1), 3–21.

Blacher, J., & Baker, B. L. (2002). *The best of AAMR: Families and mental retardation: A collection of notable AAMR journal articles across the 20th century.* Washington, DC: American Association on Mental Retardation.

*Blacher, J., Baker, B. L., & Feinfield, K. A. (1999). Leaving or launching? Continuing family involvement with children and adolescents in placement. *American Journal on Mental Retardation, 104,* 452–465.

Blacher, J., Lopez, S., Shapiro, J., & Fusco, J. (1997). Contributions to depression in Latina mothers with and without children with retardation. *Family Relations: Interdisciplinary Journal of Applied Family Studies, 46,* 325–334.

Bloom, B. L., & Naar, S. (1994). Self-report measures of family functioning: Extensions of a factorial analysis. *Family Process, 33,* 203–216.

Boyd, B. A. (2002). Examining the relationship between stress and lack of social support in mothers of children with autism. *Focus on Autism and Other Developmental Disabilities, 17,* 208–215.

Bray, J. H. (1995). Family assessment: Current issues in evaluating families. *Family Relations, 44,* 469–478.

*Bruns, D. A. (2000). Leaving home at an early age: Parents' decisions about out-of-home placement for young children with complex medical needs. *Mental Retardation, 38,* 50–60.

Burack, A., Hodapp, R. M., & Zigler, E. (1998). *Handbook of mental retardation and development.* New York: Cambridge University Press.

Burnette, D. (2000). Latino grandparents rearing grandchildren with special needs: Effects on depressive symptomatology. *Journal of Gerontological Social Work, 33*(3), 1–16.

Cahill, B. M., & Glidden, L. M. (1996). Influence of child diagnosis on family and parental functioning: Down syndrome versus other disabilities. *American Journal on Mental Retardation, 101,* 149–160.

Casper, L. M., & Bianchi, S. M. (2002). *Continuity and change in the American family.* Thousand Oaks: Sage Publications.

*Chen, S., Ryan-Henry, S., Heller, T., & Chen, E. H. (2001). Health status of mothers of adults with intellectual disability. *Journal of Intellectual Disability Research, 45,* 439–449.

*Chen, T. Y., & Tang, C. S. (1997). Stress appraisal and social support of Chinese mothers of adult children with mental retardation. *American Journal on Mental Retardation, 101,* 473–482.

Cherlin, A. J. (1992). *Marriage, divorce, remarriage* (Rev. ed.). Cambridge, Massachusetts: Harvard University Press.

Cohen, S., & Willis, T. A. (1985). Stress, social support, and the buffering hypothesis. *Psychological Bulletin, 98,* 310–357.

Coleman, M., Ganong, L., & Fine, M. (2000). Reinventing remarriage: Another decade of progress. *Journal of Marriage and the Family, 62,* 1238–1307.

Corman, H., & Kaestner, R. (1992). The effects of child health on marital status and family structure. *Demography, 29,* 389–408.

Costa, P. T., & McCrae, R. R. (1992). *Revised Personality Inventory (NEO PI-R) and NEO Five-Factor Inventory (NEO-FFI): Professional manual.* Odessa, FL: Psychological Assessment Resources.

Costigan, C. L., & Cox, M. J. (2001). Fathers' participation in family research: Is there a self-selection bias? *Journal of Family Psychology, 15,* 706–720.

Costigan, C. L., Floyd, F. J., Harter, K. S. M., & McClintock, J. C. (1997). Family process and adaptation to children with mental retardation: Disruption and resilience in family problem-solving interactions. *Journal of Family Psychology, 11,* 515–529.

Coyne, J. C., & Racioppo, M. W. (2000). Never the twain shall meet: Closing the gap between coping research and clinical intervention research. *American Psychologist, 55,* 655–664.

Craddock, A. E. (2001). Family system and family functioning: Circumplex model and FACES IV. *Journal of Family Studies, 7,* 29–39.

Crowley, S. L., & Taylor, M. J. (1994). Mothers' and fathers' perceptions of family functioning in families having children with disabilities. *Early Education and Development, 5,* 213–225.

Cuskelly, M., & Gunn, P. (1993). Maternal reports of behavior of siblings of children with Down syndrome. *American Journal on Mental Retardation, 97,* 521–529.

Cutrona, C. E., & Suhr, J. A. (1992). Controllability of stressful events and satisfaction with spouse support behaviors. *Communication Research, 19,* 154–174.

Dakof, G. A. (1996). Meaning and measurement of family: Comment on Gorman-Smith et al. (1996). *Journal of Family Psychology, 10,* 142–146.

DeFrain, J., & Olson, D. H. (1999). Contemporary family patterns and relationships. In M. Sussman, S. K. Steinmetz & G. W. Peterson (Eds.), *Handbook of marriage and the family* (2nd ed., pp. 309–326). New York: Plenum Press.

Diener, E. (2000). Subjective well-being: The science of happiness and a proposal for a national index. *American Psychologist, 55,* 34–44.

Dunst, C. J., Trivette, C. M., & Cross, A. H. (1984). Family support scale: Reliability and validity. *Journal of Individual, Family and Community Wellness, I*(4), 45–52.

Dykens, E. M. (1999). Direct effects of genetic mental retardation syndrome: Maladaptive behavior and psychopathology. In L. M. Glidden (Ed.), *International review of research in mental retardation* (pp. 1–26). San Diego: Academic Press.

*Dyson, L. (1997). Fathers and mothers of school-age children with developmental disabilities: Parental stress, family functioning, and social support. *American Journal on Mental Retardation, 102,* 267–279.

Dyson, L., Edgar, E., & Crnic, K. (1989). Psychological predictors of adjustment by siblings of developmentally disabled children. *American Journal on Mental Retardation, 94,* 292–302.

Egan, J., & Walsh, P. N. (2001). Sources of stress among adult siblings of Irish people with intellectual disability. *Irish Journal of Psychology, 22*(1), 28–38.

Emerson, E. (2003). Mothers of children and adolescents with intellectual disability: Social and economic situation, mental health status, and the self-assessed social and psychological impact of the child's difficulties. *Journal of Intellectual Disability Research, 47,* 385–399.

Farber, B. (1959). Effects of a severely mentally retarded child on family integration. *Society for the Research in Child Development Monographs, 24*(2), 1–112.

Farber, B., & Jenné, W. C. (1963). Family organization and parent–child communication: Parents and siblings of a retarded child. *Monographs of the Society for Research in Child Development, 28*(7), 1–78.

Fisman, S., Wolf, L., Ellison, D., & Freeman, T. (2000). A longitudinal study of siblings of children with chronic disabilities. *Canadian Journal of Psychiatry, 45,* 369–377.

Flaherty, E. M., & Glidden, L. M. (2000). Positive adjustment in parents rearing children with Down syndrome. *Early Education and Development, 11,* 407–422.

*Floyd, F. J., Costigan, C. L., & Phillippe, K. A. (1997). Developmental change and consistency in parental interactions with school-age children who have mental retardation. *American Journal on Mental Retardation, 101,* 579–594.

Floyd, F. J., & Gallagher, E. M. (1997). Parental stress, care demands, and use of support services for school-age children with disabilities and behavior problems. *Family Relations, 46,* 359–371.

Floyd, F. J., & Phillippe, K. A. (1993). Parental interactions with children with and without mental retardation: Behavior management, coerciveness, and positive exchange. *American Journal on Mental Retardation, 97,* 673–684.

Flynt, S. W., & Wood, T. A. (1989). Stress and coping of mothers of children with moderate mental retardation. *American Journal on Mental Retardation, 94,* 278–283.

Folkman, S., & Mokowitz, J. T. (2000). Positive affect and the other side of coping. *American Psychologist, 55,* 647–654.

Force, L. T., Botsford, A., Pisano, P. A., & Holbert, A. (2000). Grandparents raising children with and without a developmental disability: Preliminary comparisons. *Journal of Gerontological Social Work, 33*(4), 5–21.

Friedrich, W. N., & Friedrich, W. L. (1981). Psychosocial assets of parents of handicapped and non-handicapped children. *American Journal of Mental Deficiency, 85*, 551–553.

Gath, A. (1977). The impact of an abnormal child upon the parents. *British Journal of Psychiatry, 130*, 405–410.

Gibson, C. H. (1995). The process of empowerment in mothers of chronically ill children. *Journal of Advanced Nursing, 21*, 1201–1210.

Glidden, L. M. (1993). What we do *not* know about families with children who have developmental disabilities: Questionnaire on resources and stress as a case study. *American Journal on Mental Retardation, 97*, 481–495.

Glidden, L. M., & Cahill, B. M. (1998). Successful adoption of children with Down syndrome and other developmental disabilities. *Adoption Quarterly, 1*(3), 27–43.

*Glidden, L. M., & Floyd, F. J. (1997). Disaggregating parental depression and family stress in assessing families of children with developmental disabilities: A multi sample analysis. *American Journal on Mental Retardation, 102*, 250–266.

Goldberg, S., Marcovitch, S., MacGregor, D., & Lojkasek, M. (1986). Family responses to developmentally delayed preschoolers: Etiology and the father's role. *American Journal of Mental Deficiency, 90*, 610–617.

Glidden, L. M., Rogers-Dulan, J., & Hill, A. E. (1999). "The child that was meant?" or "Punishment for sin?": Religion, ethnicity, and families with children with disabilities. In L. M. Glidden (Ed.), *International review of research in mental retardation* (pp. 267–288). San Diego, CA: Academic Press.

Glidden, L. M., & Schoolcraft, S. A. (2003). Depression: Its trajectory and correlates in mothers rearing children with intellectual disability. *Journal of Intellectual Disability Research, 47*, 250–263.

Gottlieb, A. (1998). Single mothers of children with multiple disabilities: The role of sense of coherence in managing multiple challenges. In H. I. McCubbin, E. A. Thompson, A. I. Thompson, & J. E. Fromer (Eds.), *Stress, coping, and health in families* (pp. 189–204). London: Sage Publications.

Gowen, J. W., Johnson-Martin, N., Goldman, B. D., & Appelbaum, M. (1989). Feelings of depression and parenting competence of mothers of handicapped and non-handicapped infants: A longitudinal study. *American Journal on Mental Retardation, 94*, 259–271.

Grant, G., Ramcharan, P., & Goward, P. (2003). Resilience, family care, and people with intellectual disabilities. In L. M. Glidden (Ed.), *International review of research in mental retardation* (Vol. 26, pp. 135–173). Amsterdam: Academic Press.

*Grant, G., Ramcharan, P., McGrath, M., Nolan, M., & Keady, J. (1998). Rewards and gratifications among family caregivers: Towards a refined model of caring and coping. *Journal of Intellectual Disability Research, 42*, 58–71.

Guralnick, M. J. (1997). Peer social networks of young boys with developmental delays. *American Journal on Mental Retardation, 101*, 595–612.

Guralnick, M. J., Neville, B., Connor, R. T., & Hammond, M. A. (2003). Family factors associated with the peer social competence of young children with mild delays. *American Journal on Mental Retardation, 108*, 272–287.

Gutman, L. M., Sameroff, A. J., & Cole, R. (2003). Academic growth curve trajectories from 1st grade to 12th grade: Effects of multiple social risk factors and preschool child factors. *Developmental Psychology, 39*, 777–790.

Hahlweg, K., Kaiser, A., Christensen, A., Fehm-Wolfsdorf, G., & Groth, T. (2000). Self-report and observational assessment of couples' conflict: The concordance between the Communication Patterns Questionnaire and the KPI observation system. *Journal of Marriage and the Family, 62*, 61–67.

Hallahan, D. P., & Kauffman, J. M. (2003). *Exceptional learners: An introduction to special education* (9th ed.). Boston: Allyn and Bacon.

Hampson, R. B., Beavers, W. R., & Hulgus, Y. (1990). Cross-ethnic family differences: Interactional assessment of White, Black, and Mexican-American families. *Journal of Marital and Family Therapy, 16*, 307–319.

Hampson, R. B., Hulgus, Y. F., Beavers, W. R., & Beavers, J. S. (1988). The assessment of competence in families with a retarded child. *Journal of Family Psychology, 2*, 32–53.

Hannah, M. E., & Midlarsky, E. (1999). Competence and adjustment of siblings of children with mental retardation. *American Journal on Mental Retardation, 104,* 22–37.

Harris, S. L., Alessandri, M., & Gill, M. J. (1991). Training parents of developmentally disabled children. In J. L. Matson & J. A. Mulick (Eds.), *Handbook of mental retardation* (pp. 373–396). New York: Pergamon Press.

Harris, V. S., & McHale, S. M. (1989). Family life problems, daily care giving activities, and the psychological well-being of mothers of mentally retarded children. *American Journal on Mental Retardation, 94,* 231–239.

Hassiotis, A. (1997). Parents of young persons with learning disability: An application of the family adaptability and cohesion scale (FACES III). *The British Journal of Developmental Disabilities, 84,* 36–42.

Hastings, R. P. (1997). Grandparents of children with disabilities: A review. *International Journal of Disability, Development and Education, 44,* 329–340.

Hastings, R. P. (2003). Child behavior problems and partner mental health as correlates of stress in mothers and fathers of children with autism. *Journal of Intellectual Disability Research, 47,* 231–237.

*Hastings, R. P., & Brown, T. (2002). Behavior problems of children with autism, parental self-efficacy, and mental health. *American Journal on Mental Retardation 107,* 222–232.

Hastings, R. P., & Taunt, H. M. (2002). Positive perceptions in families of children with developmental disabilities. *American Journal on Mental Retardation, 107,* 116–127.

Hayden, L. C., Schiller, M., Dickstein, S., Seifer, R., Sameroff, S., Miller, I., et al. (1998). Levels of family assessment: I. Family, marital, and parent–child interaction. *Journal of Family Psychology, 12,* 7–22.

Helff, C., & Glidden, L. M. (1998). More positive or less negative? Trends in research on adjustment of families rearing children. *Mental Retardation, 36,* 457–465.

*Heller, T., Miller, A., & Factor, A. (1997). Adults with mental retardation as supports to their parents: Effects on parental care giving appraisal. *Mental Retardation, 35,* 338–346.

Henderson, S. H., Hetherington, E. M., Mekos, D., & Reiss, D. (1996). Stress, parenting, and adolescent psychopathology in non-divorced and stepfamilies: A within-family perspective. In E. M. Hetherington & E. A. Blechman (Eds.), *Stress, coping, and resiliency in children and families* (pp. 373–396). Mahwah, New Jersey: Lawrence Erlbaum Associates.

*Herman, S. E., & Marcenko, M. O. (1997). Perceptions of services and resources as mediators of depression among parents of children with developmental disabilities. *Mental Retardation, 35,* 458–467.

Hetherington, E. M., & Stanley-Hagan, M. (2002). Parenting in divorced and remarried families. In M. H. Bornstein (Ed.), *Handbook of parenting: Vol. 3. Being and becoming a parent* (2nd ed., pp. 287–315). Mahwah, New Jersey: Lawrence Erlbaum Associates.

*Hoare, P., Harris, M., Jackson, P., & Kerley, S. (1998). A community survey of children with severe intellectual disability and their families: Psychological adjustment, carer distress and the effect of respite care. *Journal of Intellectual Disability Research, 42,* 228–237.

Hodapp, R. M. (1995). Parenting children with Down syndrome and other types of mental retardation. In M. H. Bornstein (Ed.), *Handbook of parenting* (pp. 233–253). Mahwah, New Jersey: Lawrence Erlbaum Associates.

Hodapp, R. M. (1999). Indirect effects of genetic mental retardation disorders: Theoretical and methodological issues. In L. M. Glidden (Ed.), *International review of research in mental retardation* (Vol. 22, pp. 27–50). San Diego: Academic Press.

*Hodapp, R. M., Fidler, D. J., & Smith, A. (1998). Stress and coping in families of children with Smith-Magenis syndrome. *Journal of Intellectual Disability Research, 42,* 331–340.

Hodapp, R. M., Wijma, C. A., & Masino, L. L. (1997). Families of children with 5p- (cri du chat) syndrome: Familial stress and sibling reactions. *Developmental Medicine and Child Neurology, 39,* 757–761.

Holroyd, J. (1987). *Questionnaire on resources and stress for families with chronically ill or handicapped members.* Brandon, VT: Clinical Psychological Publishing Co.

Holroyd, J., & McArthur, D. (1976). Mental retardation and stress on the parents: A contrast between Down's syndrome and childhood autism. *American Journal of Mental Deficiency, 80,* 431–436.

Honig, A. S., & Winger, C. J. (1997). A professional support program for families of handi-
    capped preschoolers: Decrease in maternal stress. *The Journal of Primary Prevention, 17,*
    285–296.
Horton, T. V., & Wallander, J. L. (2001). Hope and social support as resilience factors against
    psychological distress of mothers who care for children with chronic physical conditions.
    Rehabilitation Psychology, 46, 382–399.
Hudson, A. M., Matthews, J. M., & Gavidia-Payne, S. T. (2003). Evaluation of an interven-
    tion system for parents of children with intellectual disability and challenging behavior.
    Journal of Intellectual Disability Research, 47, 238–249.
Jacob, T., & Windle, M. (1999). Family assessment: Instrument dimensionality and corre-
    spondence across family reporters. *Journal of Family Psychology, 13,* 339–354.
Janicki, M. P., McCallion, P., Grant-Griffin, L., & Kolomer, S. R. (2000). Grandparent care-
    givers I: Characteristics of the grandparents and the children with disabilities for whom
    they care. *Journal of Gerontological Social Work, 33*(3), 35–55.
Joesch, J. M., & Smtih, K. R. (1997). Children's health and their mothers' risk of divorce or
    separation. *Social Biology, 44,* 159–169.
Kelley, S. J., & Whitley, D. M. (2003). Psychological distress and physical health in grandpar-
    ents raising grandchildren: Development of an empirically based intervention model. In
    B. Hayslip, Jr. & J. H. Patrick (Eds.), *Working with custodial grandparents* (pp. 127–144).
    New York, NY: Springer Publishing Co.
Kelley, S. J., Whitley, D., Sipe, T. A., & Yorker, B. C. (2000). Psychological distress in grand-
    mother kinship care providers: The role of resources, social support, and physical health.
    Child Abuse and Neglect, 24, 311–321.
*Keogh, B. K., Garnier, H. E., Bernhiemer, L. P., & Gallimore, R. (2000). Models of child-
    family interactions for children with developmental delays: Child-driven or transactional?
    American Journal on Mental Retardation, 105, 32–46.
King, G., Cathers, T., Brown, E., Specht, J. A., Willoughby, C., Polgar, J. M., et al. (2003).
    Turning points and protective processes in the lives of people with chronic disabilities.
    Qualitative Health Research, 13, 184–206.
Kinney, J. M., McGrew, K. B., & Nelson, I. M. (2003). Grandparent caregivers to children with
    developmental disabilities: Added challenges. In B. Hayslip, Jr. & J. H. Patrick (Eds.),
    Working with custodial grandparents (pp. 93–109). New York: Springer.
*Kraemer, B. R., & Blacher, J. (2001). Transition for young adults with severe mental retar-
    dation: School preparation, parent expectations, and family involvement. *Mental Retar-
    dation, 39,* 423–436.
Krauss, M. W. (1993). Child-related and parenting stress: Similarities and differences between
    mothers and fathers of children with disabilities. *American Journal on Mental Retardation,
    97,* 393–404.
*Kuo, A. Y., Reiss, A. L., Freund, L. S., & Huffman, L. C. (2002). Family environment and cog-
    nitive abilities in girls with fragile-X syndrome. *Journal of Intellectual Disability Research,
    46,* 328–339.
Lazar, I., & Darlington, R. (1982). Lasting effects of early education: A report from the con-
    sortium for longitudinal studies. *Monographs of the Society for Research in Child Devel-
    opment, 47*(2, 3), 1–151.
Leung, P., & Erich, S. (2002). Family functioning of adoptive children with special needs:
    Implications of familial supports and child characteristics. *Children and Youth Services
    Review, 24,* 799–816.
Lovaas, O. I. (1987). Behavioral treatment and normal educational and intellectual function-
    ing in young autistic children. *Journal of Consulting and Clinical Psychology, 55,* 3–9.
Lunsky, Y., & Benson, B. A. (2001). Association between perceived social support and strain,
    and positive and negative outcome for adults with mild intellectual disability. *Journal of
    Intellectual Disability Research, 45,* 106–114.
Lunsky, Y., & Havercamp, S. M. (1999). Distinguishing low levels of social support and social
    strain: Implications for dual diagnosis. *American Journal on Mental Retardation, 104,*
    200–204.
Lynch, E. W., & Hanson, M. J. (1992). *Developing cross-cultural competence: A guide for work-
    ing with young children and their families.* Baltimore, MD: Paul H. Brookes.

MacLean, W. E. (1997). *Ellis' handbook of mental deficiency, psychological theory and research* (3rd ed.). Mahwah, New Jersey: Lawrence Erlbaum Associates.

*Magaña, S. M. (1999). Puerto Rican families caring for an adult with mental retardation: Role of familism. *American Journal on Mental Retardation, 104,* 466–482.

Manuel, J., Naughton, M. J., Balkrishnan, R., Smith, B. P., & Koman, A. (2003). Stress and adaptation in mothers of children with cerebral palsy. *Journal of Pediatric Psychology, 28,* 197–201.

Marfo, K. (1990). Maternal directiveness in interactions with mentally handicapped children: An analytical commentary. *Journal of Child Psychology and Psychiatry, 31,* 531–549.

Marfo, K., Dedrick, C. F., & Barbour, N. (1998). Mother-child interactions and the development of children with mental retardation. In J. A. Burack, R. M. Hodapp, & E. Zigler (Eds.), *Handbook of mental retardation and development* (pp. 637–668). New York: Cambridge University Press.

Martin, J. M., & Cole, D. A. (1993). Adaptability and cohesion of dyadic relationships in families with developmentally disabled children. *Journal of Family Psychology, 7,* 186–196.

Mauldon, J. (1992). Children's risk of experiencing divorce and remarriage: Do disabled children destabilize marriages? *Population Studies, 46,* 349–362.

McCallion, P., Janicki, M. P., & Grant-Griffin, L. (1997). Exploring the impact of culture and acculturation on older families care giving for persons with developmental disabilities. *Family Relations: Interdisciplinary Journal of Applied Family Studies, 46,* 347–357.

McCubbin, H. I., & Patterson, J. M. (1982). Family adaptation to crises. In H. I. McCubbin, A. E. Cauble, & J. M. Patterson (Eds.), *Family stress, coping, and social support* (pp. 26–47). Springfield, Illinois: Charles C Thomas.

McHale, S. M., & Gamble, W. C. (1989). Sibling relationships of children with disabled and non-disabled brothers and sisters. *Developmental Psychology, 25,* 421–429.

McHale, S. M., & Pawletko, T. M. (1992). Differential treatment of siblings in two family contexts. *Child Development, 63,* 68–81.

Menard, J., Schoolcraft, S. A., Glidden, L. M., & Lazarus, C. (2002, March). *Transition daily rewards and worries* [Abstract]. Poster presented at the 35th Annual Gatlinburg Conference, San Diego, CA.

*Miltiades, H. B., & Pruchno, R. (2001). Mothers of adults with developmental disability: Change over time. *American Journal on Mental Retardation, 106,* 548–561.

Mink, I. T., Meyers, C. E., & Nihira, K. (1984). Taxonomy of family life styles: II. Homes with slow-learning children. *American Journal of Mental Deficiency, 89,* 111–123.

Mink, I. T., & Nihira, K. (1987). Direction of effects: Family life styles and behavior of TMR children. *American Journal of Mental Deficiency, 92,* 57–64.

Minnes, P. (1988). Family stress associated with a developmentally handicapped child. In N. W. Bray (Ed.), *International review of research in mental retardation* (Vol 15, pp. 195–226). San Diego: Academic Press.

Minnes, P. (1998). Mental retardation: The impact upon the family. In J. A. Burack, R. M. Hodapp, & E. Zigler (Eds.), *Handbook of mental retardation and development* (pp. 693–712). New York: Cambridge University Press.

Moos, R. H., & Moos, B. S. (1986). *Family Environment Scale manual.* Palo Alto, CA: Consulting Psychologists Press.

Mulick, J. A. (2003, August). Is learning recovery in autism happening? Gains made in cognitive abilities, adaptive behavior, language, and autistic symptom severity after early intensive behavioral intervention for children with Autism. In J. A. Mulick (Chair), *Preliminary reports from the Ohio Autism Recovery Project.* Symposium conducted at the 111th Annual Convention of the American Psychological Society, Toronto, Canada.

Mulick, J. A., Hammer, D., & Dura, J. R. (1991). Assessment and management of antisocial and hyperactive behavior. In J. L. Matson & J. A. Mulick (Eds.), *Handbook of mental retardation* (pp. 397–412). New York: Pergamon Press.

Myerhoff, B., & Tufte, V. (1979). Introduction. In V. Tufte & B. Myerhoff (Eds.), *Changing images of the family* (pp. 1–23). New Haven: Yale University Press.

Nelson, W. P., & Levant, R. F. (1991). An evaluation of a skills training program for parents in stepfamilies. *Family Relations, 40,* 291–296.

Norris, F. H., & Kaniasty, K. (1996). Received and perceived social support in times of stress: A test of the social support deterioration deterrence Model. *Journal of Personality and Social Psychology, 71*, 498–511.

Olson, D. H., McCubbin, H., Barnes, H., Larsen, A., Muxen, M., & Wilson, M. (1985). *Family inventories*. Minneapolis: University of Minnesota, Family Social Science.

Olson, D. H., Sprenkle, D. H., & Russell, C. S. (1979). Circumplex model of marital and family systems: I. Cohesion and adaptability dimensions, family types, and clinical applications. *Family Process, 18*, 3–28.

Olson, D. H., Tiesel, J. W., & Gorall, D. (1996). *Family adaptability and cohesion scale IV*. Minneapolis, MN: University of Minnesota, Family Social Science.

*Olsson, M. B., & Hwang, C. (2001). Depression in mothers and fathers of children with intellectual disability. *Journal of Intellectual Disability Research, 45*, 535–543.

*Olsson, M. B., & Hwang, C. (2002). Sense of coherence in parents of children with different developmental disabilities. *Journal of Intellectual Disability Research, 46*, 548–559.

Olstad, R., Sexton, H., & Sogaard, A. J. (2001). The Finnmark study: A prospective population study of the social support buffer hypothesis, specific stressors and mental distress. *Social Psychiatry and Psychiatric Epidemiology, 36*, 582–589.

*Orsmond, G. I., & Seltzer, M. M. (2000). Brothers and sisters of adults with mental retardation: Gendered nature of the sibling relationship. *American Journal on Mental Retardation, 105*, 486–508.

Orsmond, G. I., Seltzer, M. M., Krauss, M. W., & Hong, J. (2003). Behavior problems in adults with mental retardation and maternal well-being: Examination of the direction of effects. *American Journal on Mental Retardation, 108*, 257–271.

*Padeliadu, S. (1998). Time demands and experienced stress in Greek mothers of children with Down's syndrome. *Journal of Intellectual Disability Research, 42*, 144–153.

Padula, M. A. (1995). Assessment issues in families of individuals with disabilities. In J. C. Conoley & E. B. Werth (Eds.), *Family assessment* (pp. 261–284). Omaha, NB: Buros Institute of Mental Measurements, University of Nebraska Press.

Pal, D. K., Chaudhury, G., Das, T., & Sengupta, S. (2002). Predictors of parental adjustment to children's epilepsy in rural India. *Child: Care, Health and Development, 28*, 295–300.

*Pruchno, R. A., Patrick, J. H., & Burant, C. L. (1999). Effects of formal and familial residential plans for adults with mental retardation on their aging mothers. *American Journal on Mental Retardation, 104*, 38–52.

Ramey, C. T., & Ramey, S. L. (1998). Early intervention and early experience. *American Psychologist, 53*, 109–120.

Reichman, N. E., Corman, H., & Noonan, K. (2004). Effects of child health on parents' relationship status. *Demography, 41*, 569–584.

Ricci, L. A., & Hodapp, R. M. (2003). Fathers of children with Down's syndrome versus other types of intellectual disability: Perceptions, stress and involvement. *Journal of Intellectual Disability Research, 47*, 273–284.

Risdal, D., & Singer, G. H., S. (2004). Marital adjustment in parents of children with disabilities: A historical review and meta-analysis. *Research and Practice for Persons with Severe Disabilities, 29*, 95–103.

*Roach, M. A., Orsmond, G. I., & Barratt, M. S. (1999). Mothers and fathers of children with Down syndrome: Parental stress and involvement in child care. *American Journal on Mental Retardation, 104*, 422–436.

Rodgers, A. Y. (1998). Multiple sources of stress and parenting behavior. *Child and Youth Services Review, 20*, 525–546.

*Rogers-Dulan, J. (1998). Religious connectedness among urban African American families who have a child with disabilities. *Mental Retardation, 36*, 91–103.

Rogers-Dulan, J., & Blacher, J. (1995). African American families, religion, and disability: A conceptual framework. *Mental Retardation, 33*, 226–238.

Rousey, A. M., Wild, M., & Blacher, J. (2002). Stability of measures of the home environment for families of children with severe disabilities. *Research in Developmental Disabilities, 23*, 17–35.

Sabatelli, R. M., & Bartle, S. E. (1995). Survey approaches to the assessment of family functioning: Conceptual, operational, and analytical issues. *Journal of Marriage and the Family, 57,* 1025–1039.

*Sarimski, K. (1997). Communication, social-emotional development and parenting stress in Cornelia-de-lange syndrome. *Journal of Intellectual Disability Research, 41,* 70–75.

Schoolcraft, S. A., & Glidden, L. M. (2002, March). Still happy after all these years? Family well being across the lifespan: Tracking maternal depression as children transition to adulthood [Abstract]. In J. Blacher (Chair), *Still happy after all these years? Family well-being across the lifespan.* Symposium conducted at the 35th Annual Gatlinburg Conference, San Diego, CA.

Schoolcraft, S. A., & Glidden, L. M. (2003, March). Sources of Support in Rearing Children with Developmental Disabilities [Abstract]. Poster session presented at the 36th annual Gatlinburg Conference, Annapolis, MD.

Schumm, W. R. (1990). Intimacy and family values. In J. Touliatos, B. F. Perlmutter, & M. A. Straus. *Handbook of family measurement techniques* (pp. 164–284). Newbury Park, CA: Sage Publications.

*Scorgie, K., & Sobsey, D. (2000). Transformational outcomes associated with parenting children who have disabilities. *Mental Retardation, 38,* 195–206.

Seligman, M. E. P., & Csikszentmihalyi, M. (2000). Positive psychology: An introduction. *American Psychologist, 55,* 5–14.

*Seltzer, M. M., Greenberg, J. S., Floyd, F. J., Pettee, Y., & Hong, J. (2001). Life course impacts of parenting a child with a disability. *American Journal on Mental Retardation, 106,* 265–286.

Seltzer, M. M., & Heller, T. (1997). Families and care giving across the life course: Research advances on the influence of context. *Family Relations, 46,* 321–323.

*Seltzer, M. M., Krauss, M. W., Hong, J., & Orsmond, G. I. (2001). Continuity or discontinuity of family involvement following residential transitions of adults who have mental retardation. *Mental Retardation, 39,* 181–194.

Seltzer, M. M., Krauss, M. W., & Tsunematsu, N. (1993). Adults with Down syndrome and their aging mothers: Diagnostic group differences. *American Journal on Mental Retardation, 97,* 496–508.

Sexton, D., Burrell, B., Thompson, B., & Sharpton, W. R. (1992). Measuring stress in families of children with disabilities. *Early Education and Development, 3,* 60–66.

Sgandurra, C. A. (2001). The relationship between family functioning and sibling adjustment in families with a child with a developmental disability. *Dissertation Abstracts International: Section B: The Sciences & Engineering, 62*(3-B), 1598.

Shapiro, J., Blacher, J., & Lopez, S. R. (1998). Maternal reactions to children with mental retardation. In J. A. Burack (Ed.), *Handbook of mental retardation and development* (pp. 606–636). New York: Cambridge University Press.

Sheldon, K. M., & King, L. (2001). Why positive psychology is necessary. *American Psychologist, 56,* 216–217.

Shin, J. Y. (2002). Social support for families of children with mental retardation: Comparison between Korea and the United States. *Mental Retardation, 40,* 103–118. *

Skinner, H. A. (1987). Self-report instruments for family assessment. In: T. Jacob (Ed), *Family interaction and psychopathology: Theories, methods, and findings* (pp. 427–452). New York: Plenum Press.

Skinner, D., Rodriguez, P., & Bailey, D. B., Jr. (1999). Qualitative analysis of Latino parents' religious interpretations of their child's disability. *Journal of Early Intervention, 22,* 271–285.

Skinner, H., Steinhauer, P., & Sitarenios, G. (2000). Family assessment measure (FAM) and process model of family functioning. *Journal of Family Therapy, 22,* 190–210.

*Smith, G. C. (1997). Aging families of adults with mental retardation: Patterns and correlates of service use, need, and knowledge. *American Journal on Mental Retardation, 102,* 13–26.

Snyder, D. K., Cavell, T. A., Heffer, R. W., Mangrum, L. F. (1995). Marital and family assessment: A multifaceted, multilevel approach. In R. H. Mikesell, D. D. Lusterman, & S. H. McDaniel (Eds.), *Integrating family therapy: Handbook of family psychology and systems theory* (pp. 163–182). Washington, DC: American Psychological Association.

Somerfield, M. R., & McCrae, R. R. (2000). Stress and coping research: Methodological challenges, theoretical advances, and clinical applications. *American Psychologist, 55*, 620–
625.

Steinhauer, P. (1987). The family as a small group: The process model of family functioning.
In T. Jacob (Ed.), *Family interaction and psychopathology: Theories, methods, and findings*
(pp. 67–115). New York: Plenum Press.

Stoneman, Z. (1997). Mental retardation and family adaptation. In W. E. MacLean, Jr. (Ed.),
Ellis' handbook of mental deficiency, psychological theory and research (pp. 405–437).
Mahwah, NJ: Lawrence Erlbaum Associates.

Stoneman, Z. (1998). Research on siblings of children with mental retardation: Contributions
of developmental theory and etiology. In J. A. Burack R. M. Hodapp, & E. Zigler (Eds.),
Handbook of mental retardation and development (pp. 669–692). New York: Cambridge
University Press.

*Stores, R., Stores, G., Fellows, B., & Buckley, S. (1998). Daytime behavior problems and
maternal stress in children with Down's syndrome, their siblings, and non-intellectually
disabled and other intellectually disabled peers. *Journal of Intellectual Disability Research,
42*, 228–237.

Tannock, R. (1988). Mothers' directiveness in their interactions with their children
with and without Down syndrome. *American Journal on Mental Retardation, 93*,
154–165.

Tate, D. G., & Pledger, C. (2003). An integrative conceptual framework of disability: New
directions for research. *American Psychologist, 58*, 289–295.

Touliatos, J., Perlmutter, B. F., & Straus, M. A. (1990). *Handbook of family measurement
techniques*. Newbury Park, CA: Sage Publications.

Trute, B., & Hauch, C. (1988). Building on family strength: A study of families with positive
adjustment to the birth of a developmentally disabled child. *Journal of Marital and Family
Therapy, 14*, 185–193.

Trute, B., & Hiebert-Murphy, D. (2002). Family adjustment to childhood developmental disability: A measure of parent appraisal of family impacts. *Journal of Pediatric Psychology,
27*, 271–280.

Urbano, R. C., & Hodapp, R. M. (2005, March). *Divorce in families of children with Down
syndrome: A population-based study*. Paper presented at the 38th Annual Gatlinburg
conference on Research & Theory in Intellectual & Developmental Disabilities, Annapolis,
MD.

U.S. Department of Education (2000). *Annual report to Congress on the implementation of the
Individuals with Disabilities Education Act*. Washington, DC: Author.

U.S. Department of Education (2001). *Annual report to Congress on the implementation of the
Individuals with Disabilities Education Act*. Washington, DC: Author.

Westhues, A., & Cohen, J. S. (1990). Preventing disruption of special-needs adoptions. *Child
Welfare, 69*, 141–155.

Wolf, L., Fisman, S., Ellison, D., & Freeman, T. (1998). Effects of sibling perception of differential treatment in sibling dyads with one disabled child. *Journal of the American Academy
of Child & Adolescent Psychiatry, 37*, 1317–1325.

SUGGESTED READINGS

Note: These following references were included in the *Recent Journal Sample* of 51 articles on
family assessment and were reviewed, but not cited in the preceding text.

Baker, B. L., Blacher, J., Crnic, K. A., & Edelbrock, C. (2002). Behavior problems and parenting stress in families of three year old children with and without developmental delays.
American Journal on Mental Retardation 107, 433–444.

Blacher, J., Shapiro, J., Lopez, S., & Diaz, L. (1997). Depression in Latina mothers of children
with mental retardation: A neglected concern. *American Journal on Mental Retardation,
101*, 483–496.

Clare, L., Garnier, H., & Gallimore, R. (1998). Parents' developmental expectations and child characteristics: Longitudinal study of children with developmental delays and their families. *American Journal on Mental Retardation, 103,* 117–129.

Cooney, B. F. (2002). Exploring perspectives on transition of youth with disabilities: Voices of young adults, parents, and professionals. *Mental Retardation, 40,* 425–435.

Einam, M., & Cuskelly, M. (2002). Paid employment of mothers and fathers of an adult child with multiple disabilities. *Journal of Intellectual Disability Research, 46,* 158–167.

Essex, E. L., Seltzer, M. M., & Krauss, M. W. (1999). Differences in coping effectiveness and well-being among aging mothers and fathers of adults with mental retardation. *American Journal on Mental Retardation, 104,* 545–563.

Freedman, R. I., Krauss, M. W., & Seltzer, M. M. (1997). Aging parents' residential plans for adult children with mental retardation. *Mental Retardation, 35,* 114–123.

Grissom, M. O., & Borkowski, J. G. (2002). Self-efficacy in adolescents who have siblings with or without disabilities. *American Journal on Mental Retardation, 107,* 79–90.

Hanneman, R., & Blacher, J. (1998). Predicting placement in families who have children with sever handicaps: A longitudinal analysis. *American Journal on Mental Retardation, 102,* 392–408.

Hayden, M. F., & Heller, T. (1997). Support, problem-solving/coping ability, and personal burden of younger and older caregivers of adults with mental retardation. *Mental Retardation, 35,* 364–372.

Llewellyn, G., Dunn, P., Fante, M., Turnbull, L., & Grace, R. (1999). Family factors influencing out-of-home placement decisions. *Journal of Intellectual Disability Research, 43,* 219–233.

McIntyre, L., Blacher, J., & Baker, B. (2002). Behavior/mental health problems in young adults with intellectual disability: the impact on families. *Journal of Intellectual Disability Research, 46,* 239–249.

Scott, B. S., Atkinson, L., Minton, H. L., Bowman, T. (1997). Psychological distress of parents of infants with Down syndrome. *American Journal on Mental Retardation, 102,* 161–171.

Shearn, J., & Todd, S. (1997). Parental work: An account of the day-to-day activities of parents of adults with learning disabilities. *Journal of Intellectual Disability Research, 41,* 285–301.

Shu, B., Lung, F. & Huang, C. (2002). Mental health of primary family caregivers with children with intellectual disability who receive a home care program. *Journal of Intellectual Disability Research, 46,* 257–263.

Warfield, M. E. (2001). Employment, parenting, and well-being among mother of children with disabilities. *Mental Retardation, 39,* 297–309.

IV

Prevention and Treatment

The focus of this section is on intervention at the individual or small group level. Each chapter includes information regarding the prevalence or demographics of the behavior or condition treated, a depiction of the range of available or frequently encountered treatments, an appraisal of which treatments are empirically or differentially validated, mitigating or mediating factors affecting the effectiveness of treatment, and clinical practices that alleviate mitigation.

22

Science to Practice in Intellectual Disability

The Role of Empirically Supported Treatments

SIGAN L. HARTLEY, SARAH VOSS HORRELL, and WILLIAM E. MACLEAN JR.

Developmental disabilities, including mental retardation (or intellectual disability [ID]), are severe and chronic human conditions that are likely to continue indefinitely (P. L. 104-83, 1996). Although current definitions of mental retardation (American Psychiatric Association, 2000; American Association on Mental Retardation [AAMR], 2002; World Heath Organization, 1993) make no reference to the expected duration of the condition, it is generally accepted that mental retardation is lifelong and "essentially incurable" (Doll, 1941). For the most part, children diagnosed with ID develop into adults with ID. There are no credible reports of spontaneous remission of ID. Rather there is a legacy of failed attempts to raise the intelligence of affected individuals (for reviews, see Spitz, 1986, 1999). With the exception of people who function at the margin between mild mental retardation and borderline intelligence, improvements in intellectual functioning have typically been transient or due to interventions that inadvertently result in "teaching to the test" thereby increasing scores on intellectual assessments (Spitz, 1999, p. 285). Intelligence is a trait that remains remarkably stable over time, especially when scores fall below the average range (Sattler, 2001). This is not to say that cognitive and adaptive functioning cannot improve following interventions. However, the gains are most often characterized as modest in magnitude and do not result in meaningful or

SIGAN L. HARTLEY, SARAH VOSS HORRELL, and WILLIAM E. MACLEAN JR. • Department of Psychology, University of Wyoming, Laramie, Wyoming 82071.

permanent increases in intellectual ability (Spitz, 1999), notwithstanding some reports to the contrary (e.g., Lovaas, 1987).

Intervention efforts in the field of ID are considered tertiary prevention. These efforts seek to reduce problems associated with the disability and maximize normalized participation in daily life activities as opposed to efforts that attempt to change the fundamental nature of the disorder (Odom & Kaiser, 1997). Such tertiary prevention methods occur throughout the life span (e.g., early intervention, special education, services for seniors), are conducted by a variety of professionals (e.g., educators, occupational and physical therapists, psychologists, physicians), and involve the amelioration of a variety of adaptive and maladaptive behaviors (e.g., communication, self-care, self-injurious behavior, and psychological disorders). Indeed, there is an incredible range of intervention opportunities in the field of ID. Although these interventions may result in greater sustained and meaningful improvements than do attempts to alter intellectual level, there needs to be more effort directed toward establishing their efficacy. For example, there is a massive literature on skills training and intervention for problem behaviors using single- or several-participant designs. However, these efforts have not been accompanied by group design studies that systematically portray the influences of moderating variables, incidence of side effects, penetrance of effects within groups of people with ID, and varying degrees of impairments, or range of effects obtained with faithful or manualized treatment.

In contrast, researchers in the field of ID devote a great deal of effort toward proving that particular treatments are inefficacious (Jacobson, Mulick, & Foxx, 2005). Although such a goal is clearly within the responsibilities of the profession (Jacobson, Mulick, & Schwartz, 1995), there is no agreement on how many negative findings are necessary to substantiate that an intervention is ineffective. For example, there are repeated demonstrations that facilitated communication is an ineffective treatment (Jacobson et al., 1995). Between 1992 and 1995, Jacobson et al. (1995) found 26 controlled studies and between 1995 and 2001, Mostert (2001) found a further 19 controlled studies—all of which concluded that there is no convincing evidence that facilitated communication is effective. The time spent critiquing inefficacious interventions and refuting poorly conducted studies means that less time is being devoted to examining untested, but promising interventions.

Perhaps a more general issue for the field is the difficulty in translating science to practice (MacLean, 2002). All too often, practitioners do not take full advantage of the scientific knowledge base before developing intervention programs. The use of unsubstantiated methods, such as facilitated communication, is one example of this disconnection. However, there are also instances in which practitioners appear unaware of empirical evidence regarding efficacy of particular intervention procedures that may be strongly indicated for treatment of a specific class of behaviors or disorders. For example, studies have shown that pharmacological interventions are widely used to treat behavior problems of individuals with ID despite repeated findings that pharmacotherapy alone is less effective than behavioral interventions or conjoint pharmacotherapeutic and behavioral interventions (Didden, Duker, Korzilius, 1997; Scotti, Evans, Meyer, & Walker, 1991; Sternberg, Taylor, & Babkie, 1994). Another potential difficulty, which will be discussed in a later section, is the traditional top-down strategy that researchers employ in designing research studies. Although the scientific aspects of such studies may be superb, there is an assumption that the research questions will be relevant for practitioners (Abbott, Walton, Tapia, & Greenwood, 1999). Furthermore, "without an established mechanism of synthesizing research findings, it is difficult to know what to translate to practice" (MacLean, 2002). MacLean's comments fit within a broader call in clinical psychology, special education, medicine, and other disciplines within the last decade to establish universal criteria to evaluate treatment efficacy, to develop a list of empirically supported treatments, and to distribute this list to all providers serving people with ID (Sindelar & Wilson, 1984). This chapter focuses on efforts to identify empirically supported treatments and how these efforts can be applied to the field of ID.

THE MOVEMENT TOWARD EMPIRICALLY SUPPORTED TREATMENTS

Clinical researchers from a variety of disciplines are working to establish mechanisms to evaluate the effectiveness of various intervention approaches in an effort to identify empirically supported treatments. In medicine the term is "evidence-based medicine." In physical therapy the term is "evidence-based clinical practice guidelines." Education-related fields use the term "best practices." Clinical psychology uses the term "empirically validated or empirically supported treatments." Chambless and Ollendick (2001) summarize four basic arguments, which provide the foundation for these various initiatives. First, the use of empirically based knowledge can improve patient/client care. Second, keeping up with the continuously emerging research findings relevant to one's practice is difficult for practitioners. Third, failure to remain familiar with new research findings will result in less effective clinical performance over time. Finally, practitioners should be provided with expert reviews and summaries of current research and instructions regarding how to use and access this evidence in practice (Chambless & Ollendick, 2001).

Interest in establishing and promoting empirically supported treatments also grows out of concern that practitioners might employ controversial and untested interventions that could result in harm to clients (Beutler, Moleiro, & Talebi, 2002). The growing attention to treatments such as rebirthing therapy, recovered memory, cell therapy, and similar treatments in other fields created an incentive to establish a system that would scientifically evaluate interventions and only promote those that are truly efficacious. Pressure to develop criteria to determine empirically supported treatments also comes from third party insurance companies (Beutler et al., 2002; Bohart, O'Hara, & Leitner, 1998). The increasing costs of health care in the 1980s initiated the development of a new system for managing the delivery of health services that include privately run managed care organizations (MCOs) and, more recently, managed behavioral healthcare organizations (MBHOs). MCOs, in the form of health maintenance organizations (HMOs), preferred provider organizations (PPOs), individual practice associations (IPAs), and employment assistance programs (EAPs), sought to increase the effectiveness and efficiency of health care by decreasing costs while maintaining the quality of care. The movement toward empirically supported treatments offered third party MCOs a way to hold practitioners accountable for providing the most efficacious treatments (Hayes, Barlow, & Nelson-Gray, 1999). The movement was also a logical extension of the emergence of treatment manuals, which began the call for more standardized therapy procedures in training and practice to improve quality of care (Garfield, 1996; Strupp, 2001).

CURRENT SYSTEMS FOR IDENTIFYING EMPIRICALLY SUPPORTED TREATMENTS

One of the largest efforts to establish a mechanism to evaluate and synthesize scientific findings on the effectiveness of psychological interventions comes from the American Psychological Association (APA). The Task Force on the Promotion and Dissemination of Psychological Procedures was formed in 1993 by Division 12 of the APA (Chambless & Hollon, 1998). The Task Force's purpose is to develop a system to impartially and systematically ascertain whether an intervention or treatment is efficacious (Beutler et al., 2002). The Task Force issued its first report in 1995. This document contained two different sets of criteria for determining empirically validated treatments (EVTs) and a list of treatments that met either set of criteria (see Table 22.1). The efficacy of *well-established treatments* is demonstrated by between-group designs or a large series of single case experiments in which the treatment is shown to be more effective than a placebo or alternative treatment, a treatment manual is used, more than one investigative group is involved, and the client sample is clearly described. The category of *probably efficacious treatments* differs from the previous category in that it only requires treatment comparison to a waitlist control group, does not require more than one investigatory team, and allows for a small number of single case studies.

Similar mechanisms of synthesizing and evaluating interventions have been established in other arenas. For instance, the Food and Drug Administration (FDA) regulates the pharmaceutical industry through stringent requirements regarding the evaluation and testing of prescription and over-the-counter medications (U.S. Department of Health and Human Services, 1998). The U.S. Preventive Services Task Force provides a more extensive range of types of evidence used to evaluate treatment efficacy. This scheme is presented in Table 22.2. Within the field of education, the U.S. Office of Special Education Programs (OSEP) is leading a movement to provide organizational criteria for identifying efficacious school practices (OSEP, 2003).

Table 22.1. Division 12 Task Force on the Promotion and Dissemination of Psychological Procedures Criteria for Empirically Validated Treatments

---

Well-established treatments
   I. At least two good between-group design experiments demonstrating efficacy in one or more of the following ways:
      A. Superior to pill or psychological placebo or toanother treatment.
      B. Equivalent to an already established treatment in experiments with adequate statistical power (about 30 per group; cf., Kazdin & Bass, 1989).
      OR
  II. A large series of single case design experiments (at least nine) demonstrating efficacy.
      These experiments must have
      A. Used good experimental designs and
      B. Compared the intervention to another treatment as in I.A.
      Further criteria for both I and II
 III. Experiments must be conducted with treatment manuals.
  IV. Characteristics of the client samples must be clearly specified.
   V. Effects must have been demonstrated by at least two different investigators or investigatory teams.

Probably efficacious treatments
   I. Two experiments showing the treatment is more effective than a waiting-list control group.
      OR
  II. One or more experiments meeting the well-established treatment criteria I, III, IV, but not V.
      OR
 III. A small series of single case design experiments (at least three) otherwise meeting well-established treatment criteria II, III, and IV.

Efforts to develop guidelines to evaluate empirically supported treatments are not restricted to the United States. Evidence of this movement can be seen internationally. The Cochrane Collaboration in the United Kingdom has also provided a methodology for carrying out systematic reviews of treatment practices within the medical field. Similar to other proposed guidelines these efforts rely on randomized clinical trials to provide evidence for treatment efficacy. The British National Health Service commissioned a review of psychotherapies (Roth & Fonagy, 1996), the

Table 22.2. Levels of Evidence

Level	Type of evidence
1a	Systematic review of randomized, controlled trials (RCTs)
1b	Individual RCT with narrow confidence interval
2a	Systematic review (with homogeneity) of cohort studies
2b	Individual cohort study (or low-quality RCT; e.g., <80% follow-up)
2c	Outcomes research; ecological studies
3a	Systematic review (with homogeneity) of case control studies
3b	Individual case control studies
4	Case studies
5	Expert opinions with explicit critical appraisal

Source: U.S. Preventive Services Task Force (1996).

Canadian Psychological Association's Clinical Psychology Section formed a task force to identify empirically supported treatments (Parry, 1996), and efforts to develop empirically supported treatments have also been reported in Germany (Strauss & Kaechele, 1998). As in the United States, there has been pressure within Germany to establish a mechanism to address the effectiveness of psychotherapeutic treatments. In contrast to the many efforts in the United States (e.g., APA Task Force) that evaluate the efficacy of specific treatments for specific disorders, in Germany this drive has taken the form of evaluating the general effectiveness of various therapeutic approaches (Strauss & Kaechele, 1998). Despite the existence of varying criteria used to establish empirically supported psychological interventions, there is evidence of emerging consensus as to which particular treatments have empirical support (Chambless & Ollendick, 2001).

Mechanisms for evaluating and synthesizing intervention research have also emerged within professional groups and organizations geared toward specific diagnoses. Within the arena of developmental disabilities, a two-part framework for evaluating the efficacy of treatments by the American Academy for Cerebral Palsy and Developmental Medicine (AACPDM) has been advanced (Butler et al., 1999). In contrast to many other approaches (e.g., APA Task Force), this framework evaluates multiple levels of treatment efficacy, enabling the criteria to be applicable to a broader range of research designs. On the basis of a model developed by the World Health Organization (WHO), the U.S. National Center for Medical Rehabilitation Research (NCMRR), and the U.S. Institute of Medicine (IOM), the AACPDM proposed a system that (1) classifies treatments based on the multitude of levels a disease/disorder can affect (e.g., level of cells/tissue, level of organs, level of the individual, person level, and level of the society) and a grading system (see Table 22.3), commonly referred to as Sackett's rules of evidence, (2) places findings into three different confidence groups. Sackett's grading system is based on five levels of evidence and categorizes the degree of certainty about a study's conclusions in terms of the Grades A, B, and C. Treatment outcome findings that have received empirical support by at least one Level-I study are given a grade of A, those supported by at least one Level-II study receive a B grade, and those supported by Level-III, IV, or V studies receive a C. Research receiving an A is judged to be strong and the finding is considered to be the most definitive. A grade of B means the conclusions are weaker and only tentatively support the intervention. A grade of C means the research provides only minimal evidence and is not very reliable. By making specific distinctions among interventions, and the quality and type of intervention research studies, more meaningful information is generated for practice.

Comparison of the various rating systems reveals several commonalities. First, there is a premium placed on studies of large numbers of participants randomized to treatment conditions. Typically these studies provide contrasts to a placebo condition (usually pharmacological treatments), or an alternative treatment condition. Second, assuming that large randomized controlled studies are not available, efficacy can be judged on the presence of repeated single case studies using controlled conditions. Third, the

Table 22.3. Sackett's Method for Grading Research

Level	Description
I	Large randomized trials, producing results with high probability of certainty. These include studies with positive effects that show statistical significance and studies demonstrating no effect that are large enough to avoid missing a clinically significant effect
II	Small randomized trials, producing uncertain results. These are studies which have a positive trend that is not statistically significant to demonstrate efficacy or studies showing a negative effect that are not sufficiently large to rule out the possibility of a clinically significant effect
III	Nonrandomized prospective studies of concurrent treatment and control groups, i.e., cohort comparisons between contemporaneous participants who did and did not receive the intervention
IV	Nonrandomized historical cohort comparisons between participants who did receive the intervention and earlier participants who did not
V	Case series without controls. The clinical course of a group of clients is described, but no control of confounding variables is undertaken. This is a descriptive study that can generate hypotheses for future research but does not demonstrate efficacy

Source: Sackett, Richardson, Rosenberg, and Haynes (1997).

hierarchies evident in these systems can be used to characterize the maturity of an intervention field. For example, the field of psychotherapy for mental health disorders among people with ID is much less developed than comparable literatures for typically developing people. Many of the publications considered authoritative in this area correspond to levels 2c-5 in the U.S. Preventive Services Task Force System (Table 22.2).

LIMITATIONS OF CURRENT GUIDELINES FOR EVALUATING EMPIRICALLY SUPPORTED TREATMENTS

Despite the benefits, to both consumers and practitioners, of current efforts to develop guidelines for evaluating treatment effectiveness, these systems are not problem-free. One major difficulty with current attempts is that they are not based on reviews of the entire range of interventions. Unlisted treatments are not necessarily inefficacious treatments. These treatments may simply have not been examined according to the guidelines of the organization publishing the list. This creates a situation in which practitioners may find it necessary to view lists of empirically supported treatments as a resource rather than a definite guide, and continue to examine the literature and apply their own decision rubric to evaluate other possible treatments.

In addition, many argue that efforts to evaluate and synthesize intervention research are unimportant and inherently pointless. For example, opponents of the movement feel that there are no meaningful differences in the efficacy of different psychotherapies (e.g., Garfield, 1996;

Strupp, 2001; Wampold et al., 1997). They argue that nonspecific factors (e.g., quality of therapist–client relationship, attention directed at problem) are responsible for all differences in treatment outcomes. Evidence in support of this notion is offered by the finding that nonspecific or common factors have been repeatedly shown to be among the largest contributors to outcome in psychotherapy (e.g., Lambert & Bergin, 1994; Norcross & Newman, 1992; Thompson, Gallagher, & Steinmetz Breckenridge, 1987). In rebuttal to this criticism, supporters of efforts to evaluate and synthesize intervention research argue that nonspecific factor research has only been conducted with a select population that does not include people with chronic mental illness, people with developmental disabilities, children, or adolescents. Further, they argue that although some problems (e.g., depression) are improved by several different treatments, others (e.g., obsessive–compulsive disorder) only respond to specific treatments (Chambless & Ollendick, 2001).

Additionally, current frameworks for evaluating and synthesizing findings on treatment efficacy do not encompass all areas important to the definition of an efficacious intervention. For example, follow-up and longitudinal studies within current frameworks (e.g., APA Task Force, AACPDM) are conspicuously absent. Although knowledge of immediate effects is important, insight into the long-term effects and relapse rates of interventions are just as meaningful in determining whether an intervention is efficacious. Furthermore, many of the current frameworks have been criticized for ignoring effect size and clinical significance and relying entirely on statistical significance to evaluate the efficacy of treatments (e.g., Drotar, 2002; Hayes et al., 1999; Morin, 1999; Shirk, 2004; Weisz, Chu, & Polo, 2004). Statistical significance merely conveys that an intervention affects behavior and that changes in behavior are not due to chance. It does not communicate any information pertaining to the strength of the intervention or to the proportion of treated individuals who show clinically significant benefit. This means that an intervention may reliably produce changes in behavior that are not due to chance; however, these changes may not be of great size. Moreover, statistical significance can be manipulated by sample size. Studies using large sample sizes have increased power (i.e., probability of rejecting the null hypothesis), and thereby increased probability of reaching statistical significance. In addition to the lack of criteria regarding effect size, current systems lack criteria regarding clinical significance or feasibility. Knowledge that an intervention is effective is unimportant if practitioners are unwilling or unable to effectively implement the treatment.

APPLYING EST GUIDELINES TO INTELLECTUAL DISABILITY

Aside from the general concerns with current frameworks for evaluating and identifying empirically supported treatments, current systems pose several problems for the field of ID.

Reliance on the *DSM*

One major difficulty is the reliance on the disorders presented in the *Diagnostic and Statistical Manual of Mental Disorders (DSM)* to categorize interventions. ID is considered a lifelong disorder with no known cures. Therefore, interventions used with individuals who have ID are tertiary prevention methods used to treat the associated characteristics of the disorder (e.g., stereotyped behavior, self-injurious behavior, language acquisition). The utility of reviewing treatments based on the broad category of developmental disabilities or even mental retardation is thus extremely limited. For instance, the APA's endorsement of applied behavior analysis (ABA, or behavior modification) as a well-established treatment for people with developmental disabilities does not relay information about the specific behaviors the treatment addresses. Reviewing treatments based on specific problem behaviors that are secondary symptoms to ID may be more helpful. In this way, empirically supported treatments for problems such as self-injurious behavior, paucity of social skills, and aggressive behavior, could be individually reviewed.

Broad Categories of Intervention

Another significant difficulty is that many of the current frameworks address broad categories of interventions instead of specific treatment techniques. For example, the APA Task Force's sweeping generalization that ABA is empirically supported for ID does little to guide practitioners in formulating an intervention plan for a specific behavior problem. Although research does support the conclusion that ABA in general is efficacious in reducing a number of problem behaviors among individuals with ID (e.g., Kahng, Iwata, & Lewin, 2002; Scotti et al., 1991; Sternberg et al., 1994), there are differences in the effectiveness within the genre of behavioral interventions. For instance, differential reinforcement of other behavior (DRO) and differential reinforcement of incompatible behaviors (DRI) procedures alone are less effective than other behavioral intervention procedures such as time-out, relaxation, desensitization, and response cost for reducing problem behaviors (Didden et al., 1997; Lundervold & Bourland, 1988; Scotti et al., 1991). However, there is agreement that DRO and DRI increase the overall effectiveness of an intervention when combined with other behavioral procedures (Lundervold & Bourland, 1988; Scotti et al., 1991; Sternberg et al., 1994). Reviews of empirically supported treatments generally do not narrow in on the differential effectiveness of various behavioral techniques.

Broad Categories of Individuals

Similarly, many current systems evaluate interventions for broad categories of individuals. The APA Task Force's endorsement of ABA for the broader category of individuals with developmental disabilities has limited significance in terms of decisions regarding treatments for an individual with a specific etiology or severity of ID. Individuals with a diagnosis of ID can have any one of a multitude of specific etiologies and are quite heterogeneous in intellectual and adaptive functioning. Furthermore, they can have a diverse array of behavior problems and mental health diagnoses. There is an increasing need to consider etiology in the formulation of treatment plans (Dykens & Hodapp, 1997). Systems that evaluate treatment efficacy based on the *DSM* categories of mental retardation or developmental disabilities assume that these individuals are relatively homogenous. One possible influential characteristic the APA Task Force does not address in its consideration of treatment efficacy is the level of individual impairment. A large majority of research concerning individuals who have ID predominately utilized individuals who function within the severe to profound range (e.g., Didden et al., 1997; Scotti et al., 1991). This suggests that research surrounding treatment efficacy may not be applicable to individuals with mild to moderate levels of ID. Although the work of Scotti et al. (1991) suggest that level of impairment does not significantly affect treatment efficacy, this issue deserves further attention.

Reliance on Random Controlled Trials

An additional obstacle for research within the field of ID is the heavy reliance on randomized control trials and similar large-scale studies of EST criteria. Randomized control trials pose problems for research related to disorders occurring infrequently, disorders with severe functional impairments, and populations with comorbid disorders/conditions. Randomized control trials typically require large numbers of participants, which may not be feasible for research with less prevalent disorders. Intervention research within our field is often unable to gain access to large samples of participants, and must instead rely on small sample sizes. This may mean that research within the field of ID will have a difficult time demonstrating treatment efficacy in comparison to other fields in which there are ample numbers of possible participants. However, the Research Units on Pediatric Psychopharmacology (RUPP) group is an excellent example of how various disabilities-related research teams can conduct a collaborative study using the same intervention protocol (Arnold et al., 2000). Similarly, the University Centers for Excellence in Developmental Disabilities Education, Research, and Services (UCEDD) network has conducted collaborative assessment studies under the auspices of the Social Security Administration.

An additional issue is the requirement that participants be randomly assigned to conditions within the study. Ethical concerns regarding providing immediate and appropriate care to individuals with severe needs, such as individuals with intellectual and developmental disabilities, may not permit researchers to randomly assign participants to wait-list control groups or alternative treatments. For instance, the AAMR has voiced concern that current reliance on randomized control trials will "inhibit the development and validation of new scientific knowledge in education" (AAMR, 2003). As an alternative, they advocate for the use of single-participant experimental designs to demonstrate the efficacy of treatments.

Reliance on randomized control trials and similar large-scale studies is also problematic in that relatively small differences between groups may be statistically significant yet lack clinical significance. In addition, some interventions within the field of ID may be more conducive to large sample sizes than others and therefore have an advantage in demonstrating effectiveness. For instance, the endorsement of randomized control trials for psychotherapy has been criticized on the grounds that it inadvertently favors pharmacologic, behavioral, and cognitive interventions over more interpersonal and psychoanalytic approaches because of their ability to utilize large group studies (e.g., Safran, 2001).

Not only are randomized clinical trials difficult to conduct in the field of ID research, they may also be undesirable. The APA Task Force's reliance on randomized control trials may not generalize to real-life clinical practice (e.g., Safran, 2001). Randomized control trials randomly select and assign patients, who often have less severe problems and no comorbidity, to treatments for fixed durations. In practice, patients do not randomly seek out treatments, problems are often severe and complicated by comorbidity, practitioners do not apply specific treatment durations, and treatments may not always be continuous (e.g., due to intervening life events). Therefore, although randomized control trials can achieve internal validity, they sacrifice external validity, or the ability of the findings to generalize to practice settings. These considerations are relevant not only in ID research on treatment efficacy or effectiveness, but also in research involving other disorders and conditions.

Use of Single Case Experimental Designs

Many of the criteria proposed for evaluating interventions are consistent with the current state of research methodology employed within the field of ID. Consequently, many aspects of existing frameworks can provide an adequate means through which efficacious treatments for individuals with ID can be identified. For example, many of the frameworks (e.g., APA, AACPDM) specify that demonstration of a statistically significant intervention can be achieved through well-designed single case experiments. This offers research within the field of ID, which typically involves small numbers of participants, a feasible way to evaluate interventions.

Lessening reliance on randomized controlled studies would also have the advantage of encouraging practitioners to conduct research within their practices. Currently, the majority of research that meets current guidelines for establishing empirically supported treatments emerges from research organizations and experimental laboratories largely because they have the resources to conduct large-scale studies (Hayes et al., 1999). Encouraging the use of single case designs and lessening current emphasis on large randomized controlled trials may stimulate practitioners within the field of ID to conduct research. Although the primary goal of treatment is not necessarily to advance knowledge in the field, the pursuit of one does not have to exclude the accomplishment of the other. Practitioners can still provide adequate care to clients by tailoring their interventions to clients' personal needs. Incorporating research into their practice would merely require more formalized monitoring of their treatments and efforts to share their findings with the rest of the field. The methodologies employed by many practitioners already resemble single case time-series methodology in which frequent measurements are taken across time to assess which interventions provide most benefit to clients, although measurements may often be taken less frequently or with less consistency than would be required for research purposes.

Whether these single case studies are conducted by practitioners or researchers, they will have to share several important elements in order to be critically evaluated. First, the studies must be well-designed and methodologically rigorous. Second, there is a need to describe the participants carefully including the presence of comorbid diagnoses. Third, experimental designs should employ replication techniques such as reversal designs or multiple-baseline across setting designs to provide convincing evidence of intervention efficacy. Finally, there should be greater emphasis on community-based samples, in contrast to historical reliance on institutional populations.

Need for Comparative Treatment Studies

Historically, the ID field has conducted almost no comparative studies of alternative treatments. Many current guidelines for establishing empirically supported treatments require effectiveness of a target intervention to be judged against a comparison group in the form of a placebo condition, wait-list control, or alternative treatment. The use of a wait-list control group and placebo condition is less desirable in research involving individuals with ID because of ethical concerns surrounding the withholding of therapy to individuals in need (although in practice, waits for access to skilled clinicians may exist). The most feasible option for ID research appears to be the utilization of alternative treatment comparisons. Unfortunately, in their review of intervention research concerning individuals with developmental disabilities, Scotti et al. (1991) found a trend against the use of comparison interventions in single case studies. Unless the field of ID begins encouraging the use of alternative treatment groups, intervention research will have difficulty being evaluated with current systems.

Use of Manuals

The field would also benefit from greater use of treatment manuals and practice guidelines—as suggested in many current frameworks. Many of the behavioral techniques employed in interventions for individuals with ID have not always been explained in great detail, resulting in possible confusion regarding what these interventions actually entail and difficulty in applying them to practice. Although some researchers have voiced concern that the use of treatment manuals or practice guidelines will lead to inflexible interventions that are not tailored to individual clients, research has demonstrated that the use of treatment manuals is linked with in-creased success in treatment outcome (e.g., Beutler, Machado, & Neufeldt, 1994), and can decrease the time needed to train practitioners (Rounsav-ille, O'Malley, Foley, & Weissman, 1988). In addition, treatment manuals and practice guidelines will help the field more clearly define the general principles of different interventions as well as give practitioners more de-tailed blueprints to guide their practice. Incentive to increase the use of treatment manuals or practice guidelines also comes from MCOs, which are increasingly requiring their use to keep practitioners accountable for providing effective interventions (Hayes et al., 1999). The need for treat-ment manuals, alternative treatment comparison groups, and methodolog-ically rigorous research designs has begun to be addressed within the field (e.g., Lutzker, 1993).

OBSTACLES TO OVERCOME

Although there are limitations in current systems for evaluating and synthesizing intervention research, establishing empirically supported treatments within the field of ID is a high priority. Not only will it help establish a list of efficacious treatments to ensure individuals are given potentially beneficial treatments, but it will also encourage higher stan-dards of research methodology. Despite this appeal, the movement is not universally supported. Common criticisms of the establishment of empiri-cally supported treatments include fears that third party insurance carri-ers will inappropriately use them as a basis for reimbursement decisions (e.g., Silverman, 1996), and that the movement will increase the number of malpractice suits against practitioners (e.g., Kovacs, 1996). Unfortu-nately, only time can tell if these fears are justified. Another common crit-icism of the movement is that it will limit practice flexibility (e.g., Elliot, 1998). Specifically, the emergence of established lists of efficacious treat-ments may mean that practitioners will be required to provide formulated treatments to clients instead of tailoring interventions to specific clients in specific settings with specific needs. In order for the movement toward empirically supported treatments to be fully embraced, this concern needs to be addressed.

A repeated finding in mental health services research is that prac-titioners often ignore empirical evidence and rely on their own intuition in clinical decision making (Dawes, Faust, & Meehl, 1989; Meehl, 1959). Practitioners often fall into the trap of believing that an empirical finding is irrelevant for their particular client because of the unique qualities, prob-lems, and situations of their client. They argue that findings based on large group studies or meta-analyses offer little information that can apply at the level of the individual (Dawes et al., 1989). Although there are instances in which a particular quality of a client's situation renders empirical evidence surrounding treatment efficacy inapplicable, practitioners are not good at determining when these exemptions occur. Numerous studies have found that the use of empirical evidence to guide clinical decisions is superior to decisions based solely on clinician judgments, regardless of a practitioner's experience or knowledge of the field (e.g., Dawes et al., 1989; Meehl, 1959). In order for the development of empirically supported treatments to be effective, practitioners need to be encouraged to use this knowledge to guide their practice.

Even if practitioners decide to use empirically supported treatments with their clients, they may require ongoing consultation from within their ID/DD service delivery system to provide the treatment effectively (Holburn, Jacobson, & Vietze, 2000). Accordingly, the effectiveness of ongoing consultation has a clear effect on the effectiveness of the intervention itself. This issue may be particularly important in cases in which ABA is being implemented by providers who lack training in behavioral principles.

In order for the field of ID to fully embrace the movement toward empirically supported treatments another issue that must be resolved is that of appropriateness of the intervention. Controversy surrounds intrusive interventions that are efficacious, yet may threaten or limit the rights of clients and have deleterious effects on their welfare. Although there has been a gradual decrease in the use of punishment-based interventions for self-injurious behavior over the past few decades and a dramatic increase in the use of reinforcement-based interventions (Kahng et al., 2002), aversive techniques are still present in practice and research. This issue has received great attention within the realm of psychology and education in the form of a movement toward Positive Behavioral Support. This movement embodies an effort to utilize empirically supported, socially and culturally appropriate positive behavioral interventions as an alternative to aversive and coercive interventions.

The issue of treatment appropriateness has not currently been addressed in empirically supported treatment literature; however its resolution is essential to the success of the movement in the field of ID. The need to review and list empirically supported intrusive treatments, in order to keep practitioners and clients informed of the available range of efficacious treatments, must be balanced with the need to avoid endorsing potentially harmful interventions. A predominate way the field has dealt with the issue of treatment appropriateness in the past is to abide by the tenet of the least intrusive hierarchy. This means that aversive techniques are only warranted with severe behavior problems for which less intrusive interventions have been attempted and documented as failing (Turnbull, 1981). Inclusion of this tenet into the movement toward empirically supported treatments may be a necessary step for the field of ID.

The movement toward empirically supported treatments within the field of ID is also inhibited by a lack of appropriate mechanisms to translate research findings into practice. Historically, the field has adopted a relatively passive approach to translation. In illustration of this, findings are presented at national meetings, published in good journals, and it is assumed that practitioners attend the conferences, read the articles, and implement the work. For example, the Fourth Congress of the International Association for the Scientific Study of Mental Deficiency (IASSMD) was held in Washington, DC, in 1976. The theme of this Congress was "From

Research to Practice." The participants included "most of the outstand-ing scientists and professional practitioners in the field" (Begab, 1977). Begab asserted that "effective communication between scientists of vari-ous persuasions and professional practitioners can effectively transform knowledge into practice." This relatively passive approach has limited ef-fectiveness. It assumes that practitioners will read the work found in good journals, and have the ability to translate from the study to their particular setting. This parallels the early history of generalization. After it was dis-covered that learning did not automatically generalize to new situations, Baer, Wolfe, and Risley (1968) made it clear that generalization training had to be an explicit part of the intervention plan.

Our special education colleagues have examined the conditions un-der which science is best translated into practice. Abbott et al. (1999) as-sert that traditional professional development mechanisms, such as work-shops, are ineffective in translating research to practice because they "grossly underestimate the time and effort needed to produce meaningful changes in practice (p. 339)." They also suggest

> "the traditional top-down educational research model, with the researcher targeting the problems and planning the solutions and the teachers implementing the findings with fidelity has not produced powerful interventions or impacted practice. Us-ing the top-down model, researchers very often asked and an-swered questions of little interest to practitioners and they have developed solutions so slowly that they were often out of date by the time they reached the classroom (p. 339)."

Abbott et al. propose collaborative approaches uniting researchers and practitioners in research and professional development designed to trans-late research to practice. Following Carnine's (1997) lead, they have sought to "bridge" the research to practice gap by making research more trust-worthy, useful, and accessible to classroom teachers. Abbott et al. have implemented this in Kansas City, Kansas with the Juniper Gardens Chil-dren's Project Model. Within this model, researchers enter into a relation-ship with local schools. The goal is to initiate and sustain ongoing inter-actions between classroom teachers and researchers interested in using research-validated practices in local classroom settings. Abbott et al. re-port the success of this approach in closing the gap between research and practice in general and special education classrooms. This is an example in which translation of research to practice is more likely to occur when there is an explicit plan for it.

FINAL CONSIDERATIONS

The conclusion that there has been little rigorous test of the efficacy of interventions for people with ID is inescapable. At a time when increasing effort is being directed toward the identification of empirically supported treatments, only applied behavior analysis interventions for people with intellectual disabilities have been included in published listings. Although we have devoted considerable effort to demonstrating that some controversial interventions are without scientific merit, there is a critical need for well-designed intervention studies of potentially beneficial methods. Moreover, there is a need to establish, within the field of ID, a mechanism for synthesizing research findings so that they can be easily translated to practice. This objective may be made even more difficult by the range of disciplines involved in the field of intellectual disabilities as well as the range of possible interventions. Multiple systems exist for evaluating the effectiveness of interventions such as the Division 12 Task Force on Promotion and Dissemination of Psychological Procedures and Sackett's Rules of Evidence. Perhaps initial efforts could be directed toward using an available framework for evaluating the efficacy of particular interventions. Although there are difficulties in conducting RCTs in the field of ID, the possibility exists that research consortiums can be developed to provide access to larger numbers of participants. Similarly, systematic use of single case methodology can provide comparable efficacy data regarding a range of intervention efforts.

The mental health arena is particularly well poised to make significant strides in establishing empirically supported treatments for people with ID. A consortium involving the National Institute of Neurological Disorders and Stroke (NINDS), the National Institute of Child Health and Human Development (NICHD), the National Institute on Mental Health (NIMH), the National Institutes of Health (NIH) Office of Rare Diseases, and the Joseph P. Kennedy Jr. Foundation held a recent workshop on the Emotional and Behavioral Health in Persons with Mental Retardation/Developmental Disabilities. The members of the workshop noted that there are a number of behavioral and psychosocial treatments that have been well researched in the general population, but have not been tested for efficacy in individuals with intellectual and developmental disabilities. Similarly, newer and safer medications are available for a range of emotional and behavioral disorders, yet few rigorous tests of their efficacy in individuals with intellectual and developmental disabilities have been performed. Furthermore, the participants prepared a series of recommendations of relevance to this chapter. Specifically, they proposed that the field

- Assess the effects of combining pharmacological treatments with behavioral, psychosocial, and educational interventions and/or natural supports.
- Develop innovative research designs to address the potential confounds of ongoing treatments and co-occurring conditions.
- Urge the FDA drug approval standards to include alternative research designs.
- Create a federal task force to develop and implement an interdisciplinary clinical research network.
- Place funding priority on testing promising interventions.

The time is obviously right to focus on linking science and practice.

REFERENCES

Abbott, M., Walton, C., Tapia, Y., & Greenwood, C. R. (1999). Research to practice: A "blueprint" for closing the gap in local schools. *Exceptional Children, 65,* 339–352.

American Association on Mental Retardation. (2002). *Mental retardation: Definition, classification and systems of supports* (10th ed.). Washington, DC: Author.

American Association on Mental Retardation Board of Directors. (2003). *Resolution of the AAMR on evidence-based research and intellectual disability.* Retrieved July 28, 2003, from http://www.aamr.org/Reading_Room/pdf/resolution_research.pdf

American Psychiatric Association. (2000). *Diagnostic and statistical manual of mental disorders* (4th ed., text revision). Washington, DC: Author.

Arnold, L. E., Aman, M. G., Martin, A., Collier-Crespin, A., Vitiello, B., Tierney, E., et al. (2000). Assessment in multisite randomized clinical trials of patients with autistic disorder: The Autism RUPP Network. Research Units on Pediatric Psychopharmacology. *Journal of Autism and Developmental Disorders, 30*(2), 99–111.

Baer, D. M., Wolf, M. M., & Risley, T. R. (1968). Some current dimensions of applied behavior analysis. *Journal of Applied Behavior Analysis, 1,* 91–97.

Begab, M. J. (1977). Barriers to the application of knowledge. In P. Mittler (Ed.), *Research to practice in mental retardation* (Vol. 1, pp. 1–30). Baltimore: University Park Press.

Beutler, L. E., Machado, P. P., & Neufeldt, S. S. (1994). Therapist variables. In A. E. Bergin & S. L. Garfield (Eds.), *Handbook of psychotherapy and behavioral change* (4th ed., pp. 229–269). New York: Wiley.

Beutler, L. E., Moleiro, C., & Talebi, H. (2002). How practitioners can systematically use empirical evidence in treatment selection. *Journal of Clinical Psychology, 58,* 1199–1212.

Bohart, A. C., O'Hara, M., & Leitner, L. M. (1998). Empirically violated treatments: Disenfranchisement of humanistic and other psychotherapies. *Psychotherapy Research, 8,* 141–157.

Butler, C., Chambers, H., Goldstein, M., Harris, S., Leach, J., Campbell, S., et al. (1999). Evaluating research in developmental disabilities: A conceptual framework for reviewing treatment outcomes. *Developmental Medicine and Child Neurology, 41,* 55–59.

Carnine, D. (1997). Bridging the research-to-practice gap. *Exceptional Children, 63,* 513–521.

Chambless, D. L., & Hollon, S. D. (1998). Defining empirically supported therapies. *Journal of Consulting and Clinical Psychology, 49,* 5–18.

Chambless, D. L., & Ollendick, T. H. (2001). Empirically supported psychological interventions: Controversies and evidence. *Annual Review of Psychology, 52,* 685–716.

Dawes, R. M., Faust, D., & Meehl, P. (1989). Clinical versus actuarial judgment. *Science, 243,* 1668–1674.

Didden, R., Duker, P. C., & Korzilius, H. (1997). Meta-analytic study on treatment effectiveness for problem behaviors with individuals who have mental retardation. *American Journal of Mental Retardation, 101,* 387–399.

Doll, E. A. (1941). The essentials of an inclusive concept of mental deficiency. *American Journal of Mental Deficiency, 46,* 214–219.

Drotar, D. (2002). Enhancing reviews of psychological treatments with pediatric populations: Thoughts on next steps. *Journal of Pediatric Psychology, 27,* 166–176.

Dykens, E. M., & Hodapp, R. M. (1997). Treatment issues in genetic mental retardation syndromes. *Professional Psychology: Research and Practice, 28,* 263–270.

Elliot, R. E. (1998). Editor's introduction: A guide to the empirically supported treatments controversy. *Psychotherapy Research, 8,* 115–125.

Garfield, S. L. (1996). Some problems associated with "validated" forms of psychotherapy. *Clinical Psychology: Science and Practice, 3,* 218–229.

Hayes, S. C., Barlow, D. H., & Nelson-Gray, R. O. (1999). *The scientist-practitioner: Research and accountability in the age of managed care.* MA: Allyn & Bacon.

Holburn, S., Jacobson, J. W., & Vietze, P. M. (2000). Quantifying the process and outcomes of person-centered planning. *American Journal on Mental Retardation, 105,* 402–416.

Jacobson, J. W., Mulick, J. A., & Foxx, R. M. (2005). Historical approaches to developmental disabilities. In J. W. Jacobson, J. A. Mulick, & R. M. Foxx (Eds.), *Controversial therapies for developmental disabilities: Fad, fashion, and science in professional psychology* (pp. 61–84). Mahwah, NJ: Erlbaum.

Jacobson, J. W., Mulick, J. A., & Schwartz, A. A. (1995). A history of facilitated communication: Science, pseudoscience, and antiscience. Working group on facilitated communication. *American Psychologist, 50,* 750–765.

Kahng, S., Iwata, B. A., & Lewin, A. B. (2002). Behavioral treatment of self-injury, 1964–2000. *American Journal on Mental Retardation, 107,* 212–221.

Kazdin, A. E., & Bass, D. (1989). Power to detect differences between alternative treatments in comparative psychotherapy outcome research. *Journal of Consulting and Clinical Research, 57,* 138–147.

Kovacs, A. L. (1996, Winter). We have met the enemy and he is us! APP Advance, pp. 6, 19, 20, 22.

Lambert, M. J., & Bergin, A. E. (1994). The effectiveness of psychotherapy. In A. E. Bergin & S. L. Garfield (Eds.), *Handbook of psychotherapy and behavioral change* (4th ed., pp. 143–189). New York: Wiley.

Lovaas, O. I. (1987). Behavioral treatment and normal education and intellectual functioning in young autistic children. *Journal of Consulting and Clinical Psychology, 55,* 3–9.

Lundervold, D., & Bourland, G. (1988). Quantitative analysis of treatment of aggression, self-injury, and property destruction. *Behavior Modification, 12,* 590–617.

Lutzker, J. R. (1993). Behavior analysis for developmental disabilities: The states of efficacy and comparative treatments. In T. R. Giles (Ed.), *Handbook of effective psychotherapy* (pp. 88–106). New York: Plenum.

MacLean, W. E., Jr. (2002). Challenges in translating research to practice for the field of mental retardation and developmental disabilities. *Psychology in Mental Retardation and Developmental Disabilities, 27,* 3–6.

Meehl, P. E. (1959). A comparison of clinicians with five statistical methods of identifying psychotic MMPI profiles. *Journal of Counseling Psychology, 6,* 102–109.

Morin, C. M. (1999). Empirically supported psychological treatments: A natural extension of the scientist-practitioner paradigm. *Canadian Psychology, 40,* 312–315.

Mostert, M. P. (2001). Facilitated communication since 1995: A review of published studies. *Journal of Autism and Developmental Disorders, 31,* 287–313.

Norcross, J. C., & Newman, C. F. (1992). Psychotherapy integration: Setting the context. In J. C. Norcross & M. R. Goldfried (Eds.), *Handbook of psychotherapy integration* (pp. 3–45). New York: Basic Books.

Odom, S. L., & Kaiser, A. P. (1997). Prevention and early intervention during early childhood: Theoretical and empirical bases for practice. In W. E. MacLean (Ed.), *Ellis' handbook of mental deficiency, psychological theory and research* (3rd ed., pp. 137–172). Mahwah, NJ: Erlbaum.

Office of Special Education Programs. (OSEP). U.S. Department of Education. Positive Behavior Interventions and Supports-PBIS Mission. Retrieved July 28, 2003, from http://www.pbis.org/english/

Parry, C. (1996). NHS psychotherapy services in England, Rep. 96PP0043. London: Department of Health.

P. L. 104-83. (1996). Developmental Disabilities Assistance and Bill of Rights Act Amendment of 1996.

Roth, A. D., & Fonagy, P. (1996). *What works for whom? A critical review of psychotherapy research.* New York: Guilford.

Rounsaville, B. J., O'Malley, S., Foley, S., & Weissman, M. W. (1988). Role of manual-guided training in the conduct of efficacy of interpersonal psychotherapy for depression. *Journal of Consulting and Clinical Psychology, 56,* 681–688.

Sackett, D. L., Richardson, W. S., Rosenberg, W., & Haynes, R. B. (1997). *Evidence-based medicine: How to practice and teach EBM.* New York: Livingstone.

Safran, J. D. (2001). When worlds collide: Psychoanalysis and the empirically supported treatment movement. *Psychoanalytic Dialogues, 11,* 659–681.

Sattler, J. M. (2001). *Assessment of children: Cognitive applications* (4th ed.). San Diego, CA: Sattler.

Scotti, J. R., Evans, I. M., Meyer, L. H., & Walker, P. (1991). A meta-analysis of intervention research with problem behavior: Treatment validity and standards of practice. *American Journal on Mental Retardation, 96,* 233–256.

Shirk, S. (2004). Dissemination of youth ESTs: Ready for prime time? *Clinical psychology: Science and Practice, 11,* 308–312.

Silverman, W. H. (1996). Cookbooks, manuals, and paint-by-numbers: Psychotherapy in the 90's. *Psychotherapy, 33,* 207–215.

Sindelar, P. T., & Wilson, R. J. (1984). The potential effects of meta-analysis on special education practice. *Journal of Special Education, 18,* 81–92.

Spitz, H. H. (1986). *The raising of intelligence: A selected history of attempts to raise retarded intelligence.* Hillsdale, NJ: Erlbaum.

Spitz, H. H. (1999). Attempts to raise intelligence. In M. Anderson (Ed.), *The development of intelligence* (pp. 275–293). London: Taylor & Francis.

Sternberg, L., Taylor, R. L., & Babkie, A. (1994). Correlates of interventions with self-injurious behavior. *Journal of Intellectual Disability Research, 38,* 475–485.

Strauss, B. M., & Kaechele, H. (1998). The writing on the wall: Comments on the current discussion about empirically validated treatments in Germany. *Psychotherapy Research, 8,* 158–177.

Strupp, H. H. (2001). Implications of the empirically supported treatment movement for psychoanalysis. *Psychoanalytic Dialogues, 11,* 605–619.

Thompson, L. W., Gallagher, E., & Steinmetz Breckenridge, J. (1987). Comparative effectiveness of psychotherapies for depressed elders. *Journal of Consulting and Clinical Psychology, 55,* 385–390.

Turnbull, H. R. (Ed.). (1981). *The least restrictive alternative: Principles and practices.* Washington, DC: American Association on Mental Deficiency.

U.S. Department of Health and Human Services, Center for Drug Evaluation and Research. (1998, May). *Guidance for industry: Providing clinical evidence of effectiveness for human drugs and biological products.* Retrieved June 9, 2003, from http://www.fda.gov/cder/guidance/1397fnl.pdf

U.S. Preventive Services Task Force. (1996). *Guide to clinical preventive services* (2nd ed.). Baltimore, MD: Williams& Wilkins.

Wampold, B. E., Mondin, G. W., Moody, M., Stich, F., Benson, K., Ahn, H., et al. (1997). A meta-analysis of outcome studies comparing bona fide psychotherapies: Empirically, "all must have prizes." *Psychological Bulletin, 122,* 203–215.

Weisz, J. R., Chu, B. C., & Polo, A. J. (2004). Treatment dissemination and evidence-based practice: Strengthening intervention through clinician–researcher collaboration. *Clinical Psychology: Science and Practice, 11,* 300–307.

World Health Organization. (1993). *International statistical classification of diseases and related health problems* (10th ed.). Geneva, Switzerland: Author.

23

Early Intervention

Background, Research Findings, and Future Directions

SHARON LANDESMAN RAMEY, CRAIG T. RAMEY, and ROBIN GAINES LANZI

The purpose of this chapter is to provide a general framework for understanding what early intervention is, what has been proven to work, and what the next steps should be. The first section describes the basics about early intervention—the what, when, why, and how. The second section presents research findings on what has been proven to work, including essential operating principles and key elements of effective early intervention programs. And the third section provides recommendations for future directions for early intervention research and services.

DEFINING EARLY INTERVENTION: THE BASICS OF WHAT, WHEN, WHY, AND HOW

In this section we describe the basics about early intervention services—*what* it is, *when* it begins, *why* it is important, and *how* a person can enroll.

What It Is

Early intervention refers to a systematic approach of early and continual treatment from a team of professionals focused on meeting the needs of

SHARON LANDESMAN RAMEY, CRAIG T. RAMEY, and ROBIN GAINES LANZI • Georgetown University Center on Health and Education, Georgetown University, Washington, District of Columbia 20057.

individual children and their families. Early intervention is founded on the belief that services need to begin as early in the child's life as possible, and that the child's development will be improved through individualized and specialized treatment and services. A broad range of types of early intervention treatment and services are available. These include assistive technology devices and services, audiology, family training, counseling, and home visits, health services, medical services for diagnosis or evaluation, nursing services, nutrition services, occupational therapy, physical therapy, psychological services, service coordination services, social work services, special instruction, speech-language pathology, transportation and related costs, as well as vision services. Not all children will need all types of services. Some may need only one or two of these services, typically the family training or counseling and early childhood education.

How these services are planned and coordinated depend on the specific needs of an individual child and his or her family. The planning and service coordination is generally conducted by a case manager. The treatment is provided by a host of professionals including pediatricians, pediatric neurologists, developmental pediatricians, physical therapists, speech-language therapists, social workers, psychologists, special education teachers, occupational therapists, audiologists, optometrists and ophthalmologists, nurses, nutritionists, and specialists who have received interdisciplinary or multidisciplinary training.

In every state and territory, there is a University Affiliated Program (UAP) that specializes in developmental disabilities. The U.S. Congress established these programs to provide information about developmental disabilities and supports to states and consumers. Additionally, each state has an Interagency Coordinating Council (ICC), which is an advisory group of parents, professionals, policy makers, and representatives of agencies that provide or administer early intervention.

When It Begins and How Long It Lasts

The ages when children enter early intervention programs range from birth through 5 years of age, although some begin working with pregnant women prior to the birth of their child. Services are generally provided in the home or child care environment on a weekly basis during the first 2 years of life. Federal legislation provides for a seamless transition of services from early intervention services to school-based preschool programs. The transition should begin when the child is 2 years of age and be completed when the child reaches 3 years of age. The school-based program (covered under Part B of federal legislation, see the subsection "How Funding Is Provided for Services and How Eligibility Is Determined" below for a description of funding) includes an expanded set of services including early counseling services, early identification and assessment, parent counseling and training, recreation, rehabilitation counseling services, school health services, social work services in schools, and special education.

Why It Is Important

Why is early intervention important? It is clear from over four decades of research that early intervention makes a difference in children's development (see reviews by Bryant & Maxwell, 1997; Carnegie Task Force on Meeting the Needs of Young Children report, 1994; Guralnick, 1997; Haskins, 1989; C. T. Ramey & Ramey, 1998a, 1998b, 1999). The first 5 years of life are essential in providing a solid foundation and support for enhancing and improving young children's development, especially those with developmental disabilities. During this time, children's brains have the greatest capacity to change and adapt with experience and stimulation. The earlier intervention begins, the more likely it is to produce desired outcomes for children and families. Developmental neurobiologists have shown that if children do not experience certain kinds of stimulation early in life, their brains may not be able to compensate for the critical loss (see Carnegie Task Force on Learning in the Primary Grades, 1996; Carnegie Task Force on Meeting the Needs of Young Children, 1994; C. T. Ramey & Ramey, 1998b, 1999; Shore, 1997). The scientific findings are the clearest for those children living in poverty who are at risk for cognitive and language development delays and for children who are biologically at risk due to low birth weight and premature birth (Ramey, Ramey, Lanzi, & Cotton, 2002; Ramey, Ramey, & Lanzi, 2006).

How Funding Is Provided for Services and How Eligibility Is Determined

Early intervention services are mandated through federal legislation. The Education for All Handicapped Children Act of 1975 initially mandated services for children with disabilities. The Education for All Handicapped Act Amendments of 1986 provided additional funding for children ages 3–5 and funded the creation of a system of early intervention for children ages birth through their third birthday. Early intervention services are currently funded by Part C (birth to 3 years) of the Individuals with Disabilities Act (IDEA) Amendments of 1997. Although federal legislation mandates services and provides funding, not all services are fully funded by federal dollars, services are supplemented with additional state funds. Private insurance and Medicaid are often billed for services. State and local programs must work together to raise additional dollars to meet the operating costs.

Federal legislation dictates that states define which risk conditions qualify children to receive early intervention as well as which services will be provided for specific diagnoses. The majority of states have a Child Find program to identify infants at risk for disability. There is, however, no uniform definition or criteria for determining eligibility. The state's criteria for the cutoff point for defining a child with a disability varies by state.

Although determination of eligibility varies, almost all assessments, involve tests or procedures to determine a child's mental development and performance in areas such as motor development, social-emotional development, language, and cognition. An individualized family service plan (IFSP) is required to be developed prior to the receipt of services. Both family members and the health professionals work together to identify the primary needs of the child and family, and how the needs can be best met.

RESEARCH ON EARLY INTERVENTION: WHAT HAS BEEN PROVEN TO WORK

For the past 70 years, researchers have been investigating how early intervention can improve the lives of young children and their families. In this section, we provide an overview of the origins of early intervention research and early scientific findings, a summary of five model early intervention programs, and a synthesis of findings including essential operating principles and key elements of effective early intervention programs.

Origins of Early Intervention Research and Early Scientific Findings

Grounded in learning theory, psychologists began to examine how early experiences can affect children's cognitive, social, and emotional development (e.g., Harlow, 1958; Hebb, 1949; McVicker Hunt, 1961) over seven decades ago. A series of studies in the 1930s and 1940s on infants and young children living in orphanages showed that the types of interaction and care provided to children was terribly inadequate compared to types of interaction and care provided to children in "typical" homes (S. L. Ramey & Ramey, 1999). Many of these investigators wrote about the lasting negative effects that the lack of warm, responsive care and stimulation in orphanages can have on children. Skeels and Dye's (1939) seminal work first highlighted how early experience can alter children's development, including intelligence, for children with mental retardation. This work launched a line of inquiry in animal and human research devoted to understanding what children need in order to ensure healthy growth and development. In the animal research, the type and timing of early experiences were carefully controlled and altered to determine their effects on later development. These studies revealed that deficits in social and sensory experiences produced abnormal social, emotional, and learning behavior in animals that otherwise were born healthy (cf., Sackett, Novak, & Droeker, 1999). In the human research, how children respond to nonoptimal living conditions and environments, and the extent to which early support and stimulation can alter the negative effect was studied (e.g., Bronfenbrenner, 1979; Landesman-Dwyer & Butterfield, 1983). This research showed that children, even those who have been institutionalized, can benefit from early supports but that not all children benefit in the same way.

During the early 1960s, another set of research was conducted that focused on children living in poverty and programs to prevent developmental

delay. Researchers found that rates of mild mental retardation were significantly elevated among children from impoverished backgrounds and
families (Deutsch, 1967; Garber, 1988; Zigler, 1967). Further, there was a
strong relationship between the quality of a child's home environment and
the child's intellectual and problem-solving capabilities (Cowan, Cowan,
Schultz, & Heming, 1994; Hess & Shipman, 1965; Huston, McLoyd,
& Garcia Coll, 1994; Maccoby & Martin, 1983; McVicker Hunt, 1961;
Vygotsky, 1962). Interestingly, researchers proved that very young infants
are capable of learning, which was at the time not widely accepted (Osofsky,
1979). These early educational intervention programs provided the basis
for the formation of Head Start and other federally funded programs. The
majority of these programs were conducted in university child development centers, with varying amounts and types of services. The Consortium
for Longitudinal Studies was a collaborative effort involving 11 systematic
studies that used experimental or quasi-experimental designs to determine
the efficacy of early intervention programs for children from socioeconomi-
cally deprived backgrounds (Darlington, Royce, Snipper, Murray, & Lazaar,
1980; Lazar, Darlington, Murray, Royce, & Snipper, 1982). These findings
reaffirmed that early educational supports can make a difference in children's academic and social development but what was controversial was
the "fade out" effect findings (i.e., IQ scores were improved by the end of
the project and were maintained for 3 or 4 years but declined over time).

Model Early Intervention Programs

Numerous large-scale model early intervention programs were developed during the 1970s, five of which included the gold standard design—
randomized controlled trial designs (Currie, 2000). These programs included: the *Abecedarian Project* (Campbell & Ramey, 1994; Ramey &
Campbell, 1984; Ramey, Campbell, Burchinal, Skinner, Gardner, &
Ramey, 2000), *Project Care* (Burchinal, Campbell, Bryant, Wasik, & Ramey,
1997; Ramey, Ramey, Gaines, & Blair, 1995; Wasik, Ramey, Bryant, &
Sparling, 1990), the *Infant Health and Development Program* (Infant
Health and Development Program—IHDP, 1990; Ramey et al., 1992),
the *Milwaukee Project* (Garber, 1988), and the *Perry Preschool Project*
(Schweinhart, Barnes, & Weikart, 1993; Schweinhart, Berrueta-Clement,
Barnett, Epstein, & Weikart, 1985; Weikart, Bond, & McNeil, 1978). These
five programs provided intensive, ongoing, and systematic early intervention services to children at risk for developmental disabilities and their
families. A major research component was included in all of the programs,
including the randomized controlled trial design, which enables the investigators to determine whether the treatment has a significant impact
on participants. All of these programs had minimal attrition and collected
data on children at least into middle school (see Ramey et al., 2002; Ramey
et al., 2006 for a fuller description of these programs). A brief description
of these programs is provided below.

The Abecedarian Project was a single-site randomized controlled trial
that began in 1972 in North Carolina at the Frank Porter Graham Child

Development Center. The project sought to determine if coordinated high-quality services of early childhood education, pediatric care, and family social support could improve the intellectual and educational competence of participating children. Enrollment into the program began when the babies were born; they were selected for the program based on a 13-item high-risk index (Ramey & Smith, 1977). The overwhelming majority of these children came from impoverished economic and educational backgrounds, but all were biologically healthy and had no known genetic or infectious links to mental retardation (Ramey & Campbell, 1992; Ramey & Ramey, 1998a). The intervention program was based on developmental systems theory (e.g., Bertalanffy, 1975), which postulates that instrumental and conceptual learning is facilitated through a stimulating, positive, and responsive environment (Ramey & Finklestein, 1981).

Half of the enrolled 111 families were randomly assigned to the comparison group and half were randomly assigned to the treatment group. The families participating in the comparison group received free nutritional supplements for the infants, social services, and free or low cost pediatric follow-up services. The families participating in the treatment group received the same services as the comparison group plus they participated in an educational intervention that involved full day, 5-day a week, 50 weeks per year in the child development center on the university campus. The children began participation in the preschool educational program by at least 4 months of age, prior to any developmental delays, and continued until they entered public school kindergarten (C. T. Ramey & Ramey, 1999).

Teachers in the educational component were formally trained in early childhood education and had many years of experience in the field, and demonstrated skill and competence in working with young children. Developing language competence and providing positive response-contingency learning experiences were targeted (Ramey, McGinness, Cross, Collier, & Barrie-Blackley, 1981). The *Partners for Learning* educational program was the basis for the curriculum for infants and toddlers, which included activities promoting development for cognitive-fine motor, social-self, motor, and language development (J. J. Sparling & Lewis, 1979; J. Sparling & Lewis, 1979, 1984). Additionally, a preliteracy curriculum was included for the older preschool children (Wallach & Wallach, 1976).

Findings indicate that children in the treatment group should significant higher IQ scores than children in the comparison group beginning at 18 months of age and at every assessment age thereafter through age 21. Early on, during the preschool years, children's IQ scores were 10–15 points higher in the treatment group than those in the comparison group. These differences remained at 12, 15, and 21 years in statistically significant and educationally meaningful ways, yet the differences narrowed somewhat. Strikingly, children in the treatment group continued to have significantly higher academic achievement scores in both reading and mathematics, were less likely to be placed in special education, were less likely to be retained in grade, more likely to be enrolled in higher education, and were more likely to delay the onset of parenting than those in the comparison group (Ramey et al., 2000). Amazingly, 99% of the living children were followed into adulthood for analyses.

Project CARE enrolled 63 children from economically impoverished backgrounds, including maternal education and family income. The program began in 1977 and 1978, and systematically compared two forms of intervention: a center-based program identical to the Abecedarian Project and a home-based program of weekly home visits for the first 3 years of life, followed by biweekly visits for the next 2 years. Additionally, children received a family-based intervention from infancy to school age. Children were randomly assigned to one of three treatment conditions: (1) center-based educational intervention plus home visits; (2) home visits only; or (3) control (see Wasik et al., 1990, for more details). All Project CARE children assigned to either treatment condition had a home-school resource teacher during the first 3 years of elementary school.

There were similar significant outcomes for children participating in the most intensive program (center-based educational intervention plus home visits) as children participating in the Abecedarian Project, in terms of their cognitive performance and reading and mathematics achievement through adolescence (Wasik et al., 1990). Disappointedly, the same child development outcomes were not evidenced for children participating in the home visiting only group. Additionally, significant differences were not found between those participating in the home visiting only group in terms of their home environment, parents' attitudes, or the children's or the parents' behavior as compared to those participating in the control group. The same curriculum materials were available in the child development centers and in the home-based program; however, the delivery and use of the materials may have varied greatly. The teachers in the child development centers were experienced and well-trained in early education, and were focused solely on providing a stimulating environment and a systematic curriculum. Parents, however, varied in their experiences and the changes that might have occurred in parenting behavior and in parent–child interactions may not have been early enough and intensive enough to equal what was received in center-based optimal educational care (Klerman et al., 2001).

The Infant Health and Development Program, referred to as IHDP, enrolled 985 infants who were premature (less than 37 weeks gestational age) and low birth weight (below 2500 g). Infants were born in Level III hospitals with no major congenital anomalies. The program was conducted in eight sites across the country, representing great ethnic and demographic diversity (IHDP, 1990; Ramey et al., 1992). Infants were randomly assigned to either the intervention group ($n = 377$) or to the follow-up group ($n = 608$). Infants participating in the intervention component began receiving program services at hospital discharge weekly for the first year, and biweekly until 36 months corrected age. Weekly home visits were the main early intervention component until children were 12 months corrected age. Beginning at 12 months corrected age, children attended a full-day, 5-day-per-week child development center and parents attended bimonthly parent group meetings. Children in both conditions received pediatric follow-up. The goals of the home visit program were: (1) to provide emotional, social, and practical support to parents, as adults; (2) to provide parents with developmentally timed information about their low birth weight child's development; (3) to help parents learn specific ways to foster their child's intellectual, physical, and social development; and (4) to help parents discover ways to cope with the responsibilities of caring for a developing and, initially, vulnerable child (IHDP, 1990). A major component of the home visiting program was the educational curriculum—the Early Partners Curriculum for 24–40 weeks gestational age low birth weight infants (Sparling, Lewis, & Neuwirth, 1992) and the *Partners for Learning* (Sparling & Lewis, 1984) curriculum for infants to 36 months.

There was a significant impact for participating in the project across all major child and family domains at 36 months of age. Interestingly, gains varied as a function of birth weight, maternal education, and family participation. Although all infants were low birth weight, there was a wide range in their birth weight, which related to developmental outcomes. Infants in the heavier birth weight group had higher average IQ scores by 13 points, whereas, infants in the lighter birth weight group had higher IQ scores by only 6.5 IQ points as compared to the infants in the control group. Further, among heavier low birth weight children, 23% of the children in the comparison group had IQ scores of 70 or below, compared with only 8% of the children in the intervention group (C. T. Ramey & Ramey, 1999). Mother's education made a difference as well in terms of both child and family outcomes. Children at greatest cognitive risk due to low family educational resources benefited the most in terms of children's cognitive development, adaptive and prosocial behavior, behavior problems, vocabulary, receptive language, and reasoning. Further, significant differences were revealed in terms of the home environment, mother–child interactions, and maternal problem-solving skills (Brooks-Gunn, Gross, Kraemer, Spiker, & Shapiro, 1992; Gross, Spiker, & Hayes, 1997; Landesman & Ramey, 1989; Martin, Ramey, & Ramey, 1990). Regarding family participation, the probability that a child would function at the borderline intellectual range or lower decreased significantly with higher degrees of family participation (Ramey et al., 1992).

Unlike Abecedarian and Project Care, the IHDP program was terminated when children were 3 years of age, and evidenced a somewhat disappointing pattern of cognitive results in later years. By 5 and 8 years of age, the overall IQ differences between the intervention and comparison groups were no longer educationally significant (Brooks-Gunn et al., 1992; McCarton et al., 1997). A noteworthy exception is that the *heavier* low birth weight children continued to have significantly higher IQ scores at age 5 and 8 than the children in the comparison group.

The Milwaukee Project targeted mothers who had an IQ below 75 in an economically impoverished inner-city neighborhood. Children were enrolled when they were between 3 and 6 months of age and randomly assigned to condition. Those participating in the intervention received home visits during the first 4 months of participation, and then were enrolled in a full-day, year round child development center through age 6. Mothers participated in 2 years of vocational and social education. In addition, the Milwaukee Project provided more direct support for the children's learning experiences and families than any other randomized controlled study. Those in the control group participated in assessments only. There were major significant differences in children's cognitive scores between the intervention and comparison group, beginning at 18 months of age. At 3 years of age, children in the intervention group had IQ scores 30 points higher than those in the comparison group. Additional improvements were revealed for children's verbal and expressive skills.

Cognitive gains continued at age 10, children in the treatment group had IQ scores 18 points higher than those in the control group (104 vs. 86, respectively). This, however, did not translate into differences in academic performance between the two groups. Interestingly, though, children in the intervention group were less likely to be placed in special education or referred for special services than those in the control group. Garber (1988) speculates that the school achievement differences may not have been found due to being schooled in poor quality inner city public schools (as compared to high quality schools in North Carolina) and unavoidable educational policies that may have negatively impacted children's performance. These findings highlight that children's success in school is a function of many factors, and that early intervention services must focus on all aspects of a child's life.

The *Perry Preschool Project* was conducted in an inner-city setting in Ypsilanti, Michigan, and focused on children who experienced developmental delay. The first cohort enrolled children when they were 4 years old and the second through fifth cohorts enrolled children when they were 3 years old. The program was conducted for 30 weeks with the first cohort and for 60 weeks with the remaining cohorts. There were 58 children in the intervention group and 65 children in the comparison group. Children in the intervention group received 2 years of preschool ($12\frac{1}{2}$ hr per week for 8 months) and weekly 90-min home visits to promote positive parenting skills. Teachers had solid backgrounds in teaching, including masters' degrees and training in child development, and taught classes with low child/teacher ratios (Schweinhart et al., 1985, 1993).

Findings indicate that children's developmental outcomes were enhanced by participation in the project. Children's IQ scores were significantly higher for those participating in the intervention than those in the comparison group, with an IQ difference of 95 versus 84, respectively at age 5. Unfortunately, by the age of 15, both groups revealed mean IQ's in the low 80s. However, other domains of positive school achievement as a function of participation were revealed. Seventy-one percent of those in the intervention group graduated from high school or received their GED versus 54% in the comparison group. Further, children in the intervention group experienced better academic achievement in the eighth grade and significantly higher literacy scores at age 19 than children in the control group. Differences were also evidenced in rates of grade retention and special education placement. The most striking benefits were noted in the real world application of their life trajectories, including significantly lower rates of school dropout and unemployment, higher rates of college attendance, reduced rates of teen pregnancy, higher income status, and decreased criminal activity at age 27 years.

Summary of Model Programs

Overall, the findings from these five model early intervention programs reveal significant improvements in children's cognitive development and reduced rates of mental retardation during the preschool years for children at risk for developmental disabilities. Children continued to realize gains, although at varying degrees, during their middle childhood years and when evaluated, during their early adult years. Improvements in children's IQ scores were maintained in children participating in the Abecedarian Project, Project Care, and the Milwaukee Project. Further, children participating in the early intervention programs (with the exception of some of the low birth weight IHDP children) evidenced higher school achievement (with the exception of the Milwaukee Project) and reduced rates of special education placement and grade retention than those in the control group (C. T. Ramey & Ramey, 1999). Those that participated in the Abecedarian Project treatment group, continued to show better outcomes than those in the comparison group at the 21-year follow-up, including higher mental test scores, higher reading and mathematic achievement test scores, greater numbers enrolled in college and employed in higher skill jobs, and older ages when they had their first baby (Campbell, Pungello, Burchinal, & Ramey, 2001). Similarly, participants in the Perry Preschool Project continued to show improvements in their life trajectories, including reduced rates of school dropout and unemployment, increased college attendance, reduced teen pregnancy, higher income earnings, and decreased criminal activity at the 27-year follow-up.

Synthesis of Findings: Essential Operating Principles and Key Elements of Effective Early Intervention Programs

Based on findings from the model early intervention programs, it is clear that there are at least *five essential operating principles* necessary for effective early intervention research. Program must be multidisciplinary, intergenerational, individualized for children and their families, contextually embedded in local service delivery systems, research-oriented, and organized around key concepts undergirding randomized controlled trials (Ramey et al., 2002; Ramey & Ramey, 1998b). All of the model programs were *multidisciplinary* in that they provided a wide array of services, including early childhood education, family counseling and home visits, health services, medical services, nursing services, nutrition services, social work services, special education services, and transportation. *Intergenerational* refers to the fact that all of the programs focused on both the needs of the child and the needs of the child's caregivers and family members. Service provision was *individualized* to meet the specific needs of the child and family, which enabled the program to meet in a meaningful way a broader range of children and families. Further, to ensure that the programs were *contextually embedded in the local service delivery* system, the cooperation and investment of social, health, and other existing human service agencies in the community were sought. Lastly, in order to provide a true picture of how effective the programs were in improving outcomes for children and families, a major feature of all of the programs was a *research component, including randomized controlled trial designs.*

Based on these operating principles and research findings, there are seven essential elements of effective early intervention programs (Ramey et al., 2002; Ramey, Echols, Ramey, & Newell, 2000; Ramey & Ramey, 1998a). These include: (1) timing and duration; (2) sufficient intensity; (3) direct engagement of the child; (4) multiple types of supports and services; (5) careful monitoring and responsiveness to individual needs; (6) follow-through to maintain early benefits; and (7) cultural appropriateness. Each of these elements is discussed below.

1. *Timing and Duration*: Early intervention services that begin earlier in children's development and continue longer generally produce the most positive outcomes for children. The model early intervention programs that began during the first 3 years of life and continued through the school age years revealed longer-term results, including the Abecedarian Project (Ramey, Campbell, & Bryant, 1987; Ramey, Yeates, & Short, 1984), the Milwaukee Project (Garber, 1988), Project CARE (Wasik et al., 1990), and IHDP (1990). Additionally the Brookline Early Education Project (Hauser-Cram, Pierson, Walker, & Tivnan, 1991) paralleled the model program in terms of timing and duration and found similar results. Two programs that did produce significant benefits in children but began when children were 3 years of age were the Perry Preschool Project (Schweinhart & Weikart, 1983) and the Early Training Project (Gray, Ramsey, & Klaus, 1982). The major difference in these programs is that the children were significantly delayed in their cognitive development at age 3, whereas the goal of the programs that enrolled during infancy was to prevent intellectual decline associated with early and continued impoverished language and learning environments.

   The National Head Start program has recognized the need for early intervention programs and has funded over 500 Early Head Start programs for families with infants and toddlers. There is compelling evidence that children from impoverished settings who do not receive systematic early intervention suffer a significant toll in both cognitive and social-emotional development during the second and third years of life (cf. Blair, Ramey, & Hardin, 1995; Escalona, 1982; Ramey et al., 1984). This toll is detectable in toddlers' language delays, their below average performance on tests of intellectual performance, somewhat increased behavioral problems, and deficiencies in parent–child interactions (e.g., Barnard, Bee, & Hammond, 1984; Bradley et al., 1989; Golden & Birns, 1983). Second, there is no evidence that complete "catch-up" in intellectual performance or social-emotional development is possible. Although substantial gains may be achievable later on, they are not likely to fully offset earlier delays (Campbell & Ramey, 1995; Landesman, 1990).

2. *Sufficient Intensity*: In general, the more intensive the program and the more the child and family participate in the program, the better the effects on children. Program intensity relates to the number of hours per day, days per week, and weeks per year. The majority of early intervention programs provide for only a few days per week and often are for only a few hours per day. A notable example is the Utah State Early Intervention Research Institute, which conducted 16 randomized trials of early intervention programs and found that none of the programs showed significant improvements in their treated group, as none of them provided full-day, 5-day per week programs. Another example is the Scarr and McCartney (1988) study, which offered a parent-oriented, 1-day a week intervention program. As the model programs described above demonstrated, the most effective ones have operated 5 days a week, year round, and full-day. Interestingly, Powell and Grantham-McGregor (1989) have shown that their early intervention program that offered services 3 days a week was of sufficient intensity to produce significant outcomes in children participating in the intervention program.

Intensity based on the child and family's participation in the program has been examined as well. A classic example is the IHDP in which a participation index was created based on daily, weekly, and monthly monitoring of the variations in the amount of intervention each child and family received over a 3-year period. The amount of participation, and consequently amount of services received, was shown to have a positive relationship with the child's cognitive and social development in a linear fashion (Ramey et al., 1992). Specifically, children who had the highest participation rate in the intervention showed a 9-fold reduction in rates of mental retardation than those in the control group. Further, children in the intermediate participation group showed a 4.9-fold factor reduction in rates of mental retardation, while those in the low participation group showed a 1.3-fold reduction.

3. *Direct Engagement of the Child:* Early intervention programs that work directly with the child to alter their daily learning experiences have been shown to have the greatest impact than those that focus on more indirect methods of services, including parent training or home visiting programs only. Certainly, an important component of the service must be parent intervention in which the parent is encouraged to promote their child's development and offered training on how to best do that; however, this cannot be the sole nor the primary method for imparting the services (Casto & Lewis, 1984; Madden, Levenstein, & Levenstein, 1976; Scarr & McCartney, 1988; Wasik et al., 1990). These findings are true for programs working with economically disadvantaged children, biologically vulnerable children, and for high-risk children with both environmental and biological risk conditions.

The first experimental study to examine the relative effect of indirect versus direct service provision on children's development was conducted on the *Project CARE* (Wasik et al., 1990). The combination of daily center-based intervention with weekly home visits produced the largest gains in children, whereas regular home visits without the center-based intervention did not show improvements in children's cognitive and social development, parent attitudes or behaviors, or the quality of the home environment. Remarkably, even though parents enjoyed the home visitation component, there were no differences between their child's development and those in the control group who received nutritional supplements, medical surveillance, and social services. The relative importance of home visitation in the delivery of early intervention services is brought to light through ongoing research such as this (Roberts, Wasik, Casto, & Ramey, 1991). That is not to say that parents do not play a significant and important role in the child's development, especially during these formative years. Parents are key players in ensuring children receive the best services possible and that benefits are maximized. Home visits are one mechanism for accomplishing this as evidenced by the findings of Powell and Grantham-McGregor (1989), indicating that providing at least three structured home visits per week was sufficient to enhance children's development.

4. *Multiple Types of Supports and Services*: Early intervention programs that offer a wide array of comprehensive services with multiple methods of providing services have been shown to have the greatest impact. That is to say, programs that are wider in breadth, yet flexible to meet the needs of the child and family are more beneficial to the child than those that are more narrow in focus and stringent in delivery. This principle is evidenced in the early educational interventions that have yielded larger effects, such as the Brookline Early Childhood Project, the Abecedarian Program, Project CARE, the Milwaukee Project, and the IHDP. All of these model programs have included a multipronged approach, including early childhood education in a child care center before the early years, parent services, health and social services, transportation assistance, support with meeting urgent needs, and other child and family supports. Schorr and Schorr (1988) have discussed the value of offering a broader array of services to families so that all needs are met and that the parent and child are able to focus on the child's developmental needs.

5. *Careful Monitoring and Responsiveness to Individual Needs*: Children's development and responsiveness to early intervention services are not the same—individual children respond differently to the same intervention and services. It is essential that early intervention services are cognizant of individual children's needs and their progress over time. Some children may progress at different rates and others may have different needs over time. A rigid program that only provides services and treatment through one method

may not be able to maximally meet the needs of the children. As an example, as previously described, the IHDP provided a broad-based early educational intervention for premature, low birth weight infants. Findings revealed that those at greater biological risk (indexed by very low birth weight) did *not* benefit as much from the program as did less impaired children—even though both groups showed significant gains.

In another study conducted by Cole, Dale, Mills, and Jenkins (1992) on early educational intervention for children with disabilities, the degree of the child's impairment and the form of educational intervention provided were examined. Interestingly, researchers found that young children with higher cognitive scores benefited more when they received direct instruction, whereas those with lower cognitive scores benefited more from a mediated learning approach. In the Abecedarian study, Martin et al. (1990) reported that children who showed the largest cognitive gains as compared to those in the control condition were those whose mothers had IQ scores below 70, such that children whose mothers had IQ's below 70 scored *at least* 20 points higher (mean = 32 points higher) than their own mothers *when they received intensive early educational intervention* (Landesman & Ramey, 1989; Ramey & Ramey, 1992). Similar findings were revealed in the Milwaukee Project, which only enrolled children whose mothers had IQ's below 75 and were from economically impoverished backgrounds (Garber, 1988).

6. *Follow-Through to Maintain Early Benefits*: It is essential that services provided to children do not stop with early intervention services. Numerous studies have shown that the initial positive effects of early intervention often diminish if similar high-quality services and supports are not continued. As previously discussed, there have been long-term positive outcomes for children participating in early intervention programs in terms of school achievement, grade retention, and special education placement (e.g., Campbell & Ramey, 1994; Lazar et al., 1982; Schweinhart & Weikart, 1983. Most of the programs have follow-up intervention services and supports. Other early intervention programs that do not follow the children and continue to provide for their needs, the many early childhood "gains" are not sustained throughout middle childhood and adolescence (Kagan, 1994).

Early on in children's development, their growth is rapid and amenable to many kinds of support. Their rate of development changes over time and the ability to maximize this does as well. Early intervention is the key to increasing children's growth and development but it cannot stand alone nor be the only set of services. Parents and health professionals must advocate for children to continue to receive services and work together to ensure that it happens; otherwise, many of the initial positive effects may be reduced over time.

7. *Cultural Appropriateness*: The principle of cultural congruence is a critical factor in engaging children and families and ensuring their adoption of the program in their homes, lives, and future. Intervention programs must recognize and appreciate the individual child and family's cultural beliefs, practices, and traditions, and, as much as possible, integrate them into the program. It is of paramount importance that all children and families feel appreciated and comfortable sharing who they are and what they believe. Further, it is essential that individuals and families practicing certain beliefs and traditions are not stereotyped. Cultures themselves are dynamic and not all individuals who identify with a given culture endorse all of its beliefs or normative practices (Barth, 1969). Further, within a given family, there may be numerous cultural beliefs and traditions (Lynch & Hanson, 1992). It is the role of the service providers to ensure that all are appreciated, welcomed, and encouraged to participate. This will directly affect how the child and family respond to the program and incorporate it into their lives.

FUTURE DIRECTIONS FOR EARLY INTERVENTION RESEARCH AND SERVICES

Early intervention services were developed with the belief that we can make a difference in the lives of children with developmental disabilities and mental retardation. As evidenced by the model programs and ongoing research, early intervention can produce significant and long-lasting effects if they incorporate key operating principles and certain elements. Programs must be multidisciplinary, intergenerational, individualized, and contextually embedded. Service delivery must be conducted early and often in the child's development, and conducted directly with the child as well as with the family. Further, services and supports that are comprehensive, individualized, and recognize the child's background and beliefs will have the greatest impact. Parents and service providers must work together to ensure that the child continues to receive services beyond early intervention into the school age years. We must build upon research findings and improve the provision of services as well as the integration of services.

Further, policymakers must recognize that funding makes a difference. As one cost–benefit analysis revealed (Barnett, 1985), for every dollar invested in early intervention services, seven public dollars are saved in the long-run due to better life trajectories for the children and their families, including reduced rates of school dropout and unemployment, increased college attendance, reduced teen pregnancy, increased income status, and decreased criminal activity. During this next phase of early intervention services, we must incorporate essential ingredients from model programs, expand services and supports, and reach more children for longer periods of time.

REFERENCES

Barnard, K., Bee, H., & Hammond, M. (1984). Home environment and cognitive development in a healthy, low risk sample: The Seattle Study. In A. Gottfried (Ed.), *Home environment and early cognitive development* (pp. 117–150). New York: Academic.

Barnett, W. S. (1985). Benefit–cost analysis of the Perry Preschool program and its long-term effects. *Educational Evaluation and Policy Analysis, 7,* 387–414.

Barth, F. (Ed.). (1969). *Ethnic groups and boundaries: The social organization of culture difference.* Boston: Little, Brown.

Bertalanffy, L. V. (1975). *Perspectives on general system theory.* New York: Braziller.

Blair, C., Ramey, C. T., & Hardin, M. (1995). Early intervention for low birth weight premature infants: Participation and intellectual development. *American Journal on Mental Retardation, 99,* 542–554.

Bradley, R. H., Caldwell, B. M., Rock, S. L., Ramey, C. T., Barnard, K. E., Gray, A., et al. (1989). Home environment and cognitive development in the first 3 years of life: A collaborative study involving six sites and three ethnic groups in North America. *Developmental Psychology, 25,* 217–235.

Bronfenbrenner, U. (1979). *The ecology of human development.* Cambridge, MA: Harvard University Press.

Brooks-Gunn, J., Gross, R. T., Kraemer, H. C., Spiker, D., & Shapiro, S. (1992). Enhancing the cognitive outcomes of low birth weight, premature infants: For whom is the intervention most effective? *Pediatrics, 89,* 1209–1215.

Bryant, D., & Maxwell, K. (1997). The effectiveness of early intervention for disadvantaged children. In M. Guralnick (Ed.), *The effectiveness of early intervention* (pp. 23–46). Baltimore: Brookes.

Burchinal, M. R., Campbell, F. A., Bryant, D. M., Wasik, B. H., & Ramey, C. T. (1997). Early intervention and mediating processes in cognitive performance of children of low-income African American families. *Child Development, 68,* 935–954.

Campbell, F. A., Pungello, E., Burchinal, M., & Ramey, C. T. (2001). The development of cognitive and academic abilities: Growth curves from an early childhood educational experiment. *Developmental Psychology, 37,* 231–242.

Campbell, F. A., & Ramey, C. T. (1994). Effects of early intervention on intellectual and academic achievement: A follow-up study of children from low-income families. *Child Development, 65,* 684–698.

Campbell, F. A., & Ramey, C. T. (1995). Cognitive and school outcomes for high risk African American students at middle adolescence: Positive effects of early intervention. *American Educational Research Journal, 32,* 743–772.

Carnegie Task Force on Learning in the Primary Grades. (1996). *Years of promise: A comprehensive learning strategy for America's children.* New York: Carnegie Corporation of New York.

Carnegie Task Force on Meeting the Needs of Young Children. (1994). *Starting points: Meeting the needs of our youngest children.* New York: Carnegie Corporation.

Casto, G., & Lewis, A. (1984). Parent involvement in infant and preschool programs. *Division of Early Childhood, 9,* 49–56.

Cole, K. N., Dale, P. S., Mills, P. E., & Jenkins, J. R. (1992). Effects of preschool integration for children with disabilities. *Exceptional Children, 58,* 36–45.

Cowan, P. A., Cowan, C. P., Schultz, M. S., & Heming, G. (1994). Prebirth to preschool family factors in children's adaptation to kindergarten. In R. D. Parke & S. G. Kellam (Eds.), *Exploring family relationships with other social contexts* (pp. 75–114). Hillsdale, NJ: Erlbaum.

Currie, J. (2000). Early childhood intervention programs: What do we know? Commissioned paper for the Brookings Roundtable on Children (On-line). Retrieved from September 2005 www.jcpr.org/conferences/childhoodbriefing.html

Darlington, R. B., Royce, J. M., Snipper, A. S., Murray, H. W., & Lazaar, I. (1980). Preschool programs and later school competence of children from low-income families. *Science, 208,* 202–204.

Deutsch, M. (1967). *The disadvantaged child.* New York: Basic Books.

Escalona, S. K. (1982). Babies at double hazard: Early development in infants at biologic and social risk. *Pediatrics, 70,* 670–676.

Garber, H. L. (1988). *The Milwaukee project: Preventing mental retardation in children at risk.* Washington, DC: American Association on Mental Retardation.

Golden, M., & Birns, B. (1983). Social class and infant intelligence. *Origins of Intelligence: Infancy and Early Childhood* (2nd ed.). New York: Plenum.

Gray, S. W., Ramsey, B. K., & Klaus, R. A. (1982). From 3 to 20: The Early Training Project. Baltimore, MD: University Park Press.

Gross, R. T., Spiker, D., & Hayes, C. (Eds.). (1997). *Helping low birth weight, premature babies: The Infant and Health Development Program.* Stanford, CA: Stanford University Press.

Guralnick, M. J. (Ed.). (1997). *The effectiveness of early intervention.* Baltimore: Brookes .

Harlow, H. F. (1958). The nature of love. *American Psychologist, 13,* 673–685.

Haskins, R. (1989). Beyond metaphor: The efficacy of early childhood education. *American Psychologist, 44,* 274–282.

Hauser-Cram, P., Pierson, D. E., Walker, D. K., & Tivnan, T. (1991). *Early education in the public schools.* San Fransisco: Jossey-Bass.

Hebb, D. O. (1949). *Organization of behavior.* New York: Wiley.

Hess, R. D., & Shipman, V. (1965). Early experiences and socialization of cognitive modes in children. *Child Development, 36,* 869–886.

Huston, A. C., McLoyd, V., & Garcia Coll, C. (1994). Children and poverty: Issues in contemporary research. *Child Development, 65,* 275–282.

Kagan, S. L. (1994). Defining and achieving quality in family support. In B. Weissbourd & S. L. Kagan (Eds.), *Putting families first: America's family support movement and the challenge of change* (pp. 375–400). San Francisco: Jossey-Bass.

Klerman, L. V., Ramey, S. L., Goldenberg, R. L., Marbury, S., Hou, J., & Cliver, S. P. (2001). A randomized trial of augmented prenatal services for multi-risk, Medicaid-eligible African-American women. *American Journal of Public Health, 91,* 105–111.

Landesman, S. (1990). Institutionalization re-visited: Expanding views on early and cumulative life experiences. In M. Lewis & S. Miller (Eds.), *Handbook of developmental psychopathology* (pp. 455–462). New York: Plenum.

Landesman, S., & Ramey, C. T. (1989). Developmental psychology and mental retardation: Integrating scientific principles with treatment practices. *American Psychologist, 44,* 409–415.

Landesman-Dwyer, S., & Butterfield, E. C. (1983). Mental retardation: Developmental issues in cognitive and social adaptation. In M. Lewis (Ed.), *Origins of intelligence: Infancy and early childhood* (2nd ed., pp. 479–519). New York: Plenum.

Lazar, I., Darlington, R., Murray, H., Royce, J., & Snipper, A. (1982). Lasting effects of early education: A report from the Consortium of Longitudinal Studies. *Monographs of the Society for Research in Child Development, 47* (2–3, Serial No. 195).

Lynch, E. W., & Hanson, M. J. (1992). Steps in the right direction: Implications for interventionists. *Developing cross-cultural competence: A guide for working with young children and their families* (pp. 355–370). Baltimore, MD: Brookes.

Maccoby, E., & Martin, J. (1983). Socialization in the context of the family: Parent–child interaction. In P. H. Mussen (Series Ed.) & E. M. Hetherington (Vol. Ed.), *Handbook of child psychology: Vol. 4. Socialization, personality, and social development* (pp. 1–101). New York: Wiley.

Madden, J., Levenstein, P., & Levenstein, S. (1976). Longitudinal IQ outcomes of the mother–child home program. *Child Development, 46,* 1015–1025.

Martin, S. L., Ramey, C. T., & Ramey, S. L. (1990). The prevention of intellectual impairment in children of impoverished families: Findings of a randomized trial of educational day care. *American Journal of Public Health, 80,* 844–847.

McCarton, C. M., Brooks-Gunn, J., Wallace, I. F., Bauer, C. R., Bennett, F. C., Bernbaum, J. C., et al. (1997). Results at age 8 years of early intervention for low-birth weight premature infants: The Infant Health and Development Program. *JAMA, 277,* 126–132.

McVicker Hunt, J. (1961). *Intelligence and experience.* New York: Ronald.

Osofsky, J. D. (1979). *Handbook of infant development.* New York: Wiley.

Powell, C., & Grantham-McGregor, S. (1989). Home visiting of varying frequency and child development. *Pediatrics, 84,* 157–164.

Ramey, C. T., Bryant, D. M., Wasik, B. H., Sparling, J. J., Fendt, K. H., & LaVange, L. M. (1992). Infant Health and Development Program for low birth weight, premature infants: Program elements, family participation, and child intelligence. *Pediatrics, 3,* 454–465.

Ramey, C. T., & Campbell, F. A. (1984). Preventive education for high-risk children: Cognitive consequences of the Carolina Abecedarian Project. *American Journal of Mental Deficiency, 88,* 515–523.

Ramey, C. T., & Campbell, F. A. (1992). Poverty, early childhood education, and academic competence: The Abecedarian experiment. In A. Huston (Ed.), *Children in poverty* (pp. 190–221). New York: Cambridge University Press.

Ramey, C. T., Campbell, F. A., & Bryant, D. M. (1987). Abecedarian Project. In C. Reynolds & L. Mann (Eds.), *Encyclopedia of special education* (Vol. 1, pp. 3–8). New York: Wiley.

Ramey, C. T., Campbell, F. A., Burchinal, M., Skinner, M. L., Gardner, D. M., & Ramey, S. L. (2000). Persistent effects of early childhood education on high-risk children and their mothers. *Applied Developmental Science, 4,* 2–14.

Ramey, C. T., & Finklestein, N. W. (1981). Psychosocial mental retardation: A biological and social coalescence. In M. Begab, H. Garber, & H. C. Haywood (Eds.), *Psychological influences in retarded performance* (pp. 65–92). Baltimore: University Park Press.

Ramey, C. T., McGinness, G., Cross, L., Collier, A., & Barrie-Blackley, S. (1981). The Abecedarian approach to social competence. Cognitive and linguistic intervention for disadvantaged preschoolers. In K. Borman (Ed.), *The social life of children in a changing society* (pp. 145–174). Hillsdale, NJ: Erlbaum.

Ramey, C. T., & Ramey, S. L. (1998a). Early intervention and early experience. *American Psychologist, 53,* 109–120.

Ramey, C. T., & Ramey, S. L. (1998b). Prevention of intellectual disabilities: Early interventions to improve cognitive development. *Preventive Medicine, 27,* 224–232.

Ramey, C. T., & Ramey, S. L. (1999). *Right from birth: Building your child's foundation for life.* New York: Goddard.

Ramey, C. T., Ramey, S. L., Gaines, R., & Blair, C. (1995). Two-generation early intervention programs: A child development perspective. In I. Sigel (Series Ed.) and S. Smith (Vol. Ed.), *Two-generation programs for families in poverty: A new intervention strategy: Vol. 9. Advances in applied developmental psychology* (pp. 199–228). Norwood, NJ: Ablex.

Ramey, C. T., Ramey, S. L., & Lanzi, R. G. (2006). Children health and education. In I. Sigel & A. Renninger (Eds.), *The handbook of child psychology.* Vol. 4 (pp. 864–892). Hoboken, New Jersey: Wiley & Sons.

Ramey, C. T., Ramey, S. L., Lanzi, R. G., & Cotton, J. (2002). Early interventions: Programmes, results, and differential response. In A. Slater & M. Lewis (Eds.), *Introduction to infant development* (pp. 317–336). Oxford, England: Oxford University Press.

Ramey, C. T., & Smith, B. (1977). Assessing the intellectual consequences of early intervention with high-risk infants. *American Journal of Mental Deficiency, 81,* 318–324.

Ramey, S. L., Echols, K., Ramey, C. T., & Newell, W. (2000). Understanding early intervention. In M. L. Batshaw (Ed.), *When your child has a disability: The complete sourcebook of daily and medical care* (2nd ed., pp. 78–84). Baltimore: Brookes.

Ramey, S. L., & Ramey, C. T. (1992). Early educational intervention with disadvantaged children: To what effect? *Applied and Preventive Psychology, 1,* 131–140.

Ramey, S. L., & Ramey, C. T. (1999). Early experience and early intervention for children "at risk" for developmental delay and mental retardation [Special issue]. *Mental Retardation and Developmental Disabilities Research Reviews, 5,* 1–10.

Ramey, S. L., Yeates, K. O., & Short, E. J. (1984). The plasticity of intellectual development: Insights from preventive intervention. *Child Development, 55,* 1913–1925.

Roberts, R., Wasik, B., Casto, G., & Ramey, C. T. (1991). Family support in the home: Programs, policy and social change. *American Psychologist, 46,* 281–294.

Sackett, G. P., Novak, M. F. S. X., & Kroeker, R. (1999). Early experience effects on adaptive behavior: Theory revisited. *Mental Retardation and Developmental Disabilities Research Reviews, 5*(1), 30–40.

Scarr, S., & McCartney, K. (1988). Far from home: An experimental evaluation of the mother–child home program in Bermuda. *Child Development, 59,* 531–543.

Schorr, L. B., & Schorr, D. (1988). *Within our reach: Breaking the cycle of disadvantage.* New York: Anchor.

Schweinhart, L. J., Barnes, H. V., & Weikart, D. P. (1993). Significant benefits: The High/Scope Perry Preschool Study through age 27. *Monographs of the High/Scope Educational Research Foundation* (No. 10). Ypsilanti, MI: High/Scope.

Schweinhart, L. J., Berrueta-Clement, J. R., Barnett, W. S., Epstein, A. S., & Weikart, D. P. (1985). Effects of the Perry Preschool Program on youths through age 19: A summary. *Topics in Early Childhood Special Education, 5,* 26–35.

Schweinhart, L. J., & Weikart, D. P. (1983). The effects of the Perry Preschool Program on youths through age 15, In *As the twig is bent...Lasting effects of preschool programs, Consortium for Longitudinal Studies* (pp. 71–101). Hillsdale, NJ: Erlbaum.

Shore, R. (1997). *Rethinking the brain: New insights into early development.* New York: Families and Work Institute.

Skeels, H. M., & Dye, H. A. (1939). A study of the effects of differential stimulation in mentally retarded children. *Proceedings of the American Association of Mental Deficiency, 44,* 114–136.

Sparling, J., & Lewis, I. (1979). *Learning games for threes and fours: A guide to adult/child play.* New York: Walker.

Sparling, J., & Lewis, I. (1984). *Learning games for threes and fours: A guide to adult/child play.* New York: Walker.

Sparling, J. J., & Lewis, I. (1979). Learning *games for the first three years: A guide to parent–child play.* New York: Walker.

Sparling, J. J., Lewis, I., & Neuwirth, S. (1992). *Early partners.* Lewisville, NC: Kaplan.

The Infant Health and Development Program. (1990). Enhancing the outcomes of low-birth-weight, premature infants. *JAMA, 263,* 3035–3042.

Vygotsky, L. S. (1962). *Thought and language* (E. Hanfmann & G. Vakar, Trans.). Cambridge, MA: MIT Press.

Wallach, M. A., & Wallach, L. (1976). *Teaching all children to read.* Chicago: University of Chicago Press.

Wasik, B. H., Ramey, C. T., Bryant, D. M., & Sparling, J. J. (1990). A longitudinal study of two early intervention strategies. Project CARE. *Child Development, 61,* 1682–1696.

Weikart, D. P., Bond, J. T., & McNeil, J. T. (1978). *The Ypsilanti Perry Preschool Project: Preschool years and longitudinal results through fourth grade.* Ypsilanti, MI: High/Scope Press.

Zigler, E. F. (1967). Familial mental retardation: A continuing dilemma. *Science, 155,* 292–298.

24

The System of Early Intervention for Children with Developmental Disabilities

Current Status and Challenges for the Future

MICHAEL J. GURALNICK

In both principle and practice, early intervention is now a well-established feature of service and support networks for children with documented developmental disabilities in the United States and around the world (Guralnick, 2005). In the United States, the systems nature of early intervention is firmly grounded in legislation, particularly the Education of the Handicapped Act Amendments of 1986 (P.L. 99-457). Over the years, the provisions of this act (now the Individuals with Disabilities Education Act [IDEA]) have been modified and revised in an effort to further strengthen the early intervention system, for example, IDEA Amendments of 1991 (P.L. 102-119) and the reauthorization of IDEA (P.L. 105-17; see Guralnick (1997b; Meisels & Shonkoff, 2000; Smith & McKenna, 1994, for historical accounts of this legislation). Taken together, this legislation actually created two components of an early intervention system: one focusing on infants and toddlers (birth-to-3 years of age; Part C of IDEA) and one addressing the needs of preschool children (3-to-5-year olds; Part B, section 619). Although both components will be discussed in this chapter,

MICHAEL J. GURALNICK • Center on Human Development and Disability, University of Washington, Seattle, Washington 98195-7920.

I will emphasize the early intervention system focusing on infants and toddlers.

Federal policy regarding the system serving infants and toddlers was quite clear, ". . . to develop and implement a statewide, comprehensive, coordinated, multidisciplinary, interagency system that provides early intervention services for infants and toddlers with disabilities and their families" (P.L. 105-17, Section 631). To accomplish this, incentives were provided to each state to establish a set of common components. Included among these components was the development of a proactive system to identify children in conjunction with supportive referral mechanisms and a central resource directory, the availability of a process to ensure that comprehensive and multidisciplinary evaluations and assessments occurred to help identify appropriate services and supports to be specified in an Individualized Family Service Plan (IFSP), and the existence of a service coordination mechanism to facilitate interagency activities. Administrative requirements governing each state's definition of developmental delay (the basis for eligibility), designating a lead agency responsible for the program, ensuring procedural safeguards, and establishing and maintaining professional standards were among other features of the system to be adopted by each state. When children reached 3 years of age, they were to become the responsibility of the local education agency and were provided with a free appropriate public education along with related services. Many of the same administrative requirements have applied to preschoolers, such as procedural safeguards. Although continuity between the infant and toddler and preschool systems was recognized as a critical element, and transition plans were to be put in place, the change from one component of the system to another has been nevertheless substantial, including a greater focus on children rather than on families for preschoolers (an Individualized Educational Program [IEP] is required). Moreover, there has been an overall absence of formal service coordination at the preschool level, especially for services not normally provided by school systems.

In this chapter, I examine various aspects of this system. First, I discuss the sources of continuing support for a system of early intervention programs and the core principles that have evolved to guide the system. This will be followed by a descriptive section focusing on the current status of the services provided by the system. In the next section, I consider the remaining and extensive challenges faced by the system of early intervention. In the final section, I present specific suggestions for addressing those challenges and emphasize the need to achieve greater consistency with respect to the principles and practices of early intervention.

CONTINUING SCIENTIFIC SUPPORT FOR EARLY INTERVENTION

Efforts to refine and further strengthen such a comprehensive and coordinated intervention system for children birth through 5 years of age continue to find strong support at many levels. Indeed, over time, continuing advances in the science of early childhood development and early intervention, knowledge obtained from experiences in the provision of services, and changing professional and educational philosophies have combined to influence the specific features of the system and to further strengthen its foundations. In particular, the developmental science of normative development has continued to suggest that the early years contribute in vital and sometimes extraordinary ways to children's future development (National Research Council and Institute of Medicine, 2000). From this work, critical influences, particularly family influences on children's developmental trajectories, have been thoroughly documented. Constructs such as parental sensitivity, reciprocity, affective warmth, scaffolding, and discourse-based interactions, clearly have important independent and interrelated associations with children's social and cognitive competence (Landry, Smith, Swank, Assel, & Vellet, 2001; Landry, Smith, Swank, & Miller-Loncar, 2000; National Research Council and Institute of Medicine, 2000). Similarly, the influence of more distal or contextual factors and the mechanisms through which they operate to influence early childhood development have become more completely understood. Factors associated with the availability of social support, the family's financial resources, or intergenerationally transmitted parental beliefs and attitudes about child development can be measured effectively and are linked to children's developmental patterns even when development is proceeding without concern (e.g., Bradley, Corwyn, Burchinal, McAdoo, & Coll, 2001).

Corresponding research on the developmental science of risk and disability has also continued to reveal how the developmental trajectories of children can be altered by conditions associated with a child's biological risk or disability and also when environmental risk factors reach a level where the expected course of child development is likely to be adversely affected (Guralnick, 1997a, 1998). Perhaps most important has been the growing recognition that the organization of behavior of these vulnerable children (Hodapp & Zigler, 1990), and the influences on children's development operate in a fashion similar to that of typically developing children (e.g., Hauser-Cram et al., 1999). Unique and unusual developmental patterns are certainly evident in many instances, especially when considering the heterogeneity of children with developmental disabilities, but this evolving body of research continues to emphasize the value of a developmental framework and the corresponding importance of the early years (Guralnick, 1998).

Finally, intervention science has developed in the past and continues to develop a body of knowledge strongly suggesting that the course of development for children with developmental disabilities can be altered during the early years through well-designed interventions. Given the heterogeneity of children with developmental disabilities, outcomes can be expected to vary, but effect sizes generally range from 0.50 to 0.75 *SD* for these interventions (Guralnick, 1997a; Shonkoff & Hauser-Cram, 1987). Findings indicate that having a firm structure and plan that involves both parents and children in the intervention is most effective. This certainly suggests that the planning and evaluation components that characterize the system of early intervention as represented in IDEA are essential, and further underscores the need for parental participation in early intervention to ensure its effectiveness.

Despite weaknesses in many of the experimental designs, a consensus has emerged from intervention science that early intervention is capable of producing important short-term gains in children's development. To be sure, some subgroups of children such as those with autism may respond unusually well to intensive interventions evident soon after intervention is completed (Lovaas, 1987), with gains retained many years later (McEachin, Smith, & Lovaas, 1993). Even for children with autism, however, responsiveness varies substantially (Smith, Groen, & Lynn, 2000. This variability and lack of responsiveness of certain subgroups is apparent for children with other broadly defined disabilities as well (e.g., Harris, 1997).

As might be expected, community-based intervention approaches that have emerged are diverse, combining information based on the developmental science of normative development, the developmental science of risk and disability, intervention science, and clinical experience (see Guralnick, 2001b). Taken together, although much remains to be accomplished, existing knowledge clearly provides support for the continuation and refinement of a comprehensive early intervention system. It is anticipated that as knowledge of developmental and intervention science increases, it can be more fully integrated to achieve the level of specificity and individualization required to maximize the effectiveness of an early intervention system.

CORE PRINCIPLES

Paralleling, and often interacting with, the scientific and clinical efforts that continued to generate support for the value of early intervention programs have been changes in philosophical approaches associated with early intervention. These philosophical issues have also strongly influenced the nature of the evolving system itself and have produced what might best be referred to as a set of core principles that could serve as further guides to practice. First, almost revolutionary changes occurred with respect to the values related to society's perceptions of children with disabilities. Concepts such as encouraging belongingness, respecting individual differences, and ensuring that all children were accorded the full measure of their civil rights including due process, equal protection, and minimum intrusion, became the foundation for establishing the core principle of *inclusion* (see Bailey, McWilliam, Buysse, & Wesley, 1998; Guralnick, 1978, 2001d). The complexity of the principle of inclusion notwithstanding, further legislative and related changes have continued to press the early intervention system to maximize the participation of children with developmental disabilities and their families in typical community settings and activities. For infants and toddlers this has meant that services have increasingly been provided in "natural environments" such as the home or other places common to children without disabilities (see Bruder, 2001). For preschool-age children, inclusion initiatives have centered around efforts to maximize involvement and interactions among children with and without disabilities, usually in preschool or child care programs.

Second, the powerful movement to empower families in the context of the early intervention system, to develop true and meaningful partnerships with early intervention personnel, and to orient interventions around family concerns and issues, together constituted the principle of family-centered practices in early intervention (Bruder, 2000; Dunst, 2001). Over time, the concept of family centeredness became the central feature of the larger core principle regarding the importance of maintaining a *developmental framework*. Related to this developmental framework core principle has been an awareness of the implications of cultural differences on the design of early interventions and a recognition of the extraordinary diversity of families likely to encounter the early intervention system, especially families facing considerable challenges (Hanson & Carta, 1995). This emphasized further that a focus on families and a corresponding developmental orientation must be a critical feature of any early intervention system. Of note, legislative requirements in Part C, in particular, reflected the principle of family centeredness. Indeed, one major rationale for the law was to strengthen families as a means of helping them toward meeting their child's special needs. As a consequence, in addition to multidisciplinary child focused assessments, an assessment designed to enhance the family's ability to meet their child's needs considering family resources, priorities, and concerns as identified by the family was required and continues to be emphasized in legislation.

Third, the movement to integrate and coordinate services and supports for children and families at all levels emerged in response to the already overwhelming task that generally fell to families who were attempting to organize extraordinarily diverse and separate community resources into a coherent intervention program for their children (see American Academy of Pediatrics, 1999; Bruder & Bologna, 1993). In addition, the fractionated, discipline-specific approaches to intervention that were dominant at the time the legislation was enacted were inconsistent with newer philosophies emphasizing more holistic approaches to child development and the similarities and continuities in development characterizing both children with and without disabilities (Bredekamp & Copple, 1997). Accordingly, legislation initially included, and subsequently reiterated, clear goals designed to improve integration and coordination, such as requiring a service coordinator for families, ensuring the involvement of a multidisciplinary team and, at the systems level, mandating states to coordinate resources. Consequently, as with the other core principles, this core principle of *integration and coordination* was intended to influence virtually all components and aspects of the early intervention system.

SERVICES PROVIDED BY THE EARLY
INTERVENTION SYSTEM

Today, early intervention systems are in place in all 50 U.S. states following the broad principles and practices articulated in the federal legislation. Certainly from a quantitative perspective, this system has been a success because there has been considerable growth over time in the number of children served annually, now nearing 200,000 infants and toddlers (1.8% of the 0–3 population) and nearly 600,000 preschoolers (5% of the 3- to 5-year olds—U.S. Department of Education, 2001). Moreover, in a recent report of a nationally representative sample of infants and toddlers served under Part C, it was evident that the program has been reaching families with diverse characteristics (Hebbeler et al., 2001). In fact, 42% of children entering early intervention were recipients of some form of public assistance and the children enrolled exhibited a wide range of delays and disabilities. About 20% of children entered the system within the first 6 months of life, with the average age of referral being 15.5 months. IFSPs generally were developed shortly after referral.

Efforts to examine the types, location, and intensity of services families received through the early intervention system have occurred frequently. Although differences across studies are common due to intrinsic variations among states as well as sampling and evaluation methods, a general picture has nevertheless emerged. Part C, in particular, specifies the types of services to be made available to families including assistive technology, audiology, service coordination, transportation, translation services, family counseling, family training, and genetic counseling and evaluation in addition to more conventional health and therapeutic services. A recent federal report (U.S. Department of Education, 2001) based on the *National Early Intervention Longitudinal Study* revealed extensive use of these services by families even during the first 6 months of participation in early intervention. Most notable perhaps is that 80% of families availed themselves of service coordination, reflecting the complex task facing families of integrating and coordinating the various service types. Indeed, over three-quarters of families received from two to six different services, with 10% receiving eight or more services. Family-related services, directed at addressing the needs of family members rather than principally those of the child, also occurred with reasonable frequency, but rarely exceeded 20% of the participants. Overall, the most frequently used services were special instruction, speech and language therapy, and physical and occupational therapy (Perry, Greer, Goldhammer, & Mackey-Andrews, 2001).

These service patterns are consistent with parents' expressed priorities with respect to information about their child's disability, the course of their child's development, and present and future services (Garshelis & McConnell, 1993; Mahoney & Filer, 1996). That families value these services is reflected further in work that has revealed high utilization rates of scheduled early intervention services for "exemplary" programs (Kochanek & Buka, 1998), although utilization rates are lower when statewide analyses are carried out (Perry et al., 2001).

Participation in the System

Consistent with the fact that a high proportion of families with substantial economic needs are enrolled in Part C programs is that, for the most part, sociodemographic factors do not appear to be associated with utilization rates or other service characteristics (Kochanek & Buka, 1998; Shonkoff, Hauser-Cram, Krauss, & Upshur, 1992). Clearly, the system is doing well here, apparently arranging services in a manner consistent with child and family needs (Shonkoff et al., 1992).

This is not to say, however, that family characteristics do not matter in terms of systems involvement. As might be expected, some reports suggest that service levels are linked to the time available to families to participate in and competently and actively engage the service system (Mahoney & Filer, 1996), rather than potential benefits from using additional services per se. Studies of actual parent involvement in early intervention programs do, in fact, reveal strong associations with family characteristics. Specifically, for parents already enrolled in early intervention, Gavidia-Payne and Stoneman (1997) indexed parent involvement or participation by measuring parental attendance at IFSP and IEP meetings, voluntary participation in workshops and related activities, knowledge about their child's disability, educational rights, and other relevant factors suggesting involvement, and their cooperation with the early intervention program on various projects including parent participation in goal-related activities in the home. Using this index, factors associated with greater parental involvement in early intervention included higher levels of family education, income, social supports, coping abilities, marital adjustment, and general family functioning, but lower levels of stress (hassles and depression). Not all of these factors applied to both mothers and fathers, but the pattern was clear: family well-being, including cognitive coping strategies, is associated with greater participation in early intervention programs.

Service Intensity and Location

The effect of increased parental involvement is certain to result in increased intensity of child and family services, and perhaps their quality as well. For many subgroups of children and families, intensity of services does matter (Guralnick, 1998). Recommended practices for as many as 25–40 h a week of services (National Research Council, 2001; New York State Department of Health, 1999) for children with autism, provides an indication of the potential importance of intensity for an increasingly prevalent subgroup of children with established disabilities. Even more modest intervention efforts focusing on the many influential factors on child development can have an important cumulative impact representing a considerable level of intensity of services (see Guralnick, 2001b).

Of importance is that, when the actual hours of service provided is evaluated across the system, the number turns out to be surprisingly small. In the Shonkoff et al. (1992) analysis of children participating in Part C services, the total number of service hours ranged from as little as less than 1 h to as many as 21 h a month. On average, however, approximately 7 h of service were provided monthly. Severity of a disability was associated with greater service hours, but considerable variability was the norm, even among children with severe disability. Similar patterns are seen in more recent statewide analyses (Perry et al., 2001). However, when children reach preschool age, service hours increase substantially as children participate in almost daily one-half day preschool educational programs. Service hours are also higher for those participating in specialized intervention programs, such as for many children with autism but, despite continuing legal and administrative efforts, overall service hours remain relatively modest even for that group of children (see Feinberg & Beyer, 1998).

Parents have also sought out services beyond those provided by the early intervention system for both infants and toddlers and preschoolers (Kochanek, McGinn, & Cummins, 1998; Shonkoff et al., 1992). The range of such additional services is quite extraordinary, including child care, family supports, mental health, recreation, employment, and various therapies. It is not clear the extent to which the early intervention program either recommended or helped coordinate these additional services, but it appears that many parents take the initiative to arrange these services and, in many instances, pay additional costs.

With respect to location, for infants and toddlers, most of the services are delivered in the family home, but services occur frequently in specialized centers, clinics, or offices as well (U.S. Department of Education, 2001). For preschool-age children, the dominant location for services is the child's preschool program.

Satisfaction

For the most part, families have been quite satisfied with services received as part of the early intervention system. Surveys, interviews, and questionnaires related to satisfaction do tend to elicit positive responses in general; in part because parents wish to be supportive and have often established positive relationships with program staff, and in part because there is no expectation for or awareness of other service possibilities (Harbin, McWilliam, & Gallagher, 2000; McWilliam et al., 1995). Parental concerns that do exist usually focus around the need for easily accessible information about services, informal facilitation of connections with other parents, and further refinement and enhancement of service coordination (see Harbin et al., 2000, for a discussion of these concerns).

CHALLENGES FOR THE FUTURE

It is evident that extraordinary progress has been achieved in creating a system of early intervention services and supports for children with developmental disabilities. Within a period of less than 20 years, the elements of a comprehensive early intervention system are in place in all 50 states, and services continue to expand. As might be expected, however, given the demands facing states to create a system of services for such diverse and heterogeneous groups of children and families with complex and ever changing needs, a number of important challenges remain. A special challenge has been to translate the core principles discussed earlier in this chapter into practice to effectively meet the needs of children and families. Accordingly, I discuss below the critical challenges for the future of early intervention systems in the domains of inclusion, integration and coordination, and developmental framework. In addition, I suggest that other principles and practices that are central to an early intervention system must also be addressed in order to enhance the system's effectiveness. Overall, a need exists for a coherent and commonly shared framework to guide states in the further development of a system of early intervention.

Inclusion

Recent analyses have revealed that the early intervention system has not yet been able to provide universal access to inclusive programs (see Guralnick, 2001d). Many communities simply offer few inclusive options, and those that are available frequently do not provide for maximum participation with typically developing children (e.g., Cavallaro, Ballard-Rosa, & Lynch, 1998; Kochanek & Buka, 1999). In addition, the quality of many inclusive programs is questionable (see Bricker, 2001), as it is difficult to adjust curricula to meet the highly diverse needs of children with disabilities and to do so in a nonstigmatizing manner. Moreover, how to best implement the concept of natural environments for infants and toddlers is far from clear and has even created a level of controversy narrowly focusing on service location and the role of traditional therapeutic activities. Yet, even for traditional therapies, techniques are available that enable therapists to provide effective therapies in natural settings (see Hanft & Pilkington, 2000).

Indeed, this challenge has given rise to a larger issue that is now focusing on identifying learning opportunities for children in home, educational, recreational, and community settings that can be supported through early intervention (see Bruder, 2000; Dunst, 2001). Similarly, the importance of working with families in the context of early intervention to support existing family routines is compatible with a more general approach to natural environments in particular, and inclusion in general (Bernheimer & Keogh, 1995). Certainly there is a place for specialized therapeutic services, but a major challenge remains for the early intervention system to clarify these issues, to determine ways to embed interventions in natural environments, family routines, and community activities, and, in general, to ensure the maximum participation of children and families in typical activities in home and community settings (see Guralnick, 2001a).

Integration and Coordination

Due to the involvement of numerous disciplines, service agencies, and administrative organizations in any early intervention system, a major challenge continues to exist to integrate and coordinate all the elements efficiently and effectively (see Bruder & Bologna, 1993; Roberts, Innocenti, & Goetze, 1999). Problems are frequently identified by families with respect to service coordination (see Harbin et al., 2000). Moreover, a recent analysis of service coordination models in different states as part of the *National Early Intervention Longitudinal Study* (Spiker, Hebbeler, Wagner, Cameto, & McKenna, 2000) revealed wide variations in approaches among the states studied. In some instances, service coordinators remained stable as families moved throughout various phases of the early intervention system, whereas in other instances new coordinators were assigned or selected after referral and intake. Variations were also apparent with respect to the type of agency that employed the service coordinator or whether single or multiple functions (e.g., service provision as well as coordination) were carried out by the service coordinator. Advantages and disadvantages with respect to effective service coordination are likely to be associated with each model, but perhaps the most salient result of this analysis was the heterogeneity in service coordination approaches that was found and the lack of corresponding rationales for policies or practices.

As noted, from a broad systems perspective, concerns with respect to coordination among the agencies providing services under Part C are many and have been discussed by Harbin et al. (2000). In the Spiker et al. (2000) report, service system models varied substantially with respect to the comprehensiveness of the services available and the leadership and decision-making ability of the lead agency. The report also noted that a high level of coordination and comprehensiveness was uncommon. Policy direction provided at the state level to promote interagency coordination, along with relevant training to make integration and coordination a reality, was generally absent. Indeed, this study revealed not only considerable cross-state variation for a number of early intervention system components, but considerable within-state variation as well. In fact, many states delegated administrative responsibility to local communities, including determination of the lead agency (Spiker et al., 2000). Although we have limited information about the efficiency and effectiveness of these different approaches, it appears likely that the degree of integration and coordination across and within elements of the service system varies substantially and constitutes a major challenge for the future (Roberts et al., 1999).

In addition to broad systemic concerns, integration and coordination pose challenges at other levels of the system. Interdisciplinary teams constitute one such challenge both at the level of comprehensive interdisciplinary assessments (Guralnick, 2000) and in the delivery of services (Bruder & Bologna, 1993). Team process factors, professional training issues, and incompatible administrative requirements for different providers are among the challenges to integration and coordination at this level. Models of collaborative consultation are also emerging (McWilliam, 1996) that hold the promise of integrating often duplicative and inefficient services provided by separate disciplines, many of which appear to have only limited functional utility for the child and family (Dunst, 2001; Hanft & Pilkington,

2000). Fully implementing these new models where appropriate is a major challenge for the future.

Developmental Framework

The system of early intervention has increasingly focused on families as indicated by the fact that more and more family-oriented services have been included on IFSPs, and families are becoming increasingly satisfied with their involvement and participation with professionals (Mahoney & Filer, 1996). Although operating within a developmental framework in the context of early intervention means more than simply focusing on families, it is nevertheless an essential feature.

Yet, many professionals tend to remain child-focused even during home visits (McBride & Peterson, 1997), professionals often are not sure how to approach family concerns during assessment phases (Filer & Mahoney, 1996; McWilliam, Snyder, Harbin, Porter, & Munn, 2000), and families may not be sufficiently aware of their role and influence on child developmental outcomes in the context of the intervention process, expecting that professionals will focus on children (see Kochanek & Buka, 1998). In essence, what appears to be lacking is a developmental framework that can be utilized by both parents and professionals to conceptualize, organize, and guide the implementation of a program of early intervention. I have argued elsewhere that without such a developmental framework, one that clearly articulates the role of developmental processes and influences, especially family influences, the establishment of a coherent and effective early intervention system is unlikely to occur (Guralnick, 2001c).

Although many developmental models may be appropriate, the body of knowledge of developmental science has suggested that experientially based child developmental outcomes are a function of three family patterns of interaction: (1) the quality of parent–child transactions; (2) family-orchestrated child experiences; and (3) health and safety provided by the family. The various constructs associated with these family patterns of interaction (e.g., responsivity, social support, developmentally appropriate stimulation) have been well defined and measured and linked both independently and jointly with children's development (Guralnick, 1998; National Research Council and Institute of Medicine, 2000). Under a wide range of conditions considered typical, child developmental outcomes occur in an optimal or near-optimal fashion. However, as a consequence of adverse family characteristics, such as parental mental health problems, absence of social supports, marital stress, or poverty, those family patterns of interaction are stressed to a point where nonoptimal patterns result. One consequence can be poor child developmental outcomes.

This same developmental framework applies to children with established developmental disabilities (see Guralnick, 1997a, 1998). However, in this case, characteristics of the children themselves generate stressors that take different forms but clearly also impact family patterns of interaction; that is, these circumstances create stressors in the form of information needs, interpersonal and family distress, resource needs, and confidence threats to parenting. Although the level and course of development of children with established developmental disabilities will certainly be compromised, by definition, these stressors can act to perturb the three family patterns of interaction discussed above, yielding even poorer child developmental outcomes than would otherwise occur. Accordingly, when early intervention programs assess and respond to potential stressors (in which family patterns are stressed to a point in which adverse child developmental outcomes become more likely) by providing a comprehensive and individualized set of resource supports, social supports, and information and services to families as part of the early intervention system, more optimal outcomes for children should result. Available evidence is consistent with the major features of this developmental model of family support and benefit for children at risk for developmental difficulties due to family characteristics (environmental risk), children at risk due to biological factors, and for children with established developmental disabilities (see Guralnick, 1998).

FUTURE SYSTEMS DESIGN

The future challenges associated with the core principles and related practices to the system of early intervention described above signal that a larger concern is at issue. That is, despite guidance provided by IDEA with respect to the rationale, design, and implementation of statewide early intervention systems, substantial variability is found at every level that does not appear to be in the best interests of children and families, and may adversely impact the effectiveness of these systems. The varying approaches to early intervention seem to lack corresponding rationales, differing eligibility requirements across and within states seem inconsistent with the intent of IDEA, and the lack of information connecting variations in services and supports to outcomes suggests an absence of thoughtful planning and consideration of alternatives (see Spiker et al., 2000). In general, a thorough analysis of the components of an effective and efficient system and how those components are interrelated has yet to occur. Of course, uniformity is not and should not be a goal in complex systems, but states should have well-articulated frameworks for the systems they create; arguably one's consistent with the knowledge base provided by developmental and intervention science and informed by clinical practice. I have put forward one approach referred to as the Developmental Systems Model (Guralnick, 2001c), which could be used to provide such a general framework. This systems model is summarized in the next section.

Developmental Systems Model

The major organizational features of the Developmental Systems Model generally follow standard early intervention policies and practices and include the following components: (1) screening and referral; (2) surveillance and monitoring; (3) points of access; (4) comprehensive interdisciplinary assessment; (5) establishing eligibility for the program; (6) assessing stressors; (7) developing and implementing a comprehensive program; (8) monitoring and outcome evaluations; and (9) transition planning (see Guralnick, 2001c). Other features of the overall model include decision points for the various components, a distinction between preventive intervention and early intervention, and a set of sequenced relationships among components. The overall model is consistent with the prescriptive elements defined in Part C of IDEA and is certainly compatible with early intervention efforts for preschool-age children, although the emphasis on family issues is much greater. Guidance for some of the assessment components of the model is provided by stressors affecting family patterns of interaction outlined above, and the corresponding intervention activities are responsive to the various responses to those stressors in an effort to maximize the three family patterns of interaction.

The organizational framework is guided by a set of principles including the three core principles of developmental framework, integration and coordination, and inclusion. Complementing these core principles are related principles including the importance of early detection and identification, the importance of sensitivity to cultural differences, especially in connection with their developmental implications, and the need to ensure that practices are evidence-based. A major challenge for the future is to translate this organizational framework or another well-articulated framework and set of principles into practice in typical community-based early intervention systems. A process for examining each component and developing corresponding protocols (e.g., decision rules, assessment protocols) consistent with the Developmental Systems Model that can be adopted by communities is well underway (Guralnick, 2005). The hope is to be able to integrate this framework with the developmental science of normative development, the developmental science of risk and disability, intervention science, and clinical experience to create as optimal a system as possible and, of considerable importance, one that is reasonably consistent from community-to-community.

CONCLUSION

Early intervention systems are now in place in virtually every community in the United States, providing vital services and supports to young vulnerable children and their families. The growth of the system has been quite remarkable since P.L. 99-457 was enacted in 1986. The extensive heterogeneity evident in the system is both a strength and a weakness. Its strength relates to the ability of communities to build upon existing resources and administrative arrangements to accomplish its goals. Its weakness relates to the unevenness of services and supports, not only across states but also across local communities within states. Moreover, it is difficult in many instances to identify common principles and practices; most of which can have direct effects on child and family outcomes. Challenges are most apparent for core principles relating to a developmental framework, integration and coordination, and inclusion. The need for some commonly agreed-upon framework seems to be a necessary step in the further development of a truly national and effective early intervention system. Uniformity of systems is not the goal, as communities should decide what arrangements work best for them. But agreement on common points of reference and direction for communities can serve as a framework for addressing the many systems challenges facing the early intervention community in the years ahead.

REFERENCES

American Academy of Pediatrics, Committee on Children with Disabilities. (1999). Care coordination: Integrating health and related systems of care for children with special health care needs. *Pediatrics, 104,* 978–981.

Bailey, D. B., Jr., McWilliam, R. A., Buysse, V., & Wesley, P. W. (1998). Inclusion in the context of competing values in early childhood education. *Early Childhood Research Quarterly, 13,* 27–47.

Bernheimer, L. P., & Keogh, B. K. (1995). Weaving interventions into the fabric of everyday life: An approach to family assessment. *Topics in Early Childhood Special Education, 15,* 415–433.

Bradley, F. H., Corwyn, R. F., Burchinal, M., McAdoo, H. P., & Coll, C. G. (2001). The home environments of children in the United States Part II: Relations with behavioral development through age thirteen. *Child Development, 72,* 1868–1886.

Bredekamp, S., & Copple, C. (1997). *Developmentally appropriate practice in early childhood programs* (Rev. ed.). Washington, DC: National Association for the Education of Young Children.

Bricker, D. (2001). The natural environment: A useful construct? *Infants and Young Children, 13*(4), 12–31.

Bruder, M. B. (2000). Family-centered early intervention: Clarifying our values for the new millennium. *Topics in Early Childhood Special Education, 20,* 105–115.

Bruder, M. B. (2001). Inclusion of infants and toddlers: Outcomes and ecology. In M. J. Guralnick (Ed.), *Early childhood inclusion: Focus on change* (pp. 229–251). Baltimore: Brookes.

Bruder, M. B., & Bologna, T. (1993). Collaboration and service coordination for effective early intervention. In W. Brown, S. K. Thurman, & L. F. Pearl (Eds.), *Family-centered early intervention with infants and toddlers: Innovative cross-disciplinary approaches* (pp. 103–127). Baltimore: Brookes.

Cavallaro, C. C., Ballard-Rosa, M., & Lynch, E. W. (1998). A preliminary study of inclusive special education services for infants, toddlers, and preschool-age children in California. *Topics in Early Childhood Special Education, 18,* 169–182.

Dunst, C. J. (2001). Participation of young children with disabilities in community learning activities. In M. J. Guralnick (Ed.), *Early childhood inclusion: Focus on change* (pp. 307–333). Baltimore: Brookes.

Education of the Handicapped Act Amendments of 1986, P.L. 99-457, 20, U.S.C. §1400 *et seq.*

Feinberg, E., & Beyer, J. (1998). Creating public policy in a climate of clinical indeterminacy: Lovaas as the case example du jour. *Infants and Young Children, 10*(3), 54–66.

Filer, J. D., & Mahoney, G. J. (1996). Collaboration between families and early intervention service providers. *Infants and Young Children, 9*(2), 22–30.

Garshelis, J. A., & McConnell, S. R. (1993). Comparison of family needs assessed by mothers, individual professionals, and interdisciplinary teams. *Journal of Early Intervention, 17,* 36–49.

Gavidia-Payne, S., & Stoneman, Z. (1997). Family predictors of maternal and paternal involvement in programs for young children with disabilities. *Child Development, 68,* 701–717.

Guralnick, M. J. (Ed.). (1978). *Early intervention and the integration of handicapped and nonhandicapped children.* Baltimore: University Park Press.

Guralnick, M. J. (Ed.). (1997a). *The effectiveness of early intervention.* Baltimore: Brookes.

Guralnick, M. J. (1997b). Second generation research in the field of early intervention. In M. J. Guralnick (Ed.), *The effectiveness of early intervention* (pp. 3–22). Baltimore: Brookes.

Guralnick, M. J. (1998). The effectiveness of early intervention for vulnerable children: A developmental perspective. *American Journal on Mental Retardation, 102,* 319–345.

Guralnick, M. J. (2000). Interdisciplinary team assessment for young children: Purposes and processes. In M. J. Guralnick (Ed.), *Interdisciplinary clinical assessment for young children with developmental disabilities* (pp. 3–15). Baltimore: Brookes.

Guralnick, M. J. (2001a). An agenda for change in early childhood inclusion. In M. J. Guralnick (Ed.), *Early childhood inclusion: Focus on change* (pp. 531–541). Baltimore: Brookes.

Guralnick, M. J. (2001b). Connections between developmental science and intervention science. *Zero-to-Three, 21*(5), 24–29.

Guralnick, M. J. (2001c). A developmental systems model for early intervention. *Infants and Young Children, 14*(2), 1–18.

Guralnick, M. J. (2001d). A framework for change in early childhood inclusion. In M. J. Guralnick (Ed.), *Early childhood inclusion: Focus on change* (pp. 3–35). Baltimore: Brookes.

Guralnick, M. J. (2005). (Ed.). *A developmental systems approach to early intervention.* Baltimore: Brookes.

Hanft, B. E., & Pilkington, K. O. (2000). Therapy in natural environments: The means or end goal for early intervention? *Infants and Young Children, 12*(4), 1–13.

Hanson, M. J., & Carta, J. J. (1995). Addressing the challenges of families with multiple risks. *Exceptional Children, 62,* 201–212.

Harbin, G. L., McWilliam, R. A., & Gallagher, J. J. (2000). Services for young children with disabilities and their families. In J. P. Shonkoff & S. J. Meisels (Eds.), *Handbook of early childhood intervention* (2nd ed., pp. 387–415). New York: Cambridge University Press.

Harris, S. R. (1997). The effectiveness of early intervention for children with cerebral palsy and related motor disabilities. In M. J. Guralnick (Ed.), *The effectiveness of early intervention* (pp. 327–347). Baltimore: Brookes.

Hauser-Cram, P., Warfield, M. E., Shonkoff, J. P., Krauss, M. W., Upshur, C. C., & Sager, A. (1999). Family influences on adaptive development in young children with Down syndrome. *Child Development, 70,* 979–989.

Hebbeler, K., Wagner, M., Spiker, D., Scarborough, A., Simeonsson, R., & Collier, M. (2001). *The National Early Intervention Longitudinal Study (NEILS): A first look at the characteristics of children and families entering early intervention services* (Data Report 1). Menlo Park, CA: SRI International.

Hodapp, R. M., & Zigler, E. (1990). Applying the developmental perspective to individuals with Down syndrome. In D. Cicchetti & M. Beeghly (Eds.), *Children with Down syndrome: A developmental perspective* (pp. 1–28). New York: Cambridge University Press.

Individuals with Disabilities Education Act (IDEA) Amendments of 1991, PL 102-119, 20, U.S.C. §1400 *et seq.*

Individuals with Disabilities Education Act (IDEA) Amendments of 1997, PL 105-17, 20, U.S.C. §1400 *et seq.*

Kochanek, T. T., & Buka, S. L. (1998). Patterns of service utilization: Child, maternal, and service provider factors. *Journal of Early Intervention, 21,* 217–231.

Kochanek, T. T., & Buka, S. L. (1999). Influential factors in inclusive versus non-inclusive placements for preschool children with disabilities. *Early Education and Development, 10,* 191–208.

Kochanek, T. T., McGinn, J., & Cummins, C. (1998). *Beyond early intervention: Utilization of community resources and supports by families with young children with disabilities.* Providence, RI: Early Childhood Research Institute, Rhode Island College.

Landry, S. H., Smith, K. E., Swank, P. R., Assel, M. A., & Vellet, S. (2001). Does early responsive parenting have a special importance for children's development or is consistency across early childhood necessary? *Developmental Psychology, 37,* 387–403.

Landry, S. H., Smith, K. E., Swank, P. R., & Miller-Loncar, C. L. (2000). Early maternal and child influences on children's later independent cognitive and social functioning. *Child Development, 71,* 358–375.

Lovaas, O. I. (1987). Behavioral treatment and normal educational and intellectual functioning in young autistic children. *Journal of Consulting and Clinical Psychology, 55,* 3–9.

Mahoney, G., & Filer, J. (1996). How responsive is early intervention to the priorities and needs of families. *Topics in Early Childhood Special Education, 16,* 437–457.

McBride, S. L., & Peterson, C. (1997). Home-based early intervention with families of children with disabilities: Who is doing what? *Topics in Early Childhood Special Education, 17,* 209–233.

McEachin, J. J., Smith, T., & Lovaas, O. I. (1993). Long-term outcome for children with autism who received early intensive behavioral treatment. *American Journal on Mental Retardation, 97,* 359–372.

McWilliam, R. A. (1996). A program of research on integrated versus isolated treatment in early intervention. In R. A. McWilliam (Ed.), *Rethinking pull-out services in early intervention* (pp. 71–102). Baltimore: Brookes.

McWilliam, R. A., Lang, L., Vandiviere, P., Angell, R., Collins, L., & Underdown, G. (1995). Satisfaction and struggles: Family perceptions of early intervention services. *Journal of Early Intervention, 19,* 43–60.

McWilliam, R. A., Snyder, P., Harbin, G. L., Porter, P., & Munn, D. (2000). Professionals' and families' perceptions of family-centered practices in infant–toddler services. *Early Education and Development, 11,* 519–538.

Meisels, S. J., & Shonkoff, J. P. (2000). Early childhood intervention: A continuing evolution. In J. P. Shonkoff & S. J. Meisels (Eds.), *Handbook of early childhood intervention* (2nd ed., pp. 3–31). New York: Cambridge University Press.

National Research Council. (2001). *Educating children with autism.* Committee on Educational Interventions for Children with Autism, Division of Behavioral and Social Sciences and Education. Washington, DC: National Academy Press.

National Research Council and Institute of Medicine. (2000). *From neurons to neighborhoods: The science of early child development.* Committee on Integrating the Science of Early Childhood Development. In J. P. Shonkoff & D. A. Phillips (Eds.), Board on Children, Youth, and Families, Commission on Behavioral and Social Sciences and Education. Washington, DC: National Academy Press.

New York State Department of Health. (1999). *Clinical practice guideline.* Report of the recommendations, Autism/pervasive developmental disorders, assessment and intervention for young children (age 0–3 years). New York: Author.

Perry, D. F., Greer, M., Goldhammer, K., & Mackey-Andrews, S. D. (2001). Fulfilling the promise of early intervention: Rates of delivered IFSP services. *Journal of Early Intervention, 24,* 90–102.

Roberts, R. N., Innocenti, M. S., & Goetze, L. D. (1999). Emerging issues from state level evaluations of early intervention programs. *Journal of Early Intervention, 22,* 152–163.

Shonkoff, J. P., & Hauser-Cram, P. (1987). Early intervention for disabled infants and their families: A quantitative analysis. *Pediatrics, 80,* 650–658.

Shonkoff, J. P., Hauser-Cram, P., Krauss, M. W., & Upshur, C. C. (1992). Development of infants with disabilities and their families. *Monographs of the Society for Research in Child Development, 57*(6), Serial no. 230.

Smith, B. J., & McKenna, P. (1994). Early intervention public policy: Past, present, and future. In L. J. Johnson, R. J. Gallagher, M. J. LaMontagne, J. B. Jordan, J. J. Gallagher, P. L. Hutinger, & M. B. Karnes (Eds.), *Meeting early intervention challenges* (pp. 251–264). Baltimore: Brookes.

Smith, T., Groen, A. D., & Lynn, J. W. (2000). Randomized trial of intensive early intervention for children with pervasive developmental disorder. *American Journal on Mental Retardation, 105,* 269–285.

Spiker, D., Hebbeler, K., Wagner, M., Cameto, R., & McKenna, P. (2000). A framework for describing variations in state early intervention systems. *Topics in Early Childhood Special Education, 20,* 195–207.

U.S. Department of Education. (2001). *Twenty-third annual report to Congress on the implementation of the Individuals with Disabilities Education Act.* Washington, DC: U.S. Government Printing Office.

25

Stereotypy, Self-Injury, and Related Abnormal Repetitive Behaviors

JAMES W. BODFISH

Stereotyped behavior appears to be foremost among the varieties of aberrant behavior exhibited by individuals with mental retardation and autism (Bartak & Rutter, 1976; Bodfish, Symons, Parker, Lewis, 2000; Rojahn, 1986). Stereotyped behavior (STY) and self-injurious behavior (SIB) have been the focus of considerable research and clinical attention over the past several decades. As a result, distinct changes in the conceptualization of the phenomenology, pathogenesis, and treatment of STY and SIB have occurred. Phenomenologically, STY and SIB are no longer viewed as discrete, unrelated forms of aberrant behavior but instead are now viewed as part of the spectrum of abnormal repetitive behavior that is a common feature of neurodevelopmental disorders like mental retardation and autism (Cooper & Dourish, 1990; Lewis & Bodfish, 1998). Also, models of the pathogenesis of STY and SIB have shifted from a dichotomy of "nature" (e.g., brain-based) and "nurture" (e.g., learned, environmentally mediated) to more integrated models of that encompass both biological (e.g., genetic, neurological) and behavioral (e.g., environmental, psychological) factors (Lewis et al., 1996). Finally, treatment models that were based on the early notion of brain versus behavior have now been replaced by more integrated biobehavioral approaches that emphasize the combined role of behavioral/educational interventions and biomedical treatments. These shifts in the conceptualization and treatment of STY and SIB have brought about improved prognoses for persons with mental retardation and autism who display these forms of aberrant behavior. In this chapter,

JAMES W. BODFISH • Department of Psychiatry & UNC Neurodevelopmental Disorders Research Center, University of North Carolina at Chapel Hill, Morganton, North Carolina 28655.

I will describe these current conceptualizations of the phenomenology, pathogenesis, and treatment of STY, SIB, and related repetitive behaviors in persons with mental retardation.

PHENOMENOLOGY

From "Stereotypy" to the "Spectrum of Abnormal Repetitive Behavior"

Stereotyped Movement Disorder as defined by the *DSM-IV* includes both stereotypy and self-injury—discriminable forms of behavior that tend to co-occur in neurodevelopmental disorders (Bodfish et al., 1995; Lewis et al., 1996; Powell, Bodfish, Parker, Crawford, & Lewis, 1996). Stereotyped behavior (STY) occurs in up to 50% of children and adults with nonspecific mental retardation (Bodfish et al., 1995a; Rojahn, 1986) and up to 100% of children and adults with autism (Bodfish et al., 2000; Campbell et al., 1990). Self-injurious behavior (SIB), although less prevalent than stereotypy, occurs in a sizeable percentage of cases—up to a third of children and adults with mental retardation or autism (Bartak & Rutter, 1976; Bodfish et al., 1995a, 2000). A defining feature of STY is its lack of obvious purpose or function (Cooper & Dourish, 1990; Lewis et al., 1996; see review by Mason, 1991). STY often dominates the repertoire of the individual, can significantly interfere with daily functioning, can deter learning (Watkins & Konarski, 1987), and in the case of self-injury, can lead to severe tissue damage and present a formidable challenge in terms of clinical management.

A link between STY and SIB in at least some cases has long been established as SIB is frequently coexpressed with stereotypy in individuals with mental retardation (Rojahn, 1986). More recently, research has demonstrated links between STY, SIB, and a variety of other abnormal repetitive behaviors. It is now recognized that there are strong associations between the occurrence of STY and SIB and a variety of compulsive and ritualized forms of behavior in children and adults with mental retardation (Bodfish et al., 1995a; King, 1993; Powell et al., 1996). Prior to this, the associations between stereotypy, self-injury, and other repetitive behaviors had largely gone unrecognized in persons with mental retardation. Subsequently, several studies have confirmed the association of STY or SIB and other forms of repetitive behavior in persons with developmental disability (Clarke, Boer, Chung, Sturmey, & Webb, 1996; Collacott, Cooper, Branford, & McGrother, 1998; Dyken, Leckman, & Cassidy, 1996; Feurer et al., 1998; Johnson, 1999; Murphy, Hall, Oliver, & Kissi-Debra, 1999). Shifting the focus from single response forms (e.g., stereotypy or self-injury only) to the broader spectrum of abnormal repetitive behaviors and their co-occurrence has allowed researchers to model more accurately clinical presentation while providing insights into novel mechanisms and treatments for these disorders. The concept of a spectrum of abnormal repetitive behaviors has long been a part of the formulations of a variety of psychiatric (e.g., autism, obsessive–compulsive disorder [OSD], schizophrenia) and neurological disorders (e.g., Tourettes syndrome [TS], Parkinsons disease, toxic lesions of the striatum, frontal lobe lesions; Frith & Done, 1990; Lewis, & Bodfish, 1998).

A major source of difficulty in this area is the plethora of poorly operationalized terms used to refer to the variety of symptoms, behaviors, or movements that are seen clinically. For example, a given action such as skin-picking or head-hitting may be characterized as "self-injury," "habit," "self-stimulation," "stereotypy," "mannerism," "tic," "compulsion," or "ritual." Often, the choice of terms (and thus of measurement strategies) is dictated by clinical discipline. Thus, skin-picking in a person with mental retardation observed by a behavioral psychologist would be termed a "self-injurious behavior," skin picking in a person with TS observed by a neurologist would be termed a "tic," skin-picking in a person with OSD observed by a psychiatrist would be termed a "compulsion," and skin-picking observed casually in the general population would be termed a "habit." Discipline-specific terminology has given rise to a variety of taxonomies of aberrant behavior and movement. Complicating the matter is the fact that choice of a behavioral label and the discipline it derives from is often taken as suggestive evidence for the etiology or maintaining factors for the behavior in question. For example, actions labeled as tics are presumed to be involuntary, actions labeled dyskinesias are presumed to be drug-induced, actions labeled as self-stimulatory are presumed to be maintained by the sensory consequences they generate, and actions labeled stereotypies or habits may be deemed not significant enough to warrant treatment or even be labeled as "normal." Also, the choice of terms can lead to adherence to a false dichotomy of structure versus function, as opposed to the recognition that behavior can be simultaneously brain-based and environmentally mediated.

In the absence of "gold-standard" type clinical markers of behavioral disorders (e.g., a specific gene defect, a biochemical abnormality, a biobehavioral marker, or an instrumental measure) identification of the links between a variety of forms of repetitive behavior requires the use of "orthogonal" or item-independent assessment strategies (e.g., structured clinical interviews, clinical rating scales, observational coding systems) to differentiate and measure the varieties of the repetitive behavior in question. Such an orthogonal assessment strategy provides a more objective means to catalogue and discriminate the various comorbid behaviors that may occur in conjunction with STY and SIB. Unfortunately, many of the existing instruments used to measure abnormal behavior and movement were not designed with these issues of potential comorbidity in mind. As a result, a single discrete behavior such as skin-picking might occur as a test item on multiple rating scales each purporting to measure separate clinical phenomena (see Lewis & Bodfish, 1998). For this reason, and having recognized that clinically persons with STY and SIB often display a variety of other abnormal behaviors and movements, researchers have developed standardized rating scales that are item-independent and thus can be used to examine the full variety of abnormal repetitive behaviors in persons with

STY and SIB. These include the Repetitive Behavior Scales (Bodfish et al., 2000), the Repetitive Behavior Interview (Turner, 1999), or the use of a series of separate measures of repetitive behavior from other fields such as psychiatry and child psychology (e.g., the Yale Brown Obsessive Compulsive Scale: McDougle et al., 1995; The Childhood Routines Inventory: Evans et al., 1997). Comprehensive assessment methods such as these provide clinicians and researchers alike with a way to examine the variety of abnormal repetitive behaviors that are seen clinically in persons with STY and SIB.

Varieties of Abnormal Repetitive Behavior

The term "stereotyped behavior" or "repetitive behavior" is an umbrella term used to refer to the broad and often disparate class of behaviors linked by repetition, rigidity, invariance, inappropriateness, and lack of adaptability. These include stereotyped movements, repetitive manipulation of objects, repetitive SIB, specific object attachments, compulsions, rituals and routines, an insistence on sameness, repetitive use of language, and narrow and circumscribed interests. This broad range of behavior can be subdivided into two conceptual categories: "lower order" repetitive motor actions (stereotyped movements, repetitive manipulation of objects and repetitive forms of SIB) that are characterized by repetition of movement, and more complex or "higher order" cognitive behaviors (compulsions, rituals, insistence on sameness, and circumscribed interests) that are characterized by an adherence to some rule or mental set (e.g., needing to have things "just so"; Lewis & Bodfish, 1998; Turner, 1999).

Common forms of stereotyped movement in persons with mental retardation include body rocking, hand flapping, finger flicking, and object movements like spinning and twirling. Repetitive motor movements occur in normally developing infants (Thelen, 1979) where they tend to dissipate by 2 years of age. Repetitive motor behaviors are also commonly observed in a large variety of developmental, psychiatric, neurological, and genetic conditions such as autism, nonspecific mental retardation, TS, Fragile X syndrome, Rett syndrome, Parkinson's disease, and schizophrenia (Frith & Done, 1990; Lewis & Bodfish, 1998; Turner, 1999). In persons with mental retardation and autism, the occurrence of stereotyped movements appears to be strongly, negatively related to mental age (Berkson & Davenport, 1962; Bodfish et al., 1995a; Freeman et al., 1981; Hermelin & O'Connor, 1963; Lord, 1995; Lord & Pickles, 1996; Rojahn, 1986; Szatmari, Bartolucci, & Bremner, 1989). Reasons for directly treating stereotyped movements are not always clear. The strong negative relation between IQ and stereotyped movements in persons with mental retardation indicates that STY can occur as a result of a failure to learn and develop more adaptive behaviors. Thus, clinical interventions typically focus on actively promoting adaptive behavior development to diminish the risk of development of stereotyped movements as opposed to more directly targeting STY for elimination. On the other hand, extreme forms of severe STY and the self-directed attention such severe forms of STY can entail, can constrain the ability to learn adaptive behaviors via either direct instruction or incidental social learning. In such severe cases of STY, more active and direct treatment of STY may be warranted (see also "Treatment" section).

Common forms of SIB seen in children and adults with mental retardation include head hitting/banging, self-biting (e.g., biting the hand), and skin-picking. The SIB described in autism appears to be similar in prevalence to those described for individuals with nonspecific mental retardation (Freeman et al., 1981). Furthermore, like STY, SIB in mental retardation and autism is negatively associated with IQ and positively correlated with severity of illness (Bartak & Rutter, 1976; Campbell et al., 1990; Freeman et al., 1981). Clinically, it is important to distinguish between SIB that routinely produces injury (e.g., tissue damage) and varieties of SIB that are less intense and typically do not produce injury. For obvious reasons, cases with SIB that routinely have serious SIB-related injuries require both safety and protection from harm measures (e.g., protective equipment, close supervision, etc.) and active treatment designed to significantly decrease SIB occurrences (see "Treatment" section). An accumulating body of evidence indicates that such severe injury-producing SIB can be distinguished from more benign varieties of SIB in terms of (a) greater impact forces associated with the SIB actions (Newell, Challis, & Bodfish, 2002), (b) specific body sites targeted for SIB (Symons, Butler, Sanders, Feurer, & Thompson, 1999; Symons & Thompson, 1997), and apparent peripheral sensory abnormality and associated pain insensitivity (Symons, Sutton, & Bodfish, 2001).

Although there has been little systematic study of higher order repetitive behaviors, there is at least some evidence that certain classes of this behavior are particularly characteristic of autistic spectrum conditions (Frith, 1989; Kanner, 1943; Wing & Gould, 1979). However, evidence also exists that higher order repetitive behaviors like compulsions, rituals, and routines exist in persons with nonspecific mental retardation (Bodfish et al., 1995a) and can co-occur with STY and SIB (Bodfish et al., 1995a; Powell et al., 1996). Examples of discrete forms of higher order repetitive behavior include (a) compulsive and ritualistic behavior such as ordering, washing, hoarding, checking, counting, and touching (Bartak & Rutter, 1976; Bodfish et al., 1995; Lord & Pickles, 1996); (b) personal routines such as particular patterns of dressing, eating, traveling, playing, and interacting (Bodfish et al., 2000; Kanner, 1943; Szatmari et al., 1989; Wing & Gould, 1979); (c) insistence on sameness and resistance to change (Kanner, 1943; Prior & MacMillan, 1973); and (d) restricted, circumscribed interests ranging from preoccupations with highly unusual aspects of the environment (such as the serial numbers of electrical appliances) to intense and all-absorbing interests in more common hobbies (such as trains or computers; Bartak & Rutter, 1976; Kanner, 1943). It is sometimes assumed that higher order repetitive behavior is more common in high-functioning individuals because it demands a higher level of ability. Although it is true that certain sophisticated circumscribed interests may be beyond the ability of some persons with profound mental retardation, it is probable for even individuals with severe cognitive impairments to demonstrate insistence on sameness or show very restricted patterns of interest and activity. The only study to compare levels of repetitive behavior in high- and low-ability individuals with autism reported that insistence on sameness was more commonly observed in mentally retarded, relative to normally intelligent, individuals with autism (82% vs. 42%), and both groups showed similar levels of circumscribed interests (71% vs. 84%; Bartak & Rutter, 1976).

Abnormal Repetitive Behavior: Continuum or Categories?

An age-old distinction in theories of abnormal behavior involves conceptualizations of a continuum or dimension of pathological behavior versus conceptualizations that posit the existence of distinct categories of pathological behavior. Dimensional models treat pathological behavior as a quantitative extreme along a continuum of behavior ranging from typical/normal to abnormal (Cloninger, 1987). In contrast, categorical models such as the *DSM-IV* assume that there are qualitative differences between typical and pathological behaviors. With respect to stereotypy, some theorists have proposed that there is a continuum of STY that cuts across typical development, and a variety of neurodevelopmental and neuropsychiatric disorders (Ridley, 1994). Support for this comes from observations that typically developing children exhibit motor stereotypies (Thelen, 1979), that intellectually normal adults can exhibit stereotyped mannerisms (Rafaeli-Mor, Foster, & Berkson, 1999), and that a large variety of developmental and psychiatric disorders involve motor stereotypies as part of their symptomatic expression. Although insufficient research has directly addressed this issue in STY and SIB in persons with mental retardation and autism, the few studies that have addressed this have failed to find evidence for a strong, single underlying factor of "stereotypy" that cuts across expressions of the variety of abnormal repetitive behaviors. Factor analytic studies of the variety of discrete topographies of stereotyped motor behavior in samples of persons with mental retardation do find a primary "stereotypy" factor (Rojahn, Matlock, & Tasse, 2000). However, when a larger variety of abnormal repetitive behaviors beyond just topographies of stereotyped motor behavior are sampled, factor analysis has failed to find a single strong underlying factor and instead has found a collection of factors that roughly correspond to the variety of repetitive behaviors sampled (e.g., stereotypy, compulsions, restricted interests, etc.; Berkson, Gutermuth, & Baranek, 1995). In addition, phenomenologic studies of repetitive behavior in persons with mental retardation (Bodfish et al., 1995a) and autism (Bodfish et al., 2000) have found both clusters of cases with just STY and SIB and also clusters of cases where STY and SIB co-occur with higher order repetitive behaviors such as compulsions, routines, or restricted interests.

The clinical implications of the evidence that supports distinct categories or "subtypes" of abnormal repetitive behavior in persons with mental retardation are that (a) assessment strategies are needed that sample the full variety of abnormal repetitive behaviors (both STY, SIB, and higher order repetitive behaviors), (b) that assessments should lead to formulations of specific subtypes (e.g., SIB only, SIB in conjunction with rituals and sameness), and (c) that distinct subtypes may have different associated treatments. Although at this time there is no accepted classification scheme for subtyping repetitive behavior disorders into separate clinical categories, for clinical purposes the distinction provided in the *DSM-IV* appears to be a reasonable starting point. In the *DSM-IV* classification scheme three subtypes of repetitive behaviors in person with mental retardation and/or autism are suggested: (a) Stereotyped Movement Disorder (includes clinically significant stereotyped motor behaviors); (b) Stereotyped Movement Disorder with SIB (includes severe, injurious SIB, possibly with co-occurring stereotyped motor behaviors); and (c) Pervasive Developmental Disorder/Autism Spectrum Disorder (includes clinically significant repetitive behaviors typically involving higher order repetitive behaviors along with at least some of the other diagnostic symptoms of autism such as language and socialization deficits). The notion of a cluster of cases with Stereotyped Movement Disorder is supported by research that has shown an association between the occurrence of stereotyped motor behaviors, involuntary movement disorders (such as spontaneous dyskinesia, tics), and motor performance deficits (Bodfish et al., 1997; Bodfish, Parker, Lewis, Sprague, & Newell, 2001; Newell, Inclendon, Bodfish, & Sprague, 1999; Rosenquist, Bodfish, & Thompson, 1997). The notion of a cluster of cases with severe, injurious SIB (with or without other repetitive behaviors) is supported by research that has shown that varieties of SIB can be identified on the basis of differences in body site location of SIB injury (Symons et al., 1999), intensity of SIB impact forces (Newell et al., 2002), and the association between such severe forms of SIB and altered peripheral sensory processes suggestive of pain insensitivity (Breau et al., 2003; Symons et al., 2001). The notion of a cluster of cases with largely higher order repetitive behavior and co-occurring autistic symptoms is supported by research which has shown that in some cases STY and SIB cluster with compulsive/ritualistic behaviors (Bodfish et al., 1995a; Powell et al., 1996), and also by research which has shown that nonspecific mental retardation with stereotyped motor behaviors can be distinguished from autism spectrum disorders in terms of the expressed pattern of higher order repetitive behaviors (Bartuk & Rutter, 1976; Bodfish et al., 2000; Turner, 1999; Wing & Gould, 1979).

PATHOGENESIS

As the focus of this chapter is on understanding (phenomenology) and treatment/intervention, a detailed review of pathogenic factors associated with STY and SIB will not be provided. However, complete clinical formulations of STY and SIB require at least some knowledge of the range of risk factors for these disorders. In addition, clinical treatment in this area is increasingly focusing on early intervention and prevention and such efforts will need to be guided by an understanding of risk and protective factors in STY and SIB.

Multiple Risk and Protective Factors

Like other complex behavioral disorders, the origins of STY and SIB are unlikely to involve simple etiologic distinctions like "structural/brain-based" and "functional/environmentally determined." Instead, the evidence base is clear in indicating that multiple and often co-occurring etiologic processes are involved in the pathogenesis of STY and SIB. Indeed, STY and SIB in persons with mental retardation and/or autism are first and foremost developmental disorders and so it is likely that separate pathogenic processes influence the trajectory of the development of STY and SIB at differing times during the course of development. Finally, it is important to make a distinction between the pathogenic factors responsible for the etiology of a disorder (e.g., a chromosomal aberration in a genetic disorder) and those responsible for the shaping and maintenance of the phenotypic expressions of the disorder (e.g., adaptation and learning of particular forms and functions of SIB in a genetic disorder). For these reasons, clinicians are urged not to draw simplistic single-factor formulations of STY and SIB and instead are urged to understand that multiple factors are likely to be involved in the development and expression of STY and SIB including, environmental factors, learning processes, neurobiologic factors, and genetic factors.

Environment, Adaptation, and Learning

Environmental risk factors that have been shown to influence the development of STY and SIB include early social isolation/lack of enrichment, adaptations to stress and hyper-arousal, and social learning of maladaptive responses (Mason, 1991). In animal models of STY and SIB, stereotypy is an invariant consequence of early social isolation with SIB also being expressed in some cases (Suomi & Harlow, 1971). The notion that early placement in "institutionalized" (i.e., unenriched) environments leads to STY and SIB is supported by observations that there tends to be a negative relation between the occurrence of STY and SIB and access to materials that support adaptive engagement (Berkson & Mason, 1964; Cowdery, Iwata, & Pace, 1990) and by research which has shown that high rates of STY and SIB occur in infants who are placed in orphanage settings at an early age and for protracted periods (Rutter et al., 1999).

As extensions of such environmental/adaptation pathogenic factors, many functions have been posited for abnormal repetitive behaviors including reward, stress reduction, and sensory stimulation. Several theorists have emphasized the apparently self-stimulatory" nature of stereotypies (Berkson & Davenport, 1962). This sensation/perception perspective has taken two forms. The perceptual reinforcement hypothesis (Lovaas, Koegel, Simmons, & Long, 1973) holds that stereotypies are learned, operant self-stimulatory behaviors for which the reinforcers are the perceptual stimuli automatically produced by the behavior. The sensorimotor integration hypothesis (Ornitz, 1971) holds that sensory deficits leave the individual reliant on the kinesthetic (sensorimotor) feedback derived from motor output. Other models focus on a presumed relation between STY, SIB, and internal motivational states such as increases in arousal (Hutt & Hutt, 1970) or reductions in stress (Brett & Levine, 1979). These models hold that STY can be a "coping" reaction used to modulate stress or arousal.

There is also a strong evidence that many behavior disorders, including SIB, are learned. As such, these behaviors are acquired through an individual's history of interaction with the environment and are influenced by the same types of contingencies—positive and negative reinforcement—that account for the development and maintenance of adaptive behavior (Carr, 1977; Iwata, Dorsey, Slifer, Bauman, & Richman, 1982). For example, it has been demonstrated that SIB may occur more often when demands to perform self-care, educational or vocational tasks are present than when they are absent, and that SIB rates increase when SIB leads to a removal of the demands (Iwata et al., 1982; Iwata, Pace, Kalsher, Cowdrey, & Cataldo, 1990). This indicates that SIB can be strengthened by negative reinforcement (i.e., escape/avoidance of aversive situations). Among the environmental risk factor models for the pathogenesis of SIB, this operant learning model leads directly to practical strategies for (a) identifying the motivational factors that are supporting the aberrant responding and (b) developing teaching programs where identified motivational factors are arranged to diminish the probability of aberrant behavior and maximize the occurrence of incompatible adaptive behaviors (see "Behavioral Assessment and Treatment" section).

Neurobiological Factors

From a neurobiological standpoint, conditions that produce early developmental damage to the basal ganglia and associated fronto-striatal circuits in the brain appear to be significant risk factors for the development of a variety of forms of abnormal repetitive behavior (Bodfish & Lewis, 2002). There is a confluence of evidence that implicates altered basal ganglia function in the mediation of repetitive behavior disorders. Historically, examinations of the functions of the basal ganglia have been limited to its role in motor control and movement disorders. Currently, the functions of the basal ganglia are grouped into circuits that include motor, cognitive, and behavioral/personality divisions (Alexander, Crutcher, & Delong, 1990; Visser, Bar, & Jinnah, 2000). A large number of studies using chemical lesioning and site-specific drug administration support the importance of basal ganglia structures in the mediation of drug-induced STY and SIB (Lewis et al., 1996). In addition, there is growing evidence that OSD is associated with perturbations in basal ganglia function. For example, there is a significant degree of comorbid OCD in a variety of diseases of the basal ganglia including Sydenham's Chorea, postencephalitic Parkinson's, toxic lesions of the striatum, and TS (Rapoport, 1991). Some of the repetitive behaviors that are features of autism are also observed in OCD and TS. Individuals with autism and OCD both exhibit compulsive rituals and rigidity whereas individuals with autism and TS share repetitive stereotyped motor behaviors. Further, abnormalities in the basal ganglia have been implicated in all three of these disorders on the basis of multiple converging findings from structural and functional neuroimaging studies (Graybiel & Rauch, 2000). A relationship between repetitive behaviors and basal ganglia circuitry has also been found in developmental disabilities associated with autism. In a recent MRI study of autism, caudate volume was associated with compulsions, rituals, difficulties with minor change, and complex motor mannerisms (Sears et al., 1999). Thus, findings from animal and human neurobiological studies have consistently indicated that both motor and cognitive functions of key cortico-striato-thalamo-cortical circuits within the basal ganglia are involved in the production and maintenance of stereotyped patterns of behavior. These findings support a model of repetitive behavior that is based on deficits in typical motor functions (e.g., motor control) and cognitive functions (e.g., cognitive flexibility). This model suggests that deficient motor control and cognitive flexibility can constrain the ability to inhibit prepotent responding (stereotyped movements, compulsions), orient to novelty (insistence on sameness), and generate flexible, adaptable patterns of behavior (rituals, restricted interests).

From a neurochemical perspective, numerous types of neurotransmitters, likely interacting within key fronto-striatal circuits, are known to mediate the expression of abnormal repetitive behaviors including dopamine, serotonin, opiate peptides, GABA, acetylcholine, and adenosine. Of these, the dopamine, serotonin, and opiate systems have received the most attention with respect to attempts to translate preclinical (e.g., animal model) neuropharmacological findings into the identification of psychopharmacologic compounds that could be used clinically to treat disorders associated with abnormal repetitive behaviors.

Stereotyped patterns of behavior can be induced in a number of mammalian species including humans, following administration of indirect- and direct-acting dopamine agonists (Lewis & Baumeister, 1982). Related experiments have established the importance of striatal dopamine pathways in the mediation of STY. Cytochemical lesioning of dopamine pathways using 6-OHDA makes animals supersensitive to direct-acting dopamine agonists. This behavioral "supersensitivity" is particularly apparent in rats lesioned neonatally as they exhibit more intense stereotyped and self-injurious behavior (Creese & Iverson, 1973). Further evidence for dopamine involvement in the mediation of repetitive behaviors has come from the study of the effects of early social isolation in animals (Lewis et al., 1996; Suomi & Harlow, 1971). A long-term consequence of early social deprivation is STY and SIB. The expression of these repetitive behaviors appears to be related to loss of dopamine in striatal brain areas and subsequent dopamine receptor supersensitivity (Lewis et al., 1996; Martin et al., 1991). Studies of dopamine function in persons with mental retardation and autism using both behavioral (e.g., eye blink rate, motor disorder), and biological (e.g., plasma homovanillic acid) measures of dopamine functioning, have shown that stereotypy in persons with mental retardation and autism is associated with decreased levels of dopamine functioning (Bodfish et al., 1995b; Lewis et al., 1996).

In preclinical studies of the relation between serotonin (5-hydroxytryptophan [5-HT]) and repetitive behavior, numerous studies have shown that administration of the 5-HT precursor, as well as drugs that act as direct 5-HT agonists, induces a complex behavioral syndrome that includes stereotyped motor activity (Curzon, 1990). In humans, studies have demonstrated alterations in serotonergic functioning in persons with autism and mental retardation. Elevated whole blood serotonin has been found in approximately a third of persons with autism (McBride et al., 1969), and may be a marker for severity of abnormal repetitive behaviors in persons with autism. Tryptophan is a dietary precursor of serotonin, and McDougle et al. (1996) demonstrated that tryptophan depletion produced a worsening of repetitive behaviors in autistic persons. Studies of persons with severe and profound mental retardation (but without autism) have also shown elevations in whole blood serotonin levels. Given the high-prevalence rates for abnormal repetitive behaviors in persons with autism and mental retardation, these findings of altered serotonergic functioning have led to models of serotonin mediation of repetitive behavior (Lewis & Bodfish, 1998).

In preclinical models of the relation between opiate peptides and STY and SIB it has been found that acute injections of the opiate agonist morphine into striatal areas results in intense stereotypies in rats. Also, chronic administration of morphine results in both STY and self-mutilative behavior in rodents (Iwamoto & Way, 1977). Opiate antagonists like naltrexone have also been shown to inhibit certain forms of stereotypy in movement-restricted farm animals (Dantzer, 1986). In humans, studies have shown links between SIB in persons with mental retardation and autism and alterations in biochemical markers of the opiate system (Symons, Sutton, Walker, & Bodfish, 2003).

Genetic Factors

There are a variety of specific genetic disorders that cause atypical brain development, mental retardation, and STY and SIB. These include Lesch–Nyhan syndrome, Prader–Willi syndrome, Rett syndrome, Cornelia de Lange syndrome, Smith–Magenis syndrome, and Fragile X syndrome. Across these disorders there is considerable variability with respect to both the prevalence and form of STY and SIB. At one extreme is Lesch–Nyhan syndrome where 100% of affected cases display SIB (Anderson & Ernst, 1994) that typically involves lip-biting or other forms of self-biting, but can also involve head-hitting, eye-poking, and other forms of SIB in a minority of cases (e.g., catching limbs in doorways, placing feet under wheelchairs, placing fingers in wheelchair spokes). SIB is prevalent in other genetic disorders but is not an invariant part of the phenotype. This includes Prader–Willi syndrome (60–80% of cases have skin-picking; Symons et al., 1999; Whitman & Accardo, 1987), Smith–Magenis syndrome (50–70% of cases have a variety of forms of SIB; Smith et al., 1998), Rett syndrome (30–40% of cases have a variety of forms of SIB). Various forms of SIB have also been reported to occur in association with Fragile X syndrome, although more recent studies have found this to be a relatively infrequent part of the phenotype (Symons, Clark, Hatton, Skinner, & Bailey, 2003).

INTERVENTION

The two treatment approaches for STY and SIB that have amassed the most scientific and clinical support are behavioral treatment approaches and biomedical treatment approaches (Iwata, Kahng, Wallace, & Lindberg, 2000; Lewis & Bodfish, 1998). These two approaches evolved from different theoretical orientations to STY and SIB. The focus on biomedical risk factors (i.e., genetic and neurological) lead naturally to a search for medical treatments. In contrast, the focus on environmental risk factors, operant learning, and abnormalities in behavioral development lead to an emphasis on behavioral interventions. The current standard of care for STY, SIB, and related abnormal repetitive behaviors involves a consideration of both of these treatment perspectives and the use of either one or the other or both treatment approaches that evolve from these perspectives based on specific case formulations and the use of an empirical treatment model (i.e., clinical hypothesis testing). In general, clinical experience and consensus (see Consensus Panel Report, *American Journal on Mental Retardation*, May 2000) suggests that (a) individualized behavioral treatments will be required for most cases of clinically significant repetitive behavior disorders; (b) in severe cases (e.g., risk of injury from SIB, STY, or compulsive/ritualistic/sameness behaviors that significantly interfere with learning and development or that lead to SIB or aggression when interrupted) specific medication therapy may be required; and (c) when medication therapy is required, that combined treatment with an individualized behavioral intervention is more likely to lead to optimal outcomes (i.e., medications do not work in a vacuum and behavioral approaches can promote the development of adaptive replacement behaviors).

Behavioral Assessment and Treatment

A large body of research and decades of clinical practice have established the efficacy of a variety of behavioral intervention techniques as forms of treatment for the STY, SIB, and related abnormal repetitive behaviors in persons with mental retardation and/or autistic disorders (Horner, Carr, Strain, Todd, & Reed, 2002; Iwata et al., 1994; Matson, Benavidez, Compton, Paclawskyi, & Baglio, 1996). The published behavioral treatment literature that has arisen on the basis of the operant learning model involves the application of the standardized methods of behavioral science to examine and demonstrate treatment effects. Key features of this empirical approach are (a) operational definition of observable target behaviors, (b) definition of behavioral antecedents and consequents that make explicit the functional relationship between the treatment environment and the target behavior, (c) a task analysis that explicitly defines the treatment procedure, (d) a measurement system for quantifying the acquisition, maintenance, and generalization of the target behavior. The goal of this methodology is to insure that effective elements of a treatment procedure can be reliably identified by researchers, tested in replication studies by other researchers, and then reliably and practically applied by treatment agents (e.g., parents and teachers).

Functional Analysis

The current standard of care with respect to the behavioral treatment of STY and SIB is defined more by advances in assessment methodology and practice than by specific contingency management procedures. Whereas older treatment models held that behavioral procedures could be used to decrease STY and SIB regardless of their causes, more recent changes in behavioral assessment methods allow for the design of interventions based on empirically derived clinical hypotheses regarding specific contingency arrangements that are maintaining STY or SIB (Deoln, Rodriguez-Catter, & Cataldo, 2002). This contemporary model of behavioral assessment to identify operant maintaining factors is termed "functional analysis." Whereas earlier behavior treatment efforts utilized nonspecific reinforcers and behavioral consequences, functional analysis models permit the empirical identification of patient-specific reinforcers (Fisher et al., 1992; Pace, Ivancic, Edwards, Iwata, & Page, 1985), patient-specific behavioral contingencies (Iwata et al., 1982), and patient-specific behavioral consequences (Fisher, Piazza, Bowman, Hagopian, & Langdon, 1994). Using these empirical behavioral assessment methods, highly individualized and face-valid behavioral programs can be designed as interventions for STY and SIB. Functional analysis refers to empirical demonstrations of cause–effect (functional) relationships between environment and behavior. Functional analysis approaches to assessment involve attempts to identify the specific source or sources of reinforcement that appear to be maintain STY and SIB. There are a variety of functional analysis methods that have been developed for clinical use (see Iwata et al., 2000, for an extensive review). In general, functional analysis procedures can be classified under one of three general categories: (a) experimental (functional) analyses, (b) descriptive analyses, and (c) indirect assessments.

Experimental functional analysis involves repeated observations of STY or SIB under a series of test conditions in which variables suspected of influencing the behavior are directly manipulated (Iwata et al., 1982). Rates of STY or SIB are determined under these conditions and are compared to rates observed under a control condition in which the variables of interest are absent. For example, Iwata, Dorsey, Slifer, Bauman, and Richman (1982) developed a generic functional analysis protocol in which an individual's STY or SIB is measured during three test conditions. In an "attention" condition, a therapist ignores the individual (antecedent event) except when the given target behavior (e.g., SIB) is displayed, at which time the therapist briefly delivers attention (consequent event). This "attention" condition serves as a test for sensitivity to social-positive reinforcement. In a demand or escape condition, the therapist presents academic or vocational instructional demands trials to the individual (antecedent event) except when a target behavior (e.g., SIB) is displayed, at which time the therapist briefly terminates the trial (consequent event). This "demand" condition provides a test for sensitivity to social-negative reinforcement. In an "alone" condition the individual is observed under conditions of social deprivation, in which access to leisure materials is restricted. As the occurrence of STY/SIB behavior during the alone condition is unlikely to be related to social reinforcement (positive or negative), automatic-positive reinforcement (sensory stimulation) is implicated by default. A control condition (e.g., "play") is also included wherein the variables manipulated during the test conditions are absent. Attention is available on a frequent and noncontingent basis, demands are absent, and access to leisure materials is continuous. In the most extensive experimental analysis of SIB to date, Iwata et al. (1994) summarized the results of 152 assessments and reported the following prevalence rates for different functions for SIB in persons with nonspecific mental retardation or autistic spectrum disorders: Social-positive reinforcement, 26.3%; social-negative reinforcement, 38.1%; automatic reinforcement, 25.7%; multiple controlling variables or uncontrolled outcomes, 9.9%. Thus, in approximately 50–60% of cases of SIB, a clear operant function could be identified using the functional analysis assessment method. In contrast to SIB, however, functional analysis methods have generally failed to reveal clear operant functions for STY, and their validity for examining higher order forms of abnormal repetitive behavior has not been established. However, SIB is among the most frequent forms of aberrant behavior targeted for direct treatment in this population and functional analysis methods have clearly proven their utility in the treatment of SIB.

Behavioral Treatment

Using functional analysis methods, clinicians are now able to identify the environmental determinants of SIB and, as a result, to systematically alter environmental circumstances through their behavioral treatment programs. Typically, environmental change is established through the use of a variety of reinforcement-based techniques, which produce suppression of STY or SIB in one of three general ways: modification of antecedent conditions or establishing operations, elimination reinforcement for problem behavior through extinction procedures, or strengthening of competing behaviors (Delon et al., 2002; Iwata et al., 2000). Results of a functional analysis yield information can be used to attenuate the influence of antecedent conditions or establishing operations on SIB by dictating the specific components of noncontingent reinforcement procedures. For example, the noncontingent delivery of attention to individuals whose SIB is maintained by attention (positive reinforcement) has been shown to produce rapid and clinically significant decrease in SIB (Vollmer, Iwata, Zarcone, Smith, & Mazaleski, 1993). Noncontingent reinforcement procedures can also be used to treat people displaying SIB maintained by escape from demands (negative reinforcement). This would involve either access to escape on a response-independent basis or the alteration of tasks to reduce their aversive characteristics. Finally, the noncontingent delivery of sensory stimulation may be used decrease SIB or STY maintained by sensory (automatic) reinforcement (Piazza, Adelinis, Hanley, Goh, & Delia, 2000). Results of a functional analysis can also be used to dictate the design of specific extinction procedures because they identify the source of reinforcement to be discontinued. SIB maintained by attention is extinguished by withholding attention or terminating it when SIB occurs; SIB maintained by escape is extinguished by preventing escape or avoidance of task demands when SIB occurs. Finally, treatment procedures based on the alteration of antecedent conditions and on extinction can be highly effective in reducing SIB, but they do not explicitly strengthen appropriate alternative responses. For this, some form of formal replacement behavior therapy is required and is an important component to include to help insure the maintenance of gains made by behavioral treatment procedures. Behavioral replacement is accomplished through either incidental learning procedures or established direct teaching strategies paired with the use of differential reinforcement procedures. The results of a functional analysis may be used to identify reinforcers to strengthen competing behavior in a replacement behavior program.

Although functional analysis and treatment methods have brought about significant advances in the treatment of SIB (and to a lesser extent STY and other forms of abnormal repetitive behavior), protective and restrictive procedures still seem to remain necessary to prevent harm in extreme cases. This includes the use of protective gear and clothing to prevent serious and even life-threatening injuries caused by SIB, and also the ethical and controlled therapeutic use of restrictive procedures such as restraint, seclusion/time-out, and punishment (Brown, Genel, & Riggs, 2000). However, advances in applied behavior analysis methods have also lead to the development of methods to (a) minimize the undesirable effects on quality of life and maximize treatment effects in cases where restrictive procedures are indicated, and (b) permit the systematic fading of the use of restrictive procedures over time as SIB improves (Oliver, Hall, Hales, Murphy, & Watts, 1998). In general though, apparently due to increased use of functional analysis and treatment methods coupled with a general de-emphasis on restrictive procedures in the field, the number of published reports on SIB treatment procedures that involve reinforcement have begun to significantly outnumber those that involve restrictive procedures (Delon et al., 2002).

Finally, despite clear advances in the practice of the behavioral assessment and treatment of SIB, gaps in the behavioral treatment approach exist with respect to the treatment of other forms of abnormal repetitive behavior. For example, studies on the treatment of repetitive behaviors have largely involved lower functioning individuals with nonspecific mental retardation or autism and consequently little is known about treating in relatively higher functioning persons with mental retardation and/or autistic disorders. Related to this point, the bulk of the literature on treating repetitive behaviors has focused on treating the lower order repetitive behaviors such as STY and SIB. Thus, at present we know little about effective methods for the behavioral treatment of the higher order ritualistic repetitive behaviors and general rigidity/inflexibility that are most characteristic of autism (Lewis & Bodfish, 1998; Turner, 1999).

Biomedical Treatment

There has been considerable interest in a wide range of medications for the treatment of STY, SIB, and related repetitive behaviors in persons with mental retardation and autism. In general, consistent empirical evidence and clear clinical consensus exists for three general classes of medication of the treatment of repetitive behaviors: dopaminergic medications, serotonergic medications, and opiodergic medications (Lewis & Bodfish, 1998). This is consistent with the bulk of the existing neurobiological evidence, which suggests that abnormal repetitive behavior in mental retardation and autism is mediated in part by alterations in brain dopamine, serotonin, and opiate systems (Aman, Collier-Crespin, & Lindsay, 2000; Lewis et al., 1996; Racusin, Kovner-Kline, & King, 1999). To date, there have been no "head-to-head" comparisons of the relative effectiveness of these classes of medication in the treatment of persons with mental retardation or autism, and so clinical decisions as to choice of medications within this group is largely based on the practice of empirical clinical treatment trials (i.e., clinical hypothesis testing or systematic data-based "trial and error").

Serotonin Reuptake Inhibitors (Antidepressants)

There is a reasonable body of evidence supporting the use of selective serotonin reuptake inhibitors in the treatment of older individuals with autism. This evidence includes numerous positive case series and open studies reporting improvements in adults with mental retardation and/or autistic disorders (Bodfish & Madison, 1993; Buchsbaum et al., 2001; Cook, Rowlett, Jaselskis, & Levanthal, 1992; Hellings, Kelley, Gabrielli, Kilgore, & Shah, 1996; McDougle et al., 1998; Posey, Litwiller, Koburn, & McDougle, 1999). The serotonin reuptake inhibitor (SRI) clomipramine was shown to reduce repetitive behavior to a significantly greater degree than the non-SRI comparator desipramine did but clomipramine was also associated with significant side effects in several cases (Gordon, State, Nelson, Hamburger, & Rapoport, 1993). McDougle et al. (1996) showed that fluvoxamine led to significant improvements in the overall functioning of 53% of the 16 people treated, whereas none of those in the placebo group responded. Fluvoxamine-related improvements were noted in repetitive thoughts and behaviors and associated maladaptive behaviors. In two additional placebo, double-blind studies, clomipramine produced clinically significant (>50%) reduction in a variety of repetitive behaviors in adults with pervasive developmental disorders and mental retardation. Improvements were noted in repetitive behaviors (e.g., stereotyped motor behaviors, compulsions) as measured by both direct behavioral counts and clinical ratings scales (Lewis, Bodfish, Powell, Parker, & Golden, 1996; Lewis, Bodfish, Powell, & Golden, 1995).

The evidence of the effects of SRIs in children is more equivocal as there have been no randomized controlled trials published to date in children. Published open trial studies with the less selective medication clomipramine have shown inconsistent findings and some have indicated that younger children respond less well (Brasic et al., 1994). Significant improvements have been more consistently observed in open studies of the SSRIs (DeLong, Teague, & McSwain-Kamran, 1998; Steingard, Zimnitzky, DeMaso, Bauman, & Bucci, 1997), including improvements in both repetitive behavior in children with autistic disorders. However, these effects in children have not been replicated to date under blinded, placebo-controlled conditions and concerns have been raised about the tolerability of SRIs in the pediatric populations (McDougle et al., 2000).

Opiate Antagonists (Naltrexone)

There is a reasonable body of evidence supporting the use of the opiate antagonist medication naltrexone in the treatment of SIB in persons with mental retardation and also persons with autistic spectrum disorders. Reviews of this treatment literature have indicated a large number of placebo-controlled trials in this population and that approximately 40% of SIB cases (including children and adults) examined in controlled trials of naltrexone have demonstrated a positive response (Sandman & Hetrick, 1995). The evidence is also fairly clear that naltrexone's effects appear to be specific to SIB in positive responders and that little treatment effects are seen for STY (Bodfish et al., 1997) and for other associated symptoms of autism (Gillberg, 1995). Ironically, clinical interest in naltrexone may be diminished because of this selective property despite the fact that theoretically this is a highly desirable aspect of a psychopharmacologic treatment (i.e., behavioral selectivity as opposed to myriad nonselective behavioral effects). In contrast to other drugs such as the antipsychotics that appear to nonselectively diminish mood and behavior problems, naltrexone's effects appear to be limited to SIB. Perhaps related to this property, naltrexone has also been demonstrated to have an extremely low side effect profile including no extrapyramidal (e.g., dyskinesia), metabolic (e.g., weight gain), or sedative effects.

Dopamine Antagonists (Antipsychotics)

For decades the mainstay of pharmacologic treatment for persons with mental retardation and autism was the traditional dopamine antagonists (also called "typical antipsychotics"—e.g., haloperidol, thioridazine). Although these drugs were shown to be effective in treating SIB and STY in at least some cases, their use was also clearly associated with a number of debilitating side effects in this population including tardive dyskinesia (Campbell et al., 1997). Indeed, it has been shown that individuals with STY are at an increased risk for the development of the extrapyramidal side effects of the typical antipsychotics such as dyskinesia (Bodfish, Newell, Sprague, Harper, & Lewis, 1996) and akathisia (Bodfish, Newell, Sprague,

Harper, & Lewis, 1997). Others reported that individuals with STY tended to be kept on typical antipsychotics despite a lack of compelling evidence for the efficacy of such treatment (Chadsey-Rusch & Sprague, 1989). For these reasons, and following the introduction of newer "atypical" antipsychotic medications (e.g., risperidone, olanzapine) that had superior side effect profiles, the use of the typical antipsychotics is now discouraged in this population.

There is reasonable evidence supporting the use of the atypical antipsychotics risperidone and olanzapine in the treatment of STY, SIB, and related repetitive behaviors. The evidence includes several open trials and two placebo-controlled trials of atypical antipsychotics in nonspecific mental retardation and in autism, all reporting significant improvements in at least half of the patients studied (Findling, Maxwell, & Wiznitzer, 1997; Horrigan & Barnhill, 1997; Malone, Cater, Sheikh, Choudhury, & Delaney, 2001; McCracken et al., 2002; McDougle, Holmes, Bronson, et al., 1997; McDougle, Holmes, Carlson, et al., 1998; Posey, Walsh, Wilson, & McDougle, 1999; Posey, Litwiller, et al., 1999; Potenza, Holmes, Kanes, McDougle, 1999; Zarcone et al., 2001). Although these studies provide clear evidence of the efficacy of the atypical antipsychotics in the treatment of repetitive behaviors, the evidence also suggests that this is a nonspecific effect as improvements are also seen in a wide variety of conditions (e.g., disruptive behaviors—Zarcone et al., 2001) and mood problems (e.g., irritability—McCracken et al., 2002). Further, although clearly significant with respect to improvements in behavioral problems in most cases, the atypical antipsychotics are also associated with weight gain and sedation in at least a significant minority of cases treated and for some of whom such side effects become treatment-limiting (Aman & Madrid, 1999). Although atypical antipsychotics are known to produce fewer extrapyramidal side effects (e.g., dyskinesia, akathisia, parkinsonism) than do typical antipsychotics (e.g., haloperidol, thioridazine), the acute nature of the majority of the atypical antipsychotic treatment studies in autism does not provide sufficient time to accurately evaluate potential long-term tardive effects (e.g., tardive dyskinesia).

SUMMARY

Long gone are the days when a clinician assumed simply that STY and SIB were "institutionalized" behavior and equally simply treated it with a nonspecific reinforcement program (e.g., differential reinforcement of other behavior), or a nonspecific punishment program (e.g., time out), or a nonselective drug (e.g., Mellaril). Since this time, a considerable increase in the research base on STY and SIB has occurred and with it has come considerable advances in the conceptualization of STY and SIB and also considerable increases in treatment options for these disorders in persons with mental retardation and autism. These advances in conceptualization and treatment have focused on three themes: (a) an understanding of the clinical phenomenology of STY and SIB as parts of a broader spectrum of abnormal repetitive behaviors common to a range of neurodevelopmental disorders, (b) a knowledge of the host of risk factors associated with the development and maintenance of STY and SIB including environmental factors, psychological factors, neurobiological factors, genetic factors, and their interaction, and (c) a knowledge of the advances in both behavioral assessment and treatment of STY and SIB and also the psychopharmacological assessment and treatment STY and SIB and an appreciation of how these intervention approaches can be integrated to optimize treatment outcomes. These advances have extended from research to practice where best practice clinical programs have demonstrated that these research-based advances in the conceptualization and treatment of STY, SIB, and associated repetitive behaviors can be routinely translated to treatment practices in everyday settings. Importantly, the application of these current standards of care can result in improved prognoses for persons with mental retardation and autism who exhibit STY and SIB disorders.

REFERENCES

Alexander, G. E., Crutcher, M. D., & Delong, M. R. (1990). Basal ganglia-thalamocortical circuits: Parallel substrates for motor, oculomotor, "prefrontal" and "limbic" functions. *Progress in Brain Research, 85*, 119–145.

Aman, M. G., Collier-Crespin, A., Lindsay, R. L. (2000). Pharmacotherapy of disorders in mental retardation {review}. *European Child and Adolescent Psychiatry, 9*, 98–107.

Aman, M. G., & Madrid, A. (1999). Atypical antipsychotics in persons with developmental disabilities. *Mental Retardation and Developmental Disabilities Research Reviews, 5*, 253–263.

Anderson, L. T., & Ernst, M. (1994). Self-injury in Lesch–Nyhan disease. *Journal of Autism and Developmental Disorders, 24*, 67–81.

Bartak, L., & Rutter, M. (1976). Differences between mentally retarded and normally intelligent autistic children. *Journal of Autism and Childhood Schizophrenia, 6*, 109–120.

Berkson, G., & Davenport, R. K. (1962). Stereotyped movements of mental defectives: Initial survey. *American Journal of Mental Deficiency, 66*, 849–852.

Berkson, G., Gutermuth, L., & Baranek, G. (1995). Relative prevalence and relations among stereotyped and similar behaviors. *American Journal on Mental Retardation, 100*(2), 137–145.

Berkson, G., & Mason, W. A. (1964). Stereotyped movements of mental defectives. IV. The effects of toys and the character of the acts. *American Journal of Mental Deficiencies, 68*, 511–524.

Bodfish, J. W., Crawford, T. W., Powell, S. B., Golden, R. N., & Lewis, M. H. (1995a). Compulsions in adults with mental retardation: Prevalence, phenomenology, and co-morbidity with stereotypy and self-injury. *American Journal on Mental Retardation, 100*, 183–192.

Bodfish, J. W., & Lewis, M. H. (2002). Self-injury and comorbid behavior in developmental, neurological, psychiatric, and genetic disorders. In S. Schroeder, M. Oster-Granite, & T. Thompson (Eds.), *Self-injurious behavior: Gene–brain–behavior relationships* (Vol. 2, pp. 23–39). Washington, DC: American Psychological Association Press.

Bodfish, J. W., & Madison, J. (1993). Diagnosis and fluoxetine treatment of compulsive behavior disorder of adults with mental retardation. *American Journal on Mental Retardation, 98*, 360–367.

Bodfish, J. W., McCuller, W. R., Madison, J. M., Register, M., Mailman, R. B., & Lewis M. H. (1997). Placebo, double-blind evaluation of long term Naltrexone treatment effects for adults with mental retardation and self-injury. *Journal of Developmental and Physical Disabilities, 9*, 135–152.

Bodfish, J. W., Newell, K. M., Sprague, R. L., Harper, V. N., & Lewis, M. H. (1996). Dyskinetic movement disorders among adults with mental retardation: Phenomenology & co-occurrence with stereotypy. *American Journal on Mental Retardation, 101,* 118–129.

Bodfish, J. W., Newell, K. M., Sprague, R. L., Harper, V. N., & Lewis, M. H. (1997). Akathisia in adults with mental retardation receiving maintenance neuroleptic treatment. *American Journal on Mental Retardation, 101,* 413–423.

Bodfish, J. W., Parker, D. E., Lewis, M. H., Sprague, R. L., & Newell, K. M. (2001). Stereotypy and motor control: Differences in the postural stability dynamics of persons with stereotyped and dyskinetic movement disorders. *American Journal of Mental Retardation, 106,* 123–134.

Bodfish, J. W., Powell, S. B., Golden, R. N., & Lewis, M. H. (1995b). Blink rate as an index of dopamine function in adults with mental retardation and repetitive behavior disorders. *American Journal on Mental Retardation, 99,* 335–344.

Bodfish, J. W., Symons, F. J., Parker, D. E., & Lewis, M. H. (2000). Varieties of repetitive behavior in autism: Comparisons to mental retardation. *Journal of Autism and Developmental Disorders, 30,* 237–243.

Brasic, J. R., Barnett, J. Y., Kaplan, D., Sheitman, B. B., Aisemberg, P., Lafargue, R. T., et al. (1994). Clomipramine ameliorates adventitious movements and compulsions in prepubertal boys with autistic disorder and severe mental retardation. *Neurology, 44,* 1309–1312.

Breau, L. M., Camfield, C. S., Symons, F. J., Bodfish, J. W., MacKay, A., Finley, G. A., et al. (2003). Relation between pain and self-injurious behavior in nonverbal children with severe cognitive impairments. *Journal of Pediatrics, 142,* 498–503.

Brett, L. P., & Levine, S. (1979). Schedule-induced polydipsia and pituitary–adrenal activity in rats. *Journal of Comparative Physiology and Psychology, 93,* 946–956.

Brown, R. L., Genel, M., & Rigggs, J. A. (2000). Use of seclusion and restraint in children and adolescents. *Archives of Pediatrics and Adolescent Medicine, 154,* 653–656.

Buchsbaum, M. S., Hollander, E., Haznedar, M. M., Tang, C., Speigel-Cohen, J., Wei, T. C., et al. (2001). Effect of fluoxetine on regional cerebral metabolism in autistic spectrum disorders: A pilot study. *International Journal of Neuropsychopharmacology, 4,* 119–125.

Campbell, M., Armenteros, J. L., Malone, R. P., Adams, P. B., Eisenberg, Z. W., Overall, J. E. (1997). Neuroleptic-related dyskinesias in autistic children: A prospective, longitudinal study. *Journal of American Academy of Child Adolescent Psychiatry, 36,* 835–843.

Campbell, M., Locascio, J. J., Choroco, M. C., Spencer, E. K, Malone, R. P., Kafantaris, V., et al. (1990). Stereotypies and tardive dyskinesia: Abnormal movements in autistic children. *Psychopharmacology Bulletin, 26,* 260–266.

Carr, E. G. (1977). The motivation of self-injurious behavior: A review of some hypotheses. *Psychological Bulletin, 84,* 800–816.

Chadsey-Rusch, J., & Sprague, R. L. (1989). Maladaptive behaviors associated with neuroleptic drug maintenance. *American Journal of Mental Retardation, 93,* 607–617.

Clarke, D. J., Boer, H., Chung, M. C., Sturmey, P., & Webb, T. (1996). Maladaptive behaviour in Prader–Willi syndrome in adult life. *Journal of Intellectual Disability Research, 40* (Pt 2), 159–165.

Cloninger, C. R. (1987). A systematic method for clinical description and classification of personality variants. *Archives of General Psychiatry, 44,* 573–588.

Collacott, R. A., Cooper, S. A., Branford, D., & McGrother, C. (1998). Epidemiology of self-injurious behaviour in adults with learning disabilities. *British Journal of Psychiatry, 173,* 428–432.

Cook, E. H., Rowlett, R., Jaselskis, & Levanthal, B. L. (1992). Fluoxetine treatment of children and adults with autistic disorder and mental retardation. *Journal of the American Academy of Child and Adolescent Psychiatry, 31,* 739–745.

Cooper, S. J., & Dourish, C. T. (1990). *Neurobiology of stereotyped behaviour.* Oxford: Oxford University Press.

Cowdery, G. E., Iwata, B. A., & Pace, G. M. (1990). Effects and side effects of DRO as treatment for self-injurious behavior. *Journal of Applied Behavior Analysis, 23,* 497–506.

Creese, I., & Iversen, S. D. (1973). Blockage of amphetamine induced motor stimulation and stereotypy in the adult rat following neonatal treatment with 6-hydroxydopamine. *Brain Research, 55*(2), 369–382.

Curzon, G. (1990). Stereotyped and other motor responses in 5-hydroxytryptamine receptor activation. In S. J. Cooper & C. T. Dourish (Eds.), *Neurobiology of stereotyped behaviour* (pp. 142–168). Oxford: Oxford University Press.

Dantzer, R. (1986). Behavioral, physiological and functional aspects of stereotyped behavior: A review and re-interpretation. *Journal of Animal Science, 62*, 1776–1786.

Delon, I. G., Rodriguez-Catter, V., & Cataldo, M. F. (2002). Treatment: Current standards of care and their research implications. In S. R. Schroeder, M. L. Octer-Granite, & T. Thompson (Eds.), *Self-injurious behavior: Gene–brain–behavior relationships* (pp. 81–92). Washington, DC: American Psychological Association Press.

DeLong, G. R., Teague, L. A., & McSwain-Kamran, M. (1998). Effects of fluoxetine treatment in young children with idiopathic autism. *Developmental Medicine and Child Neurology, 40*, 551–562.

Dyken, E. M., Leckman, J. F., & Cassidy, S. B. (1996). Obsessions and compulsions in Prader–Willi Syndrome. *Journal of Child Psychology and Psychiatry, 37*, 995–1002.

Evans, D. W., Leckman, J. F., Carter, A., Reznick, J. S., Henshaw, D., King, R. A., et al. (1997). Ritual, habit and perfectionism: The prevalence and development of compulsive-like behaviour in normal young children. *Child Development, 68*, 58–68.

Feurer, I. D., Dimitropoulos, A., Stone, W. L., Roof, E., Butler, M. G., & Thompson, T. (1998) The latent variable structure of the Compulsive Behaviour Checklist in people with Prader–Willi syndrome. *Journal of Intellectual Disability Research, 42*, 472–480.

Findling, R. L., Maxwell, K., & Wiznitzer, M. (1997b). An open clinical trial of risperidone monotherapy in young children with autistic disorder. *Psychopharmacology Bulletin, 33*, 155–159.

Fisher, W., Piazza, C. C., Bowman, L. G., Hagopian, L. P., & Langdon, N. A. (1994). Empirically derived consequences: A data-based method for prescribing treatments for destructive behavior. *Research in Developmental Disabilities, 15*, 133–149.

Fisher, W., Piazza, C. C., Bowman, L. G., Hagopian, L. P., Owens, J. C., & Slevin, I. (1992). A comparison of two approaches for identifying reinforcers for persons with severe and profound disabilities. *Journal of Applied Behavior Analysis, 245*, 491–498.

Freeman, B. J., Ritvo, E. R., Schroth, P. C., Tonick, I., Gurhrie, D., & Wake, L. (1981). Behavioral characteristics of high-and-low-IQ autistic children. *American Journal of Psychiatry, 138*, 25–29.

Frith, D. D., & Done, D. J. (1990). Stereotyped behaviour in madness and in health. In S. J. Cooper & C. T. Dourish (Eds.), *Neurobiology of stereotyped behaviour* (pp. 232–259). Oxford: Clarendon Press.

Frith, U. (1989). *Autism: Explaining the enigma.* Oxford: Blackwell.

Gillberg, C. (1995). Endogenous opioids and opiate antagonists in autism: Brief review of empirical findings and implications for clinicians. *Developmental Medicine and Child Neurology, 37*, 239–245.

Gordon, C. T., State, R. C., Nelson, J. E., Hamburger, S. D., & Rapoport, J. L. (1993). A double-blind comparison of clomipramine, desipramine, and placebo in the treatment of autistic disorder. *Archives of General Psychiatry, 50*, 441–447.

Graybiel, A. M., & Rauch, S. L. (2000). Toward a neurobiology of obsessive–compulsive disorder. *Neuron, 28*, 343–347.

Hellings, J. A., Kelley, L. A., Gabrielli, W. F., Kilgore, E., & Shah, P. (1996). Sertraline response in adults with mental retardation and autistic disorder. *Journal of Clinical Psychiatry, 57*, 333–336.

Hermelin, B., & O'Connnor, N. (1963). The response of self-generated behaviour of severely disturbed children and severely subnormal controls. *British Journal of Social and Clinical Psychology, 2*, 37–43.

Horner, R. H., Carr, E. G., Strain, P. S., Todd, A. W., & Reed, H. K. (2002). Problem behavior interventions for young children with autism: A research synthesis. *Journal of Autism and Developmental Disorders, 32*(5), 423–446.

Horrigan, J. P., & Barnhill, L. J. (1997). Risperidone and explosive aggressive autism. *Journal of Autism and Developmental Disorders, 27,* 313–323.

Hutt, C., & Hutt, S. (1970). Stereotypies and their relation to arousal: A study of autistic children. In S. Hutt & D. Hutt (Eds.), *Behavior studies in psychiatry* (pp. 175–204). Oxford: Pergamon Press.

Iwamoto, E. T., & Way, E. L. (1977). Circling behavior and stereotypy induced by intranigral opiate microinjection. *Journal of Pharmacology and Experimental Therapeutics, 20,* 347–359.

Iwata, B., Dorsey, M., Slifer, K., Bauman, M., & Richman, D. (1982). Toward a functional analysis of self-injury. *Analysis and Intervention in Developmental Disabilities, 2,* 3–20.

Iwata, B. A., Kahng, S., Wallace, M. D., & Lindberg, J. S. (2000). The functional analysis model of behavioral assessment. In J. Austin, & J. E. Carr (Eds.), *Handbook of applied behavior analysis.* Reno, NV: Context Press.

Iwata, B. A., Pace, G. M., Dorsey, M. F., Zarcone, J. R., Vollmer, T. R., & Smith, R. G. (1994). The functions of self-injurious behavior: An experimental epidemiological analysis. *Journal of Applied Behavior Analysis, 27,* 215–240.

Iwata, B. A., Pace, G. M., Kalsher, M. J., Cowdrey, G. E., & Cataldo, M. F. (1990). Experimental analysis and extinction of self-injurious escape behavior. *Journal of Applied Behavior Analysis, 23,* 11–27.

Johnson, K. (1999). Reliability and comorbidity of measures of repetitive movement disorders in children and adolescents with severe mental retardation. *Dissertation Abstracts International, 59*(9-B), 5066.

Kanner, L. (1943). Autistic disturbances of affective contact. *Nervous Child, 2,* 217–250.

King, B. H. (1993). Self-injury by people with mental retardation: A compulsive behavior hypothesis. *American Journal on Mental Retardation, 98,* 93–112.

Lewis, M. H., & Baumeister, A. A. (1982). Stereotyped mannerisms in mentally retarded persons: Animal modes and theoretical analyses. In N. R. Ellis (Ed.), *International review of research in mental retardation.* Academic Press: New York.

Lewis, M. H., & Bodfish, J. W. (1998). Repetitive behavior disorders in autism. Special issue: "Autism". *Mental Retardation Development Disabilities Research Review, 4,* 80–89.

Lewis, M. H., Bodfish, J. W., Powell, S. B., & Golden, R. N. (1995). Clomipramine treatment for stereotypy and related repetitive movement disorders associated with mental retardation. *American Journal on Mental Retardation , 100,* 299–312.

Lewis, M. H., Bodfish, J. W., Powell, S. B., Parker, D. E., & Golden, R. N. (1996). Clomipramine treatment for self-injurious behavior of individuals with mental retardation: A double-blind comparison with placebo. *American Journal on Mental Retardation, 100,* 654–665.

Lewis, M. H., Bodfish, J. W., Powell, S. B., Wiest, K., Darling, M., & Golden, R. N. (1996). Plasma HVA in adults with mental retardation and stereotyped behavior: Biochemical evidence for a dopamine deficiency model. *American Journal on Mental Retardation, 100,* 413–418.

Lord, C. (1995). Follow-up of 2-year-olds referred for possible autism. *Journal of Child Psychology and Psychiatry, 36,* 1365–1382.

Lord, C., & Pickles, A. (1996). Language level and nonverbal social–communicative behaviors in autistic and language-delayed children. *Journal of the Academy of Child and Adolescent Psychiatry, 35,* 1542–1550.

Lovaas, O. I., Koegel, R., Simmons, J. Q., & Long, J. S. (1973). Some generalization and follow-up measures on autistic children in behavior therapy. *Journal of Applied Behavior Analysis, 6,* 131–166.

Malone, R. P., Cater, J., Sheikh, R. M., Choudhury, M. S., & Delaney, M. A. (2001). Olanzapine versus haloperidol in children with autistic disorder: An open pilot study. *Journal of American Academy of Child Adolescent Psychiatry, 40,* 887–894.

Mason, G. (1991). Stereotypies: A critical review. *Animal Behaviour, 41,* 1015–1037.

Matson, J. L., Benavidez, D. A., Compton, L. S., Paclawskyi, T., & Baglio, C. (1996). Behavioral treatment of autistic persons: A review of research from 1980 to the present. *Research in Developmental Disabilities, 17,* 433–465.

McBride, P. A., Anderson, G. M., Hertzig, M. E., Sweeney, J. A., Kream, J., Cohen, D. J., et al. (1989). Serotonergic responsivity in male young adults with autistic disorder. Results of a pilot study. *Archives of General Psychiatry, 46*, 213–221.

McCracken, J. T., McGough, J., Shah, B., Cronin, P., Hong, D., Aman, M. G., et al. (2002). Risperidone in children with autism and serious behavioral problems. *New England Journal of Medicine, 347*(5), 314–321.

McDougle, C., Kresch, L., Goodman, W., et al. (1995). A case-controlled study of repetitive thoughts and behavior in adults with autistic disorder and obsessive-compulsive disorder. *American Journal of Psychiatry, 152*, 727–777.

McDougle, C., Naylor, S., Cohen, D., et al. (1996). Effects of tryptophan depletion in drug-free adults with autistic disorder. *Archives of General Psychiatry, 53*, 993–1000.

McDougle, C. J., Holmes, J. P., Bronson, M. R., Anderson, G. M., Volkmar, F. R., Price, L. H., et al. (1997). Risperidone treatment of children and adolescents with pervasive developmental disorders: A prospective open-label study. *Journal of the American Academy of Child and Adolescent Psychiatry, 36*, 685–693.

McDougle, C. J., Holmes, J. P., Carlson, D. C., Pelton, G. H., Cohen, D. J., & Price, L. H. (1998). A double-blind, placebo-controlled study of risperidone in adults with autistic disorder and other pervasive developmental disorders. *Archives of General Psychiatry, 55*, 633–641.

McDougle, C. J., Kresch, L. E., & Posey, D. J. (2000). Repetitive thoughts and behavior in pervasive developmental disorder: Treatment with serotonin reuptake inhibitors. *Journal of Autism and Developmental Disorders, 5*, 427–435.

McDougle, C. J., Naylor, S. T., Cohen, D. J., Volkmar, F. R., Heninger, G. R., & Price, L. H. (1996). A double-blind, placebo-controlled study of fluvoxamine in adults with autistic disorder. *Archives of General Psychiatry, 53*, 1001–1008.

Murphy, G., Hall, S., Oliver, C., & Kissi-Debra, R. (1999). Identification of early self-injurious behaviour in young children with intellectual disability. *Journal of Intellectual Disability Research, 43* (Pt 3), 149–163.

Newell, K. M., Challis, J. H., & Bodfish, J. W. (2002). Further evidence on the dynamics of self-injurious behaviors: Impact forces and limb motions. *American Journal on Mental Retardation, 107*, 60–68.

Newell, K. M., Incledon, T., Bodfish, J. W., & Sprague, R. L. (1999). The variability of stereotypic body rocking in adults with mental retardation. *American Journal on Mental Retardation, 104*, 279–288.

Oliver, C., Hall, S., Hales, J., Murphy, G., & Watts, D. (1998). The treatment of severe self-injurious behavior by the systematic fading of restraints: Effects on self-injury, self-restraint, adaptive behavior, and behavioral correlates of affect. *Research in Developmental Disabilities, 19*, 143–165.

Ornitz, E. M. (1971). Childhood autism: A disorder of sensorimotor integration. In M. Rutter (Ed.), *Infantile autism: Concepts, characteristics, and treatment*. London: Churchill Livingstone.

Pace, G. M., Ivancic, M. T., Edwards, G. L., Iwata, B. A., & Page, T. J. (1985). Assessment of stimulus preference and reinforcer value with profoundly retarded individuals. *Journal of Applied Behavior Analysis, 18*, 249–255.

Piazza, C. C., Adelinis, J. D., Hanley, G. P., Goh, H., & Delia, M. D. (2000). An evaluation of the effects of matched stimuli on behaviors maintained by automatic reinforcement. *Journal of Applied Behavior Analysis, 33*, 13–27.

Posey, D. I., Litwiller, M., Koburn, A., & McDougle, C. J. (1999). Paroxetine in autism. *Journal of the American Academy of Child and Adolescent Psychiatry, 38*, 111–112.

Posey, D. J., Walsh, K. H., Wilson, G. A., & McDougle, C. J. (1999). Risperidone in the treatment of two very young children with autism. *Journal of Child and Adolescent Psychopharmacology, 9*, 273–276.

Potenza, M. N., Holmes, J. P., Kanes, S. J., & McDougle, C. J. (1999). Olanzapine treatment of children, adolescents, and adults with pervasive developmental disorders: An open-label pilot study. *Journal of Clinical Psychopharmacology, 19*, 37–44.

Powell, S. B., Bodfish, J. W., Parker, D. E., Crawford, T. W., & Lewis, M. H. (1996). Self-restraint and self-injury: Occurrence and motivational significance. *American Journal on Mental Retardation, 101,* 41–48.

Prior, M., & MacMillan, M. (1973). Maintenance of sameness in children with Kanner's Syndrome. *Journal of Autism and Childhood Schizophrenia, 3,* 154–167.

Racusin, R., Kovner-Kline, K., & King, B. H. (1999). Selective serotonin reuptake inhibitors in intellectual disability. *Mental Retardation and Developmental Disabilities Research Reviews, 5,* 264–269.

Rafaeli-Mor, N., Foster, L., & Berkson, G. (1999). Self-reported body-rocking and other habits in college students. *American Journal on Mental Retardation, 104*(1), 1–10.

Rapoport, J. (1991). Basal ganglia dysfunction as a proposed cause of obsessive–compulsive disorder. In B. Carroll & J. Barrett (Eds.), *Psychopathology and the brain* (pp. 77–95). New York: Raven Press.

Ridley, R. M. (1994). The psychology of perseverative and stereotyped behaviour. *Progress in Neurobiology, 44,* 221–231.

Rojahn, J. (1986). Self-injurious and stereotypic behavior of non-institutionalized mentally retarded people: Prevalence and classification. *American Journal of Mental Deficiency, 91,* 268–276.

Rojahn, J., Matlock, S. T., & Tasse, M. J. (2000). The Stereotyped Behavior Scale: Psychometric properties and norms. *Research in Developmental Disabilities, 21*(6), 437–454.

Rosenquist, P. B., Bodfish, J. W., & Thompson, R. (1997). Tourette's syndrome associated with mental retardation: A single-subject, double-blind treatment study with Haloperidol. *American Journal of Mental Retardation, 101,* 497–504.

Rutter, M., Andersen-Wood, L., Beckett, C., Bredenkamp, A. J., Groothues, C., et al. (1999). Quasi-autistic patterns following severe early global privation. English and Romanian Adoptees (ERA) Study Team. *Journal of Child Psychology and Psychiatry, 40*(4), 537–549.

Sandman, C. A., & Hetrick, W. P. (1995). Opiate mechanisms in self-injury. *Mental Retardation and Developmental Disabilities Research Reviews, 1,* 130–136.

Sears, L. L., Vest, C., Mohamed, S., Bailey, J., Ranson, B. J., & Piven, J. (1999). An MRI study of the basal ganglia in autism. *Progress in Neuropsychopharmacology and Biological Psychiatry, 4,* 613–624.

Smith, A. C., Dykens, E., & Greenberg, F. (1998). Behavioral phenotype of Smith–Magenis syndrome. *American Journal of Medical Genetics, 81,* 179–185.

Steingard, R. J., Zimnitzky, B., DeMaso, D. R., Bauman, M. L., & Bucci, J. P. (1997). Sertraline treatment of transition-associated anxiety and agitation in children with autistic disorder. *Journal of Child and Adolescent Psychopharmacology, 7,* 9–15.

Suomi, S. J., & Harlow, H. F. (1971). Abnormal social behavior in young monkeys. In J. Hellmuth (Ed.), *The exceptional infant,* Vol. 2. New York: Brner-Mazel.

Symons, F. J., Butler, M. G., Sanders, M. D., Feurer, I. D., & Thompson, T. (1999). Self-injurious behavior and Prader–Willi syndrome: Behavioral forms and body locations. *American Journal on Mental Retardation, 104,* 260–269.

Symons, F. J., Clark, R. D., Hatton, D. D., Skinner, M., & Bailey, D. B., Jr. (2003). Self-injurious behavior in young boys with fragile X syndrome. *American Journal on Medical Genetics, 118*(2), 115–121.

Symons, F. J., Suttton, K. A., & Bodfish, J. W. (2001). Preliminary study of altered skin temperature at body sites associated with self-injurious behavior in adults who have developmental disabilities. *American Journal on Mental Retardation, 106,* 336–343.

Symons, F. J., Sutton, K. A., Walker, D., & Bodfish, J. W. (2003). Altered diurnal pattern of salivary substance-P in adults with developmental disabilities and chronic self-injury. *American Journal of Mental Retardation, 108,* 13–18.

Symons, F. J., & Thompson, T. (1997). Self-injurious behavior and body site preference. *Journal of Intellectual Disability Research, 41,* 456–468.

Szatmari, P., Bartolucci, G., & Bremner, R. (1989). Asperger's syndrome and autism: Comparison of early history and outcome. *Developmental Medicine and Child Neurology, 31,* 709–720.

Thelen, E. (1979). Rhythmical stereotypies in normal human infants. *Animal Behaviour, 27,* 699–715.

Turner, M. (1999). Annotation: Repetitive behavior in autism: A review of psychological research. *Journal of Child Psychology and Psychiatry, 40,* 839–849.

Visser, J. E., Bar, P. R., & Jinnah, H. A. (2000). Lesch–Nyhan disease and the basal ganglia. *Brain Research Reviews, 32,* 449–475.

Vollmer, T. R., Iwata, B. A., Zarcone, J. R., Smith, R. G., & Mazaleski, J. L. (1993). The role of attention in the treatment of attention-mediated self-injurious behavior. *Journal of Applied Behavior Analysis, 26,* 9–21.

Watkins, K. M., & Konarski, E. A., Jr. (1987). Effect of mentally retarded persons' level of stereotypy on their learning. *American Journal of Mental Deficiency,* 91(4), 361–365.

Whitman, B. Y., & Accardo, P. (1987). Emotional symptoms in Prader–Willi syndrome. *American Journal of Medical Genetics, 28,* 897–905.

Wing, L., & Gould, J. (1979). Severe impairments of social interaction and associated abnormalities in children: Epidemiology and classification. *Journal of Autism and Developmental Disorder, 9,* 11–29.

Zarcone, J. R., Hellings, J. A., Crandall, K., Reese, R. M., Marquis, J., Fleming, K., et al. (2001). Effects of risperidone on aberrant behavior of persons with developmental disabilities: I. A double-blind crossover study usi multiple measures. *American Journal on Mental Retardation,* 106(6), 525–538.

26

Assessment and Treatment Psychopathology Among People with Developmental Delays

JOHNNY L. MATSON and RINITA B. LAUD

Over the past three decades, the co-occurrence of psychopathology and intellectual disability (ID) has received a great deal of attention. Little importance was given to this population by mental health professionals prior to that time. However, both researchers and clinicians have recently been changing their priorities with respect to this problem (MacLean, 1993; Matson, Kuhn, & Mayville, 2002). Specifically, greater professional attention has focused on classification issues and conceptual models of psychopathology as they relate to ID. Consequently, more clinicians are being trained to work specifically with this population, thus increasing the number of avenues available to aid individuals with ID who have mental health service needs.

Production of research in this field has sharply increased in the past decade, particularly in the area of assessment. Numerous scales and other assessment devices have been developed, and these in turn have fostered the development of better treatments for mental illness among those with ID. For example, the Diagnostic Assessment for the Severely Handicapped II (DASH-II) (Matson et al., 1999) and the assessment of dual diagnosis (ADD) (Matson, 1997) are two scales used to screen for psychopathology in individuals with all ranges of ID. Assessment techniques have not only aided clinicians in targeting various psychiatric disorders, but they have also expanded the field of dual diagnosis by forming more accurate

JOHNNY L. MATSON and RINITA B. LAUD • Department of Psychology, Louisiana State University, Baton Rouge, Louisiana 70803.

prevalence estimates. These estimates are essential in alerting society with the fact that a large number of those afflicted with ID are in need for mental health services. Our chapter will deal with several major topics in dual diagnosis that have been discussed in the literature. These include prevalence, etiology, diagnosis, assessment, and treatment for those that are dually diagnosed.

PREVALENCE

Research conducted on the prevalence of psychiatric disorders among individuals with developmental disabilities show that the rates of psychopathology are much higher within this population than with those found in the general population (MacLean, 1993). Specifically, the numerous studies on prevalence of dual diagnosis have led to estimates ranging from less than 10% to greater than 80% (Borthwick-Duffy, 1994). Iverson and Fox (1989) found that 35.9% of their 165 adults with ID met the criteria for presence of psychopathology. Researchers have also reported that patients with ID occupy half of the inpatient mental health beds in the United States (Matson & Sevin, 1994). Estimates from the Isle of Wight, perhaps the most quoted and most prestigious of these epidemiological studies, found that the prevalence of mental illness was much higher among children with ID compared to nondisabled children (Rutter, Tizard, Yule, Graham, & Whitmore, 1976).

Although the discrepancies among the various incidence and prevalence studies is wide, the available research when taken on the whole, support three important conclusions (MacLean, 1993). First, psychiatric disorders are four to five times more prevalent in children with ID as compared with other children (Chess & Hassibi, 1970; Eaton & Menolascino, 1982; Koller, Richardson, Katz, & McLaren, 1983; Reid, 1972; Rutter, Graham, & Yule, 1970;). Second, within samples of individuals with ID, prevalence estimates of psychopathology vary widely depending on the diagnostic criteria employed (Fraser, Leudar, Gray, & Campbell, 1986), nature of the sample, (community vs. institutional—Jacobson, 1982; Leudar, Fraser, & Jeeves, 1984; Scanlon, Arick, & Krug, 1982), gender (Koller et al., 1983), age (Jacobson, 1982), level of ID (Iverson & Fox, 1989; Jacobson, 1982; Koller et al., 1983) and the manner in which the psychiatric evaluation was conducted (Iverson & Fox, 1989). With so many variables, it is easy to see how prevalence estimates may vary so widely. For example, the total population of children aged 10 and 11 years on the Isle of Wight were surveyed in 1965 and about 6 or 7% were diagnosed as having psychiatric disorders. Only 3–4 years later, the same total population was similarly surveyed when the children were 14–15-years-old. The outcome varied markedly (Graham & Rutter, 1973). For example, those children who had emotional disturbances at a younger age did not have as many antisocial problems later on life, but those who had conduct disturbances at a younger age were diagnosed as having more psychiatric problems later. It is clear that age alone can make a difference in terms of prevalence estimates. Third, the types of psychiatric disorders evident among persons with ID generally represent the full range of diagnostic classifications. However, there does appear to be some differences in prevalence of specific disorders as a function of the level of ID (Eaton & Menolascino, 1982; Jacobson, 1982; Koller et al., 1983; Lund, 1985; Phillips & Williams, 1975; Reid, 1976, 1980; Wright, 1982). Given such comprehensive investigation, there remains no question regarding the occurrence of mental disorders among some persons with ID (Iverson & Fox, 1989; Lewis & MacLean, 1982; Matson & Sevin, 1994), and that the disorders cross the broad spectrum of psychopathology.

ETIOLOGIES OF DUAL DIAGNOSIS

While prevalence has been a major focus of research in the field of ID, etiologies of dual diagnosis have received far less attention. Current etiological theories have practical implications for the treatment and prevention of dual diagnoses and suggest important directions for future research (Matson & Sevin, 1994). In many cases, it is simply not adequate to extend previous theories of mental illness to those who are dually diagnosed. There are four models of dual diagnoses characterized by Matson and Sevin (1994). The developers of each model attempt to take into account those variables specifically associated with ID which may place the handicapped person at greater risk for developing mental health problems. These four models are organic, behavior, developmental, and sociocultural.

The Organic Model

Organic models of psychopathology emphasize physiological, biochemical, and genetic factors as potential causes of psychopathology. It is quite likely that the presence of structural brain pathologies in individuals with ID increases risk of mental illness (Matson & Sevin, 1994). Specific genetic disorders have also been linked to some forms of psychopathology. For example, several authors have reported cases of affective disorders in people with Down's syndrome (Sovner, Hurley, & Labrie, 1985; Szymanski & Biederman, 1984; Warren, Holroyd, & Folstein, 1989). In addition, there is some evidence that Fragile X syndrome in boys may be associated with attention-deficit hyperactivity disorder (ADHD) (Matson & Sevin, 1994). Hagerman and Sobesky (1989) found that social anxiety was common in female clients with Fragile X. Finally, there has even been a surprising link found between epilepsy and psychopathology in individuals with ID; that is, psychiatric disorders are significantly more common in patients with a history of seizures. These data are in correlation but pose interesting questions about brain physiology which await study.

Neurotransmitter theories that are popular in the treatment of the mentally ill at large are also considered applicable when dealing with the ID population. A few preliminary studies using neuroleptics to treat psychotic symptoms in individuals with ID have also reported favorable outcomes, indicating that similar biochemical mechanisms may be at work

(Campbell, Fish, Shapiro, & Floyd, 1970; Menolascino, Wilson, Golden, & Reudrich, 1986; Varley, 1984; Wright, 1958). Specifically, neurotransmitter theories presume that either having an excess or a depletion of a certain neurotransmitter (i.e., dopamine) may cause certain psychiatric disorders. Although these findings may indicate a solid foundation supporting a neurotransmitter theory of etiology, methodological problems in many of the studies deter researchers from drawing firm conclusions.

The Behavior Model

Behavior models of psychopathology theorize that the complex interactions between an individual and his environment develop his/her behavioral repertoire. In addition, all behaviors are learned in conjunction with physiological predisposition according to the principles of classical conditioning, social learning theory, and operant psychology. Furthermore, these principles may be extended to the ID population (Matson & Sevin, 1994). Specifically, classical conditioning and social learning models in individuals with ID have been linked to anxiety disorders. Operant models appear to be linked to various forms of psychopathology, but most often that of anxiety and depression. It is hypothesized that the learning histories of individuals with ID are often characterized by failure experiences (Gardner, 1967; MacMillan, 1977), which lead to learned deficits in motivation, feelings of worthlessness, anhedonia, and symptoms of depression. Thus, according to this model, the environment as well as the individual dictates his/her behavior. Although these may contribute to the cause of psychopathology in individuals with ID, it is also likely that the phenomenon of development contributes to the etiology of dual diagnosis.

The Developmental Model

Zigler first applied the developmental model of psychopathology to individuals with ID in the 1960s (Zigler, 1969). This model postulates that there is such a phenomenon as development (Hodapp, Burack, & Zigler, 1990) and that sequences of cognitive development are universal and invariant. An individual with ID develops at a slower rate than normal, thus exhibiting characteristics that are typically displayed by normal children in an early developmental stage. In essence, behaviors that are considered pathological for a person at a given chronological age may be considered normal for a person whose developmental level is delayed. For example, psychiatric problems such as depressive symptoms, fears, and phobias are more common in the ID population. These problems, however, are also more prevalent in individuals without developmental delays, during childhood (Kennedy, 1983; Petti, 1989). Since individuals with ID clearly develop at a much slower rate than normal individuals, it is possible that this model may account for some of the behaviors typically displayed by individuals with a dual diagnosis such as frequent stereotypes and self-injury. It is imperative to also examine the sociocultural effects that individuals with ID often experience.

The Sociocultural Model

Theorists have found that a person who is classified "mentally re-tarded" is more likely to be exposed to an excessive number of negative social experiences relative to a person of normal functioning (Matson & Sevin, 1994). The considerable rejection by peers, restricted access to employment opportunities, and the labeling process may significantly affect that person's self image. It is therefore reasonable to assume that excessive exposure to economic and environmental deprivation may affect one's mental health. For example, in the general population, psychopathology has been linked to low socioeconomic status, poor family, and poor health status (Baumeister, 1988). With the additional stressors mentioned above, it seems likely that these factors would be even more detrimental for people suffering from developmental disabilities, particularly because these people may not be equipped with adequate coping measures to placate them.

DIAGNOSIS

The principle goals of diagnosis are to first identify the problem behavior(s), and determine the variables that maintain them (Matson et al., 2002). The process of diagnosing mental problems, however, is undoubtedly clouded by the presence of ID. A difficulty in extending the process of psychiatric diagnosis to people with severe ID is the traditional reliance of the process on clients' verbal report of their symptoms. To compensate for the ID clients' inability to describe symptoms, diagnosticians have had to rely heavily on direct observation and on the reports of informants such as parents, teachers, caseworkers, or staff (MacLean, 1993). Studies devoted to the ADD suggest that there is a tendency to under diagnose mental health disorders in persons with ID. This situation may be due, in part, to diagnostic overshadowing. Diagnostic overshadowing refers to the overlooking of emotional disturbances by clinicians because of the presence of significant cognitive deficits (Reiss, Levitan, & Szyszko, 1982). That is, some debilitating emotional problems may appear less significant and therefore left untreated when compared with the debilitating effects of ID (Reiss et al., 1982).

The current diagnostic reference tool for clinicians is the *Diagnostic and Statistical Manual of Mental Disorders IV—Text Revision* (American Psychiatric Association [APA], 2000), which provides specific diagnostic criteria for each psychological disorder. Although this reference tool is used worldwide, it may not be appropriate for diagnosing psychopathology in the ID population due to the reliance on self-report. For example, one diagnostic criterion for the presence of schizophrenia is "the presence of delusions or hallucinations." An individual with ID may not be able to verbally communicate or understand the concept of delusions or hallucinations, or they may not be able to verbally report their symptoms for these or other linguistic reasons. Although the latest version of the Diagnostic and Statistical Manual (DSM) contains fewer criteria that rely solely on self-report than the previous versions, methods for assessing psychopathology in people with severe development delays must be modified to improve diagnostic validity (Rush, Bowman, Eidman, & Toole, in press).

This section has provided a brief overview of possible causes for dual diagnosis. Another important area for development is the pragmatics on how to deal with these very disruptive problems, which can dramatically impede efforts at independent living. A good deal of research has been devoted to assessment and treatment. These topics will be covered next.

Assessment

The challenge of modifying methods of assessment for the ID population lies in training clinicians to focus on diagnostic criteria that can be measured and observed. Gilson and Levitas made modifications to the DSM-III-R for the purpose of assessing psychopathology in individuals with ID (primarily for adults with mild and moderate ID) (as noted by Aman, 1991a). Reportedly, the modified diagnostic criteria are useful as a screening tool to identify individuals who should be assessed further for a psychiatric disorder. However, the criteria are not intended to render a definitive diagnosis (Aman, 1991a). Although such modifications were made, individuals with developmental disabilities are still under-diagnosed in terms of psychopathology. This situation has been due in large part to the lack of adequate assessment tools designed for the ID population. However, over the past decade, there has been an emergence of scales developed specifically to screen for psychopathology in this population; thus the ability to conduct adequate assessments is improving (Rush et al., in press).

The DSM-IV-TR authors state that impairments in adaptive functioning, rather than a low IQ, are usually the presenting symptoms in individuals with ID. Adaptive functioning refers to how effectively individuals cope with common life demands and how well they meet the standards of personal independence expected of someone in their particular age group, sociocultural background, and community setting (APA, 2000). Recent advances in the assessment of individuals with developmental disabilities indicate that a multi-method approach should be utilized to assess the full range of psychopathology (i.e., mood, personality, social skills, and aberrant behavior—Reiss, 1993). Specifically, when assessing an individual with developmental disabilities, the assessment should include a review of the client's records, interviews, observations, and rating scales (Aman, 1991b; Reiss, 1993).

Review of Client Records

The first step of an assessment is typically to review the client's records. Record reviews for individuals living in a residential facility can be particularly useful, as one is often able to obtain information from the direct care staff reflecting the duration of the client's stay at the facility. Thus, patterns of behaviors and significant behavioral changes over time may be noted (Rush et al., in press). Data on past medical treatments, past behavior problems, and information on previous behavioral interventions (such as their subsequent effect on target behaviors) are all important information when assessing psychopathology in people with developmental delays. For example, if a patient has no history of maladaptive behaviors, but upon arriving at a new environment began showing signs of depression, their behaviors may be attributed to temporary adjustment issues rather than signs of chronic psychopathology. However, it is important to note that data are often inconsistent and records may not always be complete. All reviews, therefore, should be interpreted with caution.

Interviews

Following a record review, interviews are typically conducted. The interviews are designed primarily to obtain additional information concerning not only possible maladaptive behaviors, but also information regarding the individual's adaptive functioning (Rojahn & Tasse, 1996). Most interviews are done with the caregivers who know the client the best (i.e., parents, teachers, direct care-staff) and when possible, the client him or herself. However, given the limited verbal and conceptual skills of many clients, this assessment method may not be practical. Specific adaptive behavior data should include the individuals social skills (i.e., changes in interpersonal relationships, engagement in activities, etc.), communication skills (i.e., does the individual have a means of communicating), and daily living skills (changes in the ability to care for themselves, such as hygiene behaviors—Rush, et al., in press).

Observations

Observation methods play a crucial part in the assessment of psychopathology in individuals with developmental disabilities. As an assessment method it becomes more important because of the limitations noted in the previous paragraph. Before conducting an observation it is important to first identify and operationally define the behaviors one wishes to target. For example, if one is assessing an individual for depression, one may want to identify sleep patterns, eating behaviors, and mood (i.e., positive and negative affect) as the target behaviors to be observed (Rush et al., in press). In addition to identifying and defining the behaviors, it is also important to establish the rates of the behaviors. Low frequency behaviors, in particular, may not be seen during sessions, especially when the frequency is equal to or lower than once per day. High frequency behaviors, on the other hand, may be assessed in short observation periods. In addition, it is important to identify an observation schedule (continuous or sampling). A continuous schedule is one in which data is recorded throughout the day, with no interruptions. Outside of a residential facility however, this type of observation schedule may be unrealistic. Most often, a sampling schedule (where the target behavior is observed during a predefined time period or event period) is used (Rush et al., in press). Some observation methods are more time consuming and costly than others, but some of the more time consuming methods also provide rich information than others. Essentially, there are two main categories of observation methods: descriptive assessments and analogue functional analysis.

Descriptive assessments are based on direct observations in the natural environment. For example, a scatterplot analysis (Touchette, McDonald, & Langer, 1985) permits comparison of the occurrence of problem behavior with time of day and activity variables. Each occurrence of the target behavior is plotted on a grid with the time of day on the ordinate and consecutive days on the abscissa. Patterns of behavior may be identified upon examination of the grid. In addition, there is the antecedent-behavior-consequence (ABC) assessment (Bijou, Peterson, & Ault, 1968) which requires that each episode of the problem behavior and the environmental events that precede and follow the behavior be recorded. An ABC assessment is particularly useful when examining low frequency behaviors and behavior that occurs in bursts. Although descriptive assessments can be time consuming, the data can be very rich in content given that it's observed directly and in the natural environment. However, when direct observation of aberrant behavior is not possible, analogue functional analysis may provide useful information (Singh, Sood, Sonenklar, & Ellis, 1991).

Analogue functional analysis is the most empirically grueling method for determining consequences maintaining problem behaviors. The basis of this assessment is the experimental manipulation of specific variables in controlled settings. For example, during an analogue functional analysis session for attention, an experimenter presents a series of tasks to the client; 30 s of attention is then provided, contingent on the problem behavior. A control condition would also be presented. The idea would be to see if attention is reinforcing or maintaining the problem behavior. This methodology generally has been demonstrated to be highly effective in identifying variables maintaining problem behavior and in facilitating treatment selection (Iwata et al., 1994). An analogue functional assessment, however, is very time consuming and costly. In addition, when behaviors are of high intensity (i.e., risk of injury), an analogue functional analysis may not be ethically appropriate as the individual is exposed to conditions that may increase the frequency of the behavior (Sturmey, 1995; Vollmer & Smith, 1996). While the benefits of conducting analogue functional analyses generally outweigh the disadvantages, many of the limitations could be circumvented if brief yet valid functional assessments could be identified (Vollmer, Iwata, Zarcone, Smith, & Mazaleski, 1993; Yarbrough & Carr, 2000). These concerns have led to the development of functional assessment rating scales.

Functional Assessment Rating Scales

Behaviors such as aggression, self-injury, stereotypy, and property destruction are often displayed by individuals with a dual diagnosis, and these same behaviors can be treated effectively if enough information about the problem is obtained prior to the intervention. As explained above, the two main categories of observation methods are descriptive assessments and analogue functional analysis. Although these can provide rich feedback, a third way of gathering important data is by using functional assessment rating scales. For example, some individuals engage in dangerous behaviors because it frequently results in positive reinforcement, such as tangible items, or attention (Vollmer et al., 1993). Rigorous experimental analyses have confirmed that learned behavioral functions can be the reasons why a behavior is occurring for a given individual, however, many practitioners do not have the needed time, training, personnel, or resources to conduct in-vivo experimental analyses. An alternative may be to obtain as much information as possible in a short time period, and then begin testing the effects of the interventions based on hypothesized behavioral functions (Matson, Bamburg, Cherry, & Paclawskyj, 1999). In other words, gathering ratings is not necessarily sufficient to establish a basis for treatment selection, but can decrease the number of plausible hypotheses to be explored prior to selection. Rating scales are a form of indirect assessment and are administered to a third party who is most familiar with the client. Some rating scales allow clients to complete the scales themselves, assuming they have the ability to self-report. These assessments are usually interviews or checklists and are quick and easy to administer. Three functional assessment scales described below: the functional analysis checklist (FAC), the motivation assessment scale (MAS), and the questions about behavioral function (QABF).

Van Houten and Rolider (1991) presented information on the FAC. The FAC is a 15-item questionnaire covering the following subscales as functions of behavior: physical environment (e.g., crowding), adjunctive behaviors (excessive and persistent behaviors that occur as a side effect of reinforcement), transitions between activities, escape demand, and positive reinforcement. The FAC is broad in content as to the possible environmental events that may control aberrant behavior, but has been found to have poor interrater reliability when evaluated by independent researchers (Sturmey, 1994). The FAC may be completed more accurately for more salient, frequent behaviors rated by raters who are more skilled than institutional staff (Sturmey, 1994), however, it is not as widely known as the MAS.

Until recently, the MAS by Durand and Crimmins (1988) had been the most extensively evaluated psychometric instrument for functional assessment (Sturmey, 1994). The MAS is a 16-item questionnaire that addresses four subscales: attention, escape, tangibles, and sensory consequences. Initial psychometric properties seemed to be strong, however, later studies failed to replicate the robustness of the MAS (Sturmey, 1994). Newton and Sturmey (1991) scored interrater reliability ranging from 0.25 to 0.70 and the internal consistency of the scales proved to be poor. Crawford, Brockel, Schauss, and Miltenberger (1992) also found evidence that this poor reliability might be reflected in validity problems. They found that the MAS uniformly cited sensory consequences as the likely motivator for all subjects, whereas analogue baselines yielded a much more diverse range of consequences (Crawford et al., 1992). Due to the abundance of problems associated with the psychometric properties of the MAS, its use should be regarded with some caution (Spreat & Connelly, 1996; Sturmey, 1994). The QABF, which is of much more recent origin, has shown consistent results on reliability and validity tests and seems more promising (Matson, Bamburg, et al., 1999; Paclawskyj, Matson, Rush, Smalls, & Vollmer, 2000).

The QABF is a beginning point in the development of behavioral interventions. This 25-item scale is designed to address known potential behavioral functions, identified from a review of previous literature. The QABF identifies five subscales: attention, escape, nonsocial, physical, and tangible. An example of an escape item on the QABF is "Engages in the behavior when asked to do something (get dressed, brush teeth, work, etc.)." Recently researchers have shown that the QABF is a reliable tool, in terms of test-retest and interrater reliability (Paclawskyj et al., 2000). Consequently, the knowledge gained from the administration of the QABF can be used to aid in the development of a behavioral treatment plan that specifically targets the functions of the maladaptive behaviors, thereby decreasing the behaviors themselves.

As explained above, functional assessment rating scales were developed because they are considerably less expensive and less time consuming than other methods of functional analysis. This can be a great asset to researchers and clinicians. For example, when the patient is a serious danger to him or herself, it is imperative to obtain as much information about the individual as quickly as possible. What may take as long as 3 months with an analogue functional assessment procedure (i.e., honing of a causal hypothesis), the same results may be found within minutes, hours, or days with one of the functional analysis checklists mentioned above. Clearly, checklists such as the QABF are currently the most popular method of assessing the function of an individual's behavior.

Although functional analysis rating scales are used frequently worldwide, rating scales are also one of the most widely used methods for assessing psychopathology in individuals with and without developmental disabilities (Rush et al., in press). They are considerably less expensive than using the direct observation methods described above, however, it is imperative that rating scales are not used exclusively to make diagnostic decisions. The dual diagnosis rating scales described below are the psychopathology instrument for mentally retarded adults (PIMRA), the DASH-II, the aberrant behavior checklist (ABC), the ADD, and the Reiss screen for maladaptive behavior.

Rating Scales for Assessing Psychopathology

The PIMRA (Matson, Kazdin, & Senatore, 1984; Senatore, Matson, & Kazdin, 1985) was the first measure of psychopathology developed specifically for use for persons with ID. The PIMRA consists of 56 items, and conforms to the DSM-III diagnostic criteria. Validity studies examining the PIMRA suggest that test–retest reliability and internal consistency are favorable for both versions (Balboni, Battagliese, & Pedrabissi, 2000; Linaker, 1991; Matson et al. 1984; Sturmey & Ley, 1990), however, the

PIMRA does not cover the broad range of disorders in the current DSM-IV, and therefore should be considered outdated.

The DASH was originally developed to answer the need for a measure of psychopathology for individuals with severe and profound levels of MR. This scale has been revised, with the most recent version being the DASH-II. Convergent validity was established by deriving disorder subscales from individual items from the APA's Diagnostic and Statistical Manual 4th Edition (DSM-IV), and from many previous studies of this population (Matson et al., 1999). In addition, rating criteria for individual dimensions were defined in terms of specific frequency, duration, and severity levels, rather than simply presence or absence of behaviors or subjective estimates of symptom severity as in previous scale development. The DASH-II consists of 84 items representing 13 diagnostic categories: anxiety, depression, mania, autism and other pervasive developmental disorders, schizophrenia, stereotypies, self-injurious behavior, elimination disorders, eating disorders, sleep disorders, sexual disorders, organic syndromes, impulse control, and other miscellaneous behaviors. The scale is administered in interview format and subsequent studies suggest that the scale is a valid measure for screening for psychopathology in individuals with developmental delays (Matson et al., 1999; Matson & Smiraldo, 1997; Matson, Smiraldo, & Hastings, 1998; Paclawskyj, Matson, Bamburg, & Baglio, 1997). Investigations of interrater and test–retest reliability indicate that the scale possesses adequate reliability for the frequency and duration dimensions, while kappa values for items on the severity dimensions were low (Sevin, Matson, Williams, & Kirkpatrick-Sanchez, 1995). Overall, internal consistency for the scale was high (Matson, Bamburg, et al., 1999).

Another measure used to assess psychopathology among those in the severe to profound range of ID is the ABC (Aman, Singh, Stewart, & Field, 1985). The ABC consists of 58 items, all of which were empirically derived by factor analysis so that it would be statistically valid. The following subscales are identified through factor analysis: (1) Irritability, (2) Lethargy, (3) Stereotypic Behavior, (4) Hyperactivity, and (5) Inappropriate Speech. Internal consistency, test–retest reliability, and interrater reliability have all been found acceptable (Aman, 1991a). Unlike the DASH-II, the ABC was empirically derived with the specific purpose of assessing treatment effects (i.e., behavioral intervention or medication) on behavior. Internal consistency, test–retest reliability, and interrater reliability have all been found acceptable (Aman, 1991a).

Although instruments such as the DASH-II and the ABC have proven useful in screening psychopathology in individuals with severe and profound ID, a scale was needed to screen psychopathology in the mild and moderate ranges. The ADD contains 79 items and the informant is asked to rate the frequency, severity, and duration of each item in an interview style format. The following subscales are measured on the ADD: mania, depression, anxiety, posttraumatic stress disorder, substance abuse, somatoform disorders, dementia, conduct disorder, pervasive developmental disorder, schizophrenia, personality disorders, eating disorders, and sexual disorders. Preliminary investigations into the psychometric proper-ties of the ADD have indicated acceptable levels on measures of internal consistency, high inter-rater and test–retest reliability and good concur-rent validity (Matson & Bamburg, 1998; Paclawskyj et al., 1997).

In addition to the scales described above, the Reiss screen for maladap-tive behavior was also developed to identify symptoms of psychopathology in adults and adolescents (Reiss, 1988). The Reiss Screen is a 36-item in-strument that is completed by caregivers, much like the scales described above. However, the Reiss screen is different from the previous scales in that the items in the Reiss screen correspond to behavioral dimensions rather than individual behaviors. For example, a factor analysis yielded the following seven factors: (1) aggressive behavior, (2) psychosis, (3) paranoia, (4) depression (behavior signs), (5) depression (physical signs), (6) depen-dent personality disorder, and (7) avoidant personality disorder. It appears that the Reiss Screen may be most useful for identifying psychopathology in general as opposed to serving as a valid instrument for the provision of individual diagnosis (Aman, 1991b). Although Reiss (1988) reported that internal consistency and interrater reliability were adequate, other studies suggest that the subscales of the Reiss screen may lack construct validity (Sturmey & Bertman, 1994, but also see Reiss, 1997).

While quite a few scales have been designed to assess psychopathology in the ID population, there are other scales that are used in conjunction with these in order to produce a treatment plan that will best benefit the client. For example, previous studies have shown that increases in symp-toms of psychopathology predicted increases in negative social behaviors in individuals with ID (Duncan, Matson, Bamburg, Cherry, & Buckley, 1999, Singh & Winton, 1983). Additionally, social impairments have been closely linked to behavior problems such as aggression and self-injury (SIB) (Duncan et al., 1999). These findings suggest that the social competence of individuals with ID associated with co-morbid psychopathology can be en-hanced with social skills training, and this in turn may decrease maladap-tive behaviors such as aggression and SIB. The four social scales described below are the Matson evaluation of social skills in individuals with severe retardation (MESSIER), the social performance survey schedule (SPSS), the Vineland adaptive behavior scale (VABS), and the screening tool of feeding problems (STEP). The first three scales are frequently used to assess a client's social strengths and weaknesses for treatment purposes, and the last is used to screen for feeding problems.

The MESSIER (Matson, 1995) is an 85-item scale that pinpoints social behavior strengths and deficits in individuals with severe and profound ID. The MESSIER items are divided into six categories of social behavior in-cluding positive verbal, positive non-verbal, general positive, negative ver-bal, negative non-verbal, and general negative. Given that persons with ID are recognized as having rates of psychopathology four to five times higher than the general population, social skills become a particularly significant target for intervention. Specifically, the MESSIER helps in identifying pos-sible replacement behaviors, which may be viewed as the most important component of assessment.

The SPSS is a 57-item measure designed to assess strengths and deficits in higher order social skills in individuals with mild or moderate ID. The SPSS is broken up into four subscales: (1) appropriate social skills, (2) communication skills, (3) inappropriate assertion, and (4) sociopathic behavior. Much like the MESSIER, the SPSS can be an important means of identifying and addressing social skills as a significant component of a treatment program.

Finally, the VABS (Sparrow, Balla, & Cicchetti, 1984) is a widely used measure that identifies an individuals' strengths and weaknesses adaptively. The VABS has four domains: communication, daily living skills, socialization, and motor skills. These four domains can be scored separately and then integrated to form one final composite of the individuals' adaptive functioning level. Patterns of VABS domain scores have been researched in several studies and shown to bear correspondence to type of disabling condition (i.e., autism, ID, or both conditions), and to differing etiological syndromes (Hemphill, 1996; Rodrigue, Morgan, & Geffken, 1991; Szatmari, Archer, Fisman, Streiner, & Wilson, 1995), and hence these scores may complement and inform other diagnostic procedures.

As important as social and adaptive skills are to an individual's ability to integrate successfully into society, severe feeding problems displayed by individuals with developmental disabilities can greatly impede that individual's future success. One scale specifically designed to screen for feeding problems in individuals with ID is the STEP (Matson & Kuhn, 2001). The STEP is a measure designed to identify feeding and meal time behavior problems commonly exhibited by individuals with ID. The STEP separates feeding problems into five categories, including behaviors that place the individual at risk of aspiration, behaviors associated with selectively (e.g., food type selectivity, food texture selectivity), behavioral skill deficits and excesses (e.g., inability to chew, eating too rapidly), behaviors related to food refusal (e.g., pushing food away), and nutrition-related behavior problems (e.g., pica, eats too little—Matson et al., 2002). By identifying possible feeding problems and reducing them, other maladaptive behaviors that occur in synchrony may be modified in a desired direction or eliminated.

The development of appropriate and effective treatments for psychopathology is largely dependent on the accuracy of assessment to establish topography, frequency, severity, and function of the disorder and associated behaviors. The assessment process should incorporate diagnosis, functional assessment, establishment of replacement behaviors, evaluation of treatment effects, and evaluation of treatment-side effects (Matson et al., 2002). The rating scales mentioned above are all potentially useful tools utilized to assist professionals in completing the assessment process adequately and to aid in the development of well rounded treatment plans that help alleviate the occurrence of maladaptive behaviors in individuals with ID. Without reliable data on disorders, selection of target behaviors and appropriate treatment becomes a hit or miss proposition. The methods mentioned above are current state of the art tools in this regard. The remainder of this chapter will focus on the latest treatment options available for individuals with dual diagnosis individuals, and how these treatments compare in efficacy. In this section an attempt has been made to present the best data, based on methods available at present.

TREATMENT

From prevalence and case studies, it is evident that the full range of psychiatric disorders reported in the population at-large is also experienced by those with ID (Matson & Sevin, 1994). An abundance of scales addressing many assessment issues designed specifically for people with dual diagnosis have been created in the past decade, but a large void still lies in available treatment. Despite this, progress is evident and will be reviewed. The most recent treatment in the areas of depression, bipolar, anxiety, and schizophrenia will be covered next.

Major Depression

The occurrence of depression in individuals with dual diagnosis has been reported as far back as the late 19th century (Clouston, 1883; Hurd, 1888). In more recent studies, prevalence estimates of depression in the ID population have ranged from 0.9 to 3.2% (Corbett, 1979; Gotason, 1985; Lund, 1985). Yet, the literature on the identification of major depression in people with ID is limited, and it is especially limited in relation to those with moderate to profound levels of ID. Researchers have shown that the subjective complaints of major depression, such as guilt and suicidal ideations, are recognized in people with mild ID more so than in those functioning at lower levels of ID (Myers, 1998). Clearly, this limitation is due to the lack of communication skills among individuals functioning in these lower ranges. In order to treat mood disorders in these patients, clinicians must first recognize the symptoms of depression by substituting behavioral equivalents for the standard diagnostic criteria.

Major depression as described in the DSM-IV-TR (2000) is comprised of the following symptoms: depressive mood, loss of interest and/or pleasure, insomnia, impaired eating and weight changes, psychomotor retardation, psychomotor agitation, fatigue or loss of energy, diminished concentration or indecisiveness, recurrent thoughts of death, suicide, or suicide attempts, feelings of worthlessness or guilt, self-injurious behavior (SIB), and aggression. The diagnosis of major depression is made on the basis of a sustained mood change (depression or dysphoria) in conjunction with disturbances in sleep, appetite, psychomotor activity, energy, cognition, and thinking. In some cases, major depression is associated with marked anxiety, as well as panic attacks. Although it is difficult to diagnose a patient with severe ID using the criteria listed above, Sovner and Hurley (1983) propose that such criteria are adequate as long as they are used objectively and by familiar caretakers.

Dysthymic disorder is a chronic condition (of at least 2 years duration for adults, 1 year for children and adolescents) associated with depressed mood. Changes in energy level, sleep, appetite, and concentration are usually present, and other typical features include low self-esteem and feelings of hopelessness (APA, 2000). The relationship between major depression and dysthymic disorder is unclear; however, it is known that major depression may be superimposed on a dysthymic disorder. Also, in some cases, dysthymic disorder is a prodromal state, preceding bipolar disorder or recurrent major depression (Akiskal, 1983).

Very few large, controlled studies have been done regarding the treatment of depression in people with dual diagnosis. The literature consists predominantly of single case studies regarding pharmacological treatments and behavioral interventions. The study of antidepressants in particular seems to point in a multitude of directions regarding the efficacy of various drugs. For example, several researchers have published studies demonstrating the effectiveness of serotonin reuptake inhibitor antidepressants (SSRIs—Thompson, Hackenberg, & Schaal, 1991), while other studies report relative contradictions to the use of tricyclic antidepressants and monoamine oxidase inhibitors (MAOIs) (Adams, Kirowitz, & Ziskind, 1970). Mikkelsen, Albert, Emens, and Rubin (1997), Howland (1992), and yet others have reported that the anti-depressant fluoxetine appeared to be most effective (e.g., Weintraub & Evans, 1989). However, the generalizability of the studies has been limited due to lack of control. Among the most recent pharmacological studies for depression, two reports yielded positive findings for the use of antidepressant medication to treat depression (Ghaziuddin, Tsai, & Ghaziudden, 1991; Langee & Conlon, 1992). Even among the most recent studies, however, there are significant methodological flaws that preclude definitive statements about the efficacy of antidepressants for depression among those with ID (Matson et al., 2000). However, antidepressants are not the only pharmacological treatment for depression. For example, Sovner (1988) treated a 25-year-old woman with mild ID, using carbamazepine for major depressive disorder. Carbamazepine at therapeutic levels has resulted in the normalization of mood and sleep, and a decrease in SIB (Ruedrich, Des Noyers-Hurley, & Sovner, 2001).

Although quite a few studies have been conducted on pharmacological treatments for depression in the ID population, most of the studies mentioned above have not examined follow-up and drug side effects, leaving long term efficacy questionable. For example, case studies show that tricyclic antidepressants may adversely affect learning in persons with ID (Werry, 1980) and may predispose an individual with brain damage to the development of delirium (Lipowski, 1987). In addition, tricyclic antidepressants have been thought to possibly lower seizure threshold, which may be dangerous for individuals with epilepsy. Sovner et al. (1998) have recommended choosing an antidepressant based on a number of factors: a biological relative with prior good response to a particular drug, the need to determine adequacy of response via blood level side effect profiles, consideration of possible drug–drug interactions, and history of previous response to a specific medication. Essentially, given the mixed outcomes in research, the use of antidepressants appear to be a questionable intervention for individuals with ID suffering from major depression, but until further studies incorporate adequate methodological controls, it will be difficult to draw firm conclusions as to their overall or idiosyncratic value.

Behavior modification procedures are a growing area of interest when it comes to individuals with ID suffering from major depression. Specifically, individuals with mild to moderate ID have been effectively treated in single case studies and demonstrated positive treatment effects using a "package" including modeling, role playing, performance feedback, instructions, and social reinforcement for the treatment of depression (Davis, Judd, & Herrman, 1997). In one of these studies, Matson, Dettling, and Senatore (1981) reported the first case of behavioral treatment for depression for an individual with borderline to mild ID. Using an ABA design, positive self-statements and feedback regarding depressive behaviors helped to reduce symptoms of depression (i.e., suicidality). Later, Matson (1982) again demonstrated the success of behavioral modification procedures using a multiple baseline across subjects design with four depressed individuals diagnosed with mild to moderate ID. All participants showed a significant decrease in depressive behaviors. Based on this limited data, behavioral and cognitive therapy may have value in modifying depressive behaviors in individuals with mild or moderate ID, but more research is needed to assess the utility of these treatments with individuals functioning in lower intellectual ranges. It is disappointing that in the last 20 years so little attention to these issues has been given by researchers.

In addition to psychopharmacological and behavioral interventions, several groups have published case reports describing successful treatment using electroconvulsive therapy (ECT) for depression in individuals with ID. ECT is a method generally used for severely depressed patients in the population at large, for whom other forms of intervention have not been successful. Essentially, the ECT procedure consists of an electrical current that is passed through the brain, inducing a grand mal seizure. During the seizure there are a series of changes in brain waves that influence the individual's depressed affect. There are relatively few side effects, but scientists are still unsure as to why this procedure works. Although this may be a last resort for many clients, research does not fully support treatment with ECT in patients with ID, as few case reports clearly document which symptoms improve with treatment (Davis et al., 1997).

As an additional strategy for finding the right treatment for a client, it is important for the clinician to take into account specific emotional stressors that may leave the client predisposed to depression. For example, Cochran, Sran, and Varano (1977) described the "relocation syndrome" in five handicapped individuals who became depressed following transfer from a large to a smaller institution. Cohen, Conroy, Frazer, Snelbecker, and Spreat (1977) also systematically studied the effects of deinstitutionalization on 92 handicapped persons. They found the higher functioning clients became withdrawn (possibly related to depression) following their discharge into the community. Although little research has been done on the phenomenon of relocation influences on affect, it is no surprise that emotional stressors may take more a toll on those that are not as easily able to cognitively deal with them.

The need to fill the void of treatment for those individuals with ID afflicted with depression is still great, but two important conclusions may be drawn from the research to date. First, the drugs used to curb emotional problems of individuals with normal development may work with the ID population as well, however, more controlled studies are needed; and second, behavior modification procedures are of considerable merit in treating these problems (Matson, 1985). Therefore, studies which combine both behavior modification and pharmacological interventions may show the greatest promise.

Bipolar Disorder

Bipolar disorder is often characterized by recurrent episodes of mania and major depression interspersed with periods of normal affective functioning (Whybrow, Akiskal, & McKinney, 1984; Winokur, Clayton, & Reich, 1969). During the manic episodes, the individual will usually show a sharp increase in activity, and if the individual is thwarted, bursts of extreme irritation often arise. The manic person has a great deal of energy and requires few, if any, hours of sleep. If the individual is verbal, the pressure of speech is usually rapid and voluble, and the train of thought slips from one idea to another, usually described as a "flight of ideas." In addition, the manic individual is easily distracted. Depressive episodes in bipolar disorder are often associated with hypersomnia (i.e., dramatic increases in time spent sleeping) and psychomotor retardation and tend to be more frequent than in unipolar depression (Kupfer et al., 1972).

The DSM-IV-TR (2000) divides bipolar disorder into four categories: Bipolar I Disorder, Bipolar II Disorder, Cyclothymic Disorder, and Bipolar Disorder Not Otherwise Specified. Bipolar I is distinguished from Bipolar II by the presence of one or more Manic or Mixed Episodes. In Cyclothymic Disorder, there are numerous periods of hypomanic symptoms that do not meet criteria for a Manic Episode and periods of depressive symptoms that do not meet symptom or duration criteria for a Major Depressive Episode. Finally, a diagnosis of Bipolar Disorder Not Otherwise Specified may be made if there is a very rapid alternation (over days) between manic symptoms and depressive symptoms (e.g., several days of purely manic symptoms followed by several days of depressive symptoms) that do not meet minimal duration criteria for a Manic Episode or Major Depressive Episode (APA, 2000).

The prevalence of bipolar disorder among people with dual diagnosis is not low according to the literature. Much early as well as more recent research on depression of persons with ID focuses on bipolar (i.e., manic depressive illness) disorders (Carlson, 1979; Reid, 1972, 1976; Reid, Ballinger, & Heather, 1978; Roith, 1961). This focus may be due to the often greater severity of symptomology and the concomitant psychosis, as well as the overt nature of the mood swings that are associated with this disorder (Reynolds & Baker, 1988). Although the focus on bipolar disorder has increased in the past years, prevalence estimates continue to vary, and flaws in methodology limit conclusions that may be drawn.

Treatment of bipolar disorder has also been studied extensively over the past few decades. The most prevalent pharmacological breakthrough in the treatment of bipolar disorder, was the discovery of lithium. In 1949, Cade introduced the use of lithium salts to quiet agitated manic states, however, it took 20 years before a technology was developed to manage lithium's toxicity. Naylor, Donald, Poidevin, and Reid, (1974) studied 14 patients over a 2-year-period and found that lithium was useful in the treatment of patients with dual diagnosis and frequently recurring affective changes or recurrent behavioral changes. Rivenus and Harmatz (1979) described a 3-year single-blind placebo-controlled trial of lithium in five institutionalized patients with ID and bipolar disorder. They concluded that the recurrence of both manic and depressive symptoms was reduced by treatment with lithium. By contrast, Glue (1989) found lithium alone ineffective for treatment of a rapid cycling affective illness. However, he found a better response with a combination of lithium and carbamazepine. Other studies have described the efficacy of carbamazepine for treatment of mild hypomania, but do not report its effect on the depressed phase of a mood disorder. In addition, the literature also suggests valproate as an effective treatment for bipolar disorder. Specifically, Kastner, Finesmith, and Walsh (1993) reported an open trial of valproic acid in the treatment of behavioral problems and affective symptoms in individuals with ID and reported that irritability, sleep problems, aggressive orSIB, and behavior cycling improved with long-term valproic acid therapy. Finally, in a recent 10 year review of psychopharmacology in ID, one well controlled study indicated that depakote was effective in lessening symptoms associated with mania (e.g., lack of sleep; pacing) and effectively reduced the frequency and severity of self-injury (Matson et al., 2000). In essence, lithium has become the primary long-term treatment for individuals with ID and bipolar disorder for years, but due to the potential lethality of the drug, scientists are searching for a successful alternative.

The most recent developments in the treatment of bipolar disorders have been the use of newer antiepileptics, specifically lamotrigine, gabapentin, and atypical antispychotics (particularly clozapine—Buzan, Dubrovski, Firestone, & Dal Pozzo, 1998; Mikkelsen & McKenna, 1999; Pary, 1994; Ruben & Langa, 1995; Silka & Hurley, 1998). With respect to clozapine, no specifics were provided regarding treatment response, but the authors saw clozapine as safe and effective in the larger group (Ruedrich et al., 2001).

Research on behavioral interventions in the treatment of bipolar disorder in people with ID is virtually nonexistent; however, the psychotherapy for bipolar disorder and mania represents a new frontier in treatment. Interpersonal and social rhythm therapy has been a successful treatment approach with some individuals with mild ID (Frank, Matson, & Ritenour, 1997). Through this therapy, the patient is able to discuss ongoing interpersonal problems, understand the disorder and grieve the illness, and deal with the denial that occurs in many patients in the less severe ranges of ID (Ruedrich et al., 2001).

For patients in the severe to profound range of ID, a concomitant increase in aggression or self-injury may coincide with cycling (Hanzel, Johnson, Harder & Kalachnik, 1999; King & McCartney, 1999; Lowry 1997, 1998). Although the influence of stressful events has been associated with depression, it is not as strongly correlated with bipolar disorder. Nevertheless, stronger ties can be made in the individual's support group, stability can be improved in the individual's daily schedule, and the overall environment of the individual can be modulated to become less stimulating or provocating. These strategies may, in addition to behavioral programs to address aggression and self-injury, be used as augmentation of pharmacotherapy and therapeutic support (Reudrich, 1993). Undoubtedly, more research is needed to assess the utility of behavioral and cognitive therapy in persons with developmental delays and bipolar disorder, especially in those with more severe levels of ID.

Anxiety Disorders

The study of anxiety in individuals with developmental disabilities is limited; however, some investigations indicate that individuals with ID respond to stress with higher levels of anxiety than others (Cochran & Cleland, 1963; Levine, 1985; Ollendick, Oswald, & Ollendick, 1993; Reiss, 1994; Stavrakaki, 1999; Szymanski & King, 1999). Past diagnostic criteria have relied heavily on reports of subjective experience by the subject, but subjective report is often totally or partially absent in the ID population. In the DSM-IV-TR, diagnostic criteria for various anxiety disorders range from subjective report to purely observable manifestations, whether behavioral or physiological. For example, a symptom such as "fear" may manifest as agitation, screaming, crying, withdrawal, freezing, or regressive clinging behavior (Khreim & Mikkelsen, 1997). With the help of rating scales that are sensitive to individuals with ID, the gap is slowly being bridged and more individuals with dual diagnosis are receiving treatment for their anxiety.

In the DSM-IV TR, anxiety disorders are broken down into 12 distinct categories; however, in studies with the ID population, the following five categories encompass most reports in the literature thus far: generalized anxiety disorder, obsessive-compulsive disorder (OCD), panic disorder, post-traumatic stress disorder (PTSD), and phobias.

Generalized anxiety disorder is characterized by excessive worry about multiple events or activities, with the individual finding it difficult to control his or her worries (Khreim & Mikkelsen, 1997). For individuals who are unable to voice their worries, this disorder is often associated with symptoms such as difficulty concentrating, irritability, insomnia, nausea, shortness of breath, and fatigue. The diagnostic criteria in the DSM-IV TR (2000) require the presence of these symptoms for a duration of at least 6 months, on more days than not. Although previous literature does suggest this specific disorder exists among this population, studies that support its existence are scarce.

OCD is characterized by repetitive intrusive thoughts, impulses, or images that are known as obsessions; or repetitive behaviors known as compulsions that are perceived as inappropriate and cause marked anxiety or distress (APA, 2000). The behavioral manifestations of this disorder can be quite observable, such as excessive hand washing, counting, hoarding, or ordering. It is important to add, however, that these manifestations may be misinterpreted. In addition, it is not uncommon for individuals with dual diagnosis to engage in aggression or SIB when their ritualistic behavior is interrupted. Essentially, if a clinician is aware of this possible association, then these maladaptive behaviors may be decreased once the OCD is treated (Crabbe, 2001). To date, few reports in the literature cite the diagnosis of OCD among the people with developmental delays. However, whether this is a true estimate of the prevalence of this disorder, or a shortcoming of diagnostic practice remains to be seen.

Panic disorder is characterized by recurrent, unexpected panic attacks, followed by at least a 1-month period of persistent concern about having another panic attack. Research on panic disorders is sparse. In fact, the first published case of panic disorder and ID was by Khreim and Mikkelsen (1997). In this study, an individual with mild ID presenting with panic disorder without agoraphobia (fear of being in situations where escape may be difficult) was successfully treated with pharmacotherapy and psychotherapy.

Panic Disorders may be hard to identify in this population, but for the most part, the symptoms include nonspecific agitation, screaming, crying, or clinging (Khreim & Mikkelsen, 1997). Although these same symptoms may describe other anxiety disorders, generally, the manifestations of panic are easily observable, as they are more extreme in nature.

PTSD is the development of characteristic symptoms following exposure to an extreme traumatic stressor. This stressor may involve a direct experience such as witnessing an event that involves death, or an indirect experience such as learning about unexpected death. Essentially, PTSD is a condition that follows exposure to a trauma considered extremely emotional or life threatening. There are usually three clusters of symptoms associated with this disorder: first is increased arousal; second is the recurrent experiencing of the traumatic event through flashbacks, nightmares, or intrusive irresistible memories; and third is the avoidance of events, people, or situations that are related to the traumatic experience (Khreim & Mikkelsen, 1997). Although published data about this particular disorder is limited, Ryan (1994) proposes that the symptoms may be easiest to recognize in people with ID. Having said this, the general lack of professional interest in the topic has most certainly led to under-diagnosis and under-treatment of the problem when it does occur among people with ID in real world settings.

The last category of anxiety disorders cited in the literature are phobias. Vitiello and Behar (1992) suggest that phobias tend to occur more commonly in individuals with ID, relative to the general population. Phobias are usually characterized as avoidant behavioral symptoms preceded by an excessive irrational fear. Although there are many different types of phobias, the literature most often describes social and specific phobias (i.e., fear of spiders) as prevalent in this population (Crabbe, 2001). Despite this, diagnosis of phobic disorders with an individual with ID should rely on a variety of reliable observations because some characteristics of social phobia can superficially mimic withdrawal secondary to psychosis.

Although there is not a great deal of literature on the diagnosis of anxiety disorders in people with developmental delays, more research efforts have been allocated toward the treatment of these disorders. In general, the treatment of anxiety disorders in individuals with ID entails psychotherapeutic, behavioral therapy, relaxation training, and pharmacological approaches.

Psychotherapy in the treatment of anxiety disorders has received minimal attention in the literature, despite literature reviews on the general use and modification of psychotherapeutic techniques suited for persons with ID (Chandler 1989; Van Bourgandien 1989). In the treatment of adults with mild and moderate ID, Matson and Senatore (1981) have demonstrated the superiority of behavioral therapy over group psychotherapy in improving interpersonal functioning. Naturally, in individuals with more severe deficits in communication, psychotherapy (which usually relies on a great deal of self reflection) would be a very benign form of treatment. However, there is literature that indicates the importance of education, reassurance, and support during stressful times, and psychotherapy has been shown to make a difference for some individuals with dual diagnosis (Crabbe, 2001). Given the lack of literature on the topic, a great deal of additional research is warranted.

Behavior therapy applied in the treatment of an individual with dual diagnosis and an anxiety disorder has proven successful. Particularly in the treatment of specific phobias, a procedure known as systematic desensitization has been particularly successful. Systematic desensitization has been defined as "gradually exposing patients (in imagination or in vivo) to a graded hierarchy of anxiety-provoking stimuli while maintaining a state of calm through deep muscle relaxation or a variety of other methods applied to induce a countering relaxation" (Nemiah & Uhde, 1989). Essentially, if an individual was afraid of spiders, a clinician may utilize systematic desensitization by first asking the individual to think of spiders, then to look at pictures of spiders, then to draw a spider, then to see a live spider, and finally to perhaps even touch a spider. Several authors have reviewed case studies exemplifying the successful use of behavioral desensitization procedures in the treatment of phobic disorders in persons with ID (Hurley & Sovner, 1982; McNally & Ascher, 1987).

Behavior therapy also has advantages over psychotherapy in the treatment of OCD in adults with developmental delays. Matson (1982) employed an in vivo exposure technique with three adults with ID. In vivo exposure is a technique in which some form of reinforcement is used to shape appropriate behavior. In the study done by Matson (1982), there was differential reinforcement of noncompulsive ritualistic behavior by the use of tokens. When a compulsive behavior was displayed, an overcorrection procedure was implemented as a method of response prevention. This behavioral treatment, which included both operant and respondent components, was successful in these cases.

Relaxation training as a form of behavioral therapy is characterized by its focus on self-regulation strategies for reducing physiological arousal and anxiety (Crabbe, 2001). There are numerous types of techniques. However, Rickard (1986) commented on the limitations of certain relaxation training techniques for people with moderate, severe, and profound levels of ID. As a result, some techniques have been modified. For example, by using concrete images such as squeezing and letting go of a lemon, differentiation between muscle tension and relaxation in their upper extremities may be facilitated. Other forms of relaxation training include diaphragmatic breathing, imagery conditioning, biofeedback training, and can occur within the course of music therapy, art therapy, hydrotherapy, music therapy, or physical therapy.

Pharmacological treatment of anxiety disorders in the population at large has been extended to serve the ID population as well. Unfortunately, however, while there are no controlled clinical trials addressing this specific population, clinical observations and data suggest similarities in the efficacy of the same medications used in the general population in serving the people who are dually diagnosed (Khreim & Mikkelsen, 1997). Selective serotonin reuptake inhibiters (SSRIs) are known to be quite successful in the treatment of panic disorder, social phobia, generalized anxiety disorder, PTSD, and OCD (Crabbe, 2001). In addition, buspirone has proven to have well-established anxiolytic effects. Although buspirone has been used to treat generalized anxiety disorder in the ID population, it can also be used to treat panic disorder and OCD. Buspirone is considered to be a better alternative than some benzodiazepines used for anxiety disorders because they demonstrate no hard evidence of causing motor or cognitive impairment that can occur with benzodiazepines (Crabbe, 2001).

Benzodiazepines are still the most commonly prescribed anxiolytic however, despite the vast number of side effects that may occur after long term use (Khreim & Mikkelsen, 1997). They are more likely suited for treatment of short-term situational anxiety. Alprazolam (Xanax), for example, is effective in treating sudden panic attacks and agoraphobia. Clonazepam (Klonopin) is also effective in treating panic disorder, social phobia, and OCD (Khreim & Mikkelsen, 1997).

Mood stabilizers are another pharmacological treatment that has proven successful in the past. For example, mood stabilizers such as divalproex (Depakote) or carbamazepine (Tegretol) can help in cases of panic disorder, OCD, and PTSD (Khreim & Mikkelsen, 1997). Finally, a number of controlled studies in the general population have shown that clomipramine, a tricyclic psychoactive compound, has proven promising in patients with OCD (Deveaugh-Geis, Landau, & Katz, 1989; Rapoport, 1988).

Along with the use of neuroleptic medications come a number of possible side effects. It should come as no surprise then that many researchers believe that organic anxiety can be caused by the use of neuroleptics and neuroleptic withdrawal syndromes. Akathisia is an extrapyramidal side effect of antipsychotic drug therapy characterized by motor restlessness, pacing, and agitation, and is accompanied by feelings of intense anxiety, internal distress, and dysphoria (Crabbe, 2001). More recently, the term "tardive akathesia" has been used to describe a clinical phenomenon that sometimes emerges during long-term neuroleptic therapy or when the medication is tapered off or discontinued (Barnes & Braude, 1985; Crabbe, 1994; Gualtieri & Sovner, 1989). Tardive akathesia is characterized by motor restlessness, anxiety, increase in severity and frequency of maladaptive behaviors, and sleep disturbances (Branford & Hutchins, 1996; Gross, Hull, Lytton, Hill, & Piersel, 1993). The possibility of developing any form of akathisia should be taken into account by clinicians, particularly when administering neuroleptic medication. A frequent recommendation of psychopharmacological experts in ID is that neuroleptic tapering should be accomplished with minimal dosages over months to years (Crabbe, 2001), in order to diminish the likelihood of side effects.

Although many forms of treatment exist in the realm of psychopharmacology, controlled studies measuring the efficacy of these drugs in terms of long term and withdrawal effects is desperately needed. In addition, studies done on the general population suggest that psychopharmacology alone is not always sufficient; and in many cases, a combination of psychopharmacology and behavioral therapy is most successful.

Essentially, with more controlled research on anxiety disorders specific to this population on the horizon, multimodal treatment plans that incorporate the advantages of many different therapies may be the best method to enhance the lives of the people with dual diagnosis.

Schizophrenia

While historical references to schizophrenia can be traced back to ancient times (Shapiro, 1981), systematic conceptualizations of the disorder were initially formulated in the early nineteenth century, when physicians used terms such as "insanity" and "dementia" to characterize psychiatric patients. Emil Kraeplin, a German psychiatrist, is one of the most prominent figures in the development of what is now known as schizophrenia. He presented the first comprehensive description of the disorder in 1898, and made a clear distinction between schizophrenia and other mental illnesses.

Historically, dual diagnosis of schizophrenia and ID has been a source of controversy and debate in the clinical literature (Turner, 1989). Many have questioned the reliability of a diagnosis of schizophrenia in persons with ID, especially those with the inability to communicate verbally. Schizophrenia is a disturbance that lasts for at least 6 months and includes at least 1 month of the following active-phase symptoms (i.e., two or more): delusions, hallucinations, disorganized speech, and grossly disorganized or catatonic behavior (APA, 2000). Since deficits in language may hamper self-reports of delusions and hallucinations, which are two of the most common diagnostic criteria of schizophrenia, many are unsure about the reliability of a diagnosis of schizophrenia in an individual with ID. Some clinicians emphasize the need to be very cautious in diagnosing a patient with ID who displays bizarre behavioral symptoms with a psychotic disorder, because such behaviors may be due to other neurological abnormalities frequently encountered in persons with ID. However, other clinicians refute these views. Wright (1982) reported a 1.8% prevalence rate of schizophrenia in institutionalized individuals with ID, while figures at the other end of the spectrum are 14% (Eaton & Menolascino, 1982). Perhaps the most persistent prevalence rate found in the literature is 3% and this figure has become widely accepted as the most accurate rate of the number of people with schizophrenia within the ID population. Although this rate may be the most widely accepted, the main point to be made is that the reported prevalence rates for schizophrenia in the population of persons with ID generally exceed the prevalence estimates reported for those of normal intelligence, which have ranged from 0.6 to 3% (Singh & Katz, 1989).

Because research has shown that there is a very strong biological basis for schizophrenia, antipsychotic agents have been the primary treatment for this and other psychoses. In the past years, antipsychotics such as haloperidol and thioridazine have been used to reduce the number of symptoms associated with schizophrenia in individuals with ID (Menolascino et al., 1986). Unfortunately, drugs such as these (known as the typical antipsychotic drugs) have proven to have adverse side effects and may even impair some aspects of cognition (Menolascino et al., 1986). Due to medical and ethical concerns, drug treatment of schizophrenia is changing. The discovery of clozapine and other drugs, have shown better results than the previous treatments with fewer side effects (Pary, 1994). These new "non-toxic" drugs are known as atypical antipsychotics, and due to seemingly fewer adverse side effects, are quickly replacing the typical antipsychotic agents as the drugs of choice in treating schizophrenia. Some of the newer atypicals include: risperidone, olanzapine, sertindole, quetiapine, and ziprasidone.

Risperidone is more effective than a placebo and as effective as haloperidol in the treatment of chronic schizophrenia, according to Marder and Meibach (1994). Numerous studies have shown that risperidone reduces total symptom scores by as much as 20%. Olanzapine has showed similar results. A large multi-center study comparing olanzapine with haloperidol found significantly greater reductions in total and positive scores on psychiatric rating scales for olanzapine (Menolascino et al., 1986). In addition, sertindole, quetiapine and ziprasidone all have reduced symptoms significantly in patients with schizophrenia and ID (Menolascino et al., 1986). Finally, as mentioned earlier, clozapine has been successful in treating even treatment-resistant schizophrenia (Ruben & Langa, 1995). The reasons why some patients fail to respond to traditional antipsychotics include poor compliance, substance misuse, and a range of psychosocial factors. Even when these reasons are excluded or reduced, there remain 30% of patients who derive little benefit from conventional therapy (Kane & Smith, 1982). Clozapine, however, is particularly efficacious with these patients (Ruben & Langa, 1995).

The undisputed advantage of atypical over the typical antipsychotics is their lack of neurological side effects. The literature suggests that clozapine, for example, can cause relatively minor side-effects, some of which can be prevented by blood monitoring (Ruben & Langa, 1995). However, because the emergence of atypical antipsychotics is relatively new, whether these drugs have serious long-term side effects (e.g., tardive dyskinesia) has yet to be seen.

Studies on behavioral interventions for patients with schizophrenia and ID are not as numerous as the pharmacological interventions described above. However, because many of the symptoms of schizophrenia include unrealistic notions, behavioral treatments often incorporate reality based training. Other forms of social skills training are also used to help the individual cope with his or her mental illness; however, for patients with more severe forms of ID, these interventions may not offer any benefit. In any case, informing the family of the symptoms of the illness and building a support group for the client can make a difference. Often, a combined treatment package of both pharmacological and behavioral techniques achieves a profound impact on the life of the individual.

SUMMARY

The mental health of individuals with ID has become a critical clinical issue in the past few decades. Although at one time there was speculation among clinicians about whether the co-occurrence of ID and mental illness actually existed, it has now become clear that it is an abundant problem that demands immediate attention. Indeed, mental disorders are actually more common among individuals with ID than those without. Increased risk for these disorders has been linked to the presence of significant brain damage evident among individuals with ID, the co-incidence of sensory impairment and seizure disorders, aberrant behavior associated with genetic syndromes, and atypical social and emotional experiences associated with delayed development (Matson, 1985).

In the last 20 years, great strides have been made in providing mental health services to the developmentally delayed. Specifically, researchers have compiled a plethora of assessment tools that are sensitive to this particular population. With these tools, clinicians have found a way of extending the diagnostic process to include those who are not able to verbally communicate their needs. Diagnosticians are now able to rely heavily on direct observation and on the reports of informants to assess the needs of an individual with ID. Rating scales in particular have provided a means of screening individuals for psychological services, identifying the broad range of maladaptive behaviors that the people with dual diagnosis often exhibit, and ultimately helping to create a treatment plan that addresses the individual's mental health needs.

Researchers have also made great bounds in treatment options for the people with dual diagnosis. Pharmacotherapy and behavioral interventions in particular have been most utilized. Although benefits have been found for the use of many antipsychotic drugs, adverse side-effects and long-term effectiveness are two ethical issues that must be taken into consideration.

More research is still needed in order to find the most efficacious, yet least restrictive treatment for mental disorders among individuals with ID.

Despite the growing spotlight shone on this particular population, problems continue to persist in terms of conceptual as well as measurement issues. For example, the most current diagnostic manual, although an improvement from the past versions, continues to inadequately address the mental disorders occurring among the population with more severe ID. In addition, there remains some question as to whether the behavioral characteristics of persons with severe ID represent psychopathology or demonstrates deficits in behavioral competence. Thus, more controlled research is needed to establish a greater distinction between ID and coexisting mental disorders, so that one does not overshadow the other. Although steps have been taken and the road has been paved, more work is needed to ensure that the path ahead remains clear of any obstruction that may deter the scientific community from aiding those individuals with ID in need of mental health services.

REFERENCES

Adams, G. L., Kirowitz, J., & Ziskind, E. (1970). Manic depressive psychosis, mental retardation, and chromosomal rearrangement. *Archives of General Psychiatry, 23,* 305–309.

Akiskal, H. S. (1983). Dysthymic disorder: Psychopathology of proposed chronic depressive subtypes. *American Journal of Psychiatry, 140,* 11–20.

Aman, M. G. (1991a). *Assessing psychopathology and behavior problems in persons with mental retardation: A review of available instruments.* Rockville, MD: U.S. Department of Health and Human Services.

Aman, M. G. (1991b). Review and evaluation of instruments for assessing emotional and behavioral disorders. *Australia and New Zealand Journal of Developmental Disabilities, 17,* 41–57.

Aman, M. G., Singh, N. N., Stewart, A. W., & Field, C. J. (1985). The aberrant behavior checklist: A behavior rating scale for the assessment of treatment effects. *American Journal of Mental Deficiency, 89*(5), 485–491.

American Psychiatric Association. (2000). *Diagnostic and statistical manual of mental disorders* (4th ed., Text-Revision). Washington, DC: American Psychiatric Association.

Balboni, G., Battagliese, G., & Pedrabissi, L. (2000). The psychopathology inventory for mentally retarded adults: Factor structure and comparisons between subjects with or without dual diagnosis. *Research in Developmental Disabilities, 2,* 311–321.

Barnes, T. R. E., & Braude, W. M. (1985). Akathisia variants and tardive dyskinesia. *Archives of General Psychiatry, 42,* 874–878.

Baumeister, A. A. (1988). The new morbidity: Implications for prevention. In J. A. Stark, F. J. Menolascino, M. H. Albarelli, & V. C. Gray (Eds.), *Mental retardation and mental health: Classification, diagnosis, treatment, services* (pp. 71–80). New York: Springer-Verlag.

Bijou, S. W., Peterson, R. F., & Ault, M. H. (1968). A method to integrate descriptive and field studies at the level of data and empirical concepts. *Journal of Applied Behavior Analysis, 1,* 175–191.

Borthwick-Duffy, S. A. (1994). Epidemiology and prevalence of psychopathology in people with mental retardation. *Journal of Consulting and Clinical Psychology, 62,* 17–27.

Branford, D., & Hutchins, D. (1996). Tardive akathisia in people with mental retardation. *Journal of Developmental Disabilities, 8,* 117–132.

Buzan, R. D., Dubrovski S. L., Firestone, D., & Dal Pozzo, E. (1998). Use of clozapine in 10 mentally retarded adults. *Journal of Neuropsychiatry in Clinical Neuroscience, 10,* 93–95.

Campbell, M., Fish, B., Shapiro, T., & Floyd, A., Jr. (1970). Thiothixene in disturbed children. *Archives of General Psychiatry, 23,* 70–76.

Carlson, G. (1979). Affective psychosis in mental retardates. *Pediatric Clinics of North America,* 2, 499–510.

Chandler, M. (1989). Psychotherapy, in treatments of psychiatric disorders. In *A task force of the American Psychiatric Association* (pp. 108–111). Washington, DC: American Psychiatric Association.

Chess, S., & Hassibi, M. (1970). Behavior deviation in mentally retarded children. *Journal of the American Academy of Child Psychiatry,* 9, 282–297.

Clouston, T. S. (1883). *Clinical lectures on mental diseases.* London, UK: Churchill.

Cochran, J. L., & Cleland, C. C. (1963). Manifest anxiety of retardates and normals matched as to academic achievement. *American Journal of Mental Deficiency,* 67, 539–542.

Cochran, W. E., Sran, P. K., & Varano, G. A. (1977). The relocation syndrome in mentally retarded individuals. *Mental Retardation,* 15, 10–12.

Cohen, H., Conroy, J. W., Frazer, D. W., Snelbecker, G. E., & Spreat, S. (1977). Behavioral effects of interinstitutional relocation of mentally retarded residents. *American Journal of Mental Deficiency,* 82, 12–18.

Corbett, J. A. (1979). Psychiatric morbidity and mental retardation. In F. E. James & R. P. Snaith (Eds.), *Psychiatric illness and mental handicap* (pp. 11–25). London: Gaskell.

Crabbe, H. (1994). Pharmacotherapy in mental retardation. In N. Bouras (Ed.), *Mental health in mental retardation* (pp. 187–204). Cambridge, UK: Cambridge University Press.

Crabbe, H. F. (2001). Treatment of anxiety disorders in persons with mental retardation. In A. Dosen & K. Day (Eds.), *Treating mental illness and behavior disorders in children and adults with mental retardation* (pp. 227–241). Washington, DC: American Psychiatric Press.

Crawford, J., Brockel, B., Schauss, S., & Miltenberger, R. G. (1992). A comparison of methods for the functional assessment of stereotypic behavior. *Journal of the Association for Persons with Severe Handicaps,* 17(2), 77–86.

Davis, J. P., Judd, F. K., & Herrman, H. (1997). Depression in adults with intellectual disability: Part 1. A review. *Australian and New Zealand Journal of Psychiatry,* 31, 232–242.

Deveaugh-Geis, J., Landau, P., & Katz, R. J. (1989). Preliminary results from a multicenter trial of clomipramine in obsessive compulsive disorder. *Psychopharmacological Bulletin,* 25, 36–40.

Duncan, D., Matson, J. L., Bamburg, J. W., Cherry, K. E., & Buckley, T. (1999). The relationship of self-injurious behavior and aggression to social skills in persons with severe and profound learning disability. *Research in Developmental Disabilities,* 20, 441–448.

Durand, V. M., & Crimmins, D. B. (1988). Identifying the variables maintaining self-injurious behavior. *Journal of Autism and Developmental Disorders,* 18, 99–117.

Eaton, I. F., & Menolascino, F. J. (1982). Psychiatric disorders in the mentally retarded: Types, problems, and challenges. *American Journal of Mental Deficiency,* 139, 1297–1303.

Frank, C., Matson, J. L., & Ritenour, A. (1997). Inducing lifestyle regularity in recovering bipolar disorder patients: Results from the maintenance therapies in bipolar disorder protocol. *Biological Psychiatry,* 41, 1165–1173.

Fraser, W. I., Leudar, I., Gray, J., & Campbell, I. (1986). Psychiatric and behavior disturbance in mental handicap. *Journal of Mental Deficiency Research,* 30, 49–57.

Gardner, W. I. (1967). Occurrence of severe depressive reactions in the mentally retarded. *American Journal of Psychiatry,* 124, 386–388.

Ghaziuddin, M., Tsai, L., & Ghaziudden, N. (1991). Fluoxetine in autism with depression. *Journal of the American Academy of Child and Adolescent Psychiatry,* 30, 508–509.

Glue, P. (1989). Rapid cycling affective disorders in the mentally retarded. *Biological Psychiatry,* 26(3), 250–256.

Gotason, R. (1985). Psychiatric illness among the mentally retarded: A Swedish population study. *Acta Psychiatrica Scandinavia,* 71(Suppl. 318), 1–117.

Graham, P., & Rutter, M. (1973). Psychiatric disorder in the young adolescent. *Proceedings of the Royal Society of Medicine,* 66, 1226–1229.

Gross, E., Hull, H., Lytton, G., Hill, J. A., & Piersel, W. C. (1993). Case study of neuroleptic induced akathisia: Important implications for individuals with mental retardation. *American Journal of Mental Retardation,* 98, 156–164.

Gualtieri, C. T., & Sovner, R. (1989). Akathisia and tardive akathisia. *Psychiatric Aspects of Mental Retardation Reviews,* 8, 83–88.

Hagerman, R. J., & Sobesky, W. E., (1989). Psychopathology in fragile X syndrome. *American Journal of Orthopsychiatry, 59*, 142–152.

Hanzel, T. E., Johnson, J. E. G., Harder, S. R., & Kalachnik, J. E. (1999). Use of aggression to signal and measure depressive episodes with a rapid cycling bipolar disorder in an individual with mental retardation. *Mental Health Aspects of Developmental Disabilities, 2*, 122–132.

Hemphill, S. A. (1996). Characteristics of conduct-disordered children and their families: A review. *Australian Psychologist, 31*, 109–118.

Hodapp, R. M., Burack, J. A., & Zigler, E. (1990). The developmental perspective in the field of mental retardation. In R. M. Hodapp, J. A., Burack, & E. Zigler (Eds.), *Issues in the developmental approach to mental retardation* (pp. 246–271). Cambridge, UK: Cambridge University Press.

Howland, R. H. (1992). Fluoxetine treatment of depression in mentally retarded adults. *The Journal of Nervous and Mental Disease, 180*, 202–205.

Hurd, H. M. (1888). Imbecality with insanity. *Journal of Insanity, 45*, 263–371.

Hurley, A. D., & Sovner, R. (1982). Phobic behavior and mentally retarded persons. *Psychiatric Aspects of Mental Retardation Newsletter, 11*, 41–44.

Iverson, J. C., & Fox, R. A. (1989). Prevalence of psychopathology among mentally retarded adults. *Research in Developmental Disabilities, 10*, 77–83.

Iwata, B. A., Pace, G. M., Dorsey, M. F., Zarcone, J. R., Vollmer, T. R., & Smith, R. G. (1994). The functions of self-injurious behavior: An experimental epidemiological analysis. *Journal of Applied Behavior Analysis, 27*, 215–240.

Jacobson, J. W. (1982). Problem behavior and psychiatric impairment within a developmentally disabled population: Behavior frequency. *Applied Research in Mental Retardation, 3*, 121–129.

Kane, J. M., & Smith, J. M. (1982). Tardive dyskinesia: Prevalence and risk factors, 1959–1979. *Archives of General Psychiatry, 39*, 473–481.

Kastner, T., Finesmith, R., & Walsh, K. (1993). Longterm administration of valproic acid in the treatment of affective symptoms in people with mental retardation. *Journal of Clinical Psychopharmacology, 13*, 448–451.

Kennedy, W. A. (1983). Obsessive-compulsive and phobic reactions. In T. H. Ollendick & M. Hersen (Eds.), *Handbook of Child Psychopathology* (pp. 277–292). New York: Plenum Press.

Khreim, I., & Mikkelsen, E. (1997). Anxiety disorders in adults with mental retardation. *Psychiatric Annals, 27*, 175–181.

King, R., & McCartney, J. (1999). Charting for a purpose: Optimal treatment of bipolar disorder in individuals with developmental disability. *Mental Health Aspects of Developmental Disabilities, 2*, 50–58.

Koller, H., Richardson, S. A., Katz, M., & McLaren, J. (1983). Behavior disturbance since childhood among a 5-year birth cohort of all mentally retarded young adults in a city. *American Journal of Mental Deficiency, 87*, 386–395.

Kupfer, D. J., Himmelhoch, J. M., Swartzburg, M., Anderson, C., Byck, R., & Detre, T. P. (1972). Hypersomnia in manic depressive disease. *Disease of the Nervous System, 33*, 720–724.

Langee, H. R., & Conlon, M. (1992). Predictors of responses to antidepressant medication. *American Journal on Mental Retardation, 97*, 65–70.

Leudar, I., Fraser, W. I., & Jeeves, M. A. (1984). Behavior disturbance and mental handicap: Typology and longitudinal trends. *Psychological Medicine, 14*, 923–935.

Levine, H. G. (1985). Situational anxiety and everyday life experiences of mildly retarded adults. *American Journal of Mental Deficiency, 90*, 27–33.

Lewis, M. H., & MacLean, W. E., Jr. (1982). Issues in treating emotional disorders of the mentally retarded. In J. L. Matson & R. P. Barrett (Eds.), *Psychopathology in the mentally retarded* (pp. 1–36). New York: Grune & Stratton.

Linaker, O. (1991). DSM-III diagnosis compared with the factor structure of the psychopathology instrument for mentally retarded adults (PIMRA), in an institutionalized, mostly severe retarded population. *Research in Developmental Disabilities, 12*, 143–153.

Lipowski, Z. J. (1987). Delirium (acute confusional states). *Journal of the American Medical Association, 258*, 1789–1792.

Lowry, M. A. (1997). Unmasking mood disorders: Recognizing and measuring symptomatic behaviors. *The Habilitative Mental Healthcare Newsletter, 16*, 1–6.

Lowry, M. A. (1998). Assessment and treatment of mood disorders in persons with developmental disabilities. *Journal of Developmental Disabilities, 10*, 342–387.

Lund, J. (1985). The prevalence of psychiatric morbidity in mentally retarded adults. *Acta Psychiatrica Scandanavica , 72*, 563–570.

MacLean, W. E. (1993). Overview. In J. L. Matson & R. P. Barrett (Eds.), *Psychopathology in the mentally retarded* (2nd ed., pp 1–16). Needham Heights, MA: Allyn and Bacon.

MacMillan, D. L. (1977). *Mental retardation in school and society.* Boston: Little and Brown.

Marder, S. R., & Meibach, R. C. (1994). Risperidone in the treatment of schizophrenia. *American Journal of Psychiatry, 151*, 825–835.

Matson, J. L. (1982). The treatment of behavioral characteristics of depression in the mentally retarded. *Behavior Therapy, 13*, 209–218.

Matson, J. L. (1985). Emotional problems in the mentally retarded: The need for assessment and treatment. *Psychopharmacology Bulletin, 21*, 258–261.

Matson, J. L. (1995). *Manual for the matson evaluation of social skills for individuals with severe retardation.* Baton Rouge, LA: Scientific Publishers Inc.

Matson, J. L. (1997). *The assessment for dual diagnosis (ADD).* Baton Rouge, LA: Disability Consultants, LLC.

Matson, J. L., & Bamburg, J. W. (1998). Reliability of the assessment of dual diagnosis (ADD). *Research in Developmental Disabilities, 19*, 89–95.

Matson, J. L., Bamburg, J. W., Cherry, K. E., & Paclawskyj, T. R. (1999). A validity study on the questions about behavioral function (QABF) scale: Predicting treatment success for self-injury, aggression, and stereotypies. *Research in Developmental Disabilities, 20*(2), 163–175.

Matson, J. L., Bamburg, J. W., Mayville, E. A., Pinkston, J., Bielecki, J., & Kuhn, D. (2000). Psychopharmacology and mental retardation: A 10 year review (1990–1999). *Research in Developmental Disabilities, 21*, 263–296.

Matson, J. L., Dettling, J., & Senatore, V. (1981). Treating depression of a mentally retarded adult. *British Journal of Mental Subnormality, 16*, 86–88.

Matson, J. L., Gardner, W. I., Coe, D. A., & Sovner, R. (1991). A scale for evaluating emotional disorders in severely and profoundly mentally retarded persons: Development of the diagnostic assessment for the severely handicapped (DASH) scale. *British Journal of Psychiatry, 159*, 81–89.

Matson, J. L., Kazdin, A. E., & Senatore, V. (1984). Psychometric properties of the Psychopathology Instrument for mentally retarded adults (PIMRA). *Applied Research in Mental Retardation, 5*, 81–89.

Matson, J. L., & Kuhn, D. E. (2001). Identifying feeding problems in mentally retarded persons: Development and reliability of the screening tool of feeding problems (STEP). *Research in Developmental Disabilities, 22*(2),165–172.

Matson, J. L., Kuhn, D. E., & Mayville, S. B. (2002). Assessment of psychopathology and behavior problems for adults with mental retardation. *The NADD Bulletin, 5*, 19–21.

Matson, J. L., Rush, K. S., Hamilton, M., Anderson, S. J., Baglio, C. S., & Bamburg, J. (1999). The diagnostic assessment for the severely handicapped-II. *Research in Developmental Disabilities, 20*, 305–313.

Matson, J. L., & Sevin, J. A. (1994). Theories of dual diagnosis in mental retardation. *Journal of Consulting and Clinical Psychology, 62*, 6–16.

Matson, J. L., & Smiraldo, B. B. (1997). Validity of the mania subscale of the diagnostic assessment for the severely handicapped-II. *Research in Developmental Disabilities, 18*, 221–225.

Matson, J. L., Smiraldo, B. B., & Hastings, T. L. (1998). Validity of the autism/pervasive developmental disorder subscale of the diagnostic assessment for the severely handicapped-II (DASH-II). *Journal of Autism and Developmental Disabilities, 28*, 77–81.

McNally, R. J., & Ascher, L. M. (1987). Anxiety disorders in mentally retarded people. In L. Michelson & L. M. Ascher (Eds.), *Anxiety and stress disorders: Cognitive-behavioral assessment and treatment* (pp. 379–394). New York: Guilford.

Menolascino, F. J., Wilson, J., Golden, C., & Reudrich, S. L. (1986). Medication and treatment of schizophrenia in persons with mental retardation. *Mental Retardation, 24*, 277–283.

Mikkelsen, E. J., Albert, L. G., Emens, M., & Rubin, E. (1997). The efficacy of antidepressant medication for individuals with mental retardation. *Psychiatric Annals, 27,* 198–205.

Mikkelsen, G., & McKenna, L. (1999). Psychopharmacologic algorithms for adults with developmental disabilities and difficult-to-diagnose behavioral disorder. *Psychiatric Annals, 29,* 302–314.

Myers, B. A. (1998). Major depression in persons with moderate to profound mental retardation: Clinical presentation and case illustrations. *Mental Health Aspects of Developmental Disabilities, 1,* 57–68.

Naylor, G. J., Donald, J. M., Le Poidevin, D., & Reid, A. H. (1974). A double-blind trial of long-term lithium therapy in mental defectives. *British Journal of Psychiatry, 124,* 52–57.

Nemiah, J. C., & Uhde, T. W. (1989). Obsessive-compulsive disorder. In H. I. Kaplan & B. J. Sadock (Eds.), *Comprehensive textbook of psychiatry* (5th ed., pp. 1245–1254). Baltimore, MD: Williams and Wilkins.

Newton, J. T., & Sturmey, P. (1991). The motivation assessment scale: Inter-rater reliability and internal consistancy in a British sample. *Journal of Mental Deficiency Research, 35,* 472–474.

Ollendick, T. H., Oswald, D. P., & Ollendick, D. G. (1993). Anxiety disorders in mentally retarded persons. In J. L. Matson & R. Barrett (Eds.), *Psychopathology in the mentally retarded* (pp. 41–86). Boston, MA: Allyn and Bacon.

Paclawskyj, T. R., Matson, J. L., Bamburg, J. W., & Baglio, C. A. (1997). A comparison of the diagnostic assessment for the severely handicapped-II (DASH-II) and the aberrant behavior checklist (ABC). *Research in Developmental Disabilities, 18,* 289–298.

Paclawskyj, T. R., Matson, J. L., Rush, K. S., Smalls, Y., & Vollmer, T. R. (2000). Questions about behavioral function (QABF): A behavioral checklist for functional assessment of aberrant behavior. *Research in Developmental Disabilities, 21,* 223–229.

Pary, R. J. (1994). Clozapine in three individuals with mild mental retardation and treatment-refractory psychiatric disorders. *Mental Retardation, 32,* 323–327.

Petti, T. A. (1989). Depression. In T. H. Oflendick & M. Hersen (Eds.), *Handbook of child psychopathology* (2nd ed., pp. 229–246). New York: Plenum.

Phillips, I., & Williams, N. (1975). Psychotherapy and mental retardation: A study of 100 mentally retarded children: I. Psychopathology. *American Journal of Psychiatry, 132,* 1265–1271.

Rapoport, J. L. (1988). The neurobiology of obsessive-compulsive disorder. *Journal of the American Medical Association, 260,* 2888–2890.

Reid, A. H. (1972). Psychoses in adult mental defectives: I. Manic depressive psychosis. *British Journal of Psychiatry, 120,* 205–212.

Reid, A. H. (1976). Psychiatric disturbances in the mentally handicapped. *Proceedings of the Royal Society of Medicine, 69,* 509–512.

Reid, A. H. (1980). Diagnosis of psychiatric disorder in the severely and profoundly retarded patient. *Journal of the Royal Society of Medicine, 73,* 607–609.

Reid, A. H., Ballinger, B. R., & Heather, B. B. (1978). Behavioral syndromes identified by cluster analysis in a sample of 100 severely and profoundly retarded adults. *Psychological Medicine, 8,* 399–412.

Reiss, S. (1988). *Test manual for the Reiss Screen for Maladaptive Behavior.* Orland Park, IL: International Diagnostic Systems.

Reiss, S. (1993). Assessment of psychopathology in persons with mental retardation. In J. L. Matson & R. P. Barrett (Eds.). *Psychopathology in the mentally retarded* (2nd ed., pp. 17–39). Needham Heights, MA: Allyn & Bacon.

Reiss, S. (1994). *Handbook of challenging behaviors: Mental health aspects of mental retardation.* Worthington, OH: IDS Publishing.

Reiss, S. (1997). Comments on the Reiss screen for maladaptive behavior and its factor structure. *Journal of Intellectual Disability Research, 41*(4), 346–354.

Reiss, S., Levitan, G. W., & Szyszko, J. (1982). Emotional disturbance and mental retardation: Diagnostic overshadowing. *American Journal of Mental Deficiency, 86,* 567–574.

Reudrich, S. L. (1993). Treatment of bipolar mood disorder in persons with mental retardation. In R. J. Fletcher, & A. Dosen (Eds.), *Mental health aspects of mental retardation* (pp. 268–280). Lexington, MA: Lexington Books.

Reynolds, W. M., & Baker, J. A. (1988). Assessment of depression in persons with mental retardation. *American Journal on Mental Retardation, 93*, 93–103.

Rickard, H. C. (1986). Relaxation training for mentally retarded persons. *Psychiatric Aspects of Mental Retardation Reviews, 5*, 11–15.

Rivenus, T. M., & Harmatz, J. S. (1979). Diagnosis and lithium treatment of affective disorder in the retarded: Five case studies. *American Journal of Psychiatry, 136*, 551–554.

Rodrigue, J. R., Morgan, S. B., & Geffken, G. R. (1991). A comparative evaluation of adaptive behavior in children and adolescents with autism, down syndrome, and normal development. *Journal of Autism and Developmental Disabilities, 21*, 187–196.

Roith, A. J. (1961). Psychotic depression in a mongol. *Journal of Mental Subnormality, 7*, 45–47.

Rojahn, J., & Tasse, M. J. (1996). Psychopathology in mental retardation. In J. W. Jacobson & J. A. Mulick (Eds.), *Manual of diagnosis and professional practice in mental retardation* (pp. 147–156). Washington, DC: American Psychological Association.

Ruben, M., & Langa, A. (1995). Clozapine, mental retardation and severe psychiatric illness: Clinical response in the first year (letter). *Harvard Review of Psychiatry, 3*, 293–294.

Ruedrich, S. L., Des Noyers-Hurley, A., & Sovner, R. (2001). Treatment of mood disorders in mentally retarded persons. In A. Dosen & K. Day (Eds.), *Treating mental illness and behavior disorders in children and adults with mental retardation* (pp. 201–226). Washington, DC: American Psychiatric Press.

Rush, K. S., Bowman, L. G., Eidman, S. L., & Toole, L. M. (2004). Assessing psychopathology in individuals with developmental disabilities [special issue]. *Behavior Modification, 28*(5), 621–637.

Rutter, M., Graham, P., & Yule, W. (1970). *A neuropsychiatric study in childhood.* London, UK: Spastics International.

Rutter, M., Tizard, J., Yule, W., Graham, P., & Whitmore, K. (1976). Research report: Isle of Wight studies, 1964–1974. *Psychological Medicine, 6*, 313–332.

Ryan, R. (1994). Posttraumatic stress disorder in persons with developmental disabilities. *Community Mental Health Journal, 3*, 45–54.

Scanlon, C. A., Arick, J. R., & Krug, D. A. (1982). A matched sample investigation of non-adaptive behavior of severely handicapped adults across four living situations. *American Journal of Mental Deficiency, 86*, 526–532.

Senatore, V., Matson, J. L., & Kazdin, A. E. (1985). An inventory to assess psychopathology of mentally retarded adults. *American Journal of Mental Deficiency, 5*, 459–466.

Sevin, J. A., Matson, J. L., Williams, D., & Kirkpatrick-Sanchez, S. (1995). Reliability of emotional problems with the diagnostic assessment for the severely handicapped (DASH). *British Journal of Clinical Psychology, 34*, 93–94.

Shapiro, S. A. (1981). *Contemporary theories of schizophrenia: Review and synthesis.* New York: McGraw-Hill.

Silka, V. R., & Hurley, A. D. (1998). New drug therapies for bipolar disorders. *Mental Health Aspects of Developmental Disabilities, 16*, 52–54.

Singh, N., & Katz, R. C. (1989). Differential diagnosis in chronic schizophrenia and adult autism. In J. L. Matson (Ed.), *Chronic schizophrenia and adult autism* (pp. 147–180). New York: Springer.

Singh, N. N., Sood, A., Sonenklar, N., & Ellis, C. R. (1991). Assessment and diagnosis of mental illness in persons with mental retardation: Methods and measures. *Behavior Modification, 15*, 419–443.

Singh, N. N., & Winton, A. S. W. (1983). Social skills training with institutionalized severely and profoundly retarded persons. *Applied Research in Mental Retardation, 4*, 383–398.

Sovner, R. (1988). Anticonvulsant drug therapy of neuropsychiatric disorders in mentally retarded persons. In S. L. McElroy & H. G. Pope (Eds.), *Use of anticonvulsants in psychiatry* (pp. 169–181). Oxford, UK: Oxford Health Care.

Sovner, R., & Hurley, A. D. (1983). Do the mentally retarded suffer from affective illness? *Archives of General Psychiatry, 40*, 61–67.

Sovner, R., Hurley, A. D., & Labrie, R. (1985). Is mania incompatible with Down's syndrome? *British Journal of Psychiatry, 46*, 314–320.

Sovner, R., & Pary, R. J. (1993). Affective disorders in developmentally disabled persons. In J. L. Matson & R. P. Barrett (Eds.), *Psychopathology in the mentally retarded* (2nd ed., pp. 87–147). Needham Heights, MA: Allyn & Bacon.

Sovner, R., Pary, R. J., Dosen, A., Geddye, A., Hovens, J. G. F. M., Barrerra, F. J., Cantwell, D. P., & Hussey, H. R. (1998). Antidepressant drugs, in psychotropic medication and developmental disabilities. In S. Reiss & M. G. Aman (Eds.), *International consensus handbook* (pp. 179–200). Columbus, OH: Ohio State University Nisonger Center.

Sparrow, S., Balla, D., & Cicchetti, D. (1984). *Vineland adaptive behavior scales: Interview edition survey form manual.* Circle Press, MN: American Guidance Service.

Spreat, S., & Connelly, L. (1996). Reliability analysis of the motivation assessment scale. *American Journal on Mental Retardation, 100,* 528–532.

Stavrakaki, C. (1999). Depression, anxiety, and adjustment disorders in people with developmental disabilities. In N. Bouras (Ed.), *Psychiatric and behavioral disorders in developmental disabilities and mental retardation* (pp. 175–187). Chambridge, UK: Chambridge University Press.

Sturmey, P. (1994). Assessing the functions of aberrant behaviors: A review of psychometric instruments. *Journal of Autism and Developmental Disorders, 24,* 293–304.

Sturmey, P. (1995). Analog baselines: A critical review of the methodology. *Research in Developmental Disabilities, 16,* 269–284.

Sturmey, P., & Bertman, L. J. (1994). Validity of the Reiss screen for maladaptive behavior. *American Journal on Mental Retardation, 99,* 201–206.

Sturmey, P., & Ley, T. (1990). The psychopathology instrument for mentally retarded adults: Internal consistencies and relationship to behavior problems. *British Journal of Psychiatry, 156,* 428–430.

Szatmari P., Archer L., Fisman S. F., Streiner D. L., & Wilson F., J. (1995). Asperger's syndrome and autism: Differences in behavior, cognition and adaptive functioning. *Journal of the American Academy of Child and Adolescent Psychiatry, 34,* 1662–71.

Szymanski, L. S., & Biederman, J. (1984). Depression and anorexia nervosa in persons with Down's syndrome. *American Journal of Mental Deficiency, 89,* 246–251.

Szymanski, L. S., & King, B. H. (1999). Practice parameters for the assessment and treatment of children, adolescents, and adults with mental retardation and comorbid mental disorders. *Journal of the American Academy of Child Psychiatry, 38*(Suppl. 12), 5–32.

Thompson, T., Hackenberg, T., & Schaal, D. (1991). *Pharmacological treatments for behavior problems in developmental disabilities* (NIH Publication No. 91-3410). Paper presented at the Consensus Development Conference on Destructive Behavior, National Institutes on Health, Bethesda, MD.

Touchette, P. E., MacDonald, R. F., & Langer, S. N. (1985). A scatterplot for identifying stimulus control of problem behavior. *Journal of Applied Behavior Analysis, 18,* 343–351.

Turner, T. H. (1989). Schizophrenia and mental handicap: A historical review, with implications for further research. *Psychological Medicine, 19,* 301–314.

Van Bourgandien, M. E. (1989). General counseling services. In APA (Eds.),*Treatments of psychiatric disorders: A task force of the American Psychiatric Association* (pp. 104–107). Washington DC: American Psychiatric Association.

Van Houten, R., & Rolider, A. (1991). Applied behavior analysis. In J. L. Matson & J. A. Mulick (Eds.), *Handbook of mental retardation* (2nd ed., pp. 569–585). New York: Pergamon Press.

Varley, C. K. (1984). Schizophreniform psychoses in mentally retarded adolescent girls following sexual assault. *American Journal of Psychiatry, 141,* 593–595.

Vitiello, B., & Behar, D. (1992). Mental retardation and psychiatric illness. *Hospital and Community Psychiatry, 43,* 494–499.

Vollmer, T. R., Iwata, B. A., Zarcone, J. R., Smith, R. G., & Mazaleski, J. L. (1993). Within-session patterns of self-injury as indicators of behavioral function. *Research in Developmental Disabilities, 14,* 479–492.

Vollmer, T. R., & Smith, R. G. (1996). Some current themes in functional analysis research. *Research in Developmental Disabilities, 17,* 229–249.

Warren, A. C., Holroyd, S., & Folstein, M. F. (1989). Major depression in Down's syndrome. *British Journal of Psychiatry, 155,* 202–205.

Weintraub, M., & Evans, P. (1989). Bupropion: A chemically and pharmacologically unique antidepressant. *Hospital Formulary, 24*, 254–259.

Werry, J. S. (1980). Anticholinergic sedatives. In G. D. Burrows & J. B. Werry (Eds.), *Advances in human psychopharmacology* (Vol. 1, pp. 19–42). Greenwich, CT: JAI Press.

Whitaker, S. (1993). The reduction of aggression in people with learning difficulties: A review of psychological methods. *British Journal of Clinical Psychology, 32*, 1–37.

Whybrow, P. C., Akiskal, H. S., & McKinney, W. T. (1984). *Mood disorders—Towards a new psychobiology.* New York: Plenum.

Winokur, G., Clayton, P. J., & Reich, T. (1969). *Manic depressive illness.* Saint Louis, MO: C. V. Mosby.

Wright, E. C. (1982). The presentation of mental illness in mentally retarded adults. *British Journal of Psychiatry, 141*, 496–502.

Wright, W. B. (1958). Azaclonal in mental deficiency practice: A preliminary report. *Journal of Mental Science, 104*, 485–487.

Yarbrough, S. C., & Carr, E. G. (2000). Some relationships between informant assessment and functional analysis of problem behavior. *American Journal on Mental Retardation, 105*, 130–151.

Zigler, E. (1969). Developmental versus difference theories of mental retardation and the problem of motivation. *American Journal of Mental Deficiency, 73*, 536–556.

27

Aggression in Persons With Intellectual Disabilities and Mental Disorders

WILLIAM I. GARDNER

Aggression and related disruptive acts represent the most frequently occurring behavioral challenges of persons with intellectual disabilities (ID) (Eyman & Call, 1977; Jacobson, 1982; Schroeder, Rojahn, & Olenquist, 1991). Even though aggression occurs in a social context and is maintained to a major extent by social contingencies, medical, genetic, psychiatric, neuropsychiatric, and psychological conditions also are reported to represent significant contributing influences (Barnhill, 1999; Gardner, 2002a; Sheard, 1984). As an example, an increased rate of occurrence of aggression has been reported in people with ID who also have a diagnosis of a mental disorder (Borthwick-Duffy, 1994; Jacobson, 1982; Reiss & Rojahn, 1993). Additionally, referrals for mental health services for people with ID typically are initiated by presence of recurring and severe behavioral concerns involving aggression and related disruptive activities (Benson, 1985; Davidson et al., 1994). Whether primarily behavioral, psychological, psychiatric, medical, or genetic, the case formulation model selected to offer direction to diagnostic assessments and related treatment approaches thus should be sufficiently inclusive to address the range of biomedical and psychosocial conditions that may influence the frequency, severity, variability, and persistent recurrence of these acts.

WILLIAM I. GARDNER • Rehabilitation Psychology Program, University of Wisconsin–Madison, Madison, Wisconsin 53705

FEATURES OF AGGRESSION AND RELATED
DISRUPTIVE ACTS

As background for brief description and evaluation of frequently used case formulation paradigms, the conceptual, empirical, and clinical literatures addressing people with ID and mental health issues suggest that any case formulation selected should give consideration to the following features of aggression and related disruptive acts:

Aggression and related disruptive acts represent the end result of an antecedent chain of events that reflect biomedical (medical, psychiatric, neuropsychiatric, genetic) and psychological features of a person as these interact with social and physical environments. As illustrations, Lowry (1994), Lowry and Sovner (1992), and Sovner, Foxx, Lowry, and Lowry (1993) provide descriptions of the possible contributing roles of anxiety, irritability, and fluctuating mood states and the manner in which these interact with specific features of the social environments in influencing occurrence of aggression and acts of self-injury. In people with ID and a mood disorder, occurrence of problem behavioral symptoms was noted to be dependent on the presence of the specific mood states plus occurrence of various staff prompts. Different kinds of social prompts served as components of the instigating stimulus complex depending on the nature of the person's mood state. During mood states of dysphoria, staff prompts produced the problem behavior although these prompts were intended to get the person involved in activities that typically were enjoyed. During episodes of hypomania, prompts to slow the person down or focus attention produced the behavioral symptoms.

As a second illustration, Tsiouris (2001), in describing the antecedent events for occurrence of aggression in people with severe ID and mood disorders, noted "usually it was directed towards noisy consumers who invaded the isolation of others. It was also directed at staff who urged individuals to do different chores, to get ready for their program in the morning, or to participate in activities which they had previously enjoyed" (p. 118). Thus the disruptive behaviors represented the end result of the interactive influences of personal affective states and specific environmental events. As a final illustration, Lindsay, Marshall, Neilson, Quinn, and Smith (1998) studied the role of psychological central processing features in occurrence of aggressive responding. These writers evaluated the cognitive distortions of people with ID who engaged in sexually aggressive activities. Men who had been charged with exhibitionism were found to have the distorted beliefs that their victims did not object to but rather actually enjoyed the exposure experience. A case formulation that does not consider each component of these and similar transactions involving environmental, biomedical, and psychological features is incomplete and offers only a partial understanding of these human experiences.

Aggressive acts occur selectively under specific and individually varied antecedent conditions that may be identified motivationally or functionally. As noted, these antecedents consist of influential stimulus conditions that arise from a person's social and physical environments and from current psychological and biomedical features of the person. As additional illustrations of the idiosyncratic nature of these antecedent instigating conditions, O'Reilly (1995) observed that rates of aggression of a 31-year-old man with ID, when provided directives from family members and staff in both home and vocational settings, were higher following periods of sleep deprivation than following periods of more adequate sleep. The antecedent personal distress associated with sleep deprivation combined with the social directives to increase the likelihood of the aggressive acts. Berg et al. (2000), in a study involving a 9-year-old boy with developmental disabilities and autism, demonstrated that a teacher prompt to complete academic tasks that previously had been completed or mastered set the occasion for aggressive acts of hitting and pinching. Aggressive acts seldom occurred following directives to complete tasks that previously had not been completed or mastered. Thus, the type and magnitude of control of the various antecedent influences over aggressive responding is idiosyncratic to each person and thus requires a case formulation process (diagnostic activities and resulting interventions) that is individualized (e.g., Hanley, Iwata, & McCord, 2003).

Recurring acts of aggression and related disruptive behaviors, except in rare instances, represent learned behaviors that have become functional in producing various effects of value to the person (e.g., Marcus, Vollmer, Swanson, Roane, & Ringdahl, 2001; Thompson & Iwata, 2001). Recurring acts of aggression become functional in reducing, delaying, terminating, or avoiding experiences of personal distress. These activating conditions of psychological distress that initiate and provide direction to the aggressive actions may represent states of aversive affective over arousal (e.g., fear, anxiety, irritability, anger, boredom) or states of deprivation (e.g., sexual contact, social attention, sensory stimulation). Matson and Mayville (2001) demonstrated the influence of environmental or physical contingencies in understanding aggression in persons with mental retardation and a psychiatric disturbance. Using the Questions About Behavior Function Scale (Matson & Vollmer, 1995), the writers found that 75% of the sample studied of persons identified as presenting a dual diagnosis showed an environmental or physical function for their aggression. These writers concluded that, even though all persons studied had a diagnosed mental disorder, major influences in addition to features of the psychiatric disorder contributed to the functionality of the aggressive acts. Case formulations that do not attend to these multiple biomedical and psychosocial motivational sources that contribute to these functional properties of aggression will be incomplete.

As aggressive and related disruptive acts represent the end result of a sequence of antecedent controlling conditions, there are no specific treatments for aggression. Rather, interventions are selected to address the controlling conditions that influence occurrence, severity level, variation across time in occurrence and severity, and durability or strength of aggressive responding (Matson & Duncan, 1997). Antecedent conditions that set the occasion for occurrence of aggressive acts may differ from those that influence severity and variability of these acts. To illustrate, an adolescent boy's low intensity acts of aggression following attempts by peers to use his personal property without permission may become high intensity acts when these intrusions occur during periods of heightened states of personal irritability associated with psychotic delusions and sleep deprivation. As a result of these potentially multiple and individually unique sources of influence, interventions may be required to address multiple sets of controlling influences. Treatment and management approaches will be effective in influencing various features of aggressive responding only to the extent that these potentially multiple controlling conditions are identified and altered. Thus, a case formulation that does not result in diagnostically based interventions to address these controlling conditions will produce less than desired results.

CASE FORMULATION FRAMEWORKS

Review of current conceptual, empirical, and clinical literatures devoted to treatment of the conditions presumed to control aggressive responding reflects use of a range of case formulation approaches to guide research and clinical activities (Allen, 2000; Gardner, 2002a; Rush & Frances, 2000; Whitaker, 1993). In clinical settings, these frameworks are used to offer guidance in selection of the diagnostic targets and related assessment procedures as well as the resulting interventions derived from the diagnostic findings. Close review of these, however, reveals that the more commonly used frameworks address selected components of the complex biomedical and psychosocial matrix of potential influences. The *applied behavior analytic* approach primarily addresses environmental contingencies (Hutchinson, 1973; Repp & Horner, 1999), the *medical illness* approach primarily addresses medical pathologies (Gardner & Whalen, 1996; Kastner, Walsh, & Fraser, 2001), and the *mental illness* paradigm primarily addresses psychiatric disorders (Reiss & Aman, 1998). It is recognized, of course, that there are studies that report combined analysis of environmental antecedents, medical, and psychiatric factors (Baker, Blumberg, Freeman, & Wieseler, 2002; Mulick, Hammer, & Dura, 1991).

Even when influences other than those that represent the central focus of analysis and intervention are acknowledged, the transactional nature and possible reciprocal effects on each of these separate influences can be either underemphasized or ignored. As an illustration, in discussion of when a trial of psychiatric medication for behavioral concerns might be recommended, Ellis, Singh, and Singh (1997) noted that "before beginning a psychotropic medication, it must be determined that the behavior is not due to a medical condition (e.g., otitis media or migraine headache) or environmental and psychosocial factors (e.g., living conditions, peer taunting, or abuse)" (p 156). This approach reflects the view that biomedical and psychosocial influences on features of aggressive behaviors are independent. This chapter suggests a contrasting view of specifying the specific instigating, mediating, and maintaining roles that may be assumed by each of multiple sets of influences and the possible resulting significant interactive effects of these. The stimulus features of a medical condition such as those arising from a migraine headache or the cognitive, perceptual, or mood symptoms of a psychiatric condition, as examples, may influence the nature and magnitude of control exerted by environmental physical or social events (Carr, Langdon, & Yarbrough, 1999; Gardner, 2002a).

This chapter initially provides brief descriptions of the extant psychosocial and biomedical case formulation frameworks used to guide treatment selection for aggressive and related disruptive acts in persons with ID and co-occurring mental health issues. This examination is followed by description of a case formulation approach that combines features of each in construction of an integrative psychological model of aggressive responding. The chapter closes with examination of factors that require consideration in selection and evaluation of intervention programs for persons who engage in clinically significant acts of aggression.

Psychosocial Case Formulation Frameworks

The most frequently used framework in analysis and treatment of aggressive acts among persons with ID is *applied behavior analysis*. This case formulation, reflecting a radical behavioral view of human behavior, views aggressive acts as operants that are maintained by contingent environmentally based experiences (Repp & Horner, 1999). As detailed by Gardner (2002a), the application of this case formulation approach to problems of aggression and related disruptive acts, and the types of behavior modification procedures utilized, has evolved over the last few decades from one with a focus on elimination through suppression of aggressive and disruptive acts (Carr & Durand, 1985; Gardner, 1969) into a major focus on providing positive behavioral supports through altering antecedent conditions including social and physical environmental modifications, teaching functionally equivalent and alternative behaviors, and teaching more general adaptive skills (Carr, 1997; Koegel, Koegel, & Dunlap, 1996; Worsdell, Iwata, Hanley, Thompson, & Kahng, 2000).

A number of additional *behavior therapy* systems have paralleled the development of applied behavior analysis, although research on use of these systems with people with ID currently is relatively limited in scope (Cullen, 1996; O'Donohue & Krasner, 1995). While utilizing reinforcement contingencies as a major construct, these approaches have made use of a range of additional learning and related psychological models. The more notable of these involve social learning concepts and related therapy practices offered by Bandura and colleagues (Bandura, 1969, 1977, 1986; Bandura & Walters, 1963). Bandura's analysis of aggression (1973) is now largely accepted in general clinical practice of psychology and offers a range of possible intervention approaches that address potential controlling conditions. Social learning, psychological behaviorism, and related cognitive and cognitive-behavioral views (Bandura, 1986; Craighead, Craighead, Kazdin, & Mahoney, 1994; Staats, 1996) provide direction to assessment and intervention practices that have enjoyed increasing use among clinicians serving people with ID and other developmental disabilities (Gardner, 2002a). Related therapy methods include social skills training, relaxation training, contingency management, token economies, anger management training, aggression replacement training, self-management skills training, systematic desensitization procedures, cognitive-behavioral procedures, coping skills training, problem-solving, and conflict resolution procedures (Benson, 2002; Gardner, Graeber, & Cole, 1996; Matson & Duncan, 1997; Nezu & Nezu, 1994; Whitaker, 1993). These social learning and related cognitive-behavioral views of aggressive responding offer an expanded analytic and related treatment armamentarium for the clinician. With these, cognitive and emotional contributions to aggressive responding among persons with ID and mental disorders become direct targets of intervention efforts (Benson, 2002; Gardner, 2002a; Nezu, Nezu, Gill-Weiss, 1992).

Biomedical Case Formulation Frameworks

To address possible biomedical influences on aggressive responding, two case formulation approaches, the *medical illness* and the *psychiatric disorders* models are used to provide direction to medical interventions for conditions presumed to influence aggressive responding. A *medical Illness* case formulation is used to guide selection of treatment for a wide range of medical illnesses and chronic medical conditions (e.g., epileptic seizure disorders) presumed to produce personal distress that in turn combines with physical and social environmental events to influence aggressive acts in those persons prone to use aggression as a means of coping with conditions experienced as noxious. The presence of medical conditions that produce headaches, menstrual discomfort, middle ear infections, sleep difficulties, allergic reactions, skin disorders, gastrointestinal abnormalities, seizure activity, and tooth infections have been found to be correlated with increased likelihood of aggressive responding (Gardner & Whalen, 1996; Kastner et al., 2001; Mikkelsen & McKenna, 1999). Each of these conditions may produce heightened levels of internal stimuli experienced as aversive or distressing (e.g., pain, physical discomfort) that in turn may change the stimulus function of co-occurring physical and social events (Carr et al., 1999). Specifically, the presence of these stimulus conditions may change previously positive or neutral events into aversive ones or may increase the level of noxiousness of events previously viewed as noxious. These changed stimulus elements contribute to the severity levels and variability of aggressive responding (Gardner, 2002a). In a similar manner, persons with *genetic syndromes* such as Cornelia de Lange, Cri du Chat, Fragile X, Praeder–Willi, Retts, Tourettes, and Williams may present such features as hyperactivity, anxiety, hypersensitivity, proneness to strong reactions to ordinary stimuli, proneness to affective overarousal and prolonged reactions to transient stressors, panic, agitation, and emotional lability. When present, each may place the person at increased risk for experiencing heightened levels of arousal that may in turn serve as instigating antecedents for aggressive responding. When combined with deficits in functional coping skills (e.g., communication skill deficits), aggression may function as a communicative behavior (Collins & Cornish, 2002). Various writers report that acts of aggression and related disruptive acts do occur in an unusually high percentage of persons with various genetic syndromes (Barnhill, 2001; Collins & Cornish, 2002; Comings & Comings, 1985; Dykens, Hodapp, & Finucane, 2000; Einfeld, Tonge, & Florio, 1997).

In the *psychiatric disorders* case formulation framework, primary symptoms of various psychiatric syndromes are presumed to exert various influences on aggressive responding in those prone to use aggressive as a means of coping with noxious conditions (Gardner, 2002a; Reiss & Aman, 1998; Rush & Frances, 2000). As noted above for medical conditions, the presence of psychiatric symptoms also may change the stimulus functions of co-occurring social and physical events. Successful management through medication of psychiatric symptoms such as delusional thought patterns, hallucinations, heightened levels of anger or anxiety, hypomania, and dysphoric affect may serve to reduce or remove these sources of potential influence over aggressive responding. A related model, the *neurophysiological dysregulation framework*, addresses organic irritability arising from neurological or neurochemical abnormalities (e.g., head injury). Medication to address such organically induced states as irritability, hyperexcitability, and hypersensitivity may be used to reduce or remove this potential source of influence on aggressive responding (Barnhill, 1999; Sovner & Fogelman, 1996).

Summary of Case Formulation Frameworks

As is evident, while each of these psychosocial and biomedical frameworks represents a specific case formulation of some of the conditions that may influence aggressive responding in people with a dual diagnosis of ID and mental disorders, no single approach in isolation provides an adequate integrative account of the probable multiple biomedical, psychological, and environmental conditions that for any specific person may influence occurrence as well as severity, variability over time and conditions, and durability of aggressive responding. If aberrant social or physical environmental antecedent or behavioral consequence conditions are presumed to be the sole or primary conditions controlling aggressive responding, a case formulation such as an applied behavior analysis that guides assessment and related intervention practices to address these conditions may represent an efficacious approach. Even in this instance, information obtained from a functional analysis of controlling conditions will be supplemented by additional information relating to the status of alternative skills and motives that may replace or compete with the aggressive acts and motives underlying these acts. In instances in which a number of environmental, biomedical, and psychological conditions are judged to influence aggressive activity, a case formulation that addresses these multiple conditions may be required for optimal treatment program development.

AN ALTERNATIVE CASE FORMULATION

A diagnostic case formulation model is often required that reflects the complex of antecedent controlling conditions and the possible interactions among these. This paradigm should consider (a) the *salient environmental, psychological, and biomedical stimulus complex*es that precede and serve to initiate and maintain the chain of events ending in specific episodes of aggressive acts, (b) the person's current biomedical and psychological *central processing* features that serve as risk factors for engaging in these acts when confronted with an antecedent activating stimulus complex, as well as (c) proximate *consequences* that follow occurrences of aggressive and other disruptive activities and combine with motivational factors to determine their *functionality and strength.* As noted, the antecedent stimulus complex may include the arousing and activating features of a range of external physical and social environmental as well as internal psychological and biomedical conditions. These antecedent stimulus conditions are processed centrally, both neurochemically and psychologically, and transported into the motor tract as acts of aggression and related coping actions (Bradley, 2000; Ratey, 2001). The objective of a comprehensive diagnostic assessment is "to see past" specific psychosocial and biomedical conditions and to ascertain the specific role(s) served by features of each of these conditions in contributing to the *occurrence, severity, fluctuation,* and *chronic recurrence* of aggressive acts. As suggested, factors that account for frequency of occurrence may differ somewhat from those that influence severity and variability of aggression (Gardner, 2002a). Following a comprehensive assessment, informed speculation can be made about the extent of reduction in critical features of a person's aggression that may be expected following effective treatment of each or a combination of the diagnosed psychosocial and biomedical controlling conditions (Baker et al., 2002; Gardner & Sovner, 1994).

A brief description of one such case formulation model is provided. This case formulation model is described by Gardner and colleagues (Gardner, 1996, 1998, 2002a; Gardner & Sovner, 1994). This Multimodal (*bio-, psycho-,* and *socioenvironmental* modalities of influences) Contextual (*instigating, central processing,* and *maintaining* conditions that reflect three possible modalities of influence) Case Formulation approach directs the diagnostician to evaluate both psychosocial and biomedical conditions as possible contributors to occurrence, severity, variability, and habitual recurrence of aggression. This model also provides a means of combining various medical and psychiatric diagnostic insights and related diagnostically based interventions with those that involve psychological and environmental influences.

Context 1: Instigating Influences

Instigating influences consist of current external (e.g., instructional demands, conflict with peers, blocking of ritualistic or compulsive routines, staff corrective feedback, invasion of personal space) and internal (e.g., high arousal level, anger, pain-related distress, deprivation states, dysphoric mood) stimulus conditions that contribute to the occurrence, severity levels, and variability of specific aggressive and related disruptive episodes (Benson & Fuchs, 1999; Carr & Durand, 1985; Lowry & Sovner, 1992; Tsiouris, 2001). These instigating stimulus conditions are relatively varied and highly specific to each person and, when present, represent risk factors for influencing occurrence and related features of aggression for that person (McComas, Hoch, Paone, & El-Roy, 2000). Similar stimulus conditions may not represent risk factors for aggressive responding in another person. As illustrated previously, it is not unusual for these controlling antecedent conditions to consist of combinations of psychosocial and biomedical influences that vary significantly among individuals.

Context 2: Central Processing Influences

Central processing influences refer to those personal features of a biomedical and psychological nature that place a person at increased risk for aggressive behaviors (Gardner, 2002a). These features determine the influence on occurrence, severity, and variability of specific antecedent conditions such as a threatening peer, a painful headache, auditory hallucinations, a distressful level of irritability, a state of deprivation relating to valued activities or experiences, or a demanding work supervisor. Examination of these central processing influences may disclose reasons why one person is at increased risk for aggressive and related disruptive responding when another person is at minimal or no risk when both are exposed to similar antecedent conditions such as peer provocation, staff instructional demands, or heightened levels of anger arousal (e.g., Baker & Bramston, 1997; Dodge, 1993; Fuchs & Benson, 1995). Two classes of vulnerability features that place the person at increased risk for aggressive responding are of particular significance. A person's level of risk for aggressive responding when exposed to individually specific conditions of instigation is related to the type, number, and strength of these central processing vulnerability features. The initial class consists of *psychobiological* features involving (a) neurological and related neurochemical abnormalities (Barnhill, 1999), (b) psychiatric disorders and symptoms (Tuinier & Verhoeven, 1993), (c) medical abnormalities (Gedye, 1997), and (d) genetic syndromes (Dykens et al., 2000) that influence the manner in which antecedent activating events are processed by an individual.

The second class consists of two subclasses of *psychological* features. The initial psychological subclass, consisting of personal features of a cognitive, emotional/motivational, and behavioral nature, represents vulnerabilities for aggressive responding due to their *presence or excessive* nature. This initial subclass is illustrated by such personal features as (a) presence of a strong habit of aggressive responding, (b) a cognitive hostile attributional bias (Baker & Bramston, 1997), (c) cognitive distortions (Lindsay et al., 1998), and (d) a motivational inclination to enjoy sexual contact with children (Griffiths, 2002). The second subtype of psychological central processing features places the person at risk for aggressive responding as a result of the *functional absence or low strength* of these. These features include such areas as (a) deficits in skills of anger management (Benson, Rice, & Miranti, 1986; Cole, Gardner, & Karan, 1985), (b) communication skill deficits (Bird, Dores, Moniz, & Robinson, 1989), (c) problem solving skill deficits (Benson, 2002), and (d) deficits in prosocial skill alternatives to aggression (Fredericks & Nishioka-Evans, 1999). These features increase the risk of aggressive responding when a person with an inclination to use aggression as a coping response is exposed to conditions of provocation that require the deficit psychological features for alternative socially appropriate action. To illustrate, a person with a communication skill deficit who is inclined to use aggression to cope with distress-producing conditions is at increased risk for aggressive responding when exposed to situations that require some form of expressive communication. Under these conditions, acts of aggression may serve a communicative function in producing valued consequences (Carr & Durand, 1985; Schroeder, Reese, Hellings, Loupe, & Tessel, 1999). It is not unusual for a number of different central processing features to contribute to a person's aggressive acts. As an illustration, when an intrusive peer violates his personal space, an adult with severe cognitive impairments may respond immediately with a sudden surge in emotional and motor agitation followed by impulsive acts of physical aggression. Under these conditions of instigation, the adult has a number of personal characteristics that place him at high risk for aggressive and related disruptive responding. These include such features as an inclination to become hyperaroused under minor conditions of instigation, limited effective socially appropriate communicative means of expressing his distress, an impaired emotional modulation system, a strong habit of aggressive responding under conditions of distress, and limited cognitive and affective skills to inhibit these aggressive acts (Gardner, 2002b).

Context 3: Maintaining Conditions

As noted earlier, aggressive acts in most instances become functional for a person based on the type of feedback effects of these behaviors. Aggressive acts may result in the removal (termination), reduction, or avoidance of internal or external stimulus conditions experienced by the person as distressful, unpleasant, or aversive (e.g., anxiety level, taunts from peers, attempt by others to block occurrence of compulsive or ritualistic behavior, parent criticism, unwanted teacher directives) or may reduce states of deprivation through producing, maintaining, or magnifying internal or external conditions experienced as pleasant or emotionally desirable (e.g., gaining social attention, gaining access to physical, cognitive, or sensory stimulating activities, being included in a valued peer group, creating distress in others: Carr et al., 1999; Thompson & Symons, 1999). A specific contingent consequence serves to strengthen acts of aggression to the extent that the consequence addresses either the specific motivation state giving impetus to the behavior or to an equally or more powerful unmet motivational state. A motivational analysis thus represents a process of identifying individually salient motivational states ⇔ consequences dyads. Gardner (1971, 1977, 2002a) and Reiss and Havercamp (1997, 1998) describe a number of aberrant motivational features of persons with ID that may require attention in this analysis, especially in persons with significant mental health concerns. These become relevant to a specific behavioral consequence in relation to specific motivational state or states that activate the aggressive act (Gardner, 2002a). A diagnostic hypothesis that acts of aggression serve an "escape" function or a "social attention" function thus may be incomplete until the specific motivational states related to the "escape" or "attention" are described (Carr et al., 1999). With this diagnostic information, an individualized intervention program may be designed to reduce the motivational state or states or to support acquisition and/or use of alternative prosocial means of coping with the motivational conditions.

FROM DIAGNOSTICS TO INTERVENTIONS

Diagnostic findings about psychosocial and biomedical instigating, central processing, and maintaining conditions identified as influencing occurrence, severity level, variability over time in occurrence and severity, and the habitual recurrence of a person's aggression are translated into a matched set of treatment approaches. Gardner (2002a) provides a detailed description of this case formulation process for the interested reader.

Therapeutic efforts are selected to remove or minimize the influence of biomedical and psychosocial instigating and maintaining influences and to eliminate or minimize related central processing vulnerabilities. These efforts include the reduction or elimination of (a) pathological medical, psychiatric, and psychological conditions that produce or intensify distress levels and (b) impoverished and disruptive features of the social and physical environments that place a person at continued risk for aggressive acts. Treatment efforts also include programs for addressing psychological deficits, for example, through teaching anger management skills, coping communicative and other socially appropriate alternatives to aggression, and for increasing the motivation to use these newly acquired skills as adaptive functional replacements for the aggressive acts. A skill enhancement program focus to offset psychological central processing vulnerabilities is especially pertinent for those with highly restricted repertoires of coping skills. Acts of aggression may represent the most effective and efficient functional coping reactions to a range of antecedent controlling conditions. In this instance, aggression may be minimized or eliminated and treatment effects maintained following termination of interventions if these acts are replaced by equally effective and efficient functionally equivalent coping skills or by behaviors or skills that successfully compete with the aggressive behavior or with the motive associated with its occurrence (Gardner, Graeber-Whalen, & Ford, 2001; Gardner & Sovner, 1994; Horner & Day, 1991; Schroeder et al., 1999; Singh, Wahler, Adkins, & Myers, 2003).

It is not unusual that diagnostic activities would implicate a number of environmental, psychological, and biomedical features as current conditions that contribute to the occurrence, severity level, variability across time and situations, and persistent recurrence of acts of aggression and related disruptive behaviors. As a result, a staging plan would be required to prioritize and sequence the various interventions that may be required to address each of these influences (Feldman, Condillac, Tough, Hunt, & Griffiths, 2002; Gardner, 2002a; Nezu & Nezu. 1995). Staging plans are based on consideration of (a) the presumed magnitude of influence of specific interventions, (b) the need to sequentially present interventions that build on each other (i.e., the extent to which the effects of any specific intervention is dependent on the effects of earlier interventions), (c) the desirability of determining the separate effects of different interventions especially those that are intrusive or represent some risk to the physical or psychological well-being of the persons (e.g., neuroleptic medications; treatment procedures involving punishment contingencies), and (d) the projected time period in which a treatment effect should be realized. In order to evaluate the effect of specific interventions, it may be necessary to initiate only one intervention at any given time. If no treatment effect is realized within this projected time frame, the intervention should be reconsidered, modified, or even discarded. Use of this decision process is of special importance for those interventions with potential detrimental side effects or those that require considerable resources to implement and evaluate.

FOCUS OF INTERVENTIONS

Diagnostically-based interventions are selected to address the various conditions hypothesized or demonstrated to influence occurrence, severity levels, variability over time in frequency and severity, and the persistent recurrence or strength of specific acts of aggression. Thus the question of efficacy of treatment of aggression becomes a question of evaluating the efficacy of interventions that address various instigating, central processing, and maintaining conditions identified during the diagnostic assessment process as having potential influence on features of aggressive responding. If these influences reside in personal distress arising from a medical illness, evaluation would be made of the efficacy of medical treatment for the medical illness. If a controlling influence consists of a psychiatric symptom such as delusional ideation, irritability level, or a hypomanic mood state, efficacy of drug treatment for the condition producing the symptom would be assessed. If heightened levels of anger were presumed to influence aggressive acts, efficacy of treatments in reducing heightened levels of anger or in teaching alternative ways of coping with heightened anger would be considered. If a person's interpretation of the intent of the actions of others were presumed to influence acts of aggression, the usefulness of an intervention designed to modify this cognitive set would be assessed. If communication skills deficits were hypothesized to influence occurrence of aggression, the effectiveness of procedures for teaching communication skills would be assessed. If the selected interventions were successful in re-moving or reducing the presumed controlling conditions, the frequency of aggressive responding as well as severity levels and variability of these acts would be influenced to the extent that these conditions in fact served to in-fluence these features of aggressive responding. It is possible of course that a specific intervention might be highly effective in changing a presumed controlling influence (e.g., elimination of delusional ideation, reduction in anger, increase in socially-appropriate communication skills, reduction in contingent staff attention following aggressive acts, modification of a per-son's social information processing set) but have minimal or no effects on features of aggressive responding. In this event, either the presumed re-lationship did not exist or other untreated conditions were present that continued to be influential in producing the aggressive acts.

FEATURES INFLUENCING TREATMENT EFFICACY

In closing, brief attention is given to factors that influence the effi-cacy of treatments selected to modify conditions that control aggressive responding. A sampling of these features includes (a) the strength of ag-gressive responding, (b) the nature and number of antecedent controlling influences, (c) the nature and pervasiveness of differentially reinforcing consequences in the person's environment, (d) the degree to which the treatment focus is on teaching specific alternative behaviors that serve as functional replacements, and (e) the degree to which interventions are se-lected to address specific conditions presumed to be controlling influences.

Strength of Aggressive Responding

The strength of aggressive responding that reflects a person's unique reinforcement history represents a major central processing feature of an individual who uses aggression and related disruptive behaviors as coping responses (Bandura, 1973; Patterson, 1975). A specific intervention, or treatment package with several components, may be quite effective when used with an individual with low strength of aggressive responding (i.e., reinforcement history of aggressive responding is limited or acts of ag-gression previous had resulted in consequences of limited reinforcement value to the person). This same procedure or package may be relatively ineffective when used with a person who frequently engages in aggres-sive acts (i.e., rich and varied reinforcement history of aggressive respond-ing or aggressive acts have been followed systematically by consequences of high reinforcing salience to the individual). Bradley (2000) suggested that, following repeated use of aggressive responding, neural circuits are changed and thus are more resistant to treatment effects. As a result, more powerful interventions provided over repeated therapy sessions may be required for significant and enduring reduction in the probability of aggressive responding. Vitiello, Behar, Hunt, Stoff, and Ricciuti (1990) of-fered similar observations in their supposition that repeated occurrences of impulsive aggression associated with emotional states of fear or anger toward conditions of provocation may be more neurologically "hardwired" and become more automatic and habitually utilized. MacLean, Stone, and Brown (1994) noted that although intensive interventions may result in reduction in frequency and intensity of aggressive and destructive behaviors in persons with longstanding aggressive habits "... such intervention efforts have been largely ineffective in eliminating destructive behaviors. In many cases the behavior rebounds when intervention efforts are terminated" (p.68). A review of the literature on which this conclusion is based suggests that the behavioral interventions used most frequently attempted to change environmental conditions and contingencies. The results thus may reflect return to baseline environmental conditions that previously had maintained aggression and related destructive behaviors. Treatments seldom were designed to change other critical diagnostically identified central processing features. Thus, treatment efficacy may differ if different controlling conditions, especially those reflecting relevant central processing features, become the focus of treatment. The reader will recall that treatment targets refer to those conditions presumed to influence aggressive responding rather than the aggressive acts. In sum, in selection of interventions for aggressive habits of long duration, features in addition to modification of instigating conditions or changes in reinforcement contingencies may be needed for effective outcome. The research literature in behavior analysis that reports effective treatment outcomes with various combinations of antecedent and consequent environmental modifications and building of alternative functional skills and related motivational states provides one illustration of this.

Nature and Number of Antecedent Controlling Influences

Instigating events that signal occurrence of aggressive behaviors have been shown to have their origin in the external physical, social, and program environments and in covert or internal psychological, medical, and psychiatric conditions. Stimulus states emanating from any of these sources, in isolation and in combination with other events, may influence the occurrence, severity, or variability over time of acts of aggression. More specifically, depending on a person's responses to these conditions and the number of these controlling events, occurrence of any specific stimulus states may place the person at risk of heightened levels of personal distress. This distress level may serve a major instigating role for occurrence and severity levels of aggressive acts in a person inclined to use aggression as a coping attempt to reduce the noxious experience. Treatment programs that address only a limited number of the controlling antecedents may be unlikely to produce enduring treatment effects.

Further, wide individual differences in the number and type of controlling antecedents exist among persons with ID and mental health issues. Carr et al. (1999) illustrates the idiosyncratic nature of controlling events in suggesting that some children with autism are quite sensitive to loud noises. A child with this reactivity may cover her ears to reduce the personal distress produced by a noisy classroom. A teacher's prompt to uncover her ears in order to hear the classroom instruction may result in an aggressive act toward the teacher. The aggressive response in this instance resulted from a combination of the noise-produced distress and the teacher's prompt. Neither in isolation was sufficient to instigate the aggressive act. A more complete analysis of this action in addition to an audiological assessment would include a consideration of deficits as an alternative means of communicating her concern to the teacher. In sum, treatment efficacy is likely to be enhanced when interventions address the varied and multiple sets of antecedents that influence aggressive responding.

Pervasiveness and Distribution of Environmental Consequences

Treatment efficacy, as well as generalization and maintenance of treatment effects, are enhanced by treatment and posttreatment environments that systematically (a) eliminate or reduce those antecedent and maintaining conditions controlling aggressive responding and (b) include those conditions that initiate and strengthen alternative replacement or competing behaviors. If following successful treatment a person is returned to instigating and maintaining baseline conditions and has not been provided with alternative or competing skills and the motives to support their occurrence, it could be expected in most instances that aggressive responding will recur. Thus, treatment programs that hold best promise of being most efficacious have the dual objectives of (a) environmental changes conducive to occurrence and maintenance of alternatives to aggression and (b) reduction or elimination of biomedical and psychological central processing risk factors for aggressive acts. The reader will recall that psychological risk factors include skills deficits. If, in illustration, heightened anger arousal represents a major antecedent for instigation for aggressive acts, a treatment program that teaches independent use of anger management skills would enhance maintenance of treatment effects in posttreatment settings. In this instance, even if returned to pretreatment baseline conditions that produce heightened anger arousal, the person's new anger management skills would be available to interrupt the controlling influence of heightened levels of anger. This example emphasizes the value of interventions that modify both the environmental antecedents to aggressive responding and, as emphasized in the following section, also provide alternatives means of responding to sources of instigation.

Focus on Teaching Alternative Behaviors as Functional Replacements

Treatment efficacy is enhanced when attention is focused on teaching functional replacements for the aggressive acts. As one example, a relationship has been noted between deficits in expressive communication skills and prevalence of aggressive responding among persons with mental health issues. As illustration, Dura (1997) found expressive communicative difficulties and presence of psychiatric symptoms to be strong predictors of aggressive behaviors in a study of 67 adults with ID. In combination, high mental health symptoms and low expressive communicative ability were associated with the highest prevalence of aggressive responding. Numerous studies have illustrated the value of teaching effective and efficient skills of expressive communication as functional alternatives to aggressive responding. In early demonstrations, Carr and Durand (1985) taught children with developmental disabilities to use communication skills as functional alternatives when exposed to conditions that produced aggressive reactions. Bird et al. (1989) reported the successful use of communication training to teaching alternatives to aggression in an adult with autism and profound ID. Assessment suggested that the aggression was motivated by escape from demands and a desire to obtain preferred tangible items. Following acquisition and use of alternative means of communicating these needs, high rate aggressive behaviors decreased. Carr et al. (1994) and Reichle and Wacker (1993) provide excellent descriptions of successful applications of communication training as functional replacements for aggressive responding in persons with a wide range of individual differences and should be consulted for additional examples.

Focus of Interventions on Specific Controlling Influences

Although there are no specific pharmacologic treatments for aggressive behaviors, a significant percentage of persons with persistent problems of aggression become the targets of psychotropic medication administered to decrease occurrence or severity of aggressive behavior rather than for specific psychiatric or psychological symptoms that are presumed to serve as controlling influences (Matson et al., 2000; Reiss & Aman, 1998). Although a reduction in frequency or severity of aggressive responding in addition to reductions in other behaviors not targeted for change may be observed in some persons, the question of "what is being treated" remains unanswered.

The same question may be raised relative to a number of behavioral interventions including such procedures as noncontingent reinforcement, differential reinforcement procedures, punishment procedures involving overcorrection, time out, response cost and related behavior reduction techniques, providing choices, and general social skills training. Such procedures, while demonstrated to have a behavior reduction effect for some persons who use aggression as a coping behavior, typically are not diagnostically based and selected specifically to address specific antecedent, central processing, or maintaining conditions. Baker and Thyer (2000) provide illustration of this case formulation deficiency in their use of a differential reinforcement of other behavior (DRO) procedure in addressing problems of aggression and related disruptive acts in a man with cognitive impairment who attended a vocational center. Even though frequency of aggressive responding reduced following implementation of a procedure that provided a reinforcer following periods of time during which these aggressive and related disruptive behaviors were absent, no assessments of the motivational bases of the acts were conducted. Further, the program did not teach alternative means of coping with the unidentified antecedent instigating conditions controlling these aggressive and disruptive acts. Maintenance and generalization of treatment effects following withdrawal of the DRO procedures thus is highly unlikely.

CONCLUDING COMMENTS

As described, clinical approaches to treatment of acts of aggression and related disruptive behaviors reflect the specific suppositions held by a clinician relative to significant controlling conditions. These suppositions influence the selection of the case formulation framework used to determine assessment targets, assessment procedures, and the interpretations given to assessment results. Assessment findings and related interpretations of these in turn influence selection of specific treatment and management procedures to address the conditions identified as controlling influences on occurrence, severity levels, variability, and persistent recurrence of a person's aggressive acts.

A variety of case formulations currently are being used to guide the diagnostic, treatment selection, and treatment evaluation process. The medical and psychiatric illness framework guides selection of medication interventions, especially in those instances in which symptom features of medical illnesses, psychiatric disorders, neurological abnormalities, or genetic disorders are presumed to represent controlling influences on features of aggressive responding. Various behavior therapy frameworks provide direction to identification and treatment of possible cognitive, emotional, and related psychological contributors to occurrence, severity levels, and persistence of aggressive acts. Applied behavior analysis based on concepts of operant learning represents the most frequently used framework to guide management and treatment of environmental antecedents and consequences presumed to be significant controlling influences on problems of aggression in persons with mental retardation. This framework currently provides the best evidence-based practices for treatment and management of the environmental conditions controlling aggression, especially among those with more severe ID.

Although current treatment practices derived from behavioral, psychological, and biomedical case formulation frameworks have resulted in notable successful treatment outcomes, problems involving aggression and disruptive acts among persons with ID continue to represent a major clinical issue. As noted earlier, following an analysis of the treatment literatures, MacLean et al. (1994) concluded that even though intensive interventions may produce positive treatment effects "... such intervention efforts have been largely ineffective in eliminating destructive behaviors. In many cases, the behavior rebounds when intervention efforts are terminated" (p. 69).

This chapter offers a case formulation framework that emphasizes the transactional nature of environmental, biomedical, and psychological influences on aggressive responding and provides a means of combining various medical and psychiatric diagnostic insights and related diagnostically based interventions with those that involve psychological and environmental influences. As one possible approach to overcoming the difficulties of treatment maintenance, the framework recommends a major treatment focus that addresses central processing risk factors.

A final thought. Regardless of the framework used to guide clinical practice, attempts should be made to emulate the applied behavior analytic framework standard of excellence in its data- based approach to assessment of treatment effects. This objective approach to treatment efficacy is recommended as an essential central feature of all future treatment efforts, especially when potential negative side effects are possible.

REFERENCES

Allen, D. (2000). Recent research on physical aggression in persons with intellectual disabilities: An overview. *Journal of Intellectual and Developmental Disabilities, 25,* 41–57.

Baker, D. J., Blumberg, E. R., Freeman, R., & Wieseler, N. A. (2002). Can psychiatric disorders be seen as establishing operations? Integrating applied behavior analysis and psychiatry. *Mental Health Aspects of Developmental Disabilities, 5,* 118–124.

Baker, K. L., & Thyer, B. A. (2000). Differential reinforcement of other behavior in the treatment of inappropriate behavior and aggression in an adult with mental retardation at a vocational center. *Scandinavian Journal of Behaviour Therapy, 29,* 37–42.

Baker, W., & Bramston, P. (1997). Attributional and emotional determinants of aggression in people with mild intellectual disabilities. *Journal of Intellectual and Developmetnal Diabilities, 22,* 169–186.

Bandura, A. (1969). *Principles of behavior modification.* New York: Holt, Rinehart, & Winston.

Bandura, A. (1973). *Aggression: A social learning analysis.* Englewood Cliffs, NJ: Prentice-Hall.

Bandura, A. (1977). *Social learning theory.* Englewood Cliffs, NJ: Prentice-Hall.

Bandura, A. (1986). *Social foundations of thought and action: A social cognitive theory.* Englewood Cliffs, NJ: Prentice-Hall.

Bandura, A., & Walters, R. H. (1963). *Social learning and personality development.* New York: Holt, Rinehart, & Winston.

Barnhill, J. (1999). The relationships between epilepsy and violent behavior in persons with mental retardation. *The NADD Bulletin, 2,* 43–46.

Barnhill, J. (2001). Behavioral phenotypes: A glimpse into the neuropsychiatry of genes (Part II): Analysis of behavioral phenotypes-social anxiety in Fragile-X syndrome and autism. *The NADD Bulletin, 4,* 63–69.

Benson, B. A. (1985). Behavioral disorders and mental retardation: Association with age, sex, and levels of functioning in an outpatient clinic sample. *Applied Research in Mental Retardation, 6,* 79–85.

Benson, B. A. (2002). Feeling, thinking, doing: Reducing aggression through skill development. In W. I. Gardner (Ed.), *Aggression and other disruptive behavioral challenges* (pp. 293–323), Kingston, NY: NADD.

Benson, B. A., & Fuchs, C. (1999). Anger-arousing situations and coping responses of aggressive adults with intellectual disabilities. *Journal of Intellectual and Developmental Disabilities, 24,* 207–215.

Benson, B. A., Rice, C. J., & Miranti, S. V. (1986). Effects of anger management training with mentally retarded adults in group treatment. *Journal of Consulting and Clinical Psychology, 54,* 728–729.

Berg, W. K., Peck, S., Wacker, D. P., Harding, J., McComas, J., Richman, D., et al. (2000). The effects of presession exposure to attention on the results of assessments of attention as a reinforcer. *Journal of Applied Behavior Analysis, 33,* 463–478.

Bird, F., Dores, P. A., Moniz, D., & Robinson, J. (1989). Reducing severe aggressive and self-injurious behaviors with functional communication training. *American Journal of Mental Retardation, 94*, 37–48.

Borthwick-Duffy, S. A. (1994). Prevalence of destructive behaviors: A study of aggression, self-injury, and property destruction. In T. Thompson & D. B. Gray (Eds.), *Destructive behavior in developmental disabilities* (pp. 3–23), Thousand Oaks, CA: Sage.

Bradley, S. J. (2000). *Affect regulation and the development of psychopathology.* New York: Guilford.

Carr, E. G. (1997). The evolution of applied behavior analysis into positive behavior support. *Journal of the Association for Persons with Severe Handicaps, 22*, 208–209.

Carr, E. G., & Durand, V. M. (1985). Reducing behavior problems through functional communication training. *Journal of Applied Behavior Analysis, 18*, 111–126.

Carr, E. G., Langdon, N. A., & Yarbrough, S. C. (1999). Linking functional assessment to effective intervention. In A. C. Repp & R. H. Horner (Eds.), *Functional analysis of problem behavior* (pp. 7–31). Belmont, CA: Wadsworth.

Carr, E. G., Levin, L., McConnachie, G., Carlson, J. I., Kemp, D. C., & Smith, C. E. (1994). *Communication-based intervention for problem behavior.* Baltimore: Brookes.

Cole, C. L., Gardner, W. I., & Karan, O. (1985). Self-management training of mentally retarded adults presenting severe conduct difficulties. *Applied Research in Mental Retardation, 6*, 337–347.

Collins, M. S. R., & Cornish, K. (2002). A survey of the prevalence of stereotypy, self-injury and aggression in children and young adults with Cri du Chat syndrome. *Journal of Intellectual Disability Research, 46*, 133–140.

Comings, D. E., & Comings, B. G. (1985). Tourette syndrome: Clinical and psychological aspects of 250 cases. *American Journal of Human Genetics, 37*, 435–450.

Craighead, L. W., Craighead, W. E., Kazdin, A. E., & Mahoney, M. J. (1994). *Cognitive and behavioral interventions.* Boston: Allyn and Bacon.

Cullen, C. (1996). Challenging behaviours and intellectual disabilities: Assessment, analysis and treatment. *British Journal of Clinical Psychology, 35*, 153–156.

Davidson, P., Cain, N., Sloane-Reeve, J., VanSpeybroeck, A., Segel, J., Gutkin, J., et al. (1994) Characteristics of community-based individuals with mental retardation and aggressive behavioral disorders. *American Journal on Mental Retardation, 98*, 704–716.

Dodge, K. A. (1993). Social-cognitive mechanisms in the development of conduct difficulties and depression. *Annual Review of Psychology, 44*, 559–584.

Dura, J. (1997). Expressive communicative ability, symptoms of mental illness and aggressive behavior. *Journal of Clinical Psychology, 53*, 307–318.

Dykens, E. M., Hodapp, R. M., & Finucane, B. M. (2000). *Genetics and mental retardation syndromes.* Baltimore: Brookes.

Einfeld, S. L., Tonge, B. J., & Florio, T. (1997). Behavioral and emotional disturbance in individuals with Williams syndrome. *American Journal of Mental Retardation, 102*, 45–53.

Ellis, C. R., Singh, Y. N., & Singh, N. N. (1997). Use of behavior-modifying drugs. In N. N. Singh (Ed.), *Prevention and treatment of severe behavior problems* (pp. 149–176). Pacific Grove, CA: Brooks/Cole.

Eyman , R. K., & Call, T. (1977). Maladaptive behavior and community placement for mentally retarded persons. *American Journal of Mental Deficiency, 82*, 137–144.

Feldman, M. A., Condillac, R. A., Tough, S., Hunt, S., & Griffiths, D. (2002). Effectiveness of community positive behavioral intervention for persons with developmental disabilities and severe behavior disorders. *Behavior Therapy, 33*, 377–398.

Fredericks, B., & Nishioka-Evans, V. (1999). Functional assessment for a sex offender population. In A. C. Repp & R. H. Horner (Eds.), *Functional analysis of problem behavior* (pp. 279–303). Belmont, CA: Wadsworth.

Fuchs, C., & Benson, B. A. (1995). Social information processing by aggressive and nonaggressive men with mental retardation. *American Journal on Mental Retardation, 100*, 244–252.

Gardner, W. I. (1969). Use of punishment procedures with the severely retarded: A review. *American Journal of Mental Deficiency, 74*, 86–103.

Gardner, W. I. (1971). *Behavior modification in mental retardation.* London: University of London Press.

Gardner, W. I. (1977). *Learning and behavior characteristics of exceptional children and youth.* Boston: Allyn & Bacon.

Gardner, W. I. (1996). Nonspecific behavioral symptoms in persons with a dual diagnosis: A psychological model for integrating biomedical and psychosocial diagnosis and interventions. *Psychology in Mental Retardation and Developmental Disabilities, 21,* 6–11.

Gardner, W. I. (1998). Initiating the case formulation process. In D. M. Griffiths, W. I. Gardner, & J. A. Nugent (Eds.), *Behavioral supports: Individual centered interventions* (pp. 17–65). Kingston, NY: NADD.

Gardner, W. I. (2002a). *Aggression and other disruptive behavioral challenges: Biomedical and psychosocial assessment and treatment.* Kingston, NY: NADD.

Gardner, W. I. (2002b). Psychological treatment of persons with mental retardation who present emotional and behavioral challenges. In R. F. B. Gues & D. A. Flikweert (Eds.), *Behandeling van psychische en degragsproblems* (pp. 13–20). Utrecht, The Netherlands: NGBZ/NIZW.

Gardner, W. I., Graeber, J. L., & Cole, C. L. (1996). Behavior therapies: A multimodal diagnostic and intervention model. In J. W. Jacobson & J. A. Mulick (Eds.), *Manual of diagnosis and professional practice in mental retardation* (pp. 255–269). Washington, DC: American Psychological Association.

Gardner, W. I., Graeber-Whalen, J. L., & Ford, D. (2001). Behavior therapies: Individualizing interventions through treatment formulations. In A. Dosen & K. Day (Eds.), *Treating mental illness and behavior disorders in children and adults with mental retardation* (pp. 69–100). Washington, DC: American Psychiatric.

Gardner, W. I., & Sovner, R. (1994). *Self-injurious behaviors: Diagnosis and treatment.* Willow Street, PA: Vida.

Gardner, W. I., & Whalen, J. P. (1996). A multimodal behavior analytic model for evaluating the effects of medical problems on nonspecific behavioral symptoms in persons with developmental disabilities. *Behavioral Interventions, 11,* 147–161.

Gedye, A. (1997). *Behavioral diagnostic guide for developmental disabilities.* Vancouver, British Columbia, Canada: Diagnostic Books.

Griffiths, D. (2002). Sexual aggression. In W. I. Gardner (Ed.), *Aggression and other disruptive behavioral challenges: Biomedical and psychosocial assessment and treatment* (pp. 325–397). Kingston, NY: NADD.

Hanley, G. P., Iwata, B. A., & McCord, B. E. (2003). *Functional analysis of problem behavior: A review. Journal of Applied Behavior Analysis, 36,* 147–185.

Horner, R. H., & Day, H. M. (1991). The effects of response efficiency on functionally equivalent competing behaviors. *Journal of Applied Behavior Analysis, 24,* 719–732.

Hutchinson, R. R. (1973). The environmental causes of aggression. In J. K. Cole & D. D. Jensen (Eds.), *Nebraska symposium on motivation: 1972* (pp. 155–181). Lincoln, NE: University of Nebraska Press.

Jacobson, J. W. (1982). Problem behavior and psychiatric impairment in a developmentally disabled population: I. Behavior frequency. *Applied Research in Mental Retardation, 3,* 121–139.

Kastner, T., Walsh, K. K., & Fraser, M. (2001). Undiagnosed medical conditions and medication side effects presenting as behavioral/psychiatric problems in people with mental retardation. *Mental Health Aspects of Developmental Disabilities, 4,* 101–107.

Koegel, R. L., Koegel, L. K., & Dunlap, G. (1996). *Positive behavioral support.* Baltimore: Brookes.

Lindsay, W. R., Marshall, I., Neilson, C., Quinn, K., & Smith, A. H. W. (1998). The treatment of a person with a learning disability convicted of exhibitionism. *Research in Developmental Disabilities, 19,* 295–316.

Lowry, M. A. (1994). Functional assessment of problem behaviors associated with mood disorders. *The Habilitative Mental Healthcare Newsletter, 13,* 79–84.

Lowry, M. A., & Sovner, R. (1992). Severe behavior problems associated with rapid cycling bipolar disorder in two adults with profound mental retardation. *Journal of Intellectual Disability Research, 36,* 269–281.

MacLean, W. E., Stone, W. L., & Brown, W. H. (1994). Developmental psychopathology of destructive behavior. In T. Thompson & D. V. Gray (Eds.), *Destructive behavior in developmental disabilities: Diagnosis and treatment* (pp. 68–79). Thousands Oaks, CA: Sage.

Marcus, B. A., Vollmer, T. R., Swanson, V., Roane, H. R., & Ringdahl, J. E. (2001). An experimental analysis of aggression. *Behavior Modification, 25*, 189–213.

Matson, J. L., Bambury, J. W., Mayville, E. A, Pinkston, J., Bielecki, J., Kuhn, D., et al. (2000). Psychopharmacology and mental retardation: A 10 year review (1990–1999). *Research in Developmental Disabilities, 21*, 263–296.

Matson, J. L., & Duncan, D. (1997). Aggression. In N. N. Singh (Ed.), *Prevention and treatment of severe behavior problems* (pp. 217–236.). Pacific Grove, CA: Brooks/Cole.

Matson, J. L., & Mayville, E. A. (2001). The relationship of functional variables and psychopathology to aggressive behavior in persons with severe and profound mental retardation. *Journal of Psychopathology and Behavioral Assessment, 23*, 3–9.

Matson, J. L., & Vollmer, T. R. (1995). *The Questions About Behavioral Function (QABF) user's guide.* Baton Rouge, LA: Scientific.

McComas, J., Hoch, H., Paone, D., & El-Roy, D. (2000). Escape behavior during academic tasks: A preliminary analysis of idiosyncratic establishing operations. *Journal of Applied Behavior Analysis, 33*, 479–493.

Mikkelsen, E. J., & McKenna, I. (1999). Psychopharmacologic algorithms for adults for developmental disabilities and difficult-to-diagnose behavioral disorders. *Psychiatric Annuals, 29*, 302–314.

Mulick, J. A., Hammer, D., & Dura, J. R. (1991). Assessment and management of antisocial and hyperactive behavior. In J. L. Matson & J. A. Mulick (Eds.), *Handbook of mental retardation* (2nd ed., pp. 397–412). New York: Pergamon.

Nezu, C. M., & Nezu, A. M. (1994). Outpatient psychotherapy for adults with mental retardation and concomitant psychopathology: Research and clinical imperatives. *Journal of Consulting and Clinical Psychology, 62*, 34–42.

Nezu, C. M., & Nezu, A. M. (1995). Clinical decision making in everyday practice: The science in the art. *Cognitive and Behavioral Practice, 2*, 5–25.

Nezu, C. M., Nezu, A. M., & Gill-Weiss, M. J. (1992). *Psychopathology in persons with mental retardation.* Champaign, IL: Research.

O'Donohue, W., & Krasner, L. (Eds.). (1995). *Theories of behavior therapy: Exploring behavior change.* Washington, DC: American Psychological Association.

O'Reilly, M. F. (1995). Functional analysis and treatment of escape-maintained aggression correlated with sleep deprivation. *Journal of Applied Behavior Analysis, 28*, 225–226.

Patterson, G. R. (1975). *A social learning approach to family intervention: Vol. 1. Families with aggressive children.* Eugene, OR: Castalia.

Ratey, J. J. (2001). *A user's guide to the brain.* New York: Pantheon Books.

Reichle, J., & Wacker, D. P. (Eds.). (1993). *Communication and language intervention series: Vol 3. Communicative alternatives to challenging behavior: Integrating functional assessment and intervention strategies.* Baltimore: Brookes.

Reiss, S., & Aman, M. G. (1998). *Psychotropic medications and developmental disabilities: The international consensus handbook.* Columbus, OH: Ohio State University Nisonger Center.

Reiss, S., & Havercamp, S. M. (1997). Sensitivity theory and mental retardation: Why functional analysis is not enough. *American Journal of Mental Retardation, 101*, 553–566.

Reiss, S., & Havercamp, S. M. (1998). Toward a comprehensive assessment of fundamental motivation: Factor structure of the Reiss Profiles. *Psychological Assessment, 10*, 97–106.

Reiss, S., & Rojahn, J. (1993). Joint occurrence of depression and aggression in children and adults with mental retardation. *Journal of Intellectual Disability Research, 37*, 287–294.

Repp, A. G., & Horner, R. H. (Eds.). (1999). *Functional analysis of problem behavior.* Belmont, CA: Wadsworth.

Rush, A. J., & Frances, A. (2000). Treatment of psychiatric and behavioral problems in mental retardation: Expert consensus guideline series. *American Journal of Mental Retardation, 105*, 159–228.

Schroeder, S. R., Reese, R. M., Hellings, J., Loupe, J., & Tessel, R. E. (1999). The causes of self-injurious behavior and their implications. In N. A. Wieseler & R. Hanson (Eds.), *Challenging behavior in persons with mental health disorders and severe developmental disabilities* (pp. 65–87). Washington, DC: AAMR Monograph Series.

Schroeder, S. R., Rojahn, J., & Oldenquist, A. (1991). Treatment of destructive behaviors among persons with mental retardation and developmental disabilities: An overview of the problem. In *Treatment of destructive behaviors in persons with developmental disabilities* (pp. 125–172, NIMH Publication No. 9-2410). Bethesda, MD: Department of Health and Human Services.

Sheard, M. H. (1984). Clinical pharmacology of aggressive behavior. *Clinical Neuropharmacology, 7,* 173–183.

Singh, N. N., Wahler, R. G., Adkins, A. D., & Myers, R. E. (2003). Soles of the feet: A mindfulness-based self-control intervention for aggression by an individual with mild mental retardation and mental illness. *Research in Developmental Disabilities, 24,* 158–169.

Sovner, R., & Fogelman, S. (1996). Irritability and mental retardation. *Seminars in Clinical Neuropsychiatry, 1,* 105–114.

Sovner, R., Foxx, C. J., Lowry, M. J., & Lowry, M. A. (1993). Fluoretine treatment of depression and associated self-injury in two adults with mental retardation. *Journal of Intellectual Disabilities Research, 37,* 301–311.

Staats, A. W. (1996). *Behavior and personality: Psychological behaviorism.* New York: Springer .

Thompson, R. H., & Iwata, B. A. (2001). A descriptive analysis of social consequences following problem behavior. *Journal of Applied Behavior Analysis, 34,* 169–178.

Thompson, T., & Symons, F. J. (1999). Neurobehavioral mechanisms of drug action. In N. A. Wieseler & R. H. Hanson (Eds.), *Challenging behavior of persons with mental health disorders and severe developmental disabilities* (pp. 125–150). Washington, DC: American Association on Mental Retardation.

Tsiouris, J. A. (2001). Diagnosis of depression in people with severe/profound mental retardation. *Journal of Intellectual Disability Research, 45,* 115–120.

Tuinier, S., & Verhoeven, W. M. A. (1993). Psychiatry and mental retardation: Towards a behavioural pharmacological concept. *Journal of Intellectual Disabilities Research, 37,* 16–24.

Vitiello, B., Behar, D., Hunt, J., Stoff, D., & Ricciuti, A. (1990). Subtyping aggression in children and adolescents. *Journal of Neuropsychiatry, 2,* 189–192.

Whitaker, S. (1993). The reduction of aggression in people with learning difficulties: A review of psychological methods. *British Journal of Clinical Psychology, 32,* 1–37.

Worsdell, A. S., Iwata, B. A., Hanley, G. P., Thompson, R. H., & Kahng, S. W. (2000). Effects of continuous and intermittent reinforcement for problem behavior during functional communication training. *Journal of Applied Behavior Analysis, 33,* 167–179.

28

Speech and Language Deficits in Children with Developmental Disabilities

JOANNE GERENSER and BONNIE FORMAN, THURSDAY'S CHILD

Promoting effective speech, language, and communication is almost always a central issue in the treatment and education of children with mental retardation and other developmental disabilities. The range and severity of the speech–language deficits vary considerably across individuals and across disabilities.

Over the past 25 years, there have been two primary approaches used to understand the language disorders of children with developmental disabilities. The traditional approach classifies the disability by the cause or the etiology. McCormick and Schiefelbusch (1990) described five etiological categories:

1. Language and communication disorders associated with sensory disorders such as hearing and vision impairments;
2. Language and communication disorders associated with motor disorders such as cerebral palsy or spina bifida;
3. Language and communication disorders associated with central nervous system damage such as learning disabilities;
4. Language and communication disorders associated with severe emotional dysfunction such as schizophrenia or autism;
5. Language and communication disorders associated with cognitive delays such as mental retardation.

JOANNE GERENSER • The Eden II Programs, Staten Island, New York 10303.   BONNIE FORMAN, THURSDAY'S CHILD • Brooklyn, New York 11209.

One problem, however, with the etiological approach is that it does not provide the clinician with clear information as to what the individual knows about language. In addition, there is considerable overlap among the different disorders.

An alternative to the etiological approach is the descriptive developmental approach (Bloom & Lahey, 1978). The descriptive developmental approach describes rather than classifies the language disorder. More specifically, it compares the language of the child who is disabled to the language of a typically developing child. The descriptive developmental approach has resulted in interventions that are often based on the degree of mental retardation without reference to the specific etiology (Dykens, 1995).

There has been a great deal of research over the past 10 years on the learning characteristics of individuals with specific syndromes and disabilities. These learning characteristics have been discussed in terms of the implications they have for the behavioral profiles of the individuals, including the speech, language, and communication skills and deficits. Unfortunately, little of the syndrome specific information is currently integrated into clinical intervention (Mirrett, Roberts, & Price, 2003).

The focus of this chapter will be to present current information on the speech–language skills and challenges, as well as the learning characteristics of the most prevalent groups of children classified as developmentally disabled. The chapter will be divided into three sections. The first section will review fragile X syndrome (FXS) and Down syndrome (DS), the two most frequent known causes of mental retardation. The second section will provide an overview of cerebral palsy with a focus on the motor speech disorders often associated with this population. The third section will review autism and its impact on speech, language, and communication development.

The most effective treatment program for a child with a developmental disability must include both a clear description of the child's existing skills and a thorough understanding of the impact of the specific syndrome on these skills and deficits. In addition to profiles of the groups, the intervention research for each will be discussed.

GENETIC MENTAL RETARDATION SYNDROMES

DS and FXS are the two most common genetic causes of mental retardation. Studies evaluating these two populations have revealed distinct speech and language characteristics associated with each (Laws & Bishop, 2003; Roberts, Hennon, & Anderson, 2003; Roberts, Mirrett, Anderson, Burchinal, & Neele, 2002). The speech–language deficits associated with both DS and FXS cannot be fully accounted for by pure cognitive delays (Facon, Facon-Bollengier, & Grubar, 2002; Fowler, 1990). The complex neurobehavioral features of each syndrome play a significant role in the speech language development of the individual (Gibson, 1991; Sigman, 1999; Sudhalter, Cohen, Silverman, & Wolf-Schein, 1990).

Down Syndrome

Problems with speech and language may be the greatest challenges facing individuals with DS (Chapman & Heskith, 2001). Children with DS demonstrate delayed acquisition of spoken language, with slow progress across all domains of expressive language (Fabretti, Rizzuto, Vicari, & Volaterra, 1997). Vocabulary development, although delayed, is a relative strength. In fact, Byrne, Buckley, MacDonald, & Bird (1995) describe a dissociation between vocabulary and grammar, with morphology and syntax being far more challenged than vocabulary.

Despite delayed development, most individuals with DS will develop speech. The range of intelligibility, however, can be extreme, with some individuals remaining largely unintelligible. The controversy remains as to whether speech development is merely delayed (Van Borsel, 1996) or whether there are specific factors associated with DS that contribute to the speech disorder (Rondal & Edwards, 1997; Wilcox, 1988).

There are a number of factors to consider with regard to speech development in children with DS. Oral anatomical structural abnormalities are present from birth. These abnormalities include high vaulted and narrow palate as well as oral motor muscle hypotonia (Backman, Grever-Sjolander, Holm, & Johansson, 2003). In addition, there is an increased prevalence of an overbite as well as delayed eruption of primary teeth. It is crucial to secure an exam by a pediatric dentist no later than 6 months of age to address some of these issues.

To date, there are two primary approaches to address the oral motor problems. The first involves oral motor therapy, designed to strengthen the muscles of the mouth and tongue (Kumin, Goodman, & Council, 1996). The second approach involves the use of prosthetic devices such as a palatal plate (Backman et al., 2003; Carlstedt, Hernogsson, & Dahllof, 2003). A palatal plate is an individually made removable acrylic device designed to activate muscles in the mouth through a moveable ball on a stainless steel wire. Although some have found improved mouth closure and reduced tongue protrusion after the use of a palatal plate (Carlstedt et al., 2003), data on their effects on speech development and intelligibility are limited.

The speech deficits present in children with DS cannot be solely attributed to these anatomical problems. Dodd and Thompson (2001) propose that children with DS demonstrate a disorder of phonological acquisition that is not consistent with typical phonological disorders. They propose that the problems of short-term auditory memory, common in children with DS, results in incomplete phonological representation of words at the lexical level. This is reflected by the inconsistent nature of the phonological errors present in a child with DS. Furthermore, Dodd and Thompson suggest that inconsistent errors are often understood and accepted by family members and others in the environment, resulting in a persistence of these errors.

Hearing loss is another variable that may negatively affect the speech production of children with DS (Everhuis, Van Zanten, Brocoas, &

Roerdinkholder, 1992). Fluctuating otitis media is common in DS and can result in corresponding hearing loss.

In summary, speech intelligibility in children with DS is a significant issue. Clinical intervention should focus on anatomical issues such as oral motor hypotonia and other structural issues, as well as the phonological disorder often present. Consistency of word production should be a priority in treatment. The use of a "core" vocabulary approach (see Dodd, McCormack, and Woodyatt, 1994) has been demonstrated to be effective.

Although the degree of mental retardation contributes to the language disorder present in DS, it is insufficient to account for the variability (Fowler, 1990; Sigman, 1999). There have been a number of documented cases of exceptional language abilities in DS (Laws & Bishop, 2003).

There is evidence that children with DS learn differently than do other children with similar cognitive delays. These differences are present from a very early age. Research has revealed that young children with DS avoid opportunities for learning new skills, do not make use of skills that are acquired and often fail to consolidate skills that are not in their repertoires (Wishart, 1993). Problems with attending as well as deficits in short-term auditory memory contribute to these learning differences. These learning differences, in turn, affect the language development of children with DS. Attention issues reduce the amount of information that is processed. Short-term auditory problems affect syntax comprehension as well as lexical representation (Adams & Gathercole, 2000; Montgomery, 2000).

Despite significant research on the language disorder of individuals with DS, there is very little data demonstrating the efficacy of speech–language intervention for this population (Spiker & Hopmann, 1997). The use of simultaneous communication is very common with children with DS (Pueschel & Hopmann, 1993). There is some research to support the use of combined sign and spoken input to foster early language development (Clibbens, 2001; Launonen, 1996). In addition to enhancing lexical development, sign language has also been shown to enhance comprehension (Kay-Raining Bird, Gaskell, Babineau, & MacDonald, 2000) as well as improve speech intelligibility (Powell & Clibbens, 1994). Most researchers agree that signing should be viewed as a supportive system as opposed to an alternative system. Miller (1992) found that spoken words began to accelerate in children at approximately 26 months of age whereas signed words began to diminish. The benefit of sign language may be due to the relative strength of visual spatial processing in children with DS (Jarrold & Baddeley, 1997).

A focus on enhancing auditory memory skills has been recommended to address the speech–language development (Chapman, 1995). In addition to using direct instruction to enhance short-term memory, using predictable materials as well as visual information to support learning have been found to be effective (Chapman, 1995; Nadel, 1999).

One important thing that cannot be overlooked when working with children with DS is the presence of interfering or problem behavior. There is clear evidence that many children with DS develop interfering behavior such as aggression or tantrums and that these behaviors significantly compromise treatment (Capone, 2004). It is important to develop proactive plans to prevent or reduce problem behavior in order to insure best outcomes.

Fragile X Syndrome

FXS is the most common inherited cause of mental retardation (Roberts et al., 2002). Males are affected more severely by fragile X than are females (Abbeduto et al., 2003). Eighty-five percent of males with FXS demonstrate significant metal retardation. In addition, many males with FXS display characteristics consistent with autism. It has been estimated that 5–6% of children with autism test positive for FXS (Fisch, 1992) and anywhere from 7 to 25% of individuals with FXS receive a diagnosis of autism (Bailey, Hatton, & Skinner, 1998; Hagerman, 1996).

Individuals with FXS have distinct speech patterns. Repetition of sounds, words, and phrases is common (Abbeduto & Hagerman, 1997). Overall speech intelligibility varies with context. Speech intelligibility is generally good in single words yet poor for conversational speech (Roberts et al., 2003). Factors that contribute to poor speech intelligibility include oral motor problems (e.g., low muscle tone and poor lip closure) as well as rapid speech rate with marked dysfluencies and cluttering (Schopmeyer, 1992).

The syntax and vocabulary skills of individuals with FXS are generally consistent with cognitive level. Receptive language abilities are stronger than expressive skills, yet both areas decline in adolescence and adulthood (Dykens et al., 1996; Fisch et al., 1999).

Pragmatic language is most significantly affected. Individuals with FXS demonstrate perseveration of topics, difficulty answering direct questions, poor eye contact and gaze aversion, as well as tangential speech and impulsivity (Abbeduto & Hagerman, 1997; Cornish, Sudhalter, & Turk, 2004; Sudhalter & Belser, 2001). Problems with hyperarousal and executive functioning have been implicated as the primary factors underlying the language deficits of individuals with fragile X (Abbeduto & Hagerman 1997; Belser & Sudhalter, 1995). Hyperarousal is frequently manifested in difficulties with transitions and social anxiety along with a limited attention span (Cornish et al., 2004; Mirrett et al., 2003). Failure to address issues of hyperarousal and anxiety will impede progress and may result in the development of maladaptive behavior. Almost half of children with FXS attending school are described as having significant behavior problems in class (Symons, Clark, Roberts, & Bailey, 2001).

Unfortunately, as with DS, there is little empirical evidence available to support any specific intervention for individuals with FXS (Abbeduto, Evans, & Dolan, 2001). There have been some specific educational guides developed addressing syndrome specific deficits in fragile X (Braden, 1998; Scharfenaker et al., 1996). Applications of these programs, however, have not been empirically validated.

Clinical research recommends a myriad of strategies when addressing the speech and language deficits present in FXS. A team approach is considered most effective. Intervention should be provided in a structured environment with systematic behavioral teaching strategies (Mirrett et al., 2003). Efforts to decrease arousal and anxiety must be considered priority. Use of visual cues as well as the establishment of familiar routines is recommended. Speech intelligibility can be improved by reducing rate of speech, addressing oral motor issues as well as direct instruction of phonological processes (Lowe, 1992; Roberts et al., 2003).

CEREBRAL PALSY

Cerebral palsy is a disorder of motor and posture due to brain insult that occurs in the early period of brain growth (Love, 1992). The incidence and nature of speech–language disorders in people with cerebral palsy varies considerably and is influenced by many factors. Variables such as site of lesion, associated handicaps, including mental retardation, or hearing loss, as well as the cumulative effects of multiple risk factors all contribute to the speech–language deficits (Cougher, Savage, & Smith, 1992; Hardy, 1983; Rosetti, 1996). Some degree of cognitive deficits occur in approximately 50% of individuals with cerebral palsy, although motor deficits make testing difficult and often unreliable (Owens, 1993). The most common speech–language disorders present are dysarthria of speech and delayed language development.

Dysarthria is defined as a motor speech disorder resulting from disturbed neuromuscular control of the speech mechanism itself (Kent, Kent, Duffy, & Weismer, 1998). The patterns of severity of the dysarthria are dependant upon the underlying pathophysiology. For example, individuals with spastic cerebral palsy generally demonstrate low pitch and pitch breaks, hypernasal speech, and problems with respiration (Yorkston, Beukelman, Strand, & Bell, 1999). On the other hand, individuals with athetoid cerebral palsy demonstrate irregular articulation breaks, prolonged intervals between speech sounds and excessive loudness (Workinger & Kent, 1991).

The treatment for dysarthria will vary with severity. Kent et al. (1998) describes four severity groups of dysarthria. Group 1 includes individuals with speech so severely impaired that augmentative/alternative communication systems (AAC) are needed for all aspects of communication. Speakers in group 2 may need AAC to support language and communication but are intelligible enough to communicate basic needs. Group 3 includes individuals with speech that is effective for basic communication. AAC may be used for this group to support language learning. Finally, individuals in group 4 demonstrate mild problems with speech intelligibility and express themselves verbally for all aspects of communication. AAC may be considered as a backup mode of communication for this group.

There are a number of approaches to consider when treating dysarthria. The use of AAC is one frequent approach. In addition, strategies to reduce the speech impairment are employed as well as efforts to compensate behaviorally, including slowing rate and modifying respiration and prosody (Yorkston et al., 1999). Prosthetic compensation strategies are also available. These include mechanical or electrical devices designed to offset certain aspects of the impairment, including things such as a palatal lift and delayed auditory feedback (Yorkston et al., 1999).

Interventions can also be broken down into speaker strategies and listener strategies. Speaker strategies include activities such as preparing the listener, setting the topic, supplementing with gestures, and selecting a favorable environment (Hustad & Cahill, 2003). Listener preparation through the use of alphabet cues or topic cues has been shown to increase speech intelligibility (Hustad & Beukelman, 2001; 2002). Speech intelligibility can be significantly enhanced if the listener can see the speaker's mouth (Hunter, Pring, & Martin, 1991; Garcia & Dagenais, 1998).

Providing training and support to the listener can enhance speaker effectiveness. For example, training the listener to become familiar with dysarthric speech will improve comprehension (Hustad & Cahill, 2003). In addition, providing the listener with strategies such as selecting a conducive environment and maintaining topic identity can be very effective (Pennington, Jolleff, McConachie, Wisbeach, & Price, 1993).

There have been very few controlled studies examining the language development in children with cerebral palsy. It is believed, however, that the incidence of language delay is high and pervasive (Hardy, 1983). The delays present may be the result of a combination of variables, including cognitive delays, effects of unintelligible speech, and site of lesion (Feldman, Janosky, Scher, & Warehan, 1994). Young children with severe motor deficits have been found to interact less with others and when they do interact, it is often in a respondent manner (Pennington & McConachie, 2001). This type of interaction restricts the nature and quality of relationships in the environment resulting in fewer opportunities for learning. Intervention must focus on the interaction style with others and include family members in the intervention process.

AUTISM

Autism is a developmental disability characterized by deficits in social functioning, in language and communication, and in sensory perception (Gillberg, 1990; Kjelgaard & Tager-Flusberg, 2001). The behavioral characteristics of autism and related disorders vary considerably. One factor that contributes to this variability is the range of cognitive functioning within autism. Individuals with autism can demonstrate IQ scores from well above normal to severe and profound delays. It has been estimated that anywhere from 50 to 75% of individuals diagnosed with autism have IQ scores consistent with a diagnosis of mental retardation (Frith, 1989).

Deficits in speech and language are often the earliest observed symptoms of autism. The unique speech and language problems present in autism have attracted significant attention from linguists and psychologists over the past 20 years. The precise nature of these deficits, however, has not yet been delineated (for a thorough review of language and communication deficits in autism, refer to Lord & Paul, 1997).

There is a significant relationship between IQ scores and language abilities in individuals with autism. In fact, IQ itself accounts for a great deal of the heterogeneity of the language profiles found within autism. IQ scores, however, do not account for all of the language and communication deficits. There is often a clear dissociation between the language profiles and IQ scores in children with autism spectrum disorders (ASD; Kjelgaard & Tager-Flusberg, 2001).

Children with autism demonstrate learning deficits in several areas that can uniquely compromise speech and language development. The first of these areas involves joint attention. Children with ASD have significant limitations in the processing of social information and in turn, in the development of joint attention behaviors (Dawson, Meltzoff, Osterling, Rinaldi, & Brown, 1998). Impairment in joint attention in autism has been well documented (Dawson et al., 2002). Joint attention is defined as the ability to coordinate attention between an object and a person in a social context (Adamson & McArthur, 1995). These behaviors have been associated with later language development (Sigman & Ruskin, 1999). Children with ASD have problems regulating and monitoring attention to other persons in relation to objects in the environment (Charman et al., 1998). They appear less responsive to people speaking (Osterling & Dawson, 1994). Children with autism do not appear to value or process social information (Dawson, Meltzoff, Osterling, & Rinaldi, 1998).

Problems in joint attention have been implicated in many of the unique speech–language problems present in autism, including deficits in social language and intentional communication, idiosyncratic speech and neologisms, problems with theory of mind (TOM), and perspective taking as well as delayed language development (Frith, 1989; Volden & Lord, 1991; Wetherby, Prizant, & Schuler, 2000). Joint attention behaviors must be directly addressed early within intervention (Mundy, 1995; Mundy & Crowson, 1997). The use of behavioral teaching strategies has been shown to be effective in developing joint attention skills (Kasari, Freeman, & Paperalla, 2001; Whalen & Schreibman, 2003). These techniques have ranged from the more structured use of discrete trial instruction to more naturalistic behavioral teaching strategies such as natural learning paradigm and pivotal response training (Pierce & Schreibman, 1995; Whalen & Schreibman, 2003). Although developmental and social pragmatic models have been recommended for use in promoting joint attention skills, there is little empirical evidence yet to demonstrate efficacy of these procedures.

Advances in treatment procedures over the past 20 years have greatly impacted the speech development in children with autism. Prizant (1983) reviewed a great number of programs and found that nearly 50% of children with autism did not develop functional speech, despite intervention. Fifteen years later, Koegel (1995) found that, with early intervention, almost 85% of children with autism learned to communicate verbally. In general, articulation skills are relatively spared in children with ASD (Kjelgaard & Tager-Flusberg, 2001). Problems with suprasegmental aspects of speech such as prosody and rhythm, however, are quite common and can impact speech intelligibility (Fay & Schuler, 1980; Lord & Paul, 1997).

Language development in children with autism is quite variable. In general, vocabulary development may be somewhat spared with regard to labeling skills (Kjelgaard & Tager-Flusberg, 2001). Questions of impoverished underlying representation, storage, and use, however, remain (Kjelgaard & Tager-Flusberg, 2001). In addition, word use may be restricted and lexical organization may be compromised (Gerenser, 2004). Even when vocabulary development seems within normal limits, problems with abstract and figurative language are still common (Rapin & Dunn, 2003).

The most prominent problems consistent with autism lie in restricted communication skills and impaired conversation skills. Children with autism demonstrate deficits in spontaneous communication, reciprocity, and perspective taking (Lord & Paul, 1997; Loveland, McEvoy, & Tunali, 1990). Language use is typically restricted to requesting desired objects and to protest (Wetherby & Prutting, 1984). Regardless of communication level, the number of initiations and range of functions seems particularly problematic in individuals with ASD. Conversation skills are often compromised, with impaired turntaking, noncontingent utterances and lack of responding (Rapaport, Rumsey, & Sceery, 1985) In addition, the quantity and quality of gestures used in communication is extremely limited (Wetherby et al., 2000; Wetherby, Prizant, & Hutchinson, 1998).

Two other prominent issues in the speech and language of individuals with autism are the presence of echolalia as well as the unique challenges with deictic terms. Echolalia involves the repetition of what has been said. It can be immediate (repetition of what has just been said) or it can be delayed (repetition of phrases said hours or even days earlier). As a child's language develops, there is typically a reduction in the use of echolalia (McEvoy, Loveland, & Landry, 1988). Echolalia was once seen as nonfunctional and problematic (Lovaas, 1977). More recently, however, some aspects of echolalia have been shown to be quite functional and can actually play an important role in language and communication development (Prizant & Duchan, 1981; Prizant & Rydell, 1984). It is essential, especially as the child gets older, to clearly distinguish echolalia that is functional and communicative from that which is self-stimulatory and nonfunctional. There is a clear inverse relationship between the presence of high rates of self-stimulatory behavior and learning (Lovaas & Smith, 1989). Therefore, those behaviors determined to be self-stimulatory, including immediate and delayed echolalia, must be addressed programmatically to insure the learning and development of more appropriate behaviors.

The aspect of language that codes shifting reference between the speaker and the listener is referred to as deixis. Terms such as "I" and "you" or "this" and "that" depend on whether a person is a speaker or a listener. There is evidence that speakers with autism have a great deal of difficulty with deictic terms (LeCouteur et al., 1989; Lee, Hobson, & Chiat, 1994). Deficits in joint attention and perspective are the major factors that contribute to the problems with deixis in autism (Hemphill, Picardi, & Tager-Flusberg, 1991).

Due to the great variability in the language profiles within ASD, careful evaluation of each individual is essential. In addition, understanding the variables that may underlie some of the unique deficits is critical. For example, many individuals with ASD have difficulty processing transient input such as speech (Frith, 1989; Quill, 1997). This can play a significant role in the development of both receptive and expressive language. Problems with the development of joint attention adversely affects language development. Other learning characteristics that must be considered include issues of stimulus overselectivity (Lovaas, Koegel, & Schreibman, 1979), problems with motivational variables and social contingencies (Lovaas & Smith, 1989), as well as reduced observation learning and imitation skills (Rogers & Pennington, 1991).

There has been a great deal written over the past decade regarding the treatment of speech and language skills of individuals with autism (for an in-depth review of communication intervention, see Goldstein, 2002). Interventions range from behavioral approaches to developmental and social pragmatic models. A thorough review of the underlying theoretical foundations as well as in-depth overview of the actual approaches is beyond the scope of this chapter. The reader is referred to the following sources for review of the approaches: traditional behavior approach (Lovaas, 2002), natural behavior approach (Koegel, 1995), developmental (Gerber, 2003), and social-pragmatic (Prizant, Wetherby, & Rydell, 2000).

There is evidence supporting both the use of more traditional behavioral approaches such as discrete trial instruction as well as more naturalistic behavioral interventions such as natural learning paradigm to successfully address the speech–language deficits in individuals with autism (Buffington, Krantz, McClannahan, & Poulson, 1998; Koegel, O'Dell, & Dunlop, 1988; Lasky, Charlop, & Schreibman, 1988; Lovaas, 1987). The developmental model known as Developmental, Individual Difference, Relationship based (DIR) or "floortime" (Greenspan, 1997; Greenspan & Wieder, 1998), and the SCERTS model (Social-Communication, Emotional Regulation, and Transactional Support; Prizant et al., 2000) are frequently discussed in the literature as interventions for the communication deficits in individuals with autism. Although both interventions are commonly employed, little empirical support is available for either of them at this time.

The use of augmentative/alternative communication to support the speech–language development in autism has been found effective. There is evidence that the use of the Picture Exchange Communication System (PECS; Bondy & Frost, 1994), sign language, and other visual systems can enhance the speech, language, and communication of individuals with autism (Charlop-Christy, Carpenter, Le, LeBanc, & Keller, 2003; Konstantantareas, 1984; Layton & Baker, 1981).

Unfortunately, there remains considerable debate and controversy over which interventions should be used for individuals with autism. It is clear from the research that no treatment is appropriate for all individuals. The individual's strengths, deficits, and learning profile should guide the practitioner to select the intervention strategies.

CONCLUSION

There is considerable variability in the nature and severity of speech and language deficits present in children with developmental disabilities. This variability is caused by a number of factors, including the etiology of the disability, the level of mental retardation, the environment, as well as the presence of comorbid problems such as seizures, hearing loss, or motor weakness.

All treatment must begin with a thorough and complete assessment of the child's speech, language, and communication skills. The evaluation must also address the individual's interaction strategies and social skills. It will be essential to understand the individual's diagnosis (if available) and what syndrome-specific variables may affect learning and development. Finally, a preference assessment and understanding of the individual's likes and dislikes will be important for later application within the intervention program.

Although there is considerable debate as to the nature and type of intervention to use to address the speech–language deficits in individuals with developmental disabilities, there are some common components that are well agreed upon as essential for best outcome, regardless of etiology of disorder or philosophy of intervention. These include the following:

1. Begin as early as possible. It is well established that outcomes are best when intervention begins early (Harris, Handleman, Gordon, Kristoff, & Fuentes, 1991; Mahoney & Snow, 1983).
2. Provide intervention in the natural environment and include parents and family members in the intervention (Koegel, 1995; Lovaas, 1987; Owens, 1993).
3. Highlight relevant information and make it more salient (Lovaas, 2002; Owens, 1993).
4. Use overlearning and repetition as much as possible (Day & Hall, 1988).
5. Preorganize information (Owens, 1993).

REFERENCES

Abbeduto, L., Evans, J., & Dolan, T. (2001). Theoretical perspectives on language and communication problems in mental retardation and developmental disabilities. *Mental Retardation and Developmental Disabilities Research Reviews, 7*, 45–55.

Abbeduto, L., & Hagerman, R. J. (1997). Language and communication in fragile X syndrome. *Mental Retardation and Developmental Disabilities Research Review, 3*, 313–322.

Abbeduto, L., Murphy, M. M., Cawthon, S. U., Richmond, E. K., Weissman, M. D., Karadoltir, S., et al. (2003). Receptive language skills of adolescents and young adults with Down and fragile X syndrome. *American Journal of Mental Deficiency, 108*, 149–160.

Adams, A. M., & Gathercole, S. E. (2000). Limitations in working memory: Implications for language development. *International Journal of Language and Communication Disorders, 35*, 95–113.

Adamson, L., & McArthur, D. (1995). Joint attention, affect, and culture. In C. Moore, & P. Dunham (Eds.), *Joint attention: Its origins and role in development*. Hillsdale, NJ: Erlbaum.

Backman, B., Grever-Sjolander, A. C., Holm, A. K., & Johansson, I. (2003). Children with Down syndrome: Oral development and morphology after use of palatal plates between 6 and 18 months of age. *International Journal of Pediatric Dentistry, 13*, 327–335.

Bailey, D. B., Jr., Hatlon, D. D., & Skinner, M. (1998). Early developmental trajectories of males with fragile X syndrome. *American Journal of Mental Retardation, 103*, 29–39.

Belser, R. C., & Sudhalter, V. (1995). Arousal difficulties in males with fragile X syndrome: A preliminary report. *Developmental Brain Dysfunction, 8*, 270–279.

Bloom, L., & Lahey, M. (1978). *Language development and language disorders.* New York: Wiley.

Bondy, A. S., & Frost, L. A. (1994). *The picture exchange communication system: Training manual.* Cherry Hill, NJ: Pyramid.

Braden, M. (1998). *Curriculum guide for individuals with FXS.* Colorado Springs, CO: Marcia L. Braden.

Buffington, D. M., Krantz, P. J., McClannahan, L. E., & Poulson, C. L. (1998). Procedures for teaching appropriate gestural communication skills to children with autism. *Journal of Autism and Developmental Disorders, 38*, 535–545.

Byrne, A., Buckley, S., MacDonald, J., & Bird, G. (1995). Investigating the literature, language, and memory skills of children with Down syndrome. *Down Syndrome: Research and Practice, 3*, 53–58.

Capone, G. T. (2004). Down syndrome: Genetic insights and thoughts on early intervention. *Infants and Young Children, 17*, 45–58.

Carlstedt, K., Hernogsson, G., & Dahlof, G. (2003). A four-year longitudinal study of palatial plate therapy in children with Down syndrome: Effect on oral motor function, articulation, and communication preference. *Acta Odontology Scandanavia, 61*, 39–46.

Chapman, R. S. (1995). Language development in children and adolescents with Down syndrome. In P. Fletcher & B. MacWhinney (Eds.), *Handbook of child language.* Oxford: Blackwell.

Chapman, R. S., & Heskith, L. J. (2001). Language, cognition, and short term memory in individuals with Down syndrome. *Down Syndrome Research and Practice, 7*, 1–7.

Charlop-Christy, M. H., Carpenter, M., Le, L., LeBanc, L. A., & Keller, K. (2003). Using the picture exchange communication system (PECS) with children with autism: Assessment of PECS acquisition, speech, social-communicative behavior, and problem behavior. *Journal of Applied Behavior Analysis, 35*, 213–231.

Charman, T., Swettenham, J., Baron-Cohen, S., Cox, A., Baird, G., & Drew, A. (1998). An experimental investigation of social-cognitive abilities in infants with autism: Clinical implications. *Infant Mental Health Journal, 19*, 260–275.

Clibbens, J. (2001). Signing and lexical development in children with Down syndrome. *Down Syndrome Research and Practice, 7*, 101–105.

Cornish, K., Sudhalter, V., & Turk, J. (2004). Attention and language in fragile X. *Mental Retardation and Developmental Disabilities Research Review, 10*, 11–16.

Cougher, L., Savage, E., & Smith, M. F. (1992). *Cerebral palsy: The child and young person.* London: Chapman & Hall Medical.

Dawson, G., Meltzoff, A., Osterling, J., & Rinaldi, J. (1998). Neuropsychological correlates of early symptoms of autism. *Child Development, 69*, 1276–1285.

Dawson, G., Meltzoff, A. N., Osterling, J., Rinaldi, J., & Brown, E. (1998). Children with autism fail to orient to naturally occurring social stimuli. *Journal of Autism and Developmental Disorders, 28*, 479–485.

Dawson, G., Munson, J., Estes, A., Osterling, J., McPartland, J., Toth, K., et al. (2002). Neurocognitive function and joint attention abilities in young children with autism spectrum disorders versus developmental delay. *Child Development, 73*, 345–358.

Day, J. D., & Hall, L. K. (1988). Intelligence related differences in learning and transfer and enhancement of transfer among mentally retarded persons. *American Journal of Mental Retardation, 93*, 125–137.

Dodd, B., McCormack, P., & Woodyatt, G. (1994). An evaluation of an intervention program: The relationship between children's phonology and parent's communicative behavior. *American Journal of Mental Retardation, 98*, 632–645.

Dodd, B., & Thompson, L. (2001). Speech disorders in children with Down's syndrome. *Journal of Intellectual Disabilities Research, 45*, 308–316.

Dykens, E. M. (1995). Measuring behavioral phenotypes: Provocation from new genetics. *American Journal of Mental Retardation, 99*, 522–532.

Dykens, E. M., Ort, S., Cohen, I., Finucane, B., Spiridigliozzi, G., Lachiewicz, A., et al. (1996). Trajectories and profiles of adaptive behavior in males with fragile X syndrome: Multicenter studies. *Journal of Autism and Developmental Disorders, 26*, 287–301.

Everhuis, H., Van Zanten, G., Brocoas, M., & Roerdinkholder, W. (1992). Hearing loss in middle age in persons with Down syndrome. *Journal of Mental Retardation, 97*, 47–57.

Fabretti, D., Rizutto, E., Vicari, S., & Volaterra, V. (1997). A story description task in children with Down's syndrome: Lexical and morpho-syntactic abilities. *Journal of Intellectual Research, 41*, 165–179.

Facon, B., Facon-Bollengier, T., & Grubar, J. C. (2002). Chronological age, receptive vocabulary and syntax comprehension in children and adolescents with mental retardation. *American Journal of Mental Retardation, 107*, 91–98.

Fay, W., & Schuler, A. L. (1980). *Emerging language in autistic children.* Baltimore: University Park Press.

Feldman, H. M., Janosky, J. E., Scher, M. S., & Warehan, N. C. (1994). Language abilities following prematurity, preventricular brain injury, and cerebral palsy. *Journal of Communication Disorders, 27*, 71–90.

Fisch, G. S. (1992). Is autism associated with the fragile X syndrome? *American Journal of Medical Genetics, 43*, 47–55.

Fisch, G. S., Holden, J. J. A., Carpenter, N. J., Howard-Peebles, P. N., Maddalena, A., Pandya, A., et al. (1999). Age related language characteristics of children and adolescents with fragile X syndrome. *American Journal of Medical Genetics, 83*, 253–256.

Fowler, A. (1990). Language abilities in children with Down syndrome: Evidence for a specific syntactic delay. In D. Cicchetti & M. Berghly (Eds.), *Children with Down syndrome: A developmental perspective.* New York: Cambridge University Press.

Frith, U. (1989). A new look at language and communication in autism. *British Journal of Disorders of Communication, 24*, 123–150.

Garcia, J. M., & Dagenais, P. A. (1998). Dysarthric sentence intelligibility contributions of iconic gestures and message predictiveness. *Journal of Speech, Language, and Hearing Research, 41*, 1282–1293.

Gerber, S. (2003). A developmental perspective on language assessment and intervention for children on the autism spectrum. *Topics in Language Disorders, 23*, 72–95.

Gerenser, J. E. (2004). Lexical organization in children with autism. *Dissertation Abstracts International, 65*, 04B.

Gibson, D. (1991). Down syndrome and cognitive enhancement: Not like the others. In K. Marfo (Ed.), *Early intervention in transition: Current perspectives on programs for handicapped children.* New York: Praeger.

Gillberg, C. (1990). Autism and pervasive developmental disorders. *Journal of Child Psychology and Psychiatry, 31*, 99–119.

Goldstein, H. (2002). Communication intervention for children with autism: A review of treatment efficacy. *Journal of Autism and Developmental Disorders, 32*, 373–396.

Greenspan, S. (1997). *The growth of the mind and the endangered origins of intelligence.* Reading, MA: Addison Wesley Longman.

Greenspan, S., & Wieder, S. (1998). *The child with special needs: Encouraging intellectual and emotional growth.* Reading, MA: Addison Wesley Longman.

Hagerman, R. J. (1996). Physical and behavioral phenotype. In R. J. Hagerman & A. Cronister (Eds.), *Fragile X syndrome: Diagnosis, treatment, and research.* Baltimore: Johns Hopkins University Press.

Hardy, J. C. (1983). *Cerebral palsy.* Englewood Cliffs, NJ: Prentice Hall.

Harris, S., Handleman, J., Gordon, P., Kristoff, D., & Fuentes, F. (1991). Changes in cognitive and language functioning in preschool children with autism. *Journal of Autism and Developmental Disorders, 21*, 281–290.

Hemphill, L., Picardi, N., & Tager-Flusberg, H. (1991). Narrative as an index of communicative competence in mildly mentally retarded children. *Applied Psycholinguistics, 12*, 263–279.

Hunter, L., Pring, T., & Martin, S. (1991). The use of strategies to increase speech intelligibility in cerebral palsy: An experimental evaluation. *British Journal of Disorders of Communication, 26,* 163–174.

Hustad, K. C., & Beukelman, D. R. (2001). Effects of linguistic cues and stimulus cohesion on intelligibility of severely dysarthric speech. *Journal of Speech, Language, and Hearing Research, 4,* 497–510.

Hustad, K. C., & Beukelman, D. R. (2002). Listening comprehension of severely dysarthric speech: Effects of linguistic cues and stimulus cohesion. *Journal of Speech, Language, and Hearing Research, 45,* 545–558.

Hustad, K. C., & Cahill, M. A. (2003). Effects of presentation mode and repeated familiarization on intelligibility of dysarthric speech. *American Journal of Speech Language Pathology, 12,* 198–208.

Jarrold, E., & Baddeley, A. D. (1997). Short term memory for verbal and visuospatial information in Down syndrome. *Cognitive Neuropsychiatry, 2,* 101–122.

Kasari, C., Freeman, S., & Paperella, T. (2001). Early intervention in autism: Joint attention and symbolic play. In L. M. Glidden (Ed.), *International review of research on mental retardation.* New York: Academic Press.

Kay-Raining Bird, E., Gaskell, A., Babineau, M., & MacDonald, S. (2000). Novel word acquisition in children with Down syndrome: Does modality make a difference? *Journal of Communication Disorders, 33,* 241–266.

Kent, R. D., Kent, J. F., Duffy, J. R., & Weismer, P. (1998). The dysarthrias: Speech–voice profiles, related dysfunctions and neuropathology. *Journal of Medical Speech Language Pathology, 6,* 165–211.

Kjelgaard, M. M., & Tager-Flusberg, H. (2001). An investigation of language impairment in autism: Implications for genetic subgroups. *Language and Cognitive Processes, 16,* 287–308.

Koegel, L. K. (1995) Communication and language intervention. In R. L. Koegel & L. K. Koegel (Eds.), *Teaching children with autism: Strategies for initiating positive interactions and improving learning opportunities.* Baltimore: Brookes.

Koegel, R. L., O'Dell, M. C., & Dunlop, G. (1988). Producing speech use in nonverbal autistic children by reinforcing attempts. *Journal of Autism and Developmental Disorders, 18,* 525–538.

Konstantantareas, M. M. (1984). Sign language as a communication prosthesis with language impaired children. *Journal of Autism and Developmental Disorders, 14,* 9–25.

Kumin, L., Goodman, M., & Council, C. (1996). Comprehensive speech–language intervention for school aged children with Down syndrome. *Down Syndrome Quarterly, 1,* 1–8.

Lasky, K., Charlop, M., & Schreibman, L. (1988). Training parents to use the natural learning paradigm to increase their autistic children's speech. *Journal of Applied Behavior Analysis, 21,* 391–400.

Launonen, K. (1996). Enhancing communication skills of children with Down syndrome: Early use of manual signs. In S. von Tetzchner & M. H. Jensen (Eds.), *Augmentative and alternative communication: European perspectives,* London: Whurr.

Laws, G., & Bishop, D. V. M. (2003). A comparison of language abilities in adolescents with Down syndrome and children with specific language impairment. *Journal of Speech, Language, and Hearing Research, 46,* 1324–1339.

Layton, T. L., & Baker, P. S. (1981). Development of semantic–syntactic relations in an autistic child. *Journal of Autism and Developmental Disorders, 11,* 345–399.

Lee, A., Hobson, R. P., & Chiat, S. (1994). I, you, me, and autism: An experimental study. *Journal of Autism and Developmental Disorders, 24,* 155–176.

Lord, C., & Paul, R. (1997). Language and communication in autism. In D. J. Cohen & F. R. Volkmar (Eds.), *Handbook of autism and pervasive developmental disorders* (2nd ed.). New York: Wiley.

Lovaas, O. I. (1977). *The autistic child: Language development through behavior modification.* New York: Irvington Press.

Lovaas, O. I. (1987). Behavioral treatment and normal educational and intellectual functioning in young autistic children. *Journal of Consulting and Clinical Psychology, 55,* 3–9.

Lovaas, O. I. (2002). *Teaching individuals with developmental delays: Basic intervention techniques.* Austin, TX: Pro-Ed.

Lovaas, O. I., Koegel, R. I., & Schreibman, L. (1979). Stimulus overselectivity: A review of the research. *Psychological Bulletin, 86,* 1236–1254.

Lovaas, O. I., & Smith, T. (1989). A comprehensive behavioral theory of autistic children: Paradigm for research and treatment. *Journal of Behavior Therapy and Experimental Psychiatry, 20,* 17–29.

Love, R. J. (1992). *Childhood motor speech disabilities.* New York: MacMillan.

Loveland, K. A., McEvoy, R. E., & Tunali, B. (1990). Narrative storytelling in autism and Down syndrome. *British Journal of Developmental Psychology, 8,* 9–23.

Lowe, F. (1992). Speech and language therapy with the fragile X child. In B. Schopmeyer & F. Lowe (Eds.), *The fragile X child.* San Diego: Singular Publishing.

Mahoney, G., & Snow, K. (1983). The relationship of sensorimotor functioning to children's response to early language training. *Mental Retardation, 21,* 248–254.

McCormick, L., & Schiefelbusch, R. (1990). *Early language intervention.* Columbus, OH: Merrill/MacMillan.

McEvoy, R. E., Loveland, K. A., & Landry, S. H. (1988). The functions of immediate echolalia in autistic children: A developmental perspective. *Journal of Autism and Developmental Disabilities, 18,* 657–668.

Miller, J. F. (1992). Development of speech and language in children with Down syndrome. In I. T. Lott & E. E. McCoy (Eds.), *Down syndrome: Advances in medical care.* Chichester, UK: Wiley.

Mirrett, P. R., Roberts, J. E., & Price, J. (2003). Early intervention practices and communication intervention strategies for young males with fragile X syndrome. *Language, Speech, and Hearing Services in Schools, 34,* 320–331.

Montgomery, J. K. (2000). Verbal working memory and sentence comprehension in children with specific language impairment. *Journal of Speech, Language, and Hearing Research, 43,* 293–308.

Mundy, P. (1995). Joint attention and social–emotional approach behavior in children with autism. *Development and Psychopathology, 7,* 63–82.

Mundy, P., & Crowson, M. (1997). Joint attention and early social communication: Implications for research on intervention with autism. *Journal of Autism and Developmental Disorders, 27,* 653–676.

Nadel, L. (1999). Down syndrome in cognitive neuroscience perspective. In H. Tager-Flusberg (Ed.), *Neurodevelopmental disorders.* Cambridge, MA: MIT Press.

Osterling, J., & Dawson, G. (1994). Early recognition of children with autism: A study of first birthday home video tapes. *Journal of Autism and Developmental Disorders, 24,* 247–257.

Owens, R. R. (1993). Mental retardation: Difference or delay. In K. Bernstein & E. M. Tiegerman (Eds.), *Language and communication disorders in children.* Boston: Allyn & Bacon.

Pennington, L., Jolleff, N., McConachie, H., Wisbeach, A., & Price, K. (1993). *My turn to speak: A team approach to augmentative and alternative communication.* London: Institute of Child Health.

Pennington, L., & McConachie, H. (2001). Interaction between children with cerebral palsy and their mothers: The effects of intelligibility. *International Journal of Language and Communication Disorders, 36,* 371–393.

Pierce, K., & Schreibman, L. (1995). Increasing complex social behavior in children with autism: Effects of peer implemented pivotal response training. *Journal of Applied Behavior Analysis, 28,* 285–295.

Powell, G., & Clibbens, J. (1994). Actions speak louder than words: Signing and speech intelligibility in adults with Down's syndrome. *Down Syndrome Research and Practice, 2,* 127–129.

Prizant, B. M. (1983). Echolalia in autism: Assessment and intervention. *Seminars in Speech and Language, 4,* 63–67.

Prizant, B. M., & Duchan, J. F. (1981). The function of immediate echolalia in autistic children. *Journal of Speech and Hearing Disorders, 46,* 241–249.

Prizant, B. M., & Rydell, P. J. (1984). An analysis of the function of delayed echolalia in autistic children. *Journal of Speech and Hearing Research, 27*, 183–192.

Prizant, B. M., Wetherby, A. M., & Rydell, P. J. (2000). Communication intervention issues for children with autism spectrum disorders. In A. Wetherby & B. Prizant (Eds.), *Autism spectrum disorders: A transactional developmental perspective*. Baltimore: Brookes.

Pueschel, S. M., & Hopmann, M. R. (1993). Speech and language abilities of children with Down syndrome. In A. P. Kaiser & D. B. Gray (Eds.), *Enhancing children's communication: Research foundations for interventions*. London: Brookes.

Quill, K. A. (1997). Instructional considerations for young children with autism: The rationale for visually cued instruction. *Journal of Autism and Developmental Disorders, 27*, 697–714.

Rapaport, J. L., Rumsey, J. M., & Sceery, W. R. (1985). Autistic children as adults: Psychiatric, social, and behavioral outcomes. *American Academy of Child Psychology Journal, 24*, 456–474.

Rapin, I., & Dunn, M. (2003). Update on the language disorders of individuals on the autistic spectrum. *Brain and Development, 75*, 166–172.

Roberts, J., Hennon, E. A., & Anderson, K. (2003). Fragile X syndrome and speech and language. *The ASHA Leader, 8*, 6–8.

Roberts, J. E., Mirrett, P., Anderson, K., Burchinal, M., & Neele, E. (2002). Early communication, symbolic behaviors, and social profiles of young males with fragile X syndrome. *American Journal of Speech Language Pathology, 11*, 295–304.

Rogers, S. J., & Pennington, B. F. (1991). A theoretical approach to the deficits in infantile autism. *Development and Psychopathology, 3*, 137–162.

Rondal, J. A., & Edwards, S. (1997). *Language in mental retardation*. London: Whurr.

Rossetti, L. M. (1996). *Communication intervention: Birth to three*. San Diego, CA: Singular Publishing.

Scharfenaker, S., O'Connor, R., Stackhouse, T., Braden, M., Hickman, L., & Gray, K. (1996). An integrated approach to intervention. In R. J. Hagerman & A. Cronister (Eds.), *Fragile X syndrome: Diagnosis, treatment, and research*. Baltimore: Johns Hopkins University Press.

Schopmeyer, B. (1992). Speech and language characteristics in fragile X syndrome. In B. Schopmeyer & F. Lowe (Eds.), *The fragile X child*. San Diego: Singular Publishing.

Sigman, M. (1999). Developmental deficits in children with Down syndrome. In H. Tager-Flusberg (Ed.), *Constraints on language acquisition: Studies of atypical children*. Hillsdale, NJ: Erlbaum.

Sigman, M., & Ruskin, E. (1999). Continuity and change in the social competence of children with autism, Down syndrome, and developmental delays. *Monographs of the Society for Research in Child Development, 64*, 1–142.

Spiker, D., & Hopman, M. (1997). The effectiveness of early intervention for children with Down syndrome. In M. Guralnick (Ed.), *The effectiveness of early intervention*. Baltimore: Paul H. Brookes.

Sudhalter, V., & Belser, R. C. (2001). Conversational characteristics of children with fragile X syndrome: Tangential language. *American Journal of Mental Retardation, 106*, 389–400.

Sudhalter, V., Cohen, I., Silverman, W., & Wolf-Schein, E. (1999). Conversational analysis of males with fragile X syndrome, Down syndrome, and autism: Comparison of the emergence of deviant language. *American Journal of Mental Retardation, 94*, 431–441.

Symons, F. J., Clark, R. D., Roberts, J. P., & Bailey, D. B. (2001). Classroom behavior and academic engagement of elementary boys with fragile X syndrome. *Journal of Special Education, 34*, 194–202.

Van Borsel, J. (1996). Articulation in Down's syndrome adolescents and adults. *European Journal of Disorders of Communication, 31*, 415–441.

Volden, J., & Lord, C. (1991). Neologisms and idiosyncratic language in autistic speakers. *Journal of Autism and Developmental Disorders, 21*, 109–130.

Wetherby, A. M., Prizant, B. M., & Hutchinson, T. (1998). Communicative, social-affective, and symbolic profiles of young children with autism and pervasive developmental disorders. *American Journal of Speech–Language Pathology, 7*, 79–91.

Wetherby, A. M., Prizant, B. M., & Schuler, A. L. (2000). Understanding the nature of communication and language impairments. In A. M. Wetherby & B. M. Prizant (Eds.), *Autism spectrum disorders: A transactional developmental perspective*. Baltimore: Brookes.

Wetherby, A. M., & Prutting, C. A. (1984). Profiles of communicative and cognitive social abilities in autistic children. *Journal of Speech and Hearing Research, 27,* 364–377.

Whalen, C., & Schreibman, L. (2003). Joint attention training for children with autism using behavior modification procedures. *Journal of Child Psychology and Psychiatry, 44,* 456–468.

Wilcox, A. (1988). An investigation in non-fluency in Down syndrome. *British Journal of Disorders of Communication, 23,* 153–170.

Wishart, J. (1993). The development of learning difficulties in children with Down syndrome. *Journal of Intellectual Disability and Research, 32,* 389–413.

Workinger, M. S., & Kent, R. D. (1991). Perceptual analysis of the dysarthrias in children with athetoid and spastic cerebral palsy. In C. Moore & K. Yorkston (Eds.), *Dysarthria and apraxia of speech: Perspectives on management*. Baltimore: Brookes.

Yorkston, K., Beukelman, D. R., Strand, E. A., & Bell, K. R. (1999). *Management of motor speech disorders*. Austin, TX: Pro-Ed.

29

Functional Skills Training for People with Intellectual and Developmental Disabilities

PAULA K. DAVIS and RUTH ANNE REHFELDT

With the passage of the Individuals with Disabilities Education Act (originally titled the Education for All Handicapped Children Act) and the advent of normalization as a guiding philosophical premise and deinstitutionalization as prevalent public policy in the 1970s, monumental changes in the provision of services to individuals with mental retardation and similar developmental disabilities occurred. Importantly, individuals who might have once been placed in large state operated institutions at birth or shortly thereafter remained living at home and began attending public schools. At school, children with mild mental retardation often were exposed to a simplified version of the regular education curriculum (Heward, 1996). Children with more severe retardation were often exposed to a curriculum that was based on normal child development or a readiness model (Wilcox & Bellamy, 1982). Within the developmental model individuals were taught skills in the order in which they emerged in children without disabilities in the belief that those early skills were prerequisite or necessary for the attainment of skills typically learned by children later. Unfortunately, data collected on the postschool outcomes of individuals with disabilities, including mental retardation and related disabilities, revealed that they were not making transitions to adult life successfully (McDonnell, Wilcox, & Hardman, 1991). There were high rates of unemployment, with those who were employed working less than full time. Most lived with parents or

PAULA K. DAVIS and RUTH ANNE REHFELDT • Rehabilitation Institute, Southern Illinois University, Carbondale, Illinois.

with some other type of supervision. Most did not have friends outside their residential setting or immediate family members. They spent most of their time engaged in passive activities such as watching television and participated minimally in life in the community. Most had limited opportunities to make decisions regarding their lifestyle.

The purpose of an educational program for any individual, whether that person is a child, teenager, or adult, and whether or not that person has a disability, is to be practical or functional (Wehman, 1997). The curriculum should focus on teaching useful skills that assist a student in becoming as independent as possible in everyday life. As the outcome data reveal, however, traditional curriculum approaches have not been an effective foundation for preparing individuals with mental retardation to live or work in the community. As a result of these disappointing outcomes, educators now emphasize a curriculum that addresses the attainment of more typical and productive adult roles (Heward, 1996; Turnbull, Turnbull, Shank, & Leal, 1995). This contemporary curriculum is focused on teaching skills that prepare individuals to participate as independently as possible in daily life, whether at home, at work, or in the larger community. This curricular approach has been referred to as a *functional* (Wehman & Kregel, 1997), *ecological* (McDonnell, Mathot-Buckner, & Ferguson, 1996) or *life-skills* curriculum (Turnbull et al., 1995) among other terms. Regardless of the name used, the curriculum focuses on teaching skills that address the demands of life by examining the requirements of functioning in the person's current and future environments in vocational, domestic, community living, leisure, and social skill domains rather than strictly academic (e.g., reading, writing, arithmetic) or developmental domains (e.g., fine and gross motor skills, perceptual skills).

For more than 25 years, the applied behavior analytic approach has been predominant in the area of skill acquisition by individuals with mental retardation and other developmental disabilities (Cuvo & Davis, 2000). Early applications were in the areas of academic skills, verbal behavior, and discrimination tasks, among others. As the ecological or functional skills curricular approach gained predominance, the behavior analytic treatment model was applied to that content area as well. Although variation exists, there are common elements in the instructional model developed in the context of the behavior analysis of functional living skills (Cuvo & Davis, 1983). The purpose of this chapter is to describe the components of that model. Additionally, we will examine the factors that affect the selection, implementation, and effectiveness of the behavior analytic approach to skill acquisition and those that affect the selection, implementation, and effectiveness of a functional curricular approach.

A BEHAVIORAL MODEL FOR TEACHING FUNCTIONAL SKILLS

This section of the chapter will present the major steps in the development of a program to teach functional skills using an applied behavior analytic model. These steps are pertinent to both children and youth in schools as well as to adult learners served by adult developmental disabilities service agencies. Throughout this chapter we will use the term "student" to refer to the individual being taught regardless of age, and the term "teacher" to refer to the individual providing instruction regardless of training location (for a more complete description of the instructional model, see Cuvo & Davis, 1983).

Assess the Individual's Current and Future Environment

The first step in the model for teaching functional skills is to determine the skills needed by the individual to function in his or her current and future environment, including home, school or job site, and community (Brown et al., 1979). This ecological approach ensures that the skills targeted for instruction reflect actual skills needed by an individual to perform in his or her own communities. This information can be obtained by making observations in the community to determine what skills are necessary in typical settings and by conducting interviews with individuals who have knowledge of the skill requirements of specific sites (e.g., the manager of a supervised apartment, or staff providing assistance in independent living for people with disabilities).

Assess the Individual's Skills

At this stage of program development, the purpose is to determine which skills needed in the current and future environment are already present in the individual's repertoire. A number of commercially available instruments are available that provide checklists of functional skills (e.g., Inventory for Client and Agency Planning; Bruininks, Hill, Weatherman, & Woodcock, 1986). Such assessments provide a general overview of skill attainment on a variety of tasks, but they do not necessarily reflect the expectations of the individual's current or future environment, or fully capture the nuances of complex skills that may be required to function effectively with varying levels of supervision or assistance. A more sensitive way to gather performance information may be to observe individuals going about their daily routine to determine which skills are present and which are performed only with assistance or support. Additionally, if the person's current environment does not afford opportunities to perform particular skills, the teacher may probe the person's performance of the skill by providing such opportunity. This type of assessment is more likely to identify skills that have immediate usefulness than do global assessments typical of broad behavioral checklists.

Determine Instructional Goals and Objectives

The assessment is likely to identify several skill areas in need of instruction. A number of factors should be considered when selecting which to target for teaching. These include (a) the degree to which the skill will increase the individual's independence and physical and social integration, (b) the frequency with which the skill will be used, (c) the number of sites or types of settings requiring the skill, (d) the likelihood of the behavior being maintained by naturally occurring contingencies, and (e) the individual's preferences. After selecting objectives, they should be written to include a condition, behavior, and criterion (Mager, 1962; see Davis & Bates, 1997, for a description of how to write behavioral objectives for functional skills).

Consider Legal and Ethical Issues

When selecting a skill for instruction and developing the program, legal and ethical issues should be considered. Appropriate safeguards should be developed that protect the individual's health and safety. Care must be taken to balance the individual's need for instruction in a particular area and his or her right to be free from harm. For example, teaching cooking skills may involve safety concerns regarding oven and knife use that should be addressed as part of program development.

Develop Task Analysis for Ongoing Assessment and Training

Once a skill has been selected, if it involves more than a single response, it will be necessary to break the task into its component steps. The resulting task analysis can then be used to assess the individual's level of performance prior to, during, and after training. It is also a tool for the individual who will be providing training of the component steps during instructional trials (see Cuvo, 1978, for an in-depth discussion of the development of task analyses).

Select a Chaining Strategy

After the steps of the task have been specified, if the task has more than one step, the teacher must select a strategy for teaching the sequence of steps. The three strategies typically used are total or whole task training, forward chaining, and backward chaining (see Rehfeldt, 2002). The majority of studies teaching functional skills have used total task instruction (Cuvo & Davis, 2000). In total task training, the student completes every step on every trial with instruction provided as needed. When forward chaining is used, the student is taught the first step in the chain to a predetermined criterion. Then the learner completes step 1, and step 2 is taught. This two-step chain is repeated until the student performs both steps independently. Steps are added one at a time in this fashion until the student performs the entire chain independently. Backward chaining follows a similar logic, but the student learns the last step first. After meeting criterion (i.e., a predetermined level of performance consistency) the student learns the next to the last step and also completes the final step. As in forward chaining, new steps are added as the individual masters each step in training. Research examining the relative effectiveness of the various chaining strategies generally supports using total task instruction (e.g., McDonnell & McFarland, 1988; Spooner, 1984) although its effectiveness may be dependent on many factors including student characteristics, length and complexity of the skill being trained, and how many steps the student can already complete, among others. Therefore, unless the student is having difficulty learning using total task instruction, it is the recommended strategy for teaching functional skills that involve a series of steps (McDonnell et al., 1996).

Identify Training Sites and Materials

Ideally, training will be provided in the natural environment because that is the site where the behavior will be used. This has been referred to as community-based training. If it is desirable for a student to perform in more than one setting, training in multiple settings may be required (e.g., teaching shopping skills in several different markets rather than in a particular market). Sometimes for practical reasons, training is provided in artificial settings such as a classroom. In these situations, it is recommended that (a) the training environment resemble the natural environment as much as possible with respect to physical features and materials used to teach, and (b) students be tested in the natural environment to ensure that they have generalized their skills.

Determine Distribution of Trials

Another decision that the teacher must make is how frequently training trials should be provided. Should there be massed or repeated trials or should the trials be distributed across days or training sessions? Although little research has been done in this area specific to functional skill development, there appears to be an agreement among experts that distributed practice is recommended with massed practice provided for difficult steps (i.e., steps on which the student is making frequent errors; Cuvo & Davis, 2000; Storey, 2002). This recommendation is consistent with longstanding basic and applied behavioral research findings dating back to the 1960s and earlier indicating superior learning and persistence of simple and somewhat complex skills by people generally, when distributed practice is used as a principal teaching framework.

A related decision that the teacher must make is whether to use discrete trial training drills or more naturalistic or incidental teaching to establish functional skills. Discrete trial training is conducted in a highly specified and structured manner, in which the instructor chooses and presents an antecedent stimulus related to the skill of interest, and when the student responds correctly, the response is reinforced. Naturalistic or incidental teaching is loosely structured, and is incorporated into a student's ongoing routine and follows his or her interests. Variation in antecedent stimuli and responses is emphasized, and reinforcers for correct responses are tied to the student's ongoing activities (Sundberg & Partington, 1999). Some advantages of discrete trial training are that it is easy for multiple staff members to conduct in a consistent manner, and it is often easier to implement in a typical classroom or group learning setting. Some advantages of naturalistic training are that there is less need for additional generalization procedures, and the occurrence of challenging behaviors during teaching sessions is less likely (see Sundberg & Partington, 1999). However, naturalistic or incidental techniques should not rely on serendipitous occurrence of instructional opportunities; instead the occurrence of such opportunities should be specifically planned to assure that sufficient occasions for instruction occur to permit the skill to be established and refined.

Develop Stimulus Control Procedures

Provide Instructional Prompts

If the assessment reveals that the individual cannot perform the task independently, these findings indicate that the individual is not under the stimulus control of the natural discriminative stimuli (i.e., the cues in the environment that tell someone how to respond). To develop stimulus control, the teacher provides instructional prompts that serve to occasion correct responding or to correct errors and then provides reinforcement to the student after the response is performed. Commonly used instructional prompts are described below in the order considered to be least intrusive or controlling to most intrusive or controlling.

Verbal Instruction. A verbal instruction is a statement from the teacher directing the student's behavior. Verbal cues have been implemented across a continuum from those that are indirect and provide little to no response specificity to those that are highly directive and descriptive. Examples of indirect verbal instructions include questions such as "What's next?" or "What do you do after you put the kool-aid in the pitcher?" An example of a direct verbal instruction is "Stir the kool-aid into the water until you can't see any powder left."

Gesture. A gesture is any movement made by the teacher to draw attention to the next step to be performed. Gestures frequently take the form of a pointing response. For example, the teacher may point to the spoon in order to cue the student to stir the kool-aid as the next step in the task analysis.

Model. When providing a modeling prompt, the teacher is demonstrating how to perform the response to be performed. For example, the teacher stirs the kool-aid while the student watches. Although most often the modeling is provided "live," research has documented that videotaped modeling of teachers or peers, or oneself, can be effective (e.g., Rehfeldt, Dahman, Young, Cherry, & Davis, 2003) and that dolls or figures also can be used successfully as models (Page, Iwata, & Neef, 1976).

Physical Prompts. The most controlling type of prompt is one in which the teacher places his or her hands on the student's hands and guides the student's performance. For example, the teacher places his or her hands on the student's hands and guides him or her to stir the kool-aid. It should be noted that although this sequence from least intrusive (verbal) to most intrusive (physical) prompts is a common and typical hierarchy, in instances where a complex task has been largely acquired, steps have consistently been performed without prompting, and an error is made on a step, physical prompting alone may be used to return the person to the last step performed accurately and may be considered to be less intrusive than verbal instruction.

SELECT A STRATEGY TO TRANSFER STIMULUS CONTROL

When an individual is completing a behavior chain in response to teacher delivered prompts like those described above, that individual is not under the control of the naturally occurring stimuli. Therefore, the teacher needs to select a procedure for transferring stimulus control from the teacher's prompts to the natural discriminative stimuli. (Cuvo & Davis, 1998, provide an in-depth discussion of stimulus control, including problems in transferring control from the instructional environment to natural stimuli and consequences.)

Three transfer of stimulus control procedures have been used frequently in programs to teach functional skills to individuals with mental retardation and similar disabilities. One strategy for transfer, often called the "system of least prompts," is to provide the prompts in the order of least to most assistance always starting by giving the individual the opportunity to perform the step with no assistance (i.e., independently in response to the natural stimulus). The teacher provides a prompt only if the person does not respond within a few seconds or makes an error. In a prompt hierarchy using all the prompts described above, the first prompt delivered is a verbal cue, followed, as necessary, by a gesture, then a model, and finally a physical prompt. Each training trial is conducted in this fashion with the individual having the opportunity to perform each step of the task analysis with no help before the prompts are provided in increasing order of assistance.

Another transfer strategy is to provide the most intrusive prompt first (using the prompts described above, a physical prompt) without providing the individual an opportunity to perform the step independently. After a predetermined number of trials at that prompt level, the next several trials are provided with the less intensive prompt given immediately before the individual is given the opportunity to perform each step of the task analysis. Training is provided in this fashion moving through the prompt hierarchy until ultimately the individual responds independently.

In addition to fading across prompt types, it is also possible to fade within prompt types. For example, in a system of least prompts, an indirect verbal instruction might be followed by a direct verbal instruction as necessary. In contrast, partial physical guidance in which only light pressure is used to guide a student's responses could be followed by full physical guidance in which complete hand over hand assistance is provided. These examples illustrate fading within a prompt modality.

A third transfer procedure, known as time delay or prompt delay, is one in which only one prompt is used rather than a series of prompts. The prompt chosen for use is selected on the basis of the teacher's knowledge of the student's skill and the task being trained. Initially the prompt is delivered with no delay. In other words, there is no opportunity for the student to perform independently in response to the natural discriminative stimulus. After a predetermined number of sessions, a short delay (e.g., 2 s) is inserted between the natural cue and teacher's delivery of the prompt. That delay provides the student with the opportunity to perform the skill before being prompted and thus demonstrate skill acquisition. The delay period can remain constant or be progressive. Prompt delay procedures have been used less often than the other two procedures to teach response chains because the procedure is more difficult to implement when a task has multiple steps (McDonnell et al., 1996).

Identify Reinforcers

In order for the initially neutral stimuli in the environment to become discriminative for responding, reinforcement must follow correct responding, even when the responses are prompted as described above. A variety of consequences have been used to reinforce performance of functional skills, including praise, money, edibles, and tokens. If possible, when artificial reinforcers (i.e., those that are not naturally occurring as a result of task performance) are used, they should be eliminated slowly until the person is responding to the natural contingencies. (Hagopian, Long, & Rush, 2004, describe procedures for conducting reinforcer assessments, and Storey, 2002, discusses considerations when selecting reinforcers for training functional skills.)

Permanent Prompts

Some individuals may never learn to perform a task independently. In such situations it may be helpful to provide permanent prompts or cues that can remain indefinitely in the environment. Examples include color coded dials on a clothes washing machine that indicate where to turn the dial when starting the washer and picture shopping lists or cookbooks. In addition to environmental modifications, it is also possible to change the manner in which the task is done to avoid difficult steps. For example, an individual can be taught to pay a dollar more and to receive change instead of learning to count change. Permanent prompts and alternative performance strategies provide assistance to the individual or change the demands of the task so that the individual can perform without the need for a teacher to provide a prompt even when the individual is not performing "independently."

Plan for Skill Maintenance and Generalization

It is not enough for a person to learn a functional skill. That person must maintain the skill (i.e., continue to perform it after an acquisition criterion has been met) and demonstrate generalization (i.e., perform it in nontraining situations). In a carefully developed instructional program, the techniques for promoting skill maintenance and generalization will be included from the inception of the training program.

One way to promote skill maintenance is to select for training a skill that has a powerful natural reinforcer (e.g., eating the food item one has prepared may be a strong reinforcer for cooking or making a sandwich). Additionally, during training, as the skill is acquired, care should be taken to thin systematically the frequency of reinforcement provided by the teacher until it approximates the rate at which reinforcement will be available in the natural environment. (This may require that, in some cases, as one aspect of the development of a task analysis, the rate of naturally occurring reinforcement when the task is performed also be identified.) Another way to promote maintenance is to provide frequent opportunities to engage in the newly acquired skill, thereby increasing the likelihood that skill performance will be reinforced, a necessary component of skill maintenance.

To increase the likelihood that the new skill will generalize, several strategies may be useful. One is to train in the natural environment if possible. By doing this, the differences between the training environment and the natural environment are reduced. When training in the natural environment is not possible or practical, the training environment should be as similar to the criterion environment as possible. This strategy is known as programming common stimuli. For example, if students are learning simple meal preparation skills, it is important to use materials and equipment that are expected to be present in subsequent kitchen settings.

Because there is frequently a high degree of variability in the environments in which one performs functional skills, another way to ensure generalization is to provide multiple training examples that sample the various stimulus and response variations the individual is likely to encounter. The community-based job experiences in which many postsecondary students with disabilities participate in conjunction with transition planning illustrate the use of multiple training exemplars. These opportunities increase the likelihood that students will be able to successfully perform vocational skills in new settings, with that likelihood increasing as the number of exemplars, or work opportunities, increases. As another illustration, for a student who is learning to use fast food restaurants, training may be provided in several different restaurants in the community (e.g., McDonald's, Hardee's, Wendy's). To provide multiple exemplar training in a systematic fashion, general case instruction, in which the variations in the stimuli and the response requirements are carefully analyzed and then selected for instruction and testing, is recommended (see Horner, Sprague, & Wilcox, 1982, for a detailed description of this procedure as applied to functional skills).

When programming to promote generalization, it may also be helpful to train loosely, or to avoid the use of precisely controlled and repeated training formats (Sulzer-Azaroff & Mayer, 1991). In this way, it is less likely that the student's responses will come under rigid control of stimuli unique to the training situation. Stokes and Baer (1977) have provided an incisive review of these and other strategies for promoting maintenance and generalization.

Monitor Performance

Before, during, and after instruction, it is important to monitor the student's progress; monitoring of performance and progress through objective, well-defined measures is a hallmark of applied behavioral analytic methods. Progress is typically measured by using the task analysis to determine what percentage of the steps the individual is performing independently. Prior to the beginning of the program, assessment using the task analysis is conducted to determine whether or not the individual needs instruction. If results indicate that the individual could benefit from training, the task analysis is used to monitor progress towards meeting the program objective. Finally, observations after training using the task analysis are conducted to ensure that the individual is maintaining the skill and using it in all relevant situations that he or she encounters.

The social significance of the behavior change should also be evaluated (Kazdin, 1977). Such information can be obtained by comparing the performance of the students with competent peers. For example, the performance of students learning to purchase food at a fast food restaurant could be compared to that of typical customers, or for children, to peers. Social validity can also be determined by asking independent observers to rate the behavior change. For example, group home workers and those who live in the home could rate whether or not the food cooked by an individual tastes good. These different methods provide measures of the social significance of the behavior change.

FACTORS THAT AFFECT THE SELECTION, IMPLEMENTATION, AND EFFECTIVENESS OF THE APPLIED BEHAVIOR ANALYTIC MODEL AND A FUNCTIONAL CURRICULUM

Despite the abundance of empirical support for the effectiveness of the applied behavior analytic model, a number of factors can call into question the ease and appropriateness of its implementation, as well as the practicality of functional skill programming more generally. We will discuss those factors that hinder the implementation of a functional skills curriculum within the rubric of this model.

The Applied Behavior Analytic Model

Even though evidence confirms the effectiveness of this model, it is often logistically difficult to use this approach successfully to establish functional skills. The time period required for instruction is often lengthy, and, depending on the severity of a student's disability, teachers or aides must focus their attention on one student at a time. Schools and agencies that serve many students with severe developmental disabilities are not likely to have the financial resources to support the time and intensity of this form of instruction. Group-based behavioral instruction is a promising possibility, assuming teachers can provide the systematic instruction necessary to prepare students with more severe disabilities for group instruction. Koegel and Rincover (1974) demonstrated that students with severe autism and mental retardation could learn new skills in a group instruction format. This outcome was achieved through a systematic procedure of fading one-on-one assistants and increasing the number of correct responses required for reinforcement for each student. A similar procedure has been successful in teaching students to work independently on individualized tasks (Rincover & Koegel, 1977; Taubman et al., 2001; also see Reid & Favell, 1984, for a review of group instruction.) It must be noted, however, that a number of rudimentary skills must be established in the student's repertoire before he or she can benefit meaningfully from group instruction. For students with more severe disabilities, a lengthy period of intensive individualized instruction prior to group teaching will be necessary to establish such requisite skills as compliance with teacher or staff instruction, eye contact, orientation to teaching materials, and remaining in seat, for example.

Implementing the applied behavior analytic model also requires specialized training and experience that not all staff members are likely to have. Although some special education programs offer several courses and supervised fieldwork experiences in applied behavior analysis, many offer only one overview course, if that, or a course on classroom management that emphasizes behavioral principles. Staff at adult rehabilitation agencies typically come from a variety of educational backgrounds, and the probability that they have had formal prior training in applied behavior analysis is even less. Many special educators and adult services staff have received instruction in applied behavior analysis during inservice training sessions and workshops, where it may be doubtful that the amount of training provided is sufficient to guarantee the accuracy of implementation necessary for success. Thus, it appears that staff who are working with the individuals who most need systematic behavioral instruction are the least likely to have the skills to provide it. This problem is compounded by the simplicity of the skills that are the focus of a functional curriculum. Teachers and other service providers may erroneously believe that no special instructional skills are necessary to teach "simple" skills that most people without disabilities learn without formal instruction.

A technology for training behavioral skills to nonbehaviorally oriented staff does exist (e.g., Ivancic, Reid, Iwata, Faw, & Page, 1981; Parsons, Schepis, Reid, McCarn, & Green, 1987), but most studies have shown that in-services and workshops alone are not sufficient for ensuring that newly acquired job skills will be maintained or generalized (see Reid & Parsons, 2000). In other words, staff may attend a number of workshops by reputable behavior analysts, but it is doubtful that they will be able to actually demonstrate the job skills emphasized in the workshop when they return to their places of employment. Rather, staff must receive ongoing on-the-job performance feedback to correctly use their new skills. The research results are encouraging, for they suggest that given the right training and supervision, teachers and staff who have not had formal education in applied behavior analysis can acquire and maintain the skills necessary to implement the model. They are disconcerting at the same time, however, because few agencies or schools are likely to have qualified professionals on staff who can provide ongoing supervision, feedback, and technical assistance.

Another difficulty concerns the common finding that students with mental retardation and related disabilities often fail to generalize newly acquired skills to situations different from that in which the original training was provided. A student's fluency in performing a skill in the classroom setting does not guarantee that the student will be able to perform the skill as well in the presence of new settings, stimuli, or people. Generalization failures may be most keenly felt when, upon entering adulthood, individuals are not successful in job settings or living situations that are different from their original classroom learning situations. Just because the skills trained are functional in nature, they are not necessarily functional for the student who cannot use the skills in a meaningful way. A number of techniques were outlined previously for increasing the likelihood that functional skills will generalize. However, training for generalization requires rudimentary knowledge of behavioral principles, and as mentioned above, teachers and other staff often lack the expertise and creativity, and sometimes the opportunity, required to teach in this manner.

A final obstacle to the use of this model concerns common misconceptions about applied behavior analysis among the public, including many educators and other professionals, such as misconceptions about reliance on edible reinforcers and the use of aversive procedures such as overcorrection and contingent punishment to control challenging behaviors (Axelrod, 1990; see also Morris, 1985). Thus, more work is necessary in disseminating contemporary behavior analytic approaches to school and rehabilitation personnel. Contemporary approaches include the functionally based treatment of challenging behaviors (Iwata, Dorsey, Slifer, Bauman, & Richman, 1982, 1994), emphasis on stimulus control, environmental or activity schedule modifications, and differential reinforcement strategies (Koegel, Koegel, & Dunlap, 1996), and errorless teaching procedures that obviate the use of negative consequences (Conners, 1992; McIlvane, Kledaras, Iennaco, & McDonald, 1995).

FUNCTIONAL SKILLS CURRICULUM

Since the passage of the Education for All Handicapped Children Act of 1975, children with disabilities have been entitled to a free and appropriate education. Where that education should be provided has been debated since the passage of the law. In the 1980s children with mental retardation and similar disabilities were "mainstreamed" alongside children without disabilities for classes such as art and physical education but received most of their education in special education settings. In the 1990s the concept of "full inclusion" replaced mainstreaming. Advocates of full inclusion believe that children with disabilities should receive their instruction in the regular education setting alongside their nondisabled peers. This presents a dilemma to parents and educators who value inclusion but also believe that students with mental retardation are best served when they receive an education that focuses on functional skills using the instructional model presented above.

Although the debate has not been resolved, more students with disabilities are receiving their education in regular education settings and classrooms. Thus, two important goals of education for students with mental retardation appear to be in conflict. Educators must wrestle with how to provide appropriate functional education while promoting interaction among children and youth with and without disabilities. This problem can be addressed by careful arrangement of the proportion of time that children with disabilities spend in the various training locations (Sailor, 1989; Sailor et al., 1986). Sailor and his colleagues have proposed that initially elementary-age children spend relatively short periods of time in the community with most of their time spent in regular education settings. As children get older, they could spend progressively more educational time in the community. By the high school years, students with disabilities might spend the majority of their time in the community learning how to use community resources (e.g., shopping, banking) and working in a community employment site in the same way that older students without disabilities may be part of a high school vocational program that includes community jobs. Individual student factors such as age, past progress in a traditional curriculum, family and student preferences, and severity of disability should all be considered when determining at what age a student begins spending more time in the community rather than in the traditional classroom and how much time is spent in functional skills training rather than in the traditional academic curriculum.

Another factor to be considered when implementing the functional skills model is that to train skills effectively, individuals with mental retardation may require instruction in natural settings rather than in traditional classrooms to increase the likelihood that they will be able to generalize or perform a skill in the natural environment. In other words, instruction for many functional skills will be best provided in community settings such as grocery stores, laundromats, and other community sites a person will use. In addition to the likelihood that staff may not be sufficiently trained to program for generalization and that there may be concern regarding the amount of time children with disabilities spend apart from children without disabilities, as mentioned above, administrative, bureaucratic, and logistic constraints may prevent teachers from providing functional skill instruction if doing so requires instruction in the community. Getting to community sites and providing instruction there requires more time than training in a classroom situation and requires transportation that may not be readily available. There also may be added costs such as money to use a washing machine, to purchase an item from a vending machine or fast food restaurant, and to ride the public bus. When training is provided in the community, liability protection also is a practical concern for administrators of programs. Dymond (1997) has provided suggestions for overcoming obstacles to community-based training and recommends that these concerns be addressed before implementing a community-based curriculum. Thus, functional skill training often requires more time, more money, and more planning than does traditional instructional programming that may serve to deter service providers from implementing this type of curriculum.

Of critical importance to ensuring that individuals use the skills they are taught is provision of an environment that supports the ongoing use of the new skills (McDonnell et al., 1996). It is crucial that the skills that have been taught are embedded into a life routine that provides opportunities to engage in the skills as part of daily life. For example, an individual may be taught to purchase a cup of coffee at a fast food restaurant with 100% of the steps performed independently on three consecutive sessions. However, if that individual has no ready source of money, lacks community mobility skills, has no transportation, and does not have the skills to embed the activity into the daily routine, then it is unlikely that he or she will use the "functional" skill of purchasing coffee, and disuse is likely to result in diminishment or loss of that skill. To ensure regular use of the skill, the individual needs to be able to perform not only the skill of purchasing coffee but also needs the skills to complete the entire routine or have the support of family and staff to engage in the routine. Therefore, teaching a functional curriculum is necessary but not sufficient to ensure successful performance of a skill.

To address this common problem, Newton et al. (1994) have recommended that individualized habilitation plans for individuals with mental retardation and similar developmental disabilities include two types of objectives: (a) those that focus on skill acquisition (instructional objectives) and (b) those that promote opportunities to engage in activities regardless of skill level and without focus on instruction (participation objectives). By approaching treatment or educational plans from this perspective, there is greater likelihood that individuals will learn new skills as well as be supported in performing those they have previously mastered or have not and may not learn. The focus of such plans is on developing life routines rather than on the development of isolated skills. Implementing a comprehensive program of support rather than focusing solely on skill development will be necessary if the functional skills are to become truly functional for the individual. This approach is consistent with the American Association of Mental Retardation (AAMR) conceptualization of mental retardation that emphasizes the identification and provision of supports that will increase an individual's opportunity to engage in functional activities and to be integrated into one's community (AAMR, 2002). However, it should be noted that, for educational settings, development of community routines may present difficulties similar to those already noted that may affect the development of, and regular engagement in, community training opportunities.

The changes that would be required by schools to provide community-based training and the supports needed to integrate the use of the skills in community settings may be difficult to make. Perhaps a more feasible approach is for school personnel to work collaboratively with adult service providers. The educational system could provide both traditional academic content as appropriate as well as provide classroom training of functional skills. Adult service personnel could then provide after-school opportunities to use the functional skills in the community during the performance of natural life routines. Such integrated programming might reduce the burden on schools as well as result in transition planning that promotes a meaningful lifestyle for the individual.

Programming for participation with supports provided as needed is one solution to the problem that occurs when an individual cannot or has not acquired a skill. Another solution that has received little attention with individuals with mental retardation and similar disabilities is the use of assistive technology. Assistive technology includes devices that are used to improve or maintain the performance of the person with a disability. These devices can be purchased as special equipment or may be products available to everyone. Although holding great promises, assistive technology has been underutilized by individuals with mental retardation (Wehmeyer, 1998). One reason is that compared to other functional areas (e.g., mobility, communication), few devices have been developed expressly to compensate for or address the unique needs of individuals with cognitive disabilities. Lack of knowledge also has been identified as another reason for underuse of assistive technology. Families are often unaware of the existence of the technology. When they are aware, funding the purchase of devices can be an important obstacle (see Cook & Hussey, 2002, for a discussion of possible funding sources). Finally, obtaining assessment and training on assistive technology is a barrier to its use, as is access to services to adapt devices to individual needs, or maintain and revise the forms of assistance (e.g., cues) that the device provides. Training is an especially crucial factor, given that some of the devices may be difficult to use.

A final consideration in the selection and implementation of a functional curriculum may be the beliefs of the student's family. Parental attitudes in particular have been shown to influence the outcomes of educational programming (e.g., Kernan & Koegel, 1980). Some parents may be reluctant to concur that functional skills should be the primary focus of their child's education for a number of reasons. First, some parents may ignore or deny their child's limitations, and believe that if he or she is educated alongside children without disabilities in regular education classrooms, he or she will eventually function at the same level academically as the other children. Second, many parents have fears and concerns over future living and employment options that may follow from the acquisition of functional skills (see Schutz, 1986). Parents may fear the exploitation of their son or daughter in a competitive employment position, for example, and question their son's or daughter's financial security. They may believe that a traditional academic curriculum will offer greater promise of a future that is more certain. Third, parents may be unaware of the fact that persons with disabilities can live and work in the community with supports. With no awareness of such future options, parents may question the purpose of a functional curriculum and be content with their child's attendance at a school or rehabilitation program regardless of its focus. Finally, parents may actually desire a functional curriculum, but find that their perspectives differ from those of school personnel who may favor a more traditional curriculum. Many parents report feeling intimidated by school professionals (e.g., Oren, 1999) and have little knowledge of their legal rights in the development of their child's Individualized Education Program (IEP).

Some techniques have been documented for educating parents about the possibilities of integrated community living with supports. For example, Wehman (2001) advises that parents of school-age children with disabilities should be exposed to adults with disabilities who are living and working successfully in integrated community settings. These authors also suggest that teachers should bring role models to the classroom for both students and parents to meet, to instill concepts of supported living and working in students at a young age. It is also crucial that school personnel network closely with adult rehabilitation service personnel and that they work cooperatively with the child and his or her parents on the development of an individualized transition plan that prepares the child for the movement from school to adult life. School personnel can keep adult service personnel informed of the particular strengths and challenges of students who will soon be graduating, and adult service personnel can keep teachers informed of the different community living and employment options available so that schools can establish functional goals and objectives appropriately.

CONCLUSION

In conclusion, much progress has been made in the establishment of functional skills in students with mental retardation and other disabilities, and an abundance of data support the effectiveness of the applied behavior analytic model in the acquisition, generalization, and maintenance of those skills. Despite the solid scientific basis for using this model to teach functional skills, a number of challenges and barriers inhibit and sometimes prevent its widespread implementation in local educational agencies. Indeed, that so many schools or adult services agencies fail to teach functional skills or fail to do so using the scientifically validated behavioral model suggests that a large gap continues to exist between practical findings from scientific analysis and practice in educational and rehabilitation service settings. More efficient and effective means of disseminating applied behavior analysis to teachers and adult services personnel are needed. Finally, it is important to examine outcome measures for students for whom a functional skills curriculum taught using behavioral technology was the focus of their education or habilitation. We must evaluate if such individuals are living more meaningful, productive, and empowered lives in the community than did earlier generations of students. If not, further research will be necessary to determine what services and supports are necessary to ensure success.

REFERENCES

American Association on Mental Retardation. (2002). *Mental retardation: Definition, classification, and systems of supports* (10th ed.). Washington, DC: Author.

Axelrod, S. (1990). Myths that misguide our profession. In A. C. Repp & N. N. Singh (Eds.), *Perspectives on the use of nonaversive and aversive interventions for persons with developmental disabilities* (pp. 59–72). Sycamore, IL: Sycamore Publishing.

Brown, L., Branston, M. B., Hamre-Nietupski, A., Pumpian, I., Certo, N., & Gruenewald, L. (1979). A strategy for developing chronological age-appropriate and functional curricular content for severely handicapped adolescents and young adults. *Journal of Special Education, 13,* 81–90.

Bruininks, R. H., Hill, B. K., Weatherman, R. F., & Woodcock, R. W. (1986). *ICAP: Inventory for client and agency planning.* Allen, TX: DLM Teaching Resources.

Conners, F. A. (1992). Reading instruction for students with moderate mental retardation: Review and analysis of research. *American Journal of Mental Retardation, 96,* 577–597.

Cook, A. M., & Hussey, S. M. (2002). *Assistive technologies: Principles and practice.* St. Louis, MO: Mosby.

Cuvo, A. J. (1978). Validating task analyses of community living skills. *Vocational Evaluation and Work Adjustment Bulletin, 11*(4), 13–21.

Cuvo, A. J., & Davis, P. K. (1983). Behavior therapy and community living skills. In M. Hersen, R. M. Eisler, & P. M. Miller (Eds.), *Progress in behavior modification* (Vol. 14, pp. 125–172). New York: Academic Press.

Cuvo, A. J., & Davis, P. K. (1998). Establishing and transferring stimulus control: Teaching people with developmental disabilities. In J. K. Luiselli & M. J. Cameron (Eds.), *Antecedent control: Innovative approaches to behavioral support* (pp. 347–369). Baltimore: Brookes.

Cuvo, A. J., & Davis, P. K. (2000). Behavioral acquisition by persons with developmental disabilities. In J. Austin & J. E. Carr (Eds.), *Handbook of applied behavior analysis* (pp. 39–60). Reno, NV: Context Press.

Davis, P. K., & Bates, P. (1997). Transition-related IEP objectives: Ensuring their functionality, technical adequacy, and generality. *Exceptionality, 7,* 71–75.

Dymond, S. K. (1997). Community living. In P. Wehman & J. Kregel (Eds.), *Functional curriculum for elementary, middle, and secondary age students with special needs* (pp. 197–226). Austin, TX: Pro-Ed.

Hagopian, L. P., Long, E. S., & Rush, K. S. (2004). Preference assessment procedures for individuals with developmental disabilities. *Behavior Modification, 28,* 668–677.

Heward, W. L. (1996). *Exceptional children: An introduction to special education.* Englewood Cliffs, NJ: Merrill.

Horner, R. H., Sprague, J., & Wilcox, B. (1982). General case programming for community activities. In B. Wilcox & G. T. Bellamy (Eds.), *Design of high school programs for severely handicapped students* (pp. 61–98). Baltimore: Brookes.

Ivancic, M. T., Reid, D. H., Iwata, B. A., Faw, G. D., & Page, T. J. (1981). Evaluating a supervision program for developing and maintaining therapeutic staff-resident interactions during institutional care routines. *Journal of Applied Behavior Analysis, 14,* 95–107.

Iwata, B. A., Dorsey, M. F., Slifer, K. J., Bauman, K. E., & Richman, G. S. (1994). Toward a functional analysis of self-injury. *Journal of Applied Behavior Analysis, 27,* 197–209. (Reprinted from *Analysis and Intervention in Developmental Disabilities, 2,* 3–20, 1982).

Kazdin, A. E. (1977). Assessing the clinical or applied importance of behavior change through social validation. *Behavior Modification, 1*, 427–451.

Kernan, K., & Koegel, R. (1980). *Employment experiences of community-based mildly retarded adults.* Working paper No. 14, Socio-Behavioral Group, Mental Retardation Research Center, School of Medicine, University of California, Los Angeles.

Koegel, L. K., Koegel, R. L., & Dunlap, G. (1996). *Positive behavioral support: Including people with difficult behavior in the community.* Baltimore: Brookes.

Koegel, R. L., & Rincover, A. (1974). Treatment of psychotic children in a classroom environment. I. Learning in a large group. *Journal of Applied Behavior Analysis, 7*, 45–59.

Mager, R. F. (1962). *Preparing instructional objectives.* Belmont, CA: Fearon.

McDonnell, J., Mathot-Buckner, C., & Ferguson, B. (1996). *Transition programs for students with moderate/severe disabilities.* Pacific Grove, CA: Brooks/Cole.

McDonnell, J., & McFarland, S. (1988). A comparison of forward and concurrent chaining strategies in teaching laundromat skills to students with severe handicaps. *Research in Developmental Disabilities, 9*, 177–194.

McDonnell, J., Wilcox, B., & Hardman, M. L. (1991). *Secondary programs for students with developmental disabilities.* Boston, MA: Allyn and Bacon.

McIlvane, W. J., Kledaras, J. B., Iennaco, F. M., & McDonald, S. J. (1995). Some possible limits on errorless discrimination reversals in individuals with severe mental retardation. *American Journal of Mental Retardation, 99*, 430–436.

Morris, E. K. (1985). Public information, dissemination, and behavior analysis. *Behavior Analyst, 8*, 95–110.

Newton, J. S., Anderson, S. A., Ard, W. R., Jr., Horner, R. H., LeBaron, N. M., Sappington, G., et al. (1994). *A residential outcomes system operations manual.* Eugene: University of Oregon, Center on Human Development.

Oren, T. (1999). Early childhood special education. In B. T. Ogletree, M. A. Fischer, & J. B. Schulz (Eds.), *Bridging the family-professional gap: Facilitating interdisciplinary services for children with disabilities* (pp. 164–182). Springfield, IL: Charles C. Thomas.

Page, T. J., Iwata, B. A., & Neef, N. A. (1976). Teaching pedestrian skills to retarded persons: Generalization from the classroom to the natural environment. *Journal of Applied Behavior Analysis, 9*, 433–444.

Parsons, M. B., Schepis, M. M., Reid, D. H., McCarn, J. E., & Green, C. W. (1987). Expanding the impact of behavioral staff management: A large-scale, long-term application in schools serving severely handicapped students. *Journal of Applied Behavior Analysis, 20*, 139–150.

Rehfeldt, R. A. (2002). Chaining. In M. Hersen & W. Sledge (Eds.), *Encyclopedia of psychotherapy* (pp. 365–369). New York: Academic Press.

Rehfeldt, R. A., Dahman, D., Young, A., Cherry, H., & Davis, P. (2003). Using video modeling to teach simple meal preparation skills in adults with moderate and severe mental retardation. *Behavioral Interventions, 18*, 209–218.

Reid, D. H., & Favell, J. (1984). Group instruction with persons who have severe disabilities: A critical review. *Journal of the Association for Persons with Severe Handicaps, 9*, 167–177.

Reid, D. H., & Parsons, M. B. (2000). Organizational behavior management in human service settings. In J. Austin & J. E. Carr (Eds.), *Handbook of applied behavior analysis* (pp. 275–294). Reno, NV: Context Press.

Rincover, A., & Koegel, R. L. (1977). Classroom treatment of autistic children: II. Individualized instruction in a group. *Journal of Abnormal Child Psychology, 5*, 113–126.

Sailor, W. (1989). The educational, social, and vocational integration of students with the most severe disabilities. In D. K. Lipsky & A. Gartner (Eds.), *Beyond separate education* (pp. 53–74). Baltimore: Brookes.

Sailor, W., Halvorsen, A., Anderson, J., Goetz, L., Gee, K., Doering, K., et al. (1986). Community intensive instruction. In R. Horner, L. Meyer, & B. Fredericks (Eds.), *Education of learners with severe handicaps* (pp. 251–288). Baltimore: Brookes.

Schutz, R. P. (1986). Establishing a parent–professional partnership to facilitate competitive employment. In F. R. Rusch (Ed.), *Competitive employment: Issues and strategies* (pp. 289–302). Baltimore: Brookes.

Spooner, F. (1984). Comparisons of backward chaining and total task presentation in training severely handicapped persons. *Education and Training of the Mentally Retarded, 19,* 15–22.

Stokes, T. F., & Baer, D. M. (1977). An implicit technology of generalization. *Journal of Applied Behavior Analysis, 10,* 349–367.

Storey, K. (2002). Systematic instruction: Developing and maintaining skills that enhance community inclusion. In K. Storey, P. Bates, & D. Hunter (Eds.), *The road ahead: Transition to adult life for persons with disabilities* (pp. 46–64). St. Augustine, FL: Training Resource Network.

Sulzer-Azaroff, B., & Mayer, G. R. (1991). *Behavior analysis for lasting change.* Orlando, FL: Holt, Rinehart, & Winston.

Sundberg, M., & Partington, J. (1999). The need for both discrete trial and natural environment language training for children with autism. In P. M. Ghezzi, W. L. Williams, & J. E. Carr (Eds.), *Autism: Behavior analytic perspectives* (pp. 139–153). Reno, NV: Context Press.

Taubman, M., Brierley, S., Wishner, J., Baker, D., McEachin, J., & Leaf, R. (2001). The effectiveness of a group discrete trial instructional approach for preschoolers with developmental disabilities. *Research in Developmental Disabilities, 22,* 205–219.

Turnbull, A. P., Turnbull, H. R., III, Shank, M., & Leal, D. (1995). *Exceptional lives: Special education in today's schools.* Englewood Cliffs, NJ: Merrill.

Wehmeyer, M. L. (1998). National survey of the use of assistive technology by adults with mental retardation. *Mental Retardation, 36,* 44–51.

Wehman, P. (2001). *Life beyond the classroom* (3rd ed.). Baltimore: Brookes.

Wehman, P. (1997). Curriculum design. In P. Wehman & J. Kregel (Eds.), *Functional curriculum for elementary, middle, and secondary age students with special needs* (pp. 1–17). Austin, TX: Pro-Ed.

Wehman, P., & Kregel, J. (Eds.). (1997). *Functional curriculum for elementary, middle, and secondary age students with special needs.* Austin, TX: Pro-Ed.

Wilcox, B., & Bellamy, G. T. (1982). *Design of high school programs for severely handicapped students.* Baltimore: Brookes.

30

Social Skills Training for Children with Intellectual Disabilities

DENIS G. SUKHODOLSKY and ERIC M. BUTTER

Impairment in social functioning is an associated feature of intellectual disabilities (ID) and the diagnosis of mental retardation (American Association on Mental Retardation, 2002; American Psychiatric Association, 2000), and is also characteristic of many other developmental disabilities. The National Research Council's report on mental retardation and the eligibility requirements for social security benefits indicates social skills assessment as a priority (National Research Council, 2002). In particular, social skills deficits are vital to diagnosing individuals within the borderline and mild ranges of ID. For individuals whose cognitive abilities are within the borderline range, the degree of social skills impairment may often represent the difference between dependency and self-sufficiency. Therefore, interventions targeted at decreasing an individual's vulnerability through social skills development are critical components of any habilitation plan. This chapter reviews recent research on social skills deficits in children with ID, discusses selected studies of social skills training (SST), and identifies priorities for future research in this area.

Following a behavioral framework, social skills are viewed as specific behaviors that allow a person to respond to social demands and to maximize social reinforcements at home, at school, and in a variety of leisure contexts (McFall, 1982). Most definitions of social skills agree that social skills are interactive, acquired primarily through learning, and entail both initiation and inhibition of social responses (Merrell & Gimpel,

DENIS G. SUKHODOLSKY • Child Study Center, Yale University School of Medicine, New Haven, Connecticut 06520.   ERIC M. BUTTER • Columbus Children's Hospital and Columbus Children's Research Institute, The Ohio State University, Columbus, Ohio.

1998; Michelson, Sugai, Wood, & Kazdin, 1983). The adequacy of performance of a social skill is often referred to as social competency. However, a broader understanding of social competency as adequate social functioning may implicate many other individual characteristics, such as physical attributes and expressions, language, and social–emotional development (Spence, 2003).

There is no agreed-upon taxonomy of social skills. Most SST programs are based on task analysis procedures (Howell, 1985), where social tasks are broken down into small steps. For example, if one wants to throw a pizza party, the smaller steps involve making a list of people to invite, calling everyone on the list, and ordering pizza before the party. A recent review of 21 studies attempting to classify social skills identified the five most common dimensions: peer relations, self-management, school adjustment, compliance, and social initiation (Caldarella & Merrell, 1997). Particular social skills deficits may be associated with specific disorders, such as social withdrawal in depression and argumentativeness in oppositional defiant disorder. Developmental differences in social tasks and contexts also require different repertoires of social skills (Parker, Rubin, Price, & DeRosier 1995). During preschool years, most peer interactions involve shared play activities, whereas stable friendships begin to emerge during middle childhood, and the formation of complex social relationships is one of the central developmental tasks of adolescence (Berndt, 1982; LaGreca, 1997). However, patterns of social interaction and the levels of social adjustment may be relatively stable over time. For example, an individual's sociometric status evaluated in early childhood remains moderately stable (Rubin, Bukowski, & Parker, 1998) and poor peer relationships in childhood are related to social maladjustment in later life (Hartup, 1992; Howes & Phillipsen, 1998).

SOCIAL FUNCTIONING IN CHILDREN WITH INTELLECTUAL DISABILITIES

Social skills impairments are usually reflected in at least one of the three areas, including the level of a child's social interaction skills, the development and stability of peer relationships and friendships, and a child's ability to process social information. Several comprehensive reviews of social development and social skills deficits in children with ID are available (Guralnick, 1999; Kasari & Bauminger, 1998; Matson & Fee, 1991). The level of social maladjustment may be related to the severity of cognitive impairment, co-occurring psychiatric conditions, and the differences in behavioral phenotypes associated with specific etiologies. Historically, individuals with ID have been classified by the degree of intellectual impairment as mildly, moderately, severely, or profoundly mentally retarded. Social skills deficits of children with mild ID may be very subtle, and interpersonal behavior may appear similar to that of normally developing children. Moderate, severe, and profound levels of cognitive impairment are associated with increasing needs for supportive services and special assistance in education and daily living. As a result, social contexts and social skills deficits vary dramatically with the level of impairment in intellectual and adaptive functioning. Cooccurring psychiatric conditions also may be related to social maladjustment in children with developmental delays (Dekker, Nunn, & Koot, 2002). Extensive research has documented the negative impact of attention deficit hyperactivity disorder and disruptive behavior disorders on social functioning in children with ID (Aman, Pejeau, Osborne, Rojahn, & Handen, 1996; Margalit, 1993; Pearson et al., 2000). Similarly, internalizing problems, such as depression and anxiety, are associated with impaired social adjustment (Segrin, 2000; Spence, Donovan, & Brechman-Toussaint, 2000). Recently, an increasing number of studies revealed distinctive patterns of relative strengths and weaknesses in social behavior associated with the etiology of ID (Dykens & Hodapp, 2001; Fidler, Hodapp, & Dykens, 2002; Moldavsky, Lev, & Lerman-Sagie, 2001). For example, heightened sociability, including lack of stranger anxiety, has been noted in children with Williams syndrome (Klein-Tasman & Mervis, 2003), and children with Down's syndrome demonstrated better social skills than did matched controls with nonspecific ID (Walz & Benson, 2002).

Social Interaction

The social repertoires of children with ID have been found to be limited compared to those of normally developing children. One of the early findings is that children with ID initiate fewer social interactions and demonstrate fewer responses to peers than do normally developing children (Guralnick & Weinhouse, 1984; Strain, 1984). In a recent population-based study (Dekker, Koot, van der Ende, & Verhults, 2002) of 1,041 six- to eighteen-year-old children with mild and moderate ID, social problems were among the most prominent behaviors that distinguished children with disabilities from their nondisabled peers. These social problems were indicated by the parent and teacher report on the Child Behavior Checklist (CBCL; Achenbach, 1991) and included items such as "does not get along with peers," "is teased," and "withdrawn." Merrell and Holland (1997) reported data from 199 three- to five-year-old children with developmental disabilities from the national standardization sample of the Preschool and Kindergarten Behavior Scales (PKBS; Merrell, 1994). Over 25% of preschoolers with developmental disabilities were rated by parents and teachers to be 1.5 standard deviation units below their peers in the domains of social cooperation, interaction, and independence. The areas of particular social weaknesses included initiation of social interactions and socially withdrawn behavior.

The majority of studies of social interaction in children with ID utilized observational measures. Kopp, Baker, and Brown (1992) compared the play behavior of 15 preschool age children with mild cognitive delays to matched controls. Children were divided in groups of three and observed during brief periods when they were offered toys and encouraged to stay within close proximity of each other. The children's behavior was coded as not playing or engaging in solitary, parallel, or social play. Positive and negative affect was also coded. Children with ID spent more time alone and showed less social behavior during interactions. They were also more than two times less likely to laugh and smile in response to their peers. Disruptive initiation of social contact, coded as taking toys from another and throwing or pounding a toy was observed in half of the children with delays, but not at all in children without delays. However, there were no differences in the manifestations of negative affect.

An observational study of eight elementary school children with severe ID revealed that they received more social approaches than they made and tended to receive assistance when they initiated interactions (Evans, Salisbury, Palombaro, Berryman, & Hollowwod, 1992). Hughes et al. (1999) conducted a systematic observation of conversational interactions in 12 high school students with moderate ID and 12 age-matched controls. Peer interaction was observed during lunchtime over a period of 3 months for an average of 3 hr of observation per student. Students with ID ate lunch with groups of three to six students from their own classrooms and most conversations included groups rather than dyads. Interaction between students with disabilities and general education students was minimal. There were differences in the number of social interactions and content of conversations. Although children with ID engaged in fewer social interactions, there were no differences on the rating of appropriateness of social responses. Some of the most frequent conversational topics in groups of children from the general education classes included social school events, after-school activities, and jokes. These same topics were infrequently discussed by students with ID. Low frequency of social interaction was also found to be associated with reduced peer acceptance and sociometric status (Evans et al., 1992; Mu, Siegel, & Allinder, 2000). Children with ID show little developmental change in peer interactions (Beckman & Kohl, 1987; Lieber, Beckman, & Strong, 1993). However, increases in the amount of social behavior over time were found in children with mild, but not severe, ID (Guralnick & Weinhouse, 1984).

Peer Relationships and Friendships

Relatively little research has been conducted on the friendship patterns in children with ID. Field (1984) reported that only 1 out of 16 children with ID had a friend from general education class. An early sociometric study (Kronick, 1978) suggested that adolescents with ID were less likely to be named as possible friends by their nonhandicapped peers. Using Berndt's (1982) developmental model of friendships, Zetlin and Murtaugh (1988) conducted a naturalistic study of intimacy, empathy, and stability of friendships in 32 adolescents with mild ID. Compared to the age- and gender-matched group of normally developing children, children with ID were found to have fewer friends and to be twice less likely to belong to a peer group. For more than half of children with ID, contacts with friends were limited to the lunch hour, and after-school activities were infrequent. Their friendships were less stable and were characterized by lower levels of empathy. Both groups of students revealed similar levels of understanding that friendships involve sharing intimate information. However, students with ID reported a limited range of intimate topics and were more likely to discuss personal topics with adults and even strangers. Of course, there are also positive findings. For example, in a study of 310 high school students with mild ID, 95% of children reported having at least one friend (Heiman, 2000) and Siperstein and Bak (1989) reported similarity in the variability of friendship patterns among children with and without ID.

Several studies examined perceptions of quality of friendships and feelings of loneliness in children with mild ID using a self-report instrument developed by Asher, Hymel, and Renshaw (1984). The measure contains items reflecting children's feelings of loneliness, appraisals of peer relationships, and perceptions of social competences. High school and elementary school students reported greater levels of loneliness and dissatisfaction with peer relationships compared to their general education peers (Luftig, 1988; Taylor, Asher, & Williams, 1987). In a later study, boys, but not girls, with mild ID were reported to have greater feelings of loneliness compared to unimpaired controls (Williams & Asher, 1992).

Social Information Processing

Extensive empirical support has been accumulated for the social-information processing model of the development and maintenance of socially competent behavior. This model stems from social-learning formulations of Bandura (1977), as well as models of problem-solving (d'Zurilla & Goldfried, 1971) and causal attribution (Kelley, 1972). A variety of social–cognitive processes allow an individual to appraise social contexts and select responses that are likely to elicit positive responses from others. Dodge (1980) postulated a five-step sequential model that includes encoding of social cues, interpretation of cues, response search, response decision, and enactment of behavior. Disruption in any of these processes can result in dysfunctional social behaviors such as aggression and withdrawal. Correspondingly, social–cognitive processes have been targeted in psychosocial interventions for children with conduct disorder, depression, and anxiety (Kazdin, Esveldt-Dawson, French, & Unis, 1987). The majority of SST programs for normally developing children include treatment procedures that target social information processes. Examination of patterns of social information processing in children with ID is relevant to the application of SST programs that have been developed with nondisabled samples.

Research on social problem solving in children with ID has been limited to samples of elementary school children with mild levels of cognitive impairment. Difficulties in social problem solving and solution generation were associated with behavioral problems, social maladjustment, and rejection by peers (Healey & Masterpasqua, 1992; Siperstein & Leffert, 1997). Using Dodge's (1980) model, Leffert and Siperstein (1996) evaluated social cognitive processing in 50 children, ages 11–13. Two areas of relative weakness were noted: difficulty in identifying intentions of other people in ambiguous situations and avoidant strategies in contexts involving peer entry.

These deficits in social attribution and solution generation were associated with teacher ratings of withdrawal and aggressive behavior. However, in the context of peer provocation, friendly assertive strategies were chosen more often than aggressive strategies. Interpretation of social cues was also found impaired in 13 children with mild ID who were compared to groups of chronological and mental age-matched controls (Gomez & Hazeldine, 1996). In a recent study, 71 children with ID were found to provide fewer numbers of appropriate solutions to peer entry situations compared to the age-matched controls (Jacobs, Turner, Faust, & Stewart, 2002).

CHARACTERISTICS AND EVALUATION OF SST INTERVENTIONS

SST procedures commonly involve techniques of instruction, modeling, rehearsal, corrective feedback, and reinforcement for appropriate performance (Matson & Ollendick, 1988; Merrell & Gimpel, 1998; Michelson et al., 1983; Spence, 2003). The theoretical background of SST can be traced to behavioral and social-learning theories (Bandura, 1977; Skinner, 1938) as well as to early behavioral approaches to psychotherapy (Wolpe, 1958). The broad goal of SST is to train specific behaviors relevant to improving deficits in social interaction. Deficits in social information processing skills such as consequential thinking and emotion regulation are also often addressed as part of SST. SST is used in a variety of settings such as residential facilities, hospitals, and schools. It can be administered individually, in groups, or with the participation of peer mediators. SST applications vary broadly in terms of number, frequency, and duration of sessions, and sometimes treatment is conducted until the mastery criteria for performance of targeted social skills are reached. In addition to being used as a monomodal treatment, SST is often used as part of multicomponential psychosocial treatments and preventive interventions. Meta-analytic reviews of the effectiveness of SST with children and adolescents yielded estimates of effect sizes varying from $d = .20$ (Quinn, Kavale, Mathur, Rutherford, & Forness, 1999) to $d = .87$ (Schneider, 1992). Beelmann, Pfingsten, and Loesel (1994) reported moderate effects ($d = .38$) of SST for children with ID.

The development of specific social skills is a common treatment and curricular goal for students with ID. Specific skills that are taught vary as a function of a child's age, severity of cognitive impairment, and specific deficits in social interaction. The level of complexity of the targeted skills can range from basic social responses such as saying hello, making eye contact, and smiling to the development of more complex repertoires of social behavior in situations such as dating and in vocational settings (Chadsey Rusch, 1992; Mueser, Valenti-Hein, & Yarnold, 1987). The degree of emphasis on social cognitive processes in SST with children with ID also varies. Some treatments rely exclusively on the principles of operant conditioning, whereas the majority incorporate both operant and social learning models of skill acquisition. More generally, SST procedures have been used to teach interaction and play skills and often utilize board games, peer mediation, and social problem-solving strategies. Each of these elements is considered below.

SST for Interaction Skills

Studies utilizing single-participant designs demonstrated increases in basic verbal and nonverbal skills as a result of SST with children and adolescents with a wide range of ID. Matson, Kazdin, and Esveldt-Dawson (1980) provided intensive (two daily sessions for 14 weeks) training to 11- and 12-year-old boys with moderate intellectual impairment complicated by conduct problems. Six specific behaviors were targeted for intervention: physical gestures, facial expression, eye contact, number of words spoken, voice intonation, and verbal content. These behaviors were trained and assessed in the context of role-playing typical interpersonal situations such as making requests and giving compliments. Significant improvements were noted for all specific behaviors as well as the overall ratings of social skills. Generalization of skills occurred in the performance of new but similarly role-played situations. Duan and O'Brian (1998) reported on the application of SST with three adolescents with mild to moderate ID. First, the participants were trained by the therapist to use more appropriate verbal (e.g., asking questions, complimenting others) and nonverbal (e.g., eye contact, posture) conversational strategies. Then, one of the three participants was instructed to serve as a peer-tutor for the other two adolescents. Observation of social interaction at the residential facility and during recreational activities in the community showed increases across all targeted behaviors. Turner, Hersen, and Bellack (1978) reported the results of SST with a 19-year-old man with mild intellectual impairment. Specific social behaviors targeted by the intervention included eye contact, response latency, loudness of speech, number of words spoken, smiles, and physical gestures. Observations of interactions with a confederate during common social situations were used to evaluate the treatment. Steady improvement in performance of the target behaviors was demonstrated during the 6 months of training and higher rating of overall social competency was reported at the end of the treatment. Matson et al. (1988) examined the effects of a combination of primary and social reinforcement with verbal and nonverbal prompts to increase basic social skills in three adolescents with severe to profound ID. Target behaviors were identified on the basis of teacher reports of specific problem areas, whereas skill acquisition was evaluated via observational ratings of performance during the training sessions. All three participants demonstrated increases in the rates of eye contact, number of responses to questions and time stayed seated when addressed by the teacher.

Three randomized controlled studies of SST for improving interaction skills in children with ID reported inconsistent results for different informants. Jupp and Looser (1988) evaluated SST with 40 adolescents aged 13–16 years with mild ID who were randomly assigned to treatment or no-treatment conditions. An 11-session SST program consisted of videotaped

modeling, role-playing, and corrective feedback. Each session was dedicated to 1 of the 11 verbal and nonverbal conversational skills such as
asking questions and listening. Moderate improvements were shown on the
teacher ratings of competency on the 11 skills as well as the overall social
behaviors that were collected before and after the training. However, there
were no improvements in self-perception as measured by the Piers–Harris
scale (Piers, 1969). Soresi and Nota (2000) evaluated a 20-session group
SST with 20 adolescents with Down's syndrome randomly assigned to
treatment and no-treatment conditions. Standard SST procedures were
used to develop skills for initiating and maintaining conversations with
peers and adults. Group differences were reported for the observational
ratings of appropriate interactions but not for the teacher rating of social competence. Mixed results were reported from the use of eight-session
group SST program with eleven 14- to 15-year old adolescents with moderate ID (Elliott, Pring, & Bunning, 2002). Significant improvement was
noted on the teacher ratings of conversational skills and assertiveness.
However, students' self-report actually showed a decrease in perceived social skills from the baseline to the end of the treatment. These results were
interpreted as possibly showing that SST may have increased students'
awareness of their social skills deficits.

Social Play Skills in SST

Given that cooperative play is one of the main contexts for socialization
during childhood, teaching interactive play skills can be a useful strategy
to facilitate social functioning. Three studies examined SST procedures to
develop cooperative play skills with an overarching goal of improving social interaction in children of varying ages and different levels of intellectual impairment. In a 1971 study, Paloutzian, Hasazi, Streifel, and Edgar
used shaping and reinforcement to improve social play skills in 20 children
aged 3–13 with severe ID. Children were randomly assigned to treatment,
which consisted of 25 sessions of imitation training followed by 10 sessions of training in simple social interactions such as passing a beanbag
and pulling a peer in a wagon. Interactive behaviors were rated during
short intervals of free play for 3 consecutive days before and after training.
Most children were characterized as being either unoccupied or playing in
isolation during these observation intervals. After the training, children in
the treatment group were rated as being more interactive. The rate of improvement was significantly better than in the control group. This result
suggested that training in simple interactive tasks helps to elicit social behavior for children with severe ID.

Fajardo and McGourty (1983) reported a controlled study of teaching
developmentally relevant social play skills to adolescents with mild, moderate, and severe levels of ID. Adolescents with severe disabilities were taught
skills such as passing objects, appropriate touching, and using names of
others. Adolescents with moderate levels of impairment were taught turn-
taking and playing by the rules with each other during games such as
"tag" and "follow the leader." Finally, participants with mild disabilities

were instructed in appropriate social interactions during table-top spinner games. Forty-five minutes training sessions were conducted over 10 consecutive days and utilized standard procedures of modeling, physical, and verbal prompting, and various forms of reinforcement. Observational ratings during free play periods indicated that children in the treatment condition demonstrated greater improvement in the targeted social play skills than did the matched controls. However, after object rewards were faded 1 week after training, social interaction during the free play periods decreased.

Social play behaviors of preschoolers were targeted in a structured, 12-session, group-administered training program (Matson, Fee, Coe, & Smith, 1991). Twenty-eight 4- to 5-year-old children with mild to moderate ID were randomly assigned to treatment or no-treatment conditions. First, four appropriate social skills (greetings, asking for a toy, sharing a toy, and initiating play) were modeled using puppets. Then children were given opportunities to practice the skills with puppets and peers. Edible reinforcements and praise followed each child's adequate performance. Observational ratings conducted during two 30-min intervals of free play before and after SST revealed a significant increase in the frequency of targeted social skills such as using appropriate greetings and asking questions, but not in the quality of social play such as interacting verbally and playing with the same toy. This result suggests that improvement in specific social skills may not generalize to the broader categories of social interaction.

SST with Peer Mediation

Psychoeducational interventions for improving social adjustment of children with ID have also included nondisabled children (Strain & Odom, 1986). Teaching nondisabled children to engage their peers with disabilities in cooperative play and study activities resulted in positive effects on the social functioning of children with disabilities. Peers effected an increase in the quantity and quality of interactions, the development of friendships, and higher levels of peer acceptance (Haring & Breen, 1992; Hughes et al., 2002; Piercy, Wilton, & Townsend, 2002).

Two studies used single-participant designs to evaluate the effects of SST interventions in which nondisabled peers delivered instruction, modeling, and reinforcement during the training. In the first study, peer-mediated conversational skills intervention was evaluated in four adolescents with moderate intellectual impairment (Hughes, Killian, & Fischer, 1996). Targeted behaviors included initiating, responding, and maintaining eye contact during conversations. Peers who provided the training to adolescents with ID were taught to model and role-play appropriate social behavior and to provide social reinforcement. Improvement was noted on the observational ratings of the targeted behavior in different school settings, such as the lunchroom, classroom, and gym. In the second study, third grade students from general education classes were taught to provide peers with mild ID with prompts, praise, and corrective feedback regarding social skills during interactive play activities (McMahon, Wacker, Sasso, Berg, &

Newton, 1996). Social skills targeted for the intervention included asking peers to play, waiting for response, setting up games together, discussing who goes first, and taking turns appropriately. During the 10 training sessions, all four participants with ID demonstrated increases in the targeted social skills, and the quality of social interaction was rated as improved for three out of four participants. A possible advantage of peer-mediated SST is that peers can provide more realistic modeling of social skills. However, the relative effectiveness of peer modeling compared to modeling by adults, videotapes, or puppets is yet to be examined.

SST with Social Problem-Solving Training

Although social problem-solving training techniques are essential components of SST with normally developing children, relatively little is known about the relevance of these techniques for children with ID. Two randomized controlled studies and three single-participant studies evaluated treatments consisting of both traditional SST techniques and procedures focused on social information processing skills. One of the largest studies ($n = 96$) of SST for children with mild ID was conducted by Fleming and Fleming (1982). Children, aged 9–12, nominated by teachers for being excessively passive or aggressive were randomly assigned to a six-session treatment. Training was based on Goldstein's (1981) assertiveness program and included thinking about alternatives and consequences of one's social behavior before enacting a particular response. Children watched videotaped modeling vignettes, role-played assertive responses, and received corrective feedback. Compared to the attention-control condition, children who received SST showed significant improvement in the social competency of responses to videotaped situations but not during interaction with a peer confederate. A similar but longer program was evaluated by Vaughn, Ridley, and Cox (1983) with thirty 8- to 11-year-old children with mild ID. Forty sessions of training were delivered over 8 weeks and targeted social problem-solving processes including cue sensitivity, solution generation, and consequential thinking. Treatment effects were measured by observing children's behavior in 10 interpersonal situations with a peer confederate. Children who received training generated six appropriate solutions, and children in the no-treatment condition generated only three.

The combination of video feedback and self-monitoring training was found ineffective for improving social behavior in five children with mild ID and comorbid ADHD (Embregts, 2002). By contrast, teaching children to verbalize problem-solving steps resulted in increased classroom participation in two children with moderate ID (Agran, Blanchard, Wehmeyer, & Hughes, 2002). Similarly, SST with activities aimed at improving decoding of social cues and generation of social responses was shown to increase the number and quality of social interactions in two 16-year-old students with mild ID (O'Reilly & Glynn, 1995).

Use of Board Games in SST

A variety of board games and play therapy activities are available to facilitate child-focused psychosocial interventions (Gardner, 1973; Schaefer & Cangelosi, 2002). Two studies evaluated Foxx and McMorrow's (1983) *Stacking the Deck* SST game. In this game, participants draw cards with scenarios calling for specific social skills within six categories: compliments, criticism, politeness, questions and answers, confrontation, and initiating social interaction. Appropriate responses are modeled by the therapist and reinforced by allowing the participant to move the game piece. Wong, Morgan, Crowley, and Baker (1996) evaluated the effects of playing *Stacking the Deck* with three adolescents with mild to moderate ID who were hospitalized for severe behavioral problems. All three participants improved on the targeted skills during the game. However, no generalization was observed when situations similar to the ones in the game cards were staged by the confederates on the hospital unit. Similar results were reported by Langone, Clees, Oxford, Malone, and Ross (1995) for three adolescents with mild ID in the school setting. All participants demonstrated appropriate social skills during the game but not in the other environments. The results of these studies parallel the findings of other investigations of brief, structured SST protocols and suggest the need for procedures that would facilitate not only the acquisition but also the performance of socially appropriate behavior.

From Research to Practice

Behavior therapy research has been plagued by the lack of transfer or dissemination of evidence-based interventions from research to "real life" settings, where they can be used by practitioners. As a rule, SST treatment manuals developed for research purposes are not published in a format that can be easily accessed and utilized by practitioners. One notable exception is *Skillstreaming* (McGinnis & Goldstein, 1997), an empirically validated SST program that provides manualized systematic instruction to ameliorate social skill deficits. The activities of *Skillstreaming* are based upon the principles of learning and social learning paradigms, such as modeling, role playing, feedback, and transfer. Age-appropriate *Skillstreaming* programs have been developed for preschool, elementary, and high school students. These programs have been also evaluated in a variety of populations, including children with ID. Similar SST curricula for use in educational settings have been developed for children with ID (Sargent, 1991; Walker et al., 1988), but received limited empirical evaluation (Walker et al., 1983).

A vast amount of SST materials and activity kits for normally developing children are available commercially but have not been evaluated with children with ID. Some of these materials may be helpful for practitioners in the fields of mental health and education. For example, *Teaching Friendship Skills* (Huggins, 1998) is an educational curriculum for teaching social skills in the classroom. It consists of a step-by-step instructor's guide and a variety of resources including games, activities, literature units, and re-producible handouts. Another example of a useful resource is *Social Skills Stories* (Johnson & Susnik, 1996). This book consists of illustrated sto-ries for teaching simple skills such as greetings and using appropriate social space, and complex social skills such as gift giving. The extensive use of pictures and pictorial schedules that break down social behaviors into smaller steps makes this book a useful resource when teaching social skills to children with greater levels of cognitive and social impairment. Of course, these and similar resources should be used in conjunction with lit-erature that details behavioral principles and empirical support underlying SST interventions.

SUMMARY AND FUTURE DIRECTIONS

The reviewed treatment studies suggest that SST can produce improve-ment in social skills of children and adolescents with ID. The type and com-plexity of social skills targeted by the interventions varied with the level of cognitive impairment. Children with severe and profound impairment usually received training in basic social skills such as making eye contact and asking for help. Children in the mild to moderate range of ID received training in basic skills as well as in the application of these skills in situa-tions, such as conflict resolution and cooperative play. Elements of social problem-solving training were incorporated in several treatment studies of children with mild ID. SST treatments across all studies included var-ious forms of reinforcement, modeling, and behavioral rehearsal. Several studies utilized board games and peer mediators as part of SST.

The most frequently reported improvements were in the area of simple verbal and nonverbal interaction skills. It should be noted, however, that several studies included treatments that were conducted until the mastery criteria for performance of the targeted social skill were reached. Results on the generalization of social skills and on the improvement in broad ar-eas of social functioning were mixed. Some of the positive results included increased performance of targeted social skills outside treatment sessions, increased frequency of social initiation during play and leisure activities, and improved teacher ratings of social competency. Only 1 of the 20 re-viewed studies (Elliott et al., 2002) reported a decrease in children's self-perceptions of social competency following SST. This suggests that SST is unlikely to produce negative results. However, measures of perceived so-cial competence and subjective well-being should be included in the future studies of SST for children with ID.

Several limitations of the reviewed studies can be noted and ad-dressed in future research. First, samples are often not well character-ized in respect to the initial level of social skills and cooccurring psy-chiatric conditions. Most studies provided descriptive examples of social deficits and only a few studies reported pretreatment scores on standard-ized measures of social adjustment such as the Vineland Adaptive Behav-ior Scales (Sparrow, Balla, & Cicchetti, 1984). Comorbid psychopathology is also poorly characterized in the participants of SST treatment studies. At the same time, participants of the reviewed studies were reported to have major psychiatric disorders, including autism, psychotic disorders, attention-deficit/hyperactivity disorder, and conduct disorder (Duan & O'Brien, 1998; Matson et al., 1988).

A second concern pertains to the measurement and interpretation of treatment results. Outcome measures vary considerably across the studies with respect to informants and modalities. Although most studies used observational approaches to evaluate the primary outcomes, there seems to be no candidate for a "gold standard" measure. None of the studies included well-established standardized measures of social adjustment to evaluate the outcomes of SST. At least one measure of social skills for normally developing children, the Social Skills Rating Scales (SSRS; Gresham & Elliot, 1987) has been used to characterize social functioning in children with ID and it can be relevant to clinical studies of SST. Two instruments that measure social skills in children with ID, the Matson Evaluation of Social Skills with Youngsters (MESSY) and the Matson Evaluation of Social Skills for Individuals with Severe Retardation (MESSIER; Matson, LeBlanc, & Weinheimer, 1999; Matson, Rotatori, & Helsel, 1983) have adequate psychometric qualities and have been used in a number of research studies. Finally, the Socialization domain of the Vineland Adaptive Behavior Scales (Sparrow et al., 1984) has been used to characterize baseline levels of social functioning of children who participate in several of the reviewed SST studies but the change scores were not reported. Studies are needed to evaluate whether these or similar standardized instruments are sensitive to the effects of SST in children with ID.

Third, although patterns of social skill deficits have been linked to specific etiologies of mental retardation, the effects of SST have been examined in heterogeneous groups of children with ID. Only one study of the effects of SST for individuals with a specific etiology, that is, Down's syndrome, was located in the literature (Soresi & Nota, 2000). Research on the specific profiles of strengths and weaknesses in socialization should clarify treatment goals for SST with children with particular etiologies of ID. Despite the noted limitations, the reviewed literature suggests that SST can be a helpful intervention for children with ID.

REFERENCES

Achenbach, T. M. (1991). *Manual for the child behavior checklist/4-18 and 1991 profile.* Burlington: University of Vermont Press.

Agran, M., Blanchard, C., Wehmeyer, M., & Hughes, C. (2002). Increasing the problem-solving skills of students with developmental disabilities participating in special education. *Remedial and Special Education, 23,* 279–288.

Aman, M. G., Pejeau, C., Osborne, P., Rojahn, J., & Handen, B. (1996). Four-year follow-up of children with low intelligence and ADHD. *Research in Developmental Disabilities, 17,* 417–432.

American Association on Mental Retardation (AAMR). (2002). *Mental retardation: Definition, classification, and systems of supports.* Washington, DC: Author.

American Psychiatric Association (APA). (2000). *Diagnostic and statistical manual of mental disorders* (4th ed., text revision). Washington, DC: Author.

Asher, S. R., Hymel, S., & Renshaw, P. D. (1984). Loneliness in children. *Child Development, 55,* 1456–1464.

Bandura, A. (1977). *Social learning theory.* Englewood Cliffs, NJ: Prentice-Hall.

Beckman, P. J., & Kohl, F. L. (1987). Interactions of preschoolers with and without handicaps in integrated and segregated settings: A longitudinal study. *Mental Retardation, 25,* 5–12.

Beelmann, A., Pfingsten, U., & Loesel, F. (1994). Effects of training social competence in children: A meta-analysis of recent evaluation studies. *Journal of Clinical Child Psychology, 23,* 260–271.

Berndt, T. J. (1982). The features and effects of friendship in early adolescence. *Child Development, 53,* 1447–1460.

Caldarella, P., & Merrell, K. W. (1997). Common dimensions of social skills of children and adolescents: A taxonomy of positive behaviors. *School Psychology Review, 26,* 265–279.

Chadsey Rusch, J. (1992). Towards defining and measuring social skills in employment settings. *American Journal on mental Retardation, 96,* 405–418.

Dekker, M. C., Koot, H. M., van der Ende, J., & Verhults, F. C. (2002). Emotional and behavioral problems in children and adolescents with and without intellectual disability. *Journal of Child Psychology and Psychiatry, 43,* 1087–1098.

Dekker, M. C., Nunn, R., & Koot, H. M. (2002). Psychometric properties of the revised Developmental Behavior Checklist scales in Dutch children with intellectual disability. *Journal of Intellectual Disability Research, 46,* 61–75.

Dodge, K. A. (1980). Social cognition and children's aggressive behavior. *Child Development, 51,* 162–170.

Duan, D. W., & O'Brien, S. (1998). Peer-mediated social-skills training and generalization in group homes. *Behavioral Interventions, 13,* 235–247.

Dykens, E. M., & Hodapp, R. M. (2001). Research in mental retardation: Toward an etiologic approach. *Journal of Child Psychology and Psychiatry, 42,* 49–71.

d'Zurilla, T. J., & Goldfried, M. R. (1971). Problem solving and behavior modification. *Journal of Abnormal Psychology, 78,* 107–126.

Elliott, C., Pring, T., & Bunning, K. (2002). Social skills training for adolescents with intellectual disabilities: A cautionary note. *Journal of Applied Research in Intellectual Disabilities, 15,* 91–96.

Embregts, P. J. C. M. (2002). Effects of residents and direct-care staff training on responding during social interactions. *Research in Developmental Disabilities, 23,* 353–366.

Evans, I. M., Salisbury, C. L., Palombaro, M. M., Berryman, J., & Hollowood, T. M. (1992). Peer interactions and social acceptance of elementary-age children with severe disabilities in an inclusive school. *Journal of the Association for Persons with Severe Handicaps, 17,* 205–212.

Fajardo, D. M., & McGourty, D. G. (1983). Promoting social play in small groups of retarded adolescents. *Education and Training of the Mentally Retarded, 18,* 300–307.

Fidler, D. J., Hodapp, R. M., & Dykens, E. M. (2002). Behavioral phenotypes and special education: Parent report of educational issues for children with Down syndrome, Prader–Willi syndrome and Williams syndrome. *Journal of Special Education, 36,* 80–88.

Field, T. (1984). Play behavior or handicapped children who have friends. In T. Field, J. L. Roopnarine, & M. Segal (Eds.), *Friendships in normal and handicapped children* (pp. 153–163). Norwood, NJ: Ablex.

Fleming, E. R., & Fleming, D. C. (1982). Social skill training for educable mentally retarded children. *Education and Training of the Mentally Retarded, 17,* 44–50.

Foxx, R. M., & McMorrow, M. J. (1983). *Stacking the deck: A social skills game for retarded adults.* Champaign, IL: Research Press.

Gardner, R. A. (1973). *The talking, feeling, and doing game.* Cresskill, NJ: Creative Therapeutics.

Goldstein, A. P. (1981). *Psychological skill training.* Elmsford, NY: Pergamon.

Gomez, R., & Hazeldine, P. (1996). Social information processing in mild mentally retarded children. *Research in Developmental Disabilities, 17,* 217–227.

Gresham, F. M., & Elliot, S. N. (1987). The relationship between adaptive behavior and social skills: Issues in definition and assessment. *Journal of Special Education, 21,* 167–181.

Guralnick, M. J. (1999). Family and child influences on the peer-related social competence on young children with developmental delays. *Mental Retardation and Developmental Disabilities Research Reviews, 5,* 21–29.

Guralnick, M. J., & Weinhouse, E. (1984). Peer-related social interactions of developmentally delayed young children: Development and characteristics. *Developmental Psychology, 20,* 815–827.

Haring, T. G., & Breen, C. G. (1992). A peer-mediated social network intervention to enhance the social integration of persons with moderate and severe disabilities. *Journal of Applied Behavior Analysis, 25,* 319–333.

Hartup, W. W. (1992). Peer relation in early and middle childhood. In V. B. VanHasselt & M. Hersen (Eds.), *Handbook of social development: A lifespan perspective* (pp. 257–281). New York: Plenum.

Healey, K. N., & Masterpasqua, F. (1992). Interpersonal cognitive problem-solving among children with mild mental retardation. *American Journal on Mental Retardation, 96,* 367–372.

Heiman, T. (2000). Friendship quality among children in three education settings. *Journal of Intellectual and Developmental Disabilities, 25,* 1–12.

Howell, K. W. (1985). A task-analytical approach to social behavior. *Remedial and Special Education, 6,* 24–30.

Howes, C., & Phillipsen, L. (1998). Continuity in children's relations with peers. *Social Development, 7,* 340–349.

Huggins, P. (1995). *Teaching friendship skills: Primary version.* Longmont, CO: Sopris-West.

Hughes, C., Copeland, S. R., Wehmeyer, M. L., Agran, M., Cai., X., & Hwang, B. (2002). Increasing social interaction between general education high school students and their peers with mental retardation. *Journal of Developmental and Physical Disabilities, 14,* 387–402.

Hughes, C., Killian, D. J., & Fischer, G. M. (1996). Validation and assessment of a conversational interaction intervention. *American Journal on Mental Retardation, 100,* 493–509.

Hughes, C., Rodi, M. S., Lorden, S. W., Pitkin, S. E., Derer, K. R., Hwang, B., et al. (1999). Social interactions of high school students with mental retardation and their general education peers. *American Journal on Mental Retardation, 104,* 533–544.

Jacobs, L., Turner, L. A., Faust, M., & Stewart, M. (2002). Social problem solving of children with and without mental retardation. *Journal of Developmental and Physical Disabilities, 14,* 37–50.

Johnson, A. M., & Susnik, J. L. (1996). *Social skills stories: Functional picture stories for readers and nonreaders K-12.* Solana Beach, CA: Mayer-Johnson.

Jupp, J. J., & Looser, G. (1988). The effectiveness of the "CATCH" social skills training program with adolescents who are mildly intellectually disabled. *Australia and New Zealand Journal of Developmental Disabilities, 14,* 135–145.

Kasari, C., & Bauminger, N. (1998). Social and emotional development in children with mental retardation. In J. A. Burack, R. M. Hodapp, & E. Zigler (Eds.), *Handbook of mental retardation and development* (pp. 411–433). New York: Cambridge University Press.

Kazdin, A. E., Esveldt-Dawson, K., French, N. H., & Unis, A. S. (1987). Problem-solving skills training and relationship therapy in the treatment of antisocial child behavior. *Journal of Consulting and Clinical Psychology, 55,* 76–85.

Kelley, H. H. (1972). *Causal schemata and the attribution process.* Morristown, NJ: General Learning.

Klein-Tasman, B. P., & Mervis, C. B. (2003). Distinctive personality characteristics of 8-, 9-, and 10-year olds with Williams syndrome. *Developmental Neuropsychology, 23,* 271–292.

Kopp, C. B., Baker, B. L., & Brown, K. W. (1992). Social skills and their correlates: Preschoolers with developmental delays. *American Journal on Mental Retardation, 96,* 357–366.

Kronick, D. (1978). An examination of psychosocial aspects of learning disabled adolescents. *Learning Disabilities Quarterly, 1,* 86–93.

LaGreca, A. (1997). Children's problems with friends. *Psychotherapy in Practice, 3,* 1–21.

Langone, J., Clees, T. J., Oxford, M., Malone, M., & Ross, G. (1995). Acquisition and generalization of social skills by high school students with mild mental retardation. *Mental Retardation, 33,* 186–196.

Leffert, J. S., & Siperstein, G. N. (1996). Assessment of social-cognitive processes in children with mental retardation. *American Journal on Mental Retardation, 100,* 441–455.

Lieber, J., Beckman, P. J., & Strong, B. N. (1993). A longitudinal study of the social exchanges of young children with disabilities. *Journal of Early Intervention, 17,* 116–128.

Luftig, R. L. (1988). Assessment of the perceived school loneliness and isolation of mentally retarded and nonretarded students. *American Journal on Mental Retardation, 92,* 472–475.

Margalit, M. (1993). Social skills and classroom behavior among adolescents with mild mental retardation. *American Journal on Mental Retardation, 97,* 685–691.

Matson, J. L., & Fee, V. E. (1991). Social skills difficulties among persons with mental retardation. In J. L. Matson & J. A. Mulick (Eds.), *Handbook of mental retardation* (pp. 468–478). New York: Pergamon.

Matson, J. L., Fee, V. E., Coe, D. A., & Smith, D. (1991). A social skills program for developmentally delayed preschoolers. *Journal of Clinical Child Psychology, 20,* 428–433.

Matson, J. L., Kazdin, A. E., & Esveldt-Dawson, K. (1980). Training interpersonal skills among mentally retarded and socially dysfunctional children. *Behavior Research and Therapy, 18,* 419–427.

Matson, J. L., LeBlanc, L. A., & Weinheimer, B. (1999). Reliability of the Matson evaluation of social skills in individuals with severe retardation. *Behavior Modification, 23,* 647–661.

Matson, J. L., Manikam, R., Coe, D., Raymond, K., Taras, M., & Long, N. (1988). Training social skills to severely mentally retarded multiply handicapped adolescents. *Research in Developmental Disabilities, 9,* 195–208.

Matson, J. L., & Ollendick, T. H. (1988). *Enhancing children's social skills: Assessment and treatment.* New York: Pergamon.

Matson, J. L., Rotatori, A. F., & Helsel, W. J. (1983). Development of a rating scale to measure social skills in children: The Matson evaluation of social skills with youngsters (MESSY). *Behaviour Research and Therapy, 21,* 335–340.

McFall, R. M. (1982). A review and reformulation of the construct of social skills. *Behavioral Assessment, 4,* 1–33.

McGinnis, E., & Goldstein, A. P. (1997). *Skillstreaming the elementary school child: Revised edition.* Champaign, IL: Research Press.

McMahon, C. M., Wacker, D. P., Sasso, G M., Berg, W. K., & Newton, S. M. (1996). Analysis of frequency and type of interactions in a peer-mediated social skills intervention: Instructional vs. social interactions. *Education and Training in Mental Retardation and Developmental Disabilities, 31,* 339–352.

Merrell, K. W. (1994). *Preschool & Kindergarten Behavior Scales.* Austin, TX: Pro-Ed.

Merrell, K. W., & Gimpel, G. A. (1998). *Social skills of children and adolescents: Conceptualization, assessment, treatment.* Mahwah, NJ: Erlbaum.

Merrell, K. W., & Holland, M. L. (1997). Social–emotional behavior of preschool-age children with and without developmental delays. *Research in Developmental Disabilities, 18,* 393–405.

Michelson, L., Sugai, D. P., Wood., R. P., & Kazdin, A. E. (1983). *Social skills assessment and training with children: An empirically based handbook.* New York: Plenum.

Moldavsky, M., Lev, D., & Lerman-Sagie, T. (2001). Behavioral phenotypes of genetic syndromes: A reference guide for psychiatrists. *Journal of the American Academy of Child and Adolescent Psychiatry, 40,* 749–761.

Mu, K., Siegel, E. B., & Allinder, R. M. (2000). Peer interactions and sociometric status of high school students with moderate or severe disabilities in general education classrooms. *Journal of the Association for Persons with Severe Handicaps, 25,* 142–152.

Mueser, K. T., Valenti-Hein, D., & Yarnold, P. R. (1987). Dating-skills groups for the developmentally disabled: Social skills and problem-solving versus relaxation training. *Behavior Modification, 11,* 200–228.

National Research Council. (2002). *Mental retardation: Determining eligibility for social security benefits.* Washington, DC: National Academy Press.

O'Reilly, M. F., & Glynn, D. (1995). Using a process social skills training approach with adolescents with mild intellectual disabilities in a high school setting. *Education and Training in Mental Retardation and Developmental Disabilities, 30,* 187–198.

Paloutzian, R. F., Hasazi, J., Streifel., J., & Edgar, C. L. (1971). Promotion of positive social interaction in severely retarded young children. *American Journal of Mental Deficiency, 75,* 519–524.

Parker, J. G., Rubin, K. H., Price, J. M., & DeRosier, M. E. (1995). Peer relationships, child development, and adjustment: A developmental psychopathology perspective. In D. Cicchetti & D. J. Cohen (Eds.), *Developmental psychopathology: Vol. 2. Risk, disorder, and adaptation* (pp. 96–161). New York: Wiley.

Pearson, D. A., Lachar, D., Loveland, K. A., Santos, C. W., Faria, L. P., Azzam, P. N., et al. (2000). Patterns of behavioral adjustment and maladjustment in mental retardation: Comparison of children with and without ADHD. *American Journal on Mental Retardation, 105,* 236–251.

Piercy, M., Wilton, K., & Townsend, M. (2002). Promoting the social acceptance of young children with moderate–severe intellectual disabilities using cooperative-learning techniques. *American Journal on Mental Retardation, 107,* 352–360.

Piers, E. V. (1969). *Manual for the Piers–Harris Children's Self-Concept Scale.* Counselor Recordings and Tests, Nashville, TN.

Quinn, M. M., Kavale, K. A., Mathur, S. R., Rutherford, R. B., & Forness, S. R. (1999). A meta-analysis of social skills interventions for students with emotional or behavioral disorders. *Journal of Emotional and Behavioral Disorders, 7,* 54–64.

Rubin, K. H., Bukowski, W., & Parker, J. G. (1998). Peer interactions, relationships, and groups. In W. Damon (Series Ed.) & N. Eisenber (Vol. Ed.), *Handbook of child psychology: Vol. 3. Social emotional and personality development* (5th ed., pp. 619–700). New York: Wiley.

Sargent, L. R. (1991). *Social skills for school and community: Systematic instruction for children and youth with cognitive delays.* Reston, VA: Division on Mental Retardation, Council for Exceptional Children.

Schaefer, C. E., & Cangelosi, D. (Eds.). (2002). *Play therapy techniques* (2nd ed.). Northvale, NJ: Jason Aronson.

Schneider, B. H. (1992). Didactic methods for enhancing children's peer relations: A quantitative review. *Clinical Psychology Review, 12,* 363–382.

Segrin, C. (2000). Social skills deficits associated with depression. *Clinical Psychology Review, 20,* 379–403.

Siperstein, G. N., & Bak, J. J. (1989). Social relationships of adolescents with moderate mental retardation. *Mental Retardation, 27,* 5–10.

Siperstein, G. N., & Leffert, J. S. (1997). Comparison of socially accepted and rejected children with mental retardation. *American Journal on Mental Retardation, 101,* 339–351.

Skinner, B. F. (1938). *The behavior of organisms: An experimental analysis.* New York: Appleton Century Crofts.

Soresi, S., & Nota, L. (2000). A social skill training for persons with Down's syndrome. *European Psychologist, 5,* 34–43.

Sparrow, S. S., Balla, D. A., & Cicchetti, D. V. (1984). *Vineland Adaptive Behavior Scales: Interview edition.* Circle Pines, MN: American Guidance Service.

Spence, S. H. (2003). Social skills training with children and young people: Theory, evidence, and practice. *Child and Adolescent Mental Health, 8,* 84–96.

Spence, S. H., Donovan, C., & Brechman-Toussaint, M. (2000). The treatment of childhood social phobia: The effectiveness of a social skills training-based, cognitive behavioral intervention, with and without parental involvement. *Journal of Child Psychology and Psychiatry, 41,* 713–726.

Strain, P. S. (1984). Social behavior patters of nonhandicapped and developmentally disabled friend pairs in mainstream preschool. *Analysis and Intervention in Developmental Disabilities, 4,* 15–28.

Strain, P. S., & Odom, S. L. (1986). Peer social initiations: Effective intervention for social skills development of exceptional children. *Exceptional Children, 52,* 543–551.

Taylor, A. R., Asher, S. R., & Williams, G. A. (1987). The social adaptation of mainstreamed mentally retarded children. *Child Development, 58,* 1321–1334.

Turner, S. M., Hersen, M., & Bellack, A. S. (1978). Social skills training to teach prosocial behaviors in an organically impaired and retarded patient. *Journal of Behavior Therapy and Experimental Psychiatry, 9,* 253–258.

Vaughn, S. R., Ridley, C. A., & Cox, J. (1983). Evaluating the efficacy of an interpersonal skills training program with children who are mentally retarded. *Education and Training of the Mentally Retarded, 18,* 191–196.

Walker, H. M., McConnell, S., Holmes, D., Todis, B., Walker, J., & Golden, N. (1988). *The walker social skills curriculum: The ACCEPTS program.* Austin, TX: Pro-Ed.

Walker, H. M., McConnell, S., Walker, J. L., Clarke, J. Y., Todis, B., Cohen, G., et al. (1983). Initial analysis of the accepts curriculum: Efficacy of instructional and behavior management procedures for improving the social adjustment of handicapped children. *Analysis and Intervention in Developmental Disabilities, 3,* 105–127.

Walz, N. C., & Benson, B. A. (2002). Behavioral phenotypes in children with Down syndrome, Prader–Willi syndrome, or Angelman syndrome. *Journal of Developmental and Physical Disabilities, 14,* 307–321.

Williams, G. A., & Asher, S. R. (1992). Assessment of loneliness at school among children with mild mental retardation. *American Journal on Mental Retardation, 96,* 373–385.

Wolpe, J. (1958). *Psychotherapy by reciprocal inhibition.* Stanford, CA: Stanford University Press.

Wong, S. E., Morgan, C., Crowley, R., & Baker, J. N. (1996). Using a table game to teach social skills to adolescent psychiatric inpatients: Do the skills generalize? *Child and Family Behavior Therapy, 18,* 1–17.

Zetlin, A. G., & Murtaugh, M. (1988). Friendship patterns of mildly learning handicapped and nonhandicapped high school students. *American Journal on Mental Retardation, 92,* 447–454.

31

Vocational Skills and Performance

JANIS G. CHADSEY

Since the mid-1980s, employment has been identified as a critical outcome for youth with disabilities, particularly when the U.S. Department of Education, Office of Special Education and Rehabilitation (OSERS) emphasized the importance of facilitating the transition from high school to work. In 1990, specific language on the transition from school to work was included in the Individuals with Disabilities Education Act (IDEA), added to the 1997 IDEA Amendments, and recently modified in 2004 reauthorization. When students with disabilities leave high school, some will enter postsecondary educational institutions and some will enter the workforce. This chapter is about those students with mental retardation and developmental disabilities who plan to be employed once they exit the schools. With the passage of IDEA in 2004, an Individualized Education Program (IEP) team must implement by age 16 the type of coursework and experiences students will need to develop the basic skills for employment and other transition outcomes.

In recent testimony to the President's Commission on Excellence in Special Education Transition Task Force Meeting, Wehman (2002) stated that students with disabilities needed to be competitively employed *before* they leave high school. Unfortunately, recent data for adults with all disabilities (ages 18–64 years) reveal that only 32% work full or part-time compared to 81% of the population without disabilities (National Organization on Disability, 2000) and many work in segregated settings (Braddock, Rizzolo, & Hemp, 2004). A recent analysis of national data for adults with developmental disabilities showed an even bleaker picture of employment. Yamaki and Fujiura (2002) reported that only 27.6% of adults with developmental disabilities had a job compared to 75.1% of the general adult

JANIS G. CHADSEY • Department of Special Education, University of Illinois at Urbana-Champaign, Champaign, Illinois 61820.

population and only half of the adults with developmental disabilities were employed full-time compared to 80% in the general population. Additionally, of those individuals with developmental disabilities who were working, more than half earned less than $1000.00 per month while only 20% in the general population earned a similar income. It is important to note, however, that the data analyzed in the Yamiki and Fujiura (2002) study were based on 1990 and 1991 data from the Survey of Income and Program Participation (a periodic federal survey); these data were collected during the middle of a national economic recession.

The data reported above, and data from other sources (Butterworth, Gilmore, Kiernan, & Schalock, 1999; Wehman, Revell, & Kregel, 1998), illustrate that employment is not a reality for many individuals with developmental disabilities. Additionally, when it is achieved, many are not working full-time or are earning wages below the poverty line. Why aren't employment outcomes better? Wehman and Bricout (2001) have suggested that advocates and people with disabilities needed to be more effective in working together to increase work opportunities and changing the system of adult services to focus more on achieving positive employment outcomes. Aside from these suggestions and the recommendation that youth with disabilities be employed before they leave school, Wehman (2002) also advised that: (a) One-Stop Career Centers supported through the Workforce Investment Act (P. L. 105–220) be reorganized to include all youth with disabilities when they are still in high school, (b) other federal policy programs (e.g., Social Security Act, Rehabilitation Act) support competitive employment and career development alternatives for youth, (c) joint funding of career development and work experiences through federal and state agencies be encouraged, and (d) vocational rehabilitation be funded to allow their agencies to "participate earlier and more completely in the transition process" (p. 195).

Achieving employment outcomes for individuals with mental retardation and developmental disabilities is a complicated process and requires more than just teaching them vocational or work skills. When these youth are in high school, they must have full access to curricular options and learning experiences in general education (Johnson, Stodden, Emanuel, Luecking, & Mack, 2002) and be involved in a longitudinal career development process so they can make better choices about what type of work they will pursue when they leave school (Hutchins & Renzaglia, 2002). A team of individuals must be assembled to provide support to students so outcomes can be achieved, but students should be self-determined and assume a leadership role in these transition/IEP team meetings (e.g., Konrad & Test, 2004; Wehmeyer, Agran, & Hughes, 1998). As noted by Wehman (2002) and others (Johnson et al., 2002), it is essential that collaboration and system linkages occur at the local, state, and federal level. If businesses and agencies (such as rehabilitation service providers and government agencies) are involved and supportive of the transition process when students are young, positive employment outcomes are more likely to occur. After students are employed, supports (e.g., coworkers, job coaches, employers) should be in place so that success is not only achieved in the current job, but also to allow students opportunities to move up career ladders or to change jobs if their career interests change (Pumpian, Fisher, Certo, & Smalley, 1997).

The scenario described above suggests that with respect to the achievement of vocational outcomes, individuals with disabilities should no longer be viewed predominantly from a medical-model perspective where they need to be "fixed" or "cured," but instead should be viewed from a perspective where individual strengths and choices are considered within a system of supports (Unger, 2002). Employment outcomes are unlikely to be achieved just by teaching vocational skills. As noted above, supports at the local, state, and federal level are needed to make more certain that the transition from high school to world of work is achieved (cf., Certo et al., 2003).

Although a system of supports is needed to make employment a reality, students still need to assume some of the responsibility for their vocational future. They must participate actively in choosing the type of work they want and they need to learn the skills that will enable them to do the job. This chapter will focus on several specific individual intervention strategies that will help persons with developmental disabilities achieve employment outcomes. First, the types of vocational skills that may need to be learned are described. Second, strategies that teach individuals to choose the work they want to do are explored. Third, recent research on the systematic instruction of vocational skills is presented. And fourth, research focused on teaching individuals to be less dependent on direct service personnel in work settings is described. This chapter will conclude with a summary of contemporary issues and future areas of research.

VOCATIONAL SKILLS

There are two categories of skills that are essential to positive employment outcomes: work (or vocational) skills and social skills. This chapter will focus only on vocational skills, although appropriate social skills are also critical to job success (Chadsey & Beyer, 2001).

The types of vocational skills needed in job settings are occupation and site-specific. Past research (e.g., Rusch, Schutz, & Agran, 1982) has revealed several vocational skills that may be generic to some job sites (e.g., a person follows one instruction at a time), but even these generic skills should be socially validated in the job setting where individuals are going to be working before they are taught (Test, 1994). The types of vocational skills taught will vary; it may be that individuals will learn all the skills associated with an entire job or they may only learn a subset of skills associated with several job tasks within the same work setting. The specific skills taught to an individual will depend upon the employer's needs and the individual's vocational interests and strengths.

Over the years, individuals with developmental disabilities have been employed in a number of different types of jobs. Recently, a national survey of high school transition and adult-supported employment programs was conducted to identify community employment placements for individuals with disabilities (Morgan, Ellerd, Jenson, & Taylor, 2000). The results from the survey provided data on 7553 job placements and revealed that the highest frequency job placement for both youth and adults was food and beverage preparation services. The second highest frequency was in building and related service occupations (e.g., janitors). Other job placements included sales (e.g., department store clerks), production and stock clerks, domestic service (e.g., housekeepers), and personal service occupations (e.g., nurse assistants). When survey respondents were asked to list new, emerging job markets, tourism- and casino-related jobs were mentioned frequently.

The examples of job placements reported in the Morgan et al. (2000) study suggest the types of vocational skills (e.g., stocking medical supplies) that would need to be learned by someone employed in these jobs. Once specific skills are identified (e.g., through social validation and task analysis), individuals with disabilities can be taught the skills on the job site by a teacher, job coach, transition specialist, employer, or coworker (Brady & Rosenberg, 2002; Grossi, Schaaf, Steigerwald, & Mank, 2002). An important aspect of designing intervention strategies for teaching vocational skills is to make certain that the individual has an interest in learning the skills. Students in high school should have numerous opportunities to "try out" or sample jobs throughout their high school career (Hutchins & Renzaglia, 2002). However, when individuals with disabilities graduate, they should be working in jobs of their choice and their preferences and desires should drive the job placement process (Menchetti & Garcia, 2003).

CHOOSING VOCATIONAL TASKS

Choice-making skills are one of the component elements of self-determined behavior (Wehmeyer, 1999). Although space precludes a discussion of self-determination, Wehmeyer and others (e.g., Field, Martin, Miller, Ward, & Wehmeyer, 1998; Wehmeyer et al., 1998; Wehmeyer & Sands, 1998) have stressed the importance of students with disabilities being able to determine their own futures. Wehmeyer (1996) defined self-determination as "acting as the primary causal agent in one's life and making choices and decisions regarding one's quality of life free from undue external influence or interference" (p. 24).

Part of being self-determined is choosing the type of work one wants to do. Individuals, including individuals with disabilities, are more likely to be successful at their jobs if they like their jobs (Test, Carver, Ewers, Haddad, & Peron, 2000). If individuals with disabilities have a job that matches their interests, desires, and skills, it is quite likely that they will need less support from others. Mank, Cioffi, and Yovanoff (2000) have stated that the type of support selected for an employee with disabilities should be secondary to a good job match. Although there are many variables that should be considered for making a good job match (e.g., social climate, supervisor style), the assessment of specific work-task preferences is also important.

A number of research studies have been conducted to evaluate methods for assessing work-task choice. For example, Reid and his colleagues (Parsons, Reid, & Green, 1998; Reid, Parsons, & Green, 1998; Reid, Parsons, Green, & Browning, 2001) conducted several studies to determine work-task preferences. In Reid et al. (1998), three adults with severe multiple disabilities were involved in a prework assessment to see if their assessed preferences would be reflected in similar choices during actual paid employment. A series of five job tasks associated with the preparation of books and mailing advertising information for a publishing company were paired in 10 different combinations and presented individually to all of the participants. Participants were asked to choose one of two tasks and then helped as needed for 3 min until all pairs of the tasks had been presented. Then, the most preferred task and one least preferred task were assessed for comparison during actual paid employment. When the participants were given a choice of tasks during paid employment, each participant chose the task that had been identified as being most preferred during the prework assessment. Reid et al., also noted that the prework assessment provided opportunities for the participants to gain familiarity with unfamiliar tasks. In a subsequent study using prework assessment, Parsons et al. (1998) obtained similar results for an adult with profound mental retardation, deafness, and blindness.

In a related study, Reid et al. (2001) offered three adults with multiple disabilities the choice of two working conditions that varied by the availability of assistive devices. Reid et al., (2001) found that the participants chose to work more often in the condition in which their accustomed assistive device was available, which in turn decreased the amount of job coach support they needed. Reid et al. suggested that giving employees more control over their work situations could enhance self-determination.

Recently, Lattimore, Parsons, and Reid (2002) replicated their findings using prework assessment with three men with autism; however, in this study there was a twist. Two of the men seemed to prefer alternating tasks during their work time, rather than working on a single task. The results from the study showed that while these two men chose their preferred work task as their first choice, they wanted to shift to other work tasks over the course of the day.

The results from the Lattimore et al. (2002) study raised the question of whether or not a worker would want to participate in one chosen task for an extended period of time. Worsdell, Iwata, and Wallace (2002) investigated the feasibility of using "duration of engagement" as an index of preference; duration is a well-established measure of the reinforcement value of an activity. Four adults with mental retardation participated in the study, which was conducted in a sheltered workshop setting. Task engagement was defined as "manipulating materials in a manner required to complete the task, on a 10-second partial-interval basis" (p. 288). During one condition, seven assembly tasks were presented singly for 5 min each. During the multiple-stimulus assessment condition, the same seven tasks were presented in a concurrent arrangement during a 5-min session. Then, a series of 60-min test sessions were conducted under typical workshop conditions, and during each session the participants were given one of the seven tasks to complete. The results showed that all of the participants chose to engage in one task exclusively during the multiple-stimulus assessment, indicating preference for a particular task. Additionally, all the participants showed high levels of engagement during most tasks during the single-task presentation, and the data from the single-task presentation were most similar to work engagement shown during the 60-min sessions.

Most recently, Stock, Davies, Secor, and Wehmeyer (2003) conducted a preliminary study to investigate the use of a self-directed video and audio software program, called *WorkSight*, to help individuals with intellectual disabilities express their vocational preferences from among 12 possible job categories. In addition, teachers and agency staff compared the effectiveness of *WorkSight* to a widely used career assessment tool consisting of pictures, and also made predictions about which job category participants would choose most and least often when using *WorkSight*.

The results from the study revealed that participants with intellectual disabilities were able to select the job they presumably preferred using *WorkSight*, and they needed little help from others when using the program so they were self-directed. In addition, teachers and evaluators rated *WorkSight* as being more effective than the traditional career assessment tool. Finally, the *WorkSight* system was able to accurately predict the likely job preferences of the participants, which were chosen by the teachers and agency personnel.

Taken together, these studies indicate individuals with significant disabilities do make choices with regard to vocational task preferences. In addition, these studies suggest the value of using a prework preference assessment to determine which tasks from a paying job will be preferred. Lattimore et al. (2002) also showed that individuals will work for longer periods of time on preferred tasks, and both Lattimore et al., and Reid et al. (2001) suggested that more than one task might be preferred at different times over the course of a day. The important point to remember about these studies is that employees with disabilities must be involved in choosing the work they want to do. Making choices is one of the critical behaviors needed to be self-determined.

TEACHING VOCATIONAL SKILLS USING SYSTEMATIC INSTRUCTION

It is quite likely that once students or adults with disabilities start a new job, they will need to learn how to do the job. A number of different people can teach individuals with disabilities job skills. For example, direct service personnel, such as teachers, job coaches (also known as employment specialists or supported employment specialists), transition specialists, and rehabilitation professionals can teach skills. Or, people who are not direct service personnel, such as employers or coworkers, can teach vocational skills. When employers or coworkers teach work skills,

there is less dependence on paid direct service personnel because the resources that occur naturally in the work setting (e.g., coworkers) provide
the support needed. Natural supports will be discussed more fully in the
next section of this chapter.

Wehman (1997) stated that effective teaching strategies are essential
if individuals with cognitive disabilities are going to learn a job. For years,
direct service personnel have used systematic instructional procedures to
teach individuals with disabilities vocational skills (Rusch, 1986; Wehman,
1981). While a thorough discussion of systematic instructional procedures
is beyond the scope of this chapter, Test and Wood (1997) described some of
these procedures for teaching vocational skills. These procedures include:
(a) conducting work-site analyses through procedures such as observation
and task analyses; (b) assessing competencies of employees by collecting
data on the ability to do the job; (c) and using instructional procedures of
chaining and shaping, prompting, reinforcement and feedback, and fading
to teach the job.

Although there is a rich history of systematic instructional procedures
being used to teach vocational skills (e.g., Rusch, 1986), two recent studies
are described here for illustrative purposes. Using a multiple-probe design,
Wall and Gast (1999) grouped 12 students with cognitive disabilities into
six dyads to teach grocery bagging using a constant time-delay prompting
procedure. In addition to teaching the vocational skill, Wall and Gast also
examined the acquisition of incidental information (verbal presentation of
targeted nutritional facts) and observational learning of incidental information (verbal presentation of nontargeted nutritional facts) that occurred
during the instruction of the vocational skill. Over half of the sessions occurred in a supermarket and less than half occurred in a school setting
that resembled a supermarket. The results from the study showed that all
of the participants learned the vocational task of bagging groceries with
fewer than 10% errors in 6–11 sessions. In addition, participants acquired
and retained approximately 50% of the targeted and nontargeted nutritional facts through direct verbal presentation or through observation of
instruction delivered to their peers. The study is interesting, not because
the students learned the task of bagging groceries through systematic instructional procedures, but because they also acquired nutritional facts
through targeted verbal instruction and observational learning.

Maciag, Schuster, Collins, and Cooper (2000) employed a multiple-
probe design to study the effectiveness of a simultaneous prompting procedure, which was used to teach 10 adults construction of shipping
boxes. With a simultaneous prompting procedure, a controlling prompt
was paired with the task direction and implemented during all instructional trials to ensure a nearly errorless procedure. Before instructional
sessions, probe trials were used to see if correct responses occurred without the controlling prompt.

In this study, a task analysis was conducted to determine all of the
steps needed to construct the shipping boxes. The 10 participants were
grouped into five dyads so that each member received instruction on
one-half of the task analysis on an alternating basis. Two sessions were

conducted daily so that all participants received instruction on the entire task. Correct responses were reinforced with instructor-descriptive verbal praise.

The results from the study showed that the simultaneous prompting was effective for teaching the task to four of the five dyads, but criterion levels of success were not met for the fifth dyad due to time constraints. The results also showed that grouping the participants into dyads meant that two employees could be trained at one time, fewer materials were needed for training, and employees could observe one another.

These two studies illustrate how systematic instructional procedures, such as simultaneous prompts and positive reinforcement, were used to teach vocational skills. Interestingly, studies of this type do not occur frequently in the current literature. While systematic instructional procedures are still essential to teaching vocational skills, it is possible that their value has been accepted, and the basic elements (e.g., shaping, reinforcement) need little further research. It should be noted, however, that even though there are fewer studies of this type in the literature, it does not mean that these procedures are used frequently or accurately in practice, or that these procedures are infrequently attempted in practice. From a research perspective, current literature seems to focus more on topics related to self-determination, natural support strategies, technology, marketing and job development, and policy issues; these are also some of the areas of need identified by practitioners (Wehman, Barcus, & Wilson, 2002).

STRATEGIES FOR DECREASING DEPENDENCE ON PAID DIRECT SERVICE PERSONNEL

As discussed above, direct service personnel, such as job coaches or teachers, have generally been responsible for facilitating support and implementing technical skills (such as systematic instruction) so that employees with disabilities can learn and keep their jobs. However, research in the United States done by Mank and his colleagues (Mank, Cioffi, & Yovanoff, 1997a, 1997b, 1998, 1999, 2000, 2003) and a recent international study (Jenaro, Mank, Bottomley, Doose, & Tuckerman, 2002) have indicated that better outcomes (e.g., better wages and social integration) were related to employees with disabilities receiving the same type of typical treatment given to other coworkers. In these studies, "typical treatment" consisted of such things as experiencing a typical orientation process to the job, and having a similar work role, schedule, and hours as other coworkers. This research suggests that the role of paid direct service personnel may need to change. Rather than being totally responsible for an individual with a disability and providing all of the orientation, training, and supervision, direct service personnel might function more as consultants and facilitators of training and supports (Grossi, Banks, & Pinnyei, 2001; Ohtake & Chadsey, 2001). In addition, if employees with disabilities are more independent in their work, they may be more self-determined. Finally, once students leave school, they are not guaranteed support through the adult service system. If students need support, and can find it through other means (such as through coworkers), they may be more likely to achieve positive vocational outcomes.

Several studies have been conducted to suggest ways that dependence on paid direct service personnel can be reduced. These studies can be grouped into ones that use three different types of strategies: (a) those that use job coaches to supervise more than one employee, (b) those that use self-directed learning strategies, and (c) those that use typical or natural support strategies.

Supervising More Than One Employee

Parsons, Reid, Green, and Browning (2001) used a model that included off-site and on-site strategies to reduce job coach assistance to three individuals with severe cognitive and multiple disabilities. The off-site procedures involved analyzing the amount of job coach support that was needed to complete a task using on-the-job materials, and systematically reducing the support of the job coach through a combination of instructions and environmental arrangements (e.g., use of a work-adaptation device). When the on-site observations showed that the frequency of work assistance had been reduced to 20% or less of the observation intervals, a job coach was shared between two workers. The results from this study suggested that the procedure did reduce the amount of job coach assistance needed for individual workers, although the shared job coach feature of the on-site procedure was, unfortunately, not implemented during the baseline phase of the study and thus the data were only suggestive.

In another study conducted by Parsons, Reid, Green, Browning, and Hensley (2002), a shared-work program was implemented to decrease job coach assistance for three adults with severe multiple disabilities. Within this intervention, a systematic analysis was done of each worker performing an entire job task, and the steps in the job that required the most assistance were reassigned to another worker who could perform the step with less assistance. The results from the study indicated that job coach assistance was reduced and only two, rather than three, job coaches were needed on the job. During baseline, however, the reduced job coach feature was not implemented, so it cannot be stated unequivocally that the shared work program was responsible for the decreased assistance. Additionally, the shared work program required more than one person with a disability to work closely with others to perform the same job; this grouping feature (and the close presence of the job coach) could hamper social integration with coworkers (Chadsey, Linneman, Rusch, & Cimera, 1997).

Self-Directed Learning Strategies

Strategies have also been implemented to teach individuals to manage their own behavior in order to decrease their dependence on others. A self-management strategy, or self-directed learning, can be one of the features associated with self-determined behavior because individuals take responsibility for directing or managing their own behavior (Wehmeyer, 1999). There are a number of different self-directed learning strategies that can be used to increase and maintain vocational behavior, including: (a) permanent prompts (e.g., pictures, taped auditory instructions), (b) verbal rehearsal, (c) self-monitoring, and (d) self-reinforcement. Several studies that used these strategies are described below.

Christian and Poling (1997) used a multiple-baseline design across restaurant tasks to evaluate the effects of self-management procedures on productivity with two adult women with mild disabilities. The women were taught to use a timer to monitor and increase their productivity. If they finished their task before the timer went off, they rewarded themselves with self-selected reinforcers (e.g., lunch with supervisor). The results from the study showed that productivity increased and that the participants, coworkers, and supervisors viewed the procedures as being socially acceptable.

Grossi and Heward (1998) conducted another study aimed at increasing work productivity in a restaurant setting. In this study, four adult males with mild disabilities were taught a self-evaluation training package that consisted of: (a) setting production goals; (b) self-monitoring toward the goal by learning to operate a timer or stop watch and then recording that performance in a notebook; (c) self-evaluating by comparing work performance to the stated goal; and (d) verbally self-reinforcing if the goal was met. The results from the study showed the all four participants learned the self-evaluation package, and the package increased production skills over baseline levels. In addition, increased productivity did not have a negative effect on the quality of the work performed.

Mitchell, Schuster, Collins, and Gassaway (2000) used a faded auditory prompting system to teach janitorial skills to three students with mild disabilities. All of the steps of the vocational skill (e.g., cleaning a toilet) were verbally recorded on a cassette tape recorder. Students were taught to place earphones on their head, press the on switch of the cassette recorder, and listen to the first step of the task analysis of the skill. They were then instructed to turn the tape off when they heard a "beep," verbalize the step, and then complete it. They then turned the tape recorder back on to listen to the next step, and followed the procedure described above for each step, until the entire task analysis and vocational skill was completed. When criterion had been reached, a fading procedure was implemented. For the purposes of fading, the teacher had created another tape that had one (initially) or a sequence (later) of steps within the task analysis omitted; students were taught to verbalize the omitted steps and complete them. This process continued until all of the steps were omitted. The results from the study showed that all the students met criterion for the skills and generalized the skills to untrained areas without the need for the auditory prompting system.

The studies described above suggest that individuals with disabilities can learn to manage their own behavior through self-directed learning strategies. These strategies have been described as a component of the *Self-Determined Learning Model of Instruction* (SDLMI) proposed by

Agran, Blanchard, and Wehmeyer (2000). In this model, individuals are taught to set their own goals based on preferences and needs, develop and implement action plans to meet their goals, and self-evaluate their progress toward achieving their goals. This model could be used to teach individuals with disabilities to make choices about the work they want to do, assess their abilities in relation to the tasks that need to be performed, create a plan to address the skills they need to learn, implement their plan, and monitor their progress toward achieving their goals. Agran et al. (2000) demonstrated some empirical support for this model. More recently, McGlashing-Johnson, Agran, Sitlington, Cavin, and Wehmer (2003) demonstrated that the SDLMI was effective for three of four high school students with moderate-to-severe disabilities in setting their own vocational goals, developing an action plan, implementing the plan, and adjusting their goals and plans as needed.

Typical or Natural Support Strategies

Another way to decrease dependence upon paid direct service personnel is through the use of typical strategies that occur naturally in work settings (e.g., Butterworth, Hagner, Kiernan, & Schalock, 1996; Mank et al., 1999; Ohtake & Chadsey, 2001; Test & Wood, 1997). With typical or natural support strategies, supervisors or coworkers might teach or help to maintain vocational skills, thereby lessening the training responsibility of the direct service personnel. Although correlational studies have been conducted to show that natural support strategies are associated with better vocational outcomes (e.g., Jenaro et al., 2002; Mank et al., 1999), there have been few causal studies conducted to investigate this issue.

A pilot study using coworkers to provide direct job training and support to employees with disabilities was conducted in Australia (Farris & Stancliffe, 2001). In this study, 19 staff working at 11 KFC restaurants participated in a 2-day coworker training course; they provided training and support to 10 consumers with disabilities. In the comparison group, six consumers (who also worked at KFC restaurants) received support from job coaches. The two groups of individuals with disabilities did not differ significantly from one another with respect to their job-related skills and other pertinent personal characteristics.

After participation in the coworker training course, the experimental group of coworkers placed a significantly higher value on persons with disabilities than they had prior to participating in the course, but the size of this change was modest and data were not taken on the comparison group. In a direct comparison, however, employment outcomes (i.e., wages, hours, tenure) were as good for the coworker group as they were for the comparison group who had worked with job coach support. This study suggested that coworker training models may provide an alternative to the traditional job coach model, but further research is essential to clarify features of work environments conducive to, and possible parameters of effectiveness of, coworker training.

Strategies that are used to decrease dependence on direct service personnel are important because when students with disabilities leave school and enter the adult service system, they are not guaranteed paid support. The studies discussed above illustrate that there are various methods that can be tried to lessen the support provided by direct service personnel. Although descriptive research points to the promise of natural support strategies, more causal studies are needed. Additionally, self-directed learning strategies are enticing because they may help to increase self-determined behavior, but studies involving students and adults with more significant disabilities are warranted.

SUMMARY, ISSUES, AND FUTURE RESEARCH AREAS

Many students with disabilities leave school and seek employment rather than attending postsecondary education institutions. Unfortunately, the employment outcome data for students and adults with disabilities is not positive, spurring researchers and policy makers to suggest that students be placed in jobs before they leave school and that federal, state, and local governments work together to more positive transition outcomes (Wehman, 2002).

When students and adults are employed, they tend to have jobs in service industry occupations, such as restaurant and janitorial business (Morgan et al., 2000). These jobs may not always offer decent salaries nor career advancement. Research and model demonstrations are needed to show that individuals with disabilities can work in occupations other than service industries, and that career advancement is possible within an organization or in another job when preferences change. Research in these areas will require innovative practices, and may also require the development of different and unique relationships with employers. For example, Callahan (2002) suggested that customized employment should be considered as an option, especially for individuals with significant disabilities. Customized employment means that an employment opportunity for a person is individualized and meets the needs of both the employer and employee through a special negotiation that allows job developers to disclose features of a person's disability. It may include employment that is developed through job carving (i.e., carrying out selected component tasks of a job function), self-employment, or other types of entrepreneurial initiatives. Whether customized employment is tried or different innovative practices are proposed, it is essential that well-designed research and evaluation studies be conducted in order to determine the effectiveness of the practice.

As one aspect of the fulfillment of social roles, students and adults with disabilities should be self-determining, and part of that behavior is being able to select a job of choice (Wehmeyer, 1999). While there have been some promising studies involving choice of work tasks, most of these studies have been carried out with adults and have entailed limited work opportunities. Future research efforts are needed to more accurately assess vocational preferences and strengths, particularly for students who are still in high school. In order to ensure choice, students must have many opportunities to sample an array of jobs so that they can make informed decisions before they graduate (Wehman, 2002).

When a student or adult is learning a job, support may be provided by direct service personnel (e.g., job coach) or by more natural forms of support, such as coworkers. If support is provided by more natural means, direct service personnel will still be involved, but in more facilitative or consultative roles (Butterworth et al., 1996). Even in the latter case, it will still be essential for direct service personnel to be proficient in systematic instruction and self-directed learning strategies because these procedures have been used successfully to teach and maintain vocational skills (Test & Wood, 1997; Wehmeyer, 1999), and coworkers may also benefit by instruction in the use of these procedures. Although there are successful demonstrations of these strategies in the literature, further research is still necessary to determine the best methods to teach self-directed learning strategies, especially to individuals with the most significant disabilities. Additionally, future research is also needed to inform direct service personnel how they can negotiate and implement the facilitator or consultative role.

Ohtake and Chadsey (2001) described a continuum of six different types of facilitation strategies, ranging in level of intrusiveness, that direct service personnel could use to negotiate their roles with coworkers. Although these strategies may be attractive in theory, and descriptive research suggests that the least intrusive and more typical strategies are associated with better vocational outcomes (Mank et al., 2003), more research is needed. In particular, causal demonstrations are necessary to show which strategies on the continuum result in improved vocational outcomes for individuals with disabilities who have varied needs. In addition, research is necessary to identify the types of work cultures that more readily support more typical forms of support (Ohtake & Chadsey, 2001). It is possible that coworkers in some work cultures will not want to play a very big role in supporting a worker with a disability, or they may want to offer support but do not have the necessary skills to do so (West, Kregel, Hernandez, & Hock, 1997). It is also possible that workplaces characterized by certain types of employees may be more or less conducive to coworker support, or that the nature of typical jobs in some places may inhibit the extent of support that can be provided, due to the nature of tasks assigned to coworkers. The goal for researchers is to determine which type of support strategy will fit the most naturally into a work setting while still resulting in positive vocational outcomes for individuals with disabilities.

Individuals with disabilities want to work, make a decent salary, and obtain good benefits; in this respect they are no different from other Americans (National Organization on Disability, 2000). In order to achieve these outcomes, policy-makers representing federal, local, and state entities must work together to facilitate, and not hinder, the transition from school to work process. In addition, personnel, such as teachers and job coaches, must be able to implement effective practices that have been validated by research. Also, individuals with disabilities must be self-determined so that they can choose the jobs they want and guide the vocational process.

REFERENCES

Agran, M., Blanchard, C., & Wehmeyer, M. L. (2000). Promoting transition goals and self-determination through student self-directed learning: The self-determined learning model of instruction. *Education and Training in Mental Retardation and Developmental Disabilities, 35*, 351–364.

Braddock, D., Rizzolo, M. C., & Hemp, R. (2004). Most employment services growth in developmental disabilities during 1988–2002 was in segregated settings. *Mental Retardation, 42*, 317–320.

Brady, M. P., & Rosenberg, H. (2002). Modifying and managing employment practices: An inclusive model for job placement and support. In K. Storey, P. Bates, & D. Hunter (Eds.), *The road ahead: Transition to adult life for persons with disabilities* (pp. 121–136). St. Augustine, FL: Training Resource Network.

Butterworth, J., Gilmore, D. S., Kiernan, W. E., & Schalock, R. (1999). *State trends in employment services for people with developmental disabilities: Multi-year comparisons based on state MR/DD agency and vocational rehabilitation (RSA) data.* Boston: Children's Hospital, Institute for Community Inclusion.

Butterworth, J., Hagner, D., Kiernan, W. E., & Schalock, R. L. (1996). Natural supports in the workplace: Defining an agenda for research and practice. *Journal of the Association for Persons with Severe Handicaps, 21*, 103–113.

Callahan, M. (2002, September/October). Employment: From competitive to customized. *TASH Connections, 28*, 16–19.

Certo, N. J., Mautz, D., Pumpian, I., Sax, K., Smalley, K., Wade, H. A., et al. (2003). Review and discussion of a model for seamless transition to adulthood. *Education and Training in Developmental Disabilities, 38*, 3–17.

Chadsey, J., & Beyer, S. (2001). Social relationships in work settings. *Mental Retardation and Developmental Disabilities: Research Reviews, 1*, 122–127.

Chadsey, J. G., Linneman, D., Rusch, F. R., & Cimera, R. E. (1997). The impact of social integration interventions and job coaches in work settings. *Education and Training in Mental Retardation and Developmental Disabilities, 32*, 281–292.

Christian, L., & Poling, A. (1997). Using self-management procedures to improve the productivity of adults with developmental disabilities in a competitive employment setting. *Journal of Applied Behavior Analysis, 30*, 169–172.

Farris, B., & Stancliff, R. (2001). The co-worker training model: Outcomes of an open employment pilot project. *Journal of Intellectual and Developmental Disability, 26*, 143–149.

Field, S., Martin, J., Miller, R., Ward, M., & Wehmeyer, M. (1998). Self-determination for persons with disabilities: A position statement of the division on career development and transition. *Career Development for Exceptional Individuals, 21*, 113–128.

Grossi, T., Banks, B., & Pinnyei, D. (2001). Facilitating job site training and supports: The evolving role of the job coach. In P. Wehman (Ed.), *Supported employment in business: Expanding the capacity of workers with disabilities* (pp. 75–92). St. Augustine, FL: Training Resource Network.

Grossi, T., Schaaf, L., Steigerwald, M., & Mank, D. (2002). Adult employment. In K. Storey, P. Bates, & D. Hunter (Eds.), *The road ahead: Transition to adult life for persons with disabilities* (pp. 101–120). St. Augustine, FL: Training Resource Network.

Grossi, T. A., & Heward, W. L. (1998). Using self-evaluation to improve the work productivity of trainees in a community-based restaurant training program. *Education and Training in Mental Retardation and Development Disabilities, 33*, 248–263.

Hutchins, M. P., & Renzaglia, A. (2002). Career development: Developing basic work skills and employment preferences. In K. Storey, P. Bates, & D. Hunter (Eds.), *The road ahead: Transition to adult life for persons with disabilities* (pp. 65–100). St. Augustine, FL: Training Resource Network.

Jenaro, C., Mank, D., Bottomley, J., Doose, S., & Tuckerman, P. (2002). Supported employment in the international context: An analysis of processes and outcomes. *Journal of Vocational Rehabilitation, 17*, 5–21.

Johnson, D. R., Stodden, R. A., Emanuel, E. J., Luecking, R., & Mack, M. (2002). Current challenges facing secondary education and transition services: What research tells us. *Exceptional Children, 68*, 519–531.

Konrad, M., & Test, D. W. (2004). Teaching middle-school students with disabilities to use an IEP template. *Career Development for Exceptional Individuals, 27*, 101–124.

Lattimore, L. P., Parsons, M. B., & Reid, D. H. (2002). A prework assessment of task preferences among adults with autism beginning a supported job. *Journal of Applied Behavior Analysis, 35*, 85–88.

Maciag, K. G., Schuster, J. W., Collins, B. C., & Cooper, J. T. (2000). Training adults with moderate and severe mental retardation in a vocational skill using a simultaneous prompting procedure. *Education and Training in Mental Retardation and Development Disabilities, 35*, 306–316.

Mank, D., Cioffi, A., & Yovanoff, P. (1997a). Analysis of typicalness of supported employment jobs, natural supports, and wage and integration outcomes. *Mental Retardation, 35*, 185–197.

Mank, D., Cioffi, A. R., & Yovanoff, P. (1997b). Patterns of support for employees with severe disabilities. *Mental Retardation, 35*, 433–447.

Mank, D., Cioffi, A., & Yovanoff, P. (2000). Direct support in supported employment and its relation to job typicalness, co-worker involvement, and employment outcomes. *Mental Retardation, 38*, 506–516.

Mank, D., Cioffi, A., & Yovanoff, P. (2003). Supported employment outcomes across a decade: Is there evidence of improvement in the quality of implementation? *Mental Retardation, 41*, 188–197.

Mank, D. M., Cioffi, A. R., & Yovanoff, P. (1998). Employment outcomes for people with severe disabilities, opportunities for improvement. *Mental Retardation, 36*, 383–394.

Mank, D. M., Cioffi, A. R., & Yovonoff, P. (1999). The impact of coworker involvement with supported employees on wage and integration outcomes. *Mental Retardation, 37*, 383–394.

McGlashing-Johnson, J., Agran, M., Sitlington, P., Cavin, M., & Wehmer, M. (2003). Enhancing the job performance of youth with moderate to severe cognitive disabilities using the self-determined learning model of instruction. *Research and Practice for Persons with Severe Disabilities, 28*, 194–204.

Menchetti, B. M., & Garcia, L. A. (2003). Personal and employment outcomes of person-centered career planning. *Education and Training in Developmental Disabilties, 38*, 142–156.

Mitchell, R. J., Schuster, J. W., Collins, B. C., & Gassaway, L. J. (2000). Teaching vocational skills with a faded auditory prompting system. *Education and Training in Mental Retardation and Developmental Disabilities, 35*, 415–427.

Morgan, R. L., Ellerd, D. A., Jenson, K., & Taylor, M. J. (2000). A survey of community employment placements: Where are youth and adults with disabilities working? *Career Development for Exceptional Individuals, 23*, 73–86.

National Organization on Disability. (2000). *N.O.D. Harris Survey of Americans with Disabilities*. Washington, DC: Louis Harris & Associates.

Ohtake, Y., & Chadsey, J. (2001). Continuing to describe the natural support process. *Journal of the Association for Persons with Severe Handicaps, 26*, 84–95.

Parsons, M. B., Reid, D. H., & Green, C. W. (1998). Identifying work preferences prior to supported work for an individual with multiple severe disabilities including deaf-blindness. *The Journal for the Association for Persons with Severe Handicaps, 23*, 329–333.

Parsons, M. B., Reid, D. H., Green, C. W., & Browning, L. B. (2001). Reducing job coach assistance for supported workers with severe multiple disabilities: An alternative offsite/on-site model. *Research in Developmental Disabilities, 21*, 151–164.

Parsons, M. B., Reid, D. H., Green, C. W., Browning, L. B., & Hensley, M. B. (2002). Evaluation of a shared-work program for reducing assistance provided to supported workers with severe disabilities. *Research in Developmental Disabilities, 23*, 1–16.

Pumpian, I., Fisher, D., Certo, N. J., & Smallgy, K. A. (1997). Changing jobs: An essential part of career development. *Mental Retardation, 35*, 39–48.

Reid, D. H., Parsons, M. B., & Green, C. W. (1998). Identifying work preferences among individuals with severe multiple disabilities prior to beginning supported work. *Journal of Applied Behavior Analysis, 31*, 281–285.

Reid, D. H., Parsons, M. B., Green, C. W., & Browning, B. (2001). Increasing one aspect of self-determination among adults with severe multiple disabilities in supported work. *Journal of Applied Behavior Analysis, 34,* 341–344.

Rusch, F. R. (Ed.). (1986). *Competitive employment issues and strategies.* Baltimore: Brookes.

Rusch, F. R., Schutz, R. P., & Agran, M. (1982). Validating entry level survival skills for service occupations: Implications for curriculum development. *Journal of the Association for Persons with Severe Handicaps, 7,* 32–41.

Stock, S. E., Davies, D. K., Secor, R. R., & Wehmeyer, M. L. (2003). Self-directed career preference selection for individuals with intellectual disabilities: Using computer technology to enhance self-determination. *Journal of Vocational Rehabilitation, 19,* 95–103.

Test, D. (1994). Supported employment and social validity. *Journal of the Association for Persons with Severe Handicaps, 19,* 116–129.

Test, D. W., Carver, T., Ewers, L., Haddad, J., & Peron, J. (2000). Longitudinal job satisfaction of persons in supported employment. *Education and Training in Mental Retardation and Developmental Disabilities, 35,* 365–373.

Test, D. W., & Wood, W. M. (1997). Rocket science 101: What supported employment specialists need to know about systematic instruction. *Journal of Vocational Rehabilitation, 9,* 109–120.

Unger, D. D. (2002). Employers' attitudes toward persons with disabilities in the workforce: Myths or realities? *Focus on Autism and Other Developmental Disabilities, 17,* 2–10.

Wall, M. E., & Gast, D. L. (1999). Acquisition of incidental information during instruction for a response-chain skill. *Research in Developmental Disabilities, 20,* 31–50.

Wehman, P. (1981). *Competitive employment.* Baltimore: Brookes.

Wehman, P. (1997). Editorial. *Journal of Vocational Rehabilitation, 9,* 93–94.

Wehman, P. (2002). A new era: Revitalizing special education for children and their families. *Focus on Autism and Other Developmental Disabilities, 17,* 194–197.

Wehman, P., Barcus, M., & Wilson, K. (2002). A survey of training and technical assistance needs of community-based rehabilitation providers. *Journal of Vocational Rehabilitation, 17,* 39–46.

Wehman, P., & Bricout, J. (2001). Supported employment: New directions for the new millennium. In P. Wehman (Ed.), *Supported employment in business: Expanding the capacity of workers with disabilities* (pp. 3–22). St. Augustine, FL: Training Resource Network.

Wehman, P., Revell, G., & Kregel, J. (1998). Supported employment: A decade of rapid growth and impact. *American Rehabilitation, 24,* 31–43.

Wehmeyer, M. L. (1996). Self-determination as an educational outcome: Why is it important to children and adults with disabilities? In D. J. Sands & M. Wehmeyer (Eds.), *Self determination across the life span: Independence and choice for people with disabilities* (pp. 15–34). Baltimore: Brookes.

Wehmeyer, M. L. (1999). A functional model of self-determination: Describing development and implementing instruction. *Focus on Autism and Other Developmental Disabilities, 14,* 53–61.

Wehmeyer, M. L., Agran, M., & Hughes, C. (1998). *Teaching self-determination to students with disabilities: Basic skills for successful transition.* Baltimore: Brookes.

Wehmeyer, M. L., & Sands, D. J. (1998). *Making it happen: Student involvement in education planning, decision making, and instruction.* Baltimore: Brookes.

West, M. D., Kregel, J., Hernandez, A., & Hock, T. (1997). Everybody's doing it: A national study on the use of natural supports in supported employment. *Focus on Autism and Other Developmental Disabilities, 12,* 175–181.

Worsdell, A. S., Iwata, B. A., & Wallace, M. D. (2002). Duration-based measures of preference for vocational tasks. *Journal of Applied Behavior Analysis, 35,* 287–290.

Yamaki, K., & Fujiura, G. T. (2002). Employment and income status of adults with developmental disabilities living in the community. *Mental Retardation, 40,* 132–141.

32

Sex Offending Behavior

CHRISTINE MAGUTH NEZU, ARTHUR M. NEZU, TAMARA L. KLEIN, and MARY CLAIR

Sex offending behavior in persons with intellectual disabilities (ID) is a serious problem with significant consequences for the victims, offenders, and their social communities (Barron, Hassiots, & Banes, 2002; Nezu, Nezu, & Dudek, 1998). A growing awareness of such problems in people with ID, as well as heightened societal and cultural sensitivity to the occurrence of sex offenses, requires effective solutions with regard to assessment and treatment.

DEFINING SEX OFFENDING

Sex offending is a broad and *psycho-legal* term that identifies a person as a *sex offender* if it is determined that he or she has committed a sex offense (Lanyon, 2001). Examples of sex offenses defined by the law include sexual conduct with a minor and forcible, nonconsensual sexual acts toward an adult, including sexual acts involving an individual who is deemed unable to give consent for sexual acts. Although many sex offenders may be diagnosed or identified as exhibiting deviant sexual interests, the presence of such interests is not the same as actually engaging in a sex offending behavior. For example, some people with paraphilias, defined as recurrent, intense, sexually arousing fantasies, urges, or behaviors that are consensually specified as deviant and result in distress, do not actually engage in behaviors consistent with their urges (Hall, 1996; Lanyon, 2001). It is also possible for a person to legally offend but not to be diagnosed with a specific paraphilia, such as exhibitionism or pedophilia. Moreover, people who sexually offend may be diagnosed with additional disorders, including mood or anxiety disorders, personality disorders, brain injury, or ID.

CHRISTINE MAGUTH NEZU, ARTHUR M. NEZU, TAMARA L. KLEIN, and MARY CLAIR • Drexel University.

Thus, sex offenders represent a heterogeneous population for which few generalizations can be made regarding etiology, assessment, or treatment, which can be broadly applied to all offenders.

SEX OFFENDERS WITH INTELLECTUAL DISABILITIES

Although the prevalence of people with developmental disabilities (DD) in the total population of known sex offenders is estimated to be between 10 and 15% (Murphy, Coleman, & Haynes, 1983) and much higher if people with borderline intellectual functioning are included in this estimate, there is no support for a direct or causal association between intellectual functioning and sex offending behavior. Despite this report by Murphy and colleagues of a slightly higher percentage of offenders with DD than would be expected from population statistics on prevalence of DD more generally, this increased prevalence may be due to other variables such as the decreased likelihood of people with DD or ID being able to evade detection and arrest in contrast with their peers. Observations from other investigations support this idea. For example, Van Dyke, McBrien, and Mattheis (1996) report that problems such as genital exposure, public masturbation, and deviant fantasies are no more common in people with ID than in the general population. McCurry et al. (1998) conducted an investigation of the relation between cognitive functioning and sex offending behavior and found few differences between the participants with and without ID or DD.

Despite the similar rates and types of sex offenses in offenders with DD when compared to other sex offenders, the availability and investigation of effective treatment programs has lagged far behind those for their nondisabled cohorts (Lindsay, 2002; Timms & Goreczny, 2002). Taken together, the current data suggest that there are significant numbers of offenders with DD who are often poorly identified and inadequately treated, and consequently may pose a risk to the public (Barron et al., 2002). It is important to understand what diathetic factors may contribute to the development of sex offending behavior in people with ID so that effective interventions can be developed, researched, and made available to the population. This requires an integration of existing scientific knowledge concerning both sex offending and DD. One area that has surfaced as a possible etiologic factor is the way in which people with ID have historically been sexually acculturated.

CHALLENGES OF SEXUAL BEHAVIOR FOR PEOPLE WITH INTELLECTUAL DISABILITIES

Due to a history of institutionalization, the sexual lives of people with ID have historically been under society's control (Kempton & Kahn, 1991; Pitceathly & Chapman, 1985; Woodill, 1992). Well into the first half of this century people with ID were seen as criminal and sexually promiscuous (Kempton & Kahn, 1991; Lumley & Scotti, 2001). Control of all sexual activity and sterilization was viewed as important to the prevention of further criminality and sexually promiscuous behavior. No education in sexuality or treatment for sexual disorders was provided (Woodill, 1992).

It was not until the 1960s, consistent with the civil rights movement, that the sexual rights of people with ID began to receive societal support. The philosophy of normalization was adopted as the deleterious consequences of institutional life were exposed. Following a nationwide deinstitutionalization movement in the 1970s, people with ID were in a position to receive increased access to sexual expression. Despite several decades of this nationwide trend toward community integration, caregivers' negative bias and desire to control sexual activities may still serve as obstacles to the sexual expression of people with ID. Segregated facilities, strict supervision of sexual activities, minimal privacy, lack of opportunities for sex education, and rules against close contact between consenting adults may be the result of caregivers' desire to control sexual expression in the population (Jurkowski & Amado, 1993). Additionally, the lives of people with ID may be unfairly restricted due to the fears of others regarding issues of pregnancy, parenting, HIV, and sexual abuse. Currently, many agencies that support community residences have no specifically stated policies regarding consensual sexual activity.

One explanation for continued community control may be found in stereotypic views concerning the sexuality of people with DD that have historically existed. In one view, people with ID are seen as having uncontrollable sexual desires (Szollos & McCabe, 1995; Williams, 1991). An alternative view is that they are innocent and naïve people who have no sexual desires (Szollos & McCabe, 1995; Williams, 1991; Zuker-Weiss, 1994). Zuker-Weiss (1994) has proposed a third more accurate view of sexuality. This view proposes that people with ID are individuals in the process of development who have equal rights to sexual expression as those of nondisabled adults. Unfortunately, this view is not widely accepted or disseminated to the pubic at large, to providers of DD services, or to people with DD. For example, the small body of research that has focused on how people with ID view their own sexuality reveals that they hold sexual attitudes that are often incorrect and negative regarding expression of their sexuality (Szollos & McCabe, 1995). These views have been attributed to the finding that residential staff serving people with ID may also hold negative attitudes regarding the sexuality of their clients. Additionally, parents often express fear of the topic. Szollos and McCabe (1995) have reported that caregivers of people with DD significantly overestimate their clients' knowledge, experience, and feelings concerning sexuality. Without the support from family or caregiving systems to provide accurate and effective sexual educative experiences, the sexual knowledge that an individual inadvertently learns can be subject to significant distortion and misinterpretation (Jurkowski & Amado, 1993).

Historically, sex education programs for people with ID were not sought until a "problem" was identified (e.g., a possible or suspected sex offense).

Additionally, much of the content of the available programs was directed toward the physical or biological aspects of sex (Chivers & Mathieson, 2000; Jurkowski & Amado, 1993; Williams, 1991), and less on issues of intimacy, sensuality, sexual dysfunction, or exploitation. One possible reason for this is that biological "facts" about sex are easier to teach than are adaptive interpersonal behaviors and social or sexual competency. Finally, sexual dysfunction is rarely targeted as a therapeutic focus in people with ID despite a reported rate of sexual problems for 40% of women and 20% of men with ID (Szollos & McCabe; 1995).

When people with ID are poorly educated and the victims of sexual exploitation or abuse, they often lack the access to legal support or psychotherapy treatment alternatives that is available to nondisabled people. In their review of the extant psychotherapy research concerning people with DD, Prout and Nowak-Drabick (2003) reported that people with mild ID are significantly less likely to be provided with needed psychotherapy services. Moreover, cognitive limitations, expressive speech deficits, and limited adaptive skills can further complicate their symptoms and create challenges to psychological evaluation for this population (Nezu, Nezu, & Gill-Weiss, 1992). Finally, people with ID are more likely to have a personal history of exploitation and victimization due to the effects of impoverished residential environments or the frustrations of ill-trained caregivers (Schoen & Hoover, 1990). When people who have experienced sexual, physical, or emotional abuse do not have the opportunity to receive effective remediating experiences (e.g., interventions designed to help them understand their own feelings associated with the event, opportunity to obtain an objective perception of what has happened to them, or learn ways to cope with related problems), the likelihood that a former victim may become a future offender is increased. Thus, social–sexual education and availability of early psychotherapy interventions for people with ID who are in need of such services may be important sources of primary prevention of sex offending behavior.

SEX OFFENDING VULNERABILITY IN PEOPLE WITH INTELLECTUAL DISABILITIES

Despite an increase in research focused on inappropriate sexual behaviors that have been perpetrated by people with ID, the empirical research is very limited. However, guidelines for assessment and treatment can be developed through an integration of the existing literature with regard to sex offender vulnerability across populations, reported characteristics of sex offenders with ID, and the literature that provides support for the efficacy of psychotherapy for people with ID.

Over the years several behavioral explanatory models of sexual aggression have been proposed. The first models were based upon theories of conditioning and deviant arousal (Maguire, Carlisle, & Young, 1965). This "sexual motivational conditioning" model proposed that deviant sexual behavior occurs because the offender's early deviant sexual fantasies are paired with masturbation. Behavioral clinicians believed that it was the association of this masturbation-linked sexual arousal and fantasy that strengthened deviant sexual preferences. This view emphasized the idea that the offender's behavior was continually reinforced through further conditioning. However, research has shown that deviant arousal cannot be the only explanation (Blader & Marshall, 1989). As indicated earlier, there are men who experience deviant arousal, but do not carry through with their behavior and commit a sexual offense.

Other models attempt to explain sex offending by focusing on the aggressive or coercive aspect of the behavior, listing emotional dyscontrol and poor coping skills as problems related to offending (Marshall & Barbaree, 1990). Some of these models have focused on lack of social competency or the role of learning through aggressive models. Consistent with social cognitive processing theories, the sex offender is seen as a person who lacks social and interpersonal skills, and uses sexual aggression to solve their personal problems (Marshall, Anderson, & Fernandez, 1999; McFall, 1990; Nezu et al., 1998). Other models that may help to explain sex offending focus more on interpersonal vulnerabilities that result from the offender's developmental antecedents (history), such as the offender's own history of abuse or unpredictable and neglectful family backgrounds. These developmental theories suggest that offenders may have poor ability to form interpersonal attachments to other people (Hall, 1996; Prentky, Knight, & Lee, 1997). For example, a given offender may learn to cope with his own history of physical or sexual abuse, through attributions that he is alone in a world where he must fight and control others, before he is hurt or victimized. As such, he may have no desire to change, and this can significantly interfere with treatment progress (Tierny & McCabe, 2002). If this coping style exists, additional factors such as alcohol or drug abuse, which further reduce behavioral control of impulses, can serve to increase one's potential to sexually offend.

At present, there is no clear consensus as to what "causes" sex offending. However, there is a strong consensus that many of these risk factors combine to form a general *vulnerability* to committing a sex offense (Marshall et al., 1999). The term vulnerability refers to the idea that various cognitive and behavioral theories provide us with an understanding of different pathways or factors of vulnerability that lead to offending behavior. Therefore, "vulnerability" can be defined as composed of attitudes, beliefs, cognitive and behavioral skill deficits, behavior patterns, and emotions, all of which are tied to learning. When deficits are present in any one or a combination of these areas, it can lead to an increased offending risk.

Some of the best scientific data concerning vulnerability for offense risk comes from researchers who have investigated the factors that are present if someone is likely to commit a sex offense in the future. These risk prediction studies have reported that some specific vulnerability factors have been statistically linked to the risk of committing a later offense (Hanson & Bussiere, 1998). Possible vulnerability factors that have received scientific support in the research literature regarding sex offenders in general include deviant sexual preferences (Barbaree & Marshall, 1989; Hanson & Bussiere, 1998); a past behavior pattern of sex offending with a range of victims (Prentky et al., 1997); marital status as single or alone (Marques, Day, Nelson, & West, 1994); negative characteristics of an early home environment (Berger, Knutson, Mehm, & Perkins, 1988; Dhawan & Marshall, 1996; Seghorn, Prentky, & Boucher, 1987); social incompetence (Abel, Blanchard, & Becker, 1978; Marshall, Earls, Segal, & Drake, 1983); poor problem-solving (McMurran, Egan, Richardson, & Ahmadi, 1999; Nezu et al., 1998); poor stress or emotional management (Groth, Burgess, & Holstrom, 1977; Marques et al., 1994; Marshall et al., 1983); cognitive distortions such as use of minimization and denial (Abel et al., 1989; Ward, Hudson, & Marshall, 1995); avoidance and impulsivity (Hastings, Anderson, & Hemphill, 1997; Prentky & Knight, 1991); psychopathic characteristics and empathy deficits (Rice, Chaplin, Harris, & Couts, 1994); and lack of motivation to change, or nonadherence to treatment (Garland & Dougher, 1991; Marshall et al., 1999). It is worth noting that some of these risk factors are characteristics that cannot be changed (e.g., past behavior, marital status) whereas others represent changeable characteristics that are amenable to treatment (e.g., cognitive distortions, social problem solving).

VULNERABILITY FOR SEX OFFENSE IN PEOPLE WITH INTELLECTUAL DISABILITIES

Many of the same vulnerability factors have also specifically been reported with regard to offenders with ID. For example, Day (1994) reported that overall the offense pattern of the sex offender with ID is similar to nondisabled sex offenders such that both are characterized by sexual naiveté, poor impulse control, and lack of relationship skills. Schilling and Schinke (1989) described sex offenders with DD as sexually naïve, socially isolated, preferring the company of younger children, possessing histories of delinquent behavior, lacking knowledge about sex, having limited experience in socially desirable sexual conduct, and lacking opportunities to engage in appropriate sexual contact. Hayes (1991) reported that sex offenders with ID typically have confused self-concepts, poor peer relations, a lack of sexual and socio-sexual knowledge, negative early sexual experience, a lack of personal power, and greater social skills deficits. Of the existing theories regarding the etiology of sexual offending behavior in people with ID, the two general categories under which many vulnerabilities can be categorized are *deviance* and *deficits*.

DEVIANCE VULNERABILITY

Theoretically rooted in sexual conditioning behavioral theories, one path to sexual offending is deviant sexual desires (Marshall et al., 1999).

This view has been supported through repeated observation of a relation between phallometrically assessed fantasies and sexually deviant behavior (Prentky & Knight, 1991). However, there have been no published studies regarding the deviant arousal characteristics of sex offenders with ID.

Our own clinical experience suggests that, as is the case with nondisabled offenders, arousal patterns are quite heterogeneous and are functionally related to sex offending behavior. Further research needs to be conducted to evaluate the presence of support for these clinical hypotheses. We are concerned that the present lack of research in the area of deviant fantasies and arousal in this population may lead clinicians to focus away from deviant response patterns despite the fact that, for any given individual, such patterns may be significant and should be identified as a clinical target of treatment.

In addition to deviant fantasies, the literature concerning nondisabled offenders has supported the presence of other characteristic deviant cognitions associated with sex offending risk (Bumby, 1996; Garland & Dougher, 1991). These include a tendency toward self-serving bias, and frequent use of denial, minimization, and rationalization to justify offense. These deviant thought patterns have also been observed in sex offenders with ID (Nezu et al., 1998).

Due to the difficulty in determining whether behavior is sexually deviant or sexually inappropriate, Hingsburger, Griffiths, and Quinsey (1991) have developed the term *counterfeit deviance* to describe behavior that is topographically deviant but found to be causally related to other factors. This view of other factors as the important causal link to deviant sexual behavior is focused on deficit vulnerabilities.

DEFICIT VULNERABILITY

The deficit view of sex offending behavior that is linked to problems of social incompetence, poor interpersonal skills, and poor coping skills has strong support in the literature on nondisabled offenders (Marshal et al., 1999). There may be few differences between populations with regard to the nature of these deficits. For example, Murphy et al. (1983) found that sex offenders with ID have similar deficits in social skills. Demetral (1993) indicated that five factors account for sex offending behavior. These included lack of information about sexual expression, a history of victimization, poor assertiveness and social skills, limited social opportunities, and medication side effects.

MULTIPLE VULNERABILITY FACTORS

Murphy, Coleman, and Abel (1983) proposed a model of sex offending that addresses the need for therapeutic focus on both deviant and deficit vulnerabilities. This model proposes that sex offenders with ID who are likely to re-offend possess (1) an excess of deviant arousal or a deficit in nondeviant arousal and (2) social skills deficits, including hetero-social skills, assertiveness skills, empathy skills, social competence, and sexual knowledge. Hayes (1991) also supports a model that encompasses both types of vulnerability and states the causal influences for inappropriate sexual behaviors are the same for intellectually and nonintellectually disabled populations. These include (1) arousal toward an inappropriate sex object or method of sexual expression; (2) deficits in social skills and assertiveness; (3) lack of appropriate sexual knowledge; and (4) a pattern of cognitive distortion.

Sex offending is not limited to one particular causal factor. In his theory of sex offending, Hall (1996) proposes that the decision to respond in a sexually aggressive manner may be based on a combination of risk characteristics such as cognitive distortions about the potential victim and specific situations in which affective states (e.g., anger and hostility) become so compelling and powerful that they overcome inhibitions that typically prevent the expression of the behavior. Hall describes an additional factor as present in the genesis of offending behavior. Specifically, he views early experiences as having long-term impact and as capable of creating learned patterns that set the stage for later sexual aggression. Factors such as poor socialization experiences, abuse, punishment, and neglect, as well as other developmental learning factors can increase vulnerability to aggressive sexual behavior. The concept of this additional factor may be especially important for people with ID because longstanding developmental deficits in social information processing ability have been associated with aggression in recent studies (Basquil, Nezu, Nezu, & Klein, 2004; Fuchs & Benson, 1995).

Vulnerability factors appear to synergistically interact to lead to sex offending behavior. Each component can affect the intensity of other components and thus, increase the likelihood of sexually aggressive behavior. Because no single vulnerability factor has been associated with directly "causing" sex offending, all vulnerability factors that have been empirically identified need to be assessed for each individual. An individual case approach to assessment and treatment can highlight the particular vulnerability factors that are operating that may increase risk of offense in each case. As a result of such an assessment, a treatment approach focused on changing the various specific vulnerability factors can be designed in a prescriptive, multicomponent treatment package.

ASSESSMENT OF SEX OFFENDING VULNERABILITY FACTORS IN PEOPLE WITH INTELLECTUAL DISABILITIES

Consistent with the practice parameters for assessment of people with intellectual disability and comorbid behavioral disorder, a comprehensive diagnostic assessment should be conducted with intellectually disabled offenders (Bernet & Dulcan, 1999; Nezu et al., 1992).

Assessment data should be summarized consistent with a behavioral case formulation model (see Nezu, Nezu, Peacock, & Girdwood, 2004). Case formulation can be viewed as a set of hypotheses, generally framed by a particular personality theory or psychotherapy orientation, regarding what variables serve as causes, triggers, and maintaining factors (Eells, 1997). It is a description of a patient's behavioral difficulties and symptoms of distress, as well as an organizing mechanism to help the clinician understand how such complaints came into being, how various symptoms coexist, what environmental or intrapersonal stimuli trigger such problems, and why such symptoms persist. Assessment of IQ and adaptive behavior should be a common and integral component of this evaluation. We briefly describe various additional areas of assessment below.

ASSESSMENT OF SEXUAL DEVIANCE

With regard to deviant sexual arousal, several different measures have been described and recommended as applicable for people with DD. The *Abel Assessment for Sexual Interest* (Abel, Huffman, Warberg, & Holland, 1998) is an instrument that includes both a self-report interview and a measure of visual reaction time to stimulus slides. This test requires additional investigation in order to determine its usefulness for people with ID. The *Multiphasic Sex Inventory II* (MSI-II; Nichols & Molinder, 1996) is a self-report measure of sexually deviant cognitive and behavioral characteristics that may be useful for men who admit their deviancy (Lanyon, 2001). The use of card sort measures, which depict pictures of various sexual stimuli as a way to assess individual offender preferences and arousal patterns, has been suggested in the clinical literature (Griffiths, Quinsey, & Hingsburger, 1989). However, data to support the reliability and validity of these assessment procedures is lacking (Lanyon, 2001). Penile plethysmography (PPG) is traditionally the most popular approach for assessing sexual arousal, and has been recommended for people with developmental disabilities (Caparulo, 1991; Griffiths et al., 1989; Haaven & Schlank, 2001; Lanyon, 2001; Nezu et al., 1998; see also Card & Byrne, 1997; Lalumiere & Eerls, 1992).

ASSESSMENT OF COGNITIVE DISTORTIONS

Assessment of cognitive distortions, denial, justification, and minimization of offenses can be conducted through interviews (Lanyon, 2001) or self-report questionnaires (Abel et al., 1989). Additionally, standardized tests, such as the MSI II include several scales aimed at identifying a tendency to lie or patterns of self-serving bias. However, the existing measures have not been specifically tested with people with ID.

ASSESSMENT OF SOCIAL AND SEXUAL SKILLS

With regard to specific measures of social and sexual knowledge, Carparulo (1991) recommends using the *Socio-Sexual Knowledge and*

Attitude Test (SSKAT; Wish, McCombs, & Edmondson, 1980) to assess an individual's knowledge and attitudes about sex. The SSKAT is specifically designed for use with people who may not be verbally proficient. Griffiths et al. (1989) recommend that social skills be assessed through questionnaires, naturalistic observations, simulated role-playing, and videotapes. Other useful measures include those developed by Edwards (1979) and Johnson (1981). Common standardized measures regarding social skills that may be used to assess social adaptive skills include the *Social Behavior Inventory for the Developmentally Disabled* (Tymchuk, 1984). Goldfried and D'Zurilla (1969) developed a behavior analytic method of assessment that employs simulated role-play of relevant skill areas that require assessment. In our own clinic we have developed role play measures, based upon the Goldfried and D'Zurilla methodology.

Offenders with impoverished problem solving abilities may rely more frequently on denial and sexually deviant fantasies as a way of coping with the day-to-day problems (McMurran et al., 1999; Nezu et al., 1998; O'Connor, 1996). As a way to assess the various components of the problem-solving process, Nezu et al. (1998) recommend the *Social Problem-Solving Inventory—Revised* (SPSI-R Technical Manual; D'Zurilla, Nezu, & Maydeu-Olivares, 2002). The SPSI-R is a 52-item, multidimensional, self-report measure of social problem-solving ability with robust psychometric characteristics. In addition to a total score, the instrument provides scores on five subscales derived from factor analysis.

In cases where self-report is unreliable, or cognitive deficits interfere with an offender's ability to provide valid responses to the SPSI-R, a *Problem-Solving Task for Persons with ID—Adapted for Sex Offenders* was developed by two of the authors to evaluate the product of one's problem-solving efforts (PST-Sex Offenders; Nezu, Nezu, Good, & Saad, 1997). This behavioral measure was specifically designed to assess the problem solving abilities of intellectually disabled sex offenders.

Several areas of vulnerability, such as affective instability, and additional coping deficits can be assessed through instruments that have been developed for people with ID and comorbid psychopathology (e.g., the *Psychopathology Inventory for Mentally Retarded Adults*, Matson, 1988, and the *Reiss Screen for Maladaptive Behavior*, Reiss, 1988; see also Reiss, 1993). The *Reiss Profile of Fundamental Goals and Motivation Sensitivities for Persons with Mental Retardation* (Reiss & Havercamp, 2001) is a measure of motivation in people with cognitive disabilities and can aid in facilitating compatible relationships, diagnosing certain disorders, setting therapy goals, and conducting functional analyses.

There may be occasions when it is useful to include assessment measures in one's case formulation that have been helpful to the assessment of various clinical problems, but have not been specifically tested with developmentally disabled populations. When measures that have not been specifically developed for the population are used we recommend caution when interpreting the results. One instrument that has received much support in assessment of nondisabed populations is *The Psychopathy Checklist Revised* (PCL:R; Hare, 1991). This is a semi-structured interview that can assess for the presence of symptoms typically associated with psychopathy.

However, more research is required for its use with disabled populations, in particular because of concerns more generally about unreliable self-report (Nezu et al., 1998).

During the assessment process it is also imperative to establish a collaborative relationship with public safety and correctional services personnel. As part of the preliminary survey, it is important to review the police records and any available files (Griffiths et al., 1989). Many times, offenders will lie or minimize their offense, and it is useful to have the records available to indicate the interviewer's knowledge of the event. For similar reasons, it is also important to have a person identified who knows the person well and can serve as a collateral contact for relevant information. Assessment of the environment is essential. Information gleaned from this assessment will assist in determining the level of supervision required, and may also provide insight into whether treatment will be successfully implemented in the home milieu (Griffiths et al., 1989).

CLINICAL CASE FORMULATION

Once assessment across areas of possible sex offending vulnerability is complete, a behavioral case formulation approach can provide a clinical map with which to guide treatment as well as specific recommendations for determining an individual's level of risk for re-offense and required level of supervised community risk management (Nezu et al., 2004).

Treatment design flows directly from an individual's unique case formulation. Because the literature concerning treatment outcome for sex offenders with ID is sparse, any interventions that have received empirical support in the literature that address identified targets of vulnerability should be considered. Different interventions that address the same goal, as well as ways to adapt interventions for people with DD require further decision-making efforts. We provide a brief summary of the extant research concerning interventions for offenders with DD below.

TREATMENT OF SEX OFFENDING BEHAVIOR IN PEOPLE WITH INTELLECTUAL DISABILITIES

The empirical research concerning treatment outcome for sexual offenders with ID is extremely limited. To date, we are aware of no published controlled and randomized trials of specific treatment protocols for offenders with DD. Most studies consist of case reports, single-participant designs, and clinical program descriptions. A summary of intervention strategies that have been reported as useful for the population with regard to the various areas of vulnerability indicate that cognitive behavior therapy (CBT) programs show promise as potentially effective interventions.

With respect to treatment of deviant arousal, respondent conditioning techniques were among the first therapies reported for sex offenders with ID. Techniques that were used commonly included satiation, covert sensitization, and overt reconditioning techniques (Lund, 1992; O'Connor, 1997; Schilling & Schinke, 1989; Stermac & Sheridan, 1993).

With respect to treatment entailing operant-based strategies, Wong, Gaydos, and Fuqua (1982) reported the use of in vivo community training and contingency management to reduce inappropriate social behavior toward peers. La Vigna and Donnellan (1986) proposed the use of non-aversive procedures that focus on instructional control, manipulation of antecedents, fading, and positive reinforcement to increase adaptive social sexual behavior. Additionally, Sulzer-Azaroff and Mayer (1991) reported that positive reinforcement maintained long-term gains when alternative sexually adaptive behavior was paired with the positive reinforcement.

However, the most impressive clinical treatment programs for sex offenders with ID provide descriptions of multicomponent treatment programs and consist of CBT strategies aimed at most of the previously identified areas of vulnerability. This is not surprising in that a recent meta-analytic investigation of psychotherapy outcome research for people with dual diagnosis supported the effectiveness of CBT for this population (Prout & Nowak-Drabik, 2003). Others suggest that the literature support for CBT lacks the breadth necessary to formulate such conclusions (Cullen, 1996).

Recently, Lindsay reported a successful series of CBT studies of group therapy for aggression and anger in offenders with ID (Lindsay, Marshall, Neilson, Quinn, & Smith, 1998; Lindsay, Neilson, & Morrison, 1998; Lindsay, Olley, Baillie, & Smith, 1999; Lindsay, Olley, Jack, Morrison, & Smith, 1998). Lindsay's investigations consisted of open trials of treatments designed to reduce problems such as child molestation, stalking, and exhibitionism. Additionally, Griffiths et al. (1989) provide a description of a successful CBT program that included covert sensitization to decrease deviant arousal, behavioral techniques such as masturbatory reconditioning to increase arousal to appropriate stimuli, social skills training, and sex education. Finally, Lund (1992) reported positive outcomes for a multicomponent residential treatment program. Individual counseling included anger management, discussion of sexually inappropriate behavior, cognitive restructuring, processing their own abuse (when appropriate), victim empathy, and problem-solving. Social skills training and sex education were provided in a group format. In addition, token economy systems and behavioral contracting were used for maladaptive behaviors. It is important to note that although common and well-studied CBT therapeutic components are implemented in these studies, the procedures are typically simplified in their structure and application with patients.

Problem-solving appears to be an important part of a multicomponent treatment package for sexual offenders with ID (Griffiths et al., 1989; Lund, 1992; Nezu et al., 1998; O'Connor, 1997). Nezu et al. (1998) found that including a problem-solving intervention as a component of more comprehensive treatment played an important part for reducing risk in a clinical case report on CBT for a offender with ID. In another study, problem-solving was empirically supported as a way to reduce inappropriate social behavior and decrease impulsivity in patients with dual diagnosis (Nezu, Nezu, & Arean, 1991) without specific sex offending problems.

Some authors have underscored the importance of the social milieu with regard to treatment planning. For example, O'Connor (1997) described several programs that have advocated for the importance of social support in relapse prevention programs and Demetral (1994) reported that coping strategies learned as part of treatment are more likely to be used effectively by participants if positive social support is in place. Day (1988) further reported four factors indicative of favorable outcomes for sexual offenders with ID: stable residential placement, regular occupation, regular supervision, and support in the community.

RESIDENTIAL TREATMENT FOR SEX OFFENDING BEHAVIOR

Only a few residential treatment programs have been described in the treatment literature for sex offenders with DD. Haaven, Little, and Petre-Miller (1990) developed a residential *Social Skills Program* (SSP) program at Oregon State Hospital to serve as "a unique treatment alternative for adjudicated intellectually disabled offenders with limited adaptive skills who need both intensive treatment and a controlled safe environment" (p. 11). Treatment was described as occurring in three stages: the orientation stage (60–90 days duration), the "in-house" treatment stage (9–36 months duration), and the transition training stage (6–9 months duration). After the transition stage is complete, the participants are supervised while on parole and are mandated to have continued supervision of outpatient treatment for 12–24 months in the community. To our knowledge, no systematic program evaluation or comparative evaluation with other treatments has been reported.

With regard to another residential treatment program, Xenitidis, Henry, Russell, Ward, and Murphy (1999) reported results from the *Mental Impairment Evaluation and Treatment Service* (MIETS), an inpatient unit on the grounds of the Bethlem Royal Hospital. The unit provides multidisciplinary assessment and treatment to people with ID who exhibit challenging behaviors. Sexually challenging behaviors follow aggression as the most common challenging behaviors in this unit. Therapeutic interventions are based according to individual needs and include behavioral, pharmacological, psychological, or social approaches. Although 82.5% of the patients were admitted from noncommunity settings such as hospitals, special hospitals, and prisons, following the MIETS intervention 84.2% of the MIETS patients were placed in community settings. All of those who were originally from community placements were returned to the community.

Over the last few decades as treatment emphasis for people with dual diagnoses has shifted from custodial care to community placement, there has also been a greater emphasis on community treatments for people with ID who have committed a sexual offense. As a result of this shift, more of these people receive treatment for their sexual offending behavior through day-treatment or outpatient clinics while maintaining their residential community placements, than in the past (Lindsay et al., 2002).

Lindsay et al. (2002) propose an optimal service model that combines the benefits of inpatient assessment and treatment with those of outpatient assessment and treatment. This service model proposes a stepped approach, such that each treatment participant receives the appropriate treatment and level of supervision necessary. Cognitive behavioral treatment includes group treatment for sex offending behaviors, psychiatric consultation, treatment for concomitant mental illness, anger and anxiety management, alcohol and sex education, treatment for the offenders own past victimization, and daily and community living skills training. The goal of this service model is community placement and treatment and the majority of offenders are able to receive treatment while maintaining their community placement. Because most offenders will eventually live in the community, treatment focused on their adaptation to this social milieu is important.

AN OUTPATIENT MODEL FOR SEX OFFENDING TREATMENT

During the past 12 years, at our university, we have developed an outpatient assessment and treatment program for sex offenders with ID that provides an integration of the assessment and treatment models described thus far. The program, *Project STOP*, provides assessment and treatment to men with ID who have been convicted or identified as at risk for sex offending behavior. Treatment is based upon a multicomponent, cognitive–behavioral model of treatment, and employs an individualized case formulation approach to treatment.

We recently evaluated the outcome of treatment provided through *Project STOP* for men who were referred for treatment over the past 3 years. Our evaluation included a pre- and posttreatment assessment of patient behavior change (e.g., the amount of specific progress in treatment goals and changes in clinical target behaviors), as well as clinician ratings of treatment motivation, participation and attendance, and current level of offense risk. Our data also included the patient rate of reoffense. Although all treatment was based on a cognitive–behavioral model, we wanted to know whether or not a patients' diagnosis or mode of treatment (individual, group, family, or combined) affected their treatment progress toward clinical goals.

DESCRIPTION OF THE CLINICAL POPULATION

The records of 25 patients who were actively engaged in treatment indicated that the problem behaviors for which the men were referred included stalking, incest, child molestation, child rape, adult rape, other sexual assault, exhibitionism, and sexual threat. Diagnoses, consistent with *DSM-IV* (*Diagnostic and Statistical Manual*; American Psychiatric Association [APA], 1994), were varied. Axis I diagnoses included paraphilia, dysthymia, voyeurism, generalized anxiety disorder, schizophrenia, oppositional disorder, and pedophilia. In addition to the presence of DD, Axis II diagnoses included nonspecific personality disorder, dependent personality disorder, passive personality disorder, narcissistic personality disorder, and antisocial personality disorder.

DESCRIPTION OF CLINICAL SERVICES

The type of treatment provided to patients included individual, group, and family therapy at our clinic. Additionally, the treatment was based upon a broadly defined, cognitive–behavioral approach. For each patient, the treatment was individually planned and based upon the patient's assessment and behavioral case formulation. Our assessment methods included clinical interview, traditional psychological testing, adaptive behavior assessment, self-report and informant-report questionnaires, role-play measures designed to assess different areas of psychological, emotional, and behavioral areas of vulnerability, forensic assessment of psychopathic characteristics, functional analysis of behavior, and measures of deviant sexual arousal (e.g., PPG, Abel Assessment).

The primary treatment approaches prescribed at *Project STOP* included applied behavior analysis, behavioral accelerating and decelerating procedures, behavioral staff and family consultation, behavior therapy techniques such as relaxation, and masturbatory conditioning, and many cognitive–behavior therapy (CBT) techniques. CBT techniques included problem-solving therapy, anger management, stress management, cognitive restructuring, interpersonal skills training, social and sexual education, and functional family therapy, that is, with a strong emphasis on skills development and improved self-control. For example, depending upon the patient's individual case formulation, he may learn relaxation techniques to decrease anger arousal or use of self-instruction strategies to increase self-control, and his family may learn how to reinforce these skills at home. Moreover, family members may learn how they inadvertently excuse or minimize the patient's sexually aggressive behavior, and the importance of changing their own expectations toward patient improvement.

Group treatment was aimed at providing specific adaptive, rehabilitative, and coping skills in the context of peer participation, feedback, and support. These groups included (a) a group designed to increase basic social skills; (b) a clinical "mapping group" that helped patients to identify and change patterns or "maps" of their offense behaviors; and (c) a problem-solving coping skills group that provided patients with training to increase adaptive skills and better manage problems they face in everyday life, as well as self-control of aggressive or sexually inappropriate urges.

Our prescriptive and individualized treatment planning is based upon a scientific and problem-solving approach to decision-making (Nezu et al., 2004). Treatment decisions for specific clinical targets are consistent with expert consensus guidelines (Rush & Frances, 2000).

PROGRAM EFFECTIVENESS

Regarding the overall effectiveness of the program, we found significant improvement across a number of areas. With regard to the pre- and postscores of treated patients, their adaptive behavior increased, as well as ratings of motivation and levels of participation in treatment. Although significant change in identified clinical target behaviors showed strong trends of improvement for most of the patients, these changes were not statistically significant for the group as a whole, and are consistent with our findings that the course of treatment for offenders with ID or DD is typically far more extended, involving many more therapeutic episodes, than is typical for offenders who are nondisabled (Nezu et al., 1998).

RE-OFFENSE RATE

Recidivism rates over the past 3 years for Project STOP remain low. One patient committed another sexual offense, indicating a recidivism rate of approximately 4%. This is consistent with the rates associated with the treatment program over the past 12 years. Three other patients were reincarcerated for short periods of time due to violating probation, and upon their release, returned to treatment.

Possible reasons for low recidivism may include (1) an individualized, case formulation approach to treatment that focuses clinical targets based upon each sex offender's personal vulnerability factors; (2) a multiple treatment approach that incorporates individual, group, and family CBT strategies matched to these vulnerability factors; (3) the operation of a contingency management system in the clinic that resulted in a high adherence rates; and (4) extension of treatment to beyond 2 years. We found that patients in combined treatments seem to have the most improvement. For example, patients in combined treatments such as individual and family, or group and individual, therapy had the most improvement in many areas, although no specific combination was associated with the best outcome.

Finally, for about 35% of our patients, their level of offense risk increased in the first few months of treatment, before it started to reduce. This was not surprising, because when many offenders first enter treatment, they are resistant to facing their problem behaviors. Treatment progress occurred slowly and where changes in the clinical target behavior significantly improved, the change occurred over 2 or more years.

SUMMARY

There is a dearth of research findings to guide the clinician who is faced with assessment and, especially, treatment of sex offending behavior in people with ID. However, the studies and program reports that do exist suggest that one promising framework through which to guide treatment is through a multicomponent, CBT approach that is based upon individual case formulation. Whether the initial treatment is delivered in a residential or ambulatory environment, generalization of new skills to the community environment appears to be an inevitable and necessary part of treatment. Additionally, contingency management systems that are designed to increase the likelihood of continued attendance of outpatient therapy sessions may further boost treatment outcomes. This treatment approach appears to be an effective strategy in reducing reoffense rates and improving behavioral skills for sex offenders who are living in the community. For example, within *Project STOP*, attendance was extremely high, changes in adaptive and target behaviors occurred, and repeat offending behavior (recidivism) was very low.

Future areas of research require continued exploration of how various vulnerability factors interact to increase risk of sex offending behavior. Finally, well-controlled studies are needed that investigate whether or not changes in specific vulnerability factors (e.g., emotion regulation, social and sexual education, anger management, social problem solving) actually result in lowered sex offending risk, as well as the nature of simplifications of conventional CBT procedures that are associated with greater reduction of risk. Program effectiveness studies should make every attempt to capture the mechanisms of action responsible for change, including the specific nature of the CBT procedures and complementary interventions that are implemented. Careful attention should be given to insuring the integrity of the treatment provided in such investigations.

REFERENCES

Abel, G. G., Blanchard, E. B., & Becker, J. V. (1978). An integrated treatment program for rapists. In R. T. Rada (Ed.), *Clinical aspects of the rapist* (pp. 161–214). New York: Grune & Stratton.

Abel, G. G., Gore, D. K., Holland, C., Camp, N., Becker, J., & Rathner, J. (1989). The measurement of cognitive distortions of child molesters. *Annals of Sex Research, 2,* 135–152.

Abel, G. G., Huffman, J., Warberg, B., & Holland, C. L. (1998). Visual reaction time and plethysmography as measures of sexual interest in child molesters. *Sexual Abuse: A Journal of Research and Treatment, 10,* 81–95.

American Psychiatric Association. (1994). *Diagnostic and statistical manual of mental disorders* (4th ed.). Washington, DC: Author.

Barbaree, H. E., & Marshall, W. L. (1989). Erectile responses among heterosexual child molesters, father–daughter incest offenders, and matched offenders: Five distinct age preference profiles. *Canadian Journal of Behavioral Science, 21,* 70–82.

Barron, P., Hassiotis, A., & Banes, J. (2002). Offenders with intellectual disability: The size of the problem and therapeutic outcomes. *Journal of Intellectual Disability Research, 46,* 454–463.

Basquil, M., Nezu, C. M., Nezu, A. M., & Klein, T. L. (2004). Aggression-related hostility bias and social problem-solving deficits in adult males with mental retardation. *American Journal on Mental Retardation, 109,* 255–263.

Berger, A. M., Knutson, J. F., Mehm, J. G., & Perkins, K. A. (1988). The self-report of punitive childhood experiences of young adults and adolescents. *Child Abuse and Neglect, 12,* 251–262.

Bernet, W., & Dulcan, M. K. (1999). Practice parameters for the assessment and treatment of children, adolescents, and adults with mental retardation and comorbid mental disorders. *Child and Adolescent Psychiatry, 38*(Suppl.), 5S–31S.

Blader, J. C., & Marshall, W. L. (1989). Is assessment of sexual arousal in rapists worthwhile? A critique of current methods and a response-compatible approach. *Clinical Psychology Review, 9*, 569–587.

Bumby, K. M. (1996). Assessing the cognitive distortions of child molesters and rapists: Development and validation of MOLEST and RAP scales. *Sexual Abuse: A Journal of Research and Treatment, 8*, 37–54.

Caparulo, F. (1991). Identifying the developmentally disabled sex offenders. *Sexuality and Disability, 9*, 311–322.

Card, R. D., & Byrne, P. M. (1997). *The sensitivity and specificity of a newly developed set of DDMR phallometric stimulus materials.* Presented at the meeting of the Association for the Treatment of Sexual Abusers, Arlington, VA.

Chivers, J., & Mathieson, S. (2000). Training in sexuality and relationships: An Australian model. *Sexuality and Disability, 18*(1), 73–80.

Cullen, C. (1996). Challenging behaviour and intellectual disability: Assessment, analysis and treatment. *British Journal of Clinical Psychology, 35*, 153–156.

Day, K. (1988). A hospital-based treatment programme for male mentally handicapped offenders. *British Journal of Psychiatry, 153*, 635–644.

Day, K. (1994). Male mentally handicapped sex offenders. *British Journal of Psychiatry, 165*, 630–639.

Demetral, G. D. (1993). Assessing counterfeit deviance in persons with developmental disabilities: An ecological assessment inventory. *The Habilitative Mental Healthcare Newsletter, 12*, 1–7.

Demetral, G. D. (1994). Diagrammatic assessment of ecological integration of sex offenders with mental retardation in community residential facilities. *Mental Retardation, 32*, 141–145.

Dhawan, S., & Marshall, W. L. (1996). Sexual abuse histories of sexual offenders. *Sexual Abuse: A Journal of Research and Treatment, 8*, 7–15.

D'Zurilla, T. J., Nezu, A. M., & Maydeu-Olivares, A. (2002). *The Social Problem Solving Inventory revised (SPSI-R): Manual.* North Tonawanda, NY: MHS.

Edwards, J. P. (1979). *Edwards assessment of social–sexual skills.* Portland, OR: Ednick Communications.

Eells, T. D. (1997). Psychotherapy case formulation: History and current status. In T. D. Eells (Ed.), *Handbook of psychotherapy case formulation* (pp. 1–25). New York: Guilford Press.

Fuchs, C., & Benson, B. A. (1995). Social information processing by aggressive and nonaggressive men with mental retardation. *American Journal on Mental Retardation, 3*, 244–252.

Garland, R. J., & Dougher, M. J. (1991). Motivational interventions in the treatment of sex offenders. In W. R. Miller & M. S. Rollnick (Eds.), *Motivational interviewing: Preparing people to change addictive behavior* (pp. 303–313). New York: Guilford Press.

Goldfried, M. R., & D'Zurilla, T. J. (1969). A behavior-analytic model for assessing competence. In C. D. Spielberger (Ed.), *Current topics in clinical and community psychology* (Vol. 1, pp. 151–196). New York: Academic Press.

Griffiths, D. M, Quinsey, V. L., & Hingsburger, D. (1989). *Changing inappropriate sexual behavior: A community-based approach for persons with developmental disabilities.* Baltimore: Brookes.

Groth, A. N., Burgess, A. W., & Holstrom, L. L. (1977). Rape: Power, anger, and sexuality. *American Journal of Psychiatry, 134*, 1239–1243.

Haaven, J., Little, R., & Petre,-Miller, D. (1990). *Treating intellectually disabled sex offenders: A model residential program.* Orwell, VT: Safer Society Press.

Haaven, J., & Schlank, A. (2001). The challenge of treating the sex offender with developmental disabilities. In A. Schlank (Ed.), *The sexual predator: Vol.2. Legal issues, clinical issues, and special populations* (pp. 13.1–13.19). Kingston, NJ: Civic Research Institute.

Hall, G. C. N. (1996). *Theory-based assessment, treatment, and prevention of sexual aggression.* New York: Oxford University Press.

Hanson, R. K., & Bussiere, M. T. (1998). Predicting relapse: A meta-analysis of sexual offender recidivism studies. *Journal of Consulting and Clinical Psychology, 66,* 348–362.

Hare, R. D. (1991). *The Revised Psychopathy Checklist.* Toronto, Ont.: Multi-Health Systems.

Hastings, T., Anderson, S. J., & Hemphill, P. (1997). Comparisons of daily stress, coping, problem behavior, and cognitive distortions in adolescent sexual offenders and conduct-disordered youth. *Sexual Abuse: A Journal of Research and Treatment, 9,* 29–42.

Hayes, S. (1991). Sex offenders. *Australian and New Zealand Journal of Developmental Disabilities, 17,* 221–227.

Hingsburger, D., Griffiths, D., & Quinsey, V. (1991). Detecting counterfeit deviance: Differentiating sexual deviance from sexual inappropriateness. *Habilitative Mental Health Newsletter, 10,* 51–54.

Johnson, P. R. (1981). *Sexuality Development Index (videotape package).* Calgary: University of Alberta.

Jurkowski, E., & Amado, A. N. (1993). Affection, love, intimacy, and sexual relationships. In A. N. Amado (Ed.), *Friendships and community connections between people with and without developmental disabilities* (pp. 129–152). Baltimore: Brookes.

Kempton, W., & Kahn, E. (1991). Sexuality and people with intellectual disabilities: A historical perspective. *Sexuality and Disability, 9*(2), 93–112.

Lalumiere, M. L., & Eerls, C. M. (1992). Voluntary control of penile response as a function of stimulus duration and instructions. *Behavioral Assessment, 14,* 121–132.

Lanyon, R. I. (2001). Psychological assessment procedures in sex offending. *Professional Psychology: Research and Practice, 32,* 253–260.

La Vigna, G. W., & Donnellan, A. (1986). *Alternatives to punishment: Solving behavior problems with non-aversive strategies.* New York: Irvington.

Lindsay, W. R. (2002). Integration of recent reviews on offenders with intellectual disabilities. *Journal of Applied Research in Intellectual Disabilities, 15,* 111–119.

Lindsay, W. R., Marshall, I., Neilson, C., Quinn, K., & Smith, A. H. (1998). The treatment of men with a learning disability convicted of exhibitionism. *Research on Developmental Disabilities, 19,* 295–316.

Lindsay, W. R., Neilson, C. Q., & Morrison, F. (1998). The treatment of six men with learning disability convicted of sex offenses with children. *British Journal of Clinical Psychology, 37,* 83–98.

Lindsay, W. R., Olley, S., Baillie, N., & Smith, H. (1999). Treatment of adolescent sex offenders with intellectual disabilities. *Mental Retardation, 37,* 201–211.

Lindsay, W. R., Olley, S., Jack, C., Morrison, F., & Smith, A. H. (1998). The treatment of two stalkers with intellectual disabilities using a cognitive approach. *Journal of Applied Research in Intellectual Disabilities, 11,* 333–334.

Lindsay, W. R., Smith, H. W., Law, J., Quinn, K., Anderson, A., Smith, A., et al. (2002). A treatment service for sex offenders and abuser with intellectual disability: Characteristics of referrals and evaluation. *Journal of Applied Research in Intellectual Disabilities, 15,* 166–174.

Lumley, V. A., & Scotti, J. R. (2001). Supporting the sexuality of adults with mental retardation: Current status and future directions. *Journal of Positive Behavior Interventions, 3,* 109–119.

Lund, C. A. (1992). Long term treatment of sexual behavior problems in adolescent and adult developmentally disabled persons. *Annals of Sex Research, 5,* 5–31.

Maguire, R. J., Carlisle, J. M., & Young, B. G. (1965). Sexual deviations as conditioned behaviour: A hypothesis. *Behaviour Research and Therapy, 2,* 185–190.

Marques, J. D., Day, D. M., Nelson, C., & West, M. A. (1994). Effects of cognitive–behavioral treatment on sex offender recidivism: Preliminary results of a longitudinal study. *Criminal Justice and Behavior, 21,* 28–54.

Marshall, W. L., Anderson, D., & Fernandez, Y. (1999). *Cognitive behavioural treatment of sexual offenders.* West Sussex, UK: Wiley.

Marshall, W. L., & Barbaree, H. E. (1990). An integrated theory of the etiology of sexual offending. In W. L. Marshall, D. R. Laws, & H. E. Barbaree (Eds.), *Handbook of sexual assault: Issues, theories, and treatment of the offender* (pp. 209–229). New York: Plenum.

Marshall, W. L., Earls, C. M., Segal, Z. V., & Drake, J. (1983). A behavioral program for the assessment and treatment of sexual aggressors. In K. Craig & R. McMahon (Eds.), *Advances in clinical behavior therapy* (pp.148–174). New York: Brunner/Mazel.

Matson, J. L. (1988). *The PIMRA manual*. Orland Park, IL: International Diagnostic Systems.

McCurry, C., McClellan, J., Adams, J., Norrei, M., Storck, M., Eisner, A., & Breiger, D. (1998). Sexual behavior associated with low verbal IQ in youth who have severe mental illness. *Mental Retardation, 36*, 23–30.

McFall, R. M. (1990). The enhancement of social skills: An information-processing analysis. In W. L. Marshall, D. R. Laws, & H. E. Barbaree (Eds.), *Handbook of sexual assault: Issues, theories, and treatment of the offender* (pp. 311–327). New York: Plenum.

McMurran, M., Egan, V., Richardson, C., & Ahmadi, S. (1999). Social problem-solving in mentally disordered offenders: A brief report. *Criminal Behaviour and Mental Health, 9*, 315–322.

Murphy, W., Coleman, E., & Abel, G. (1983). Human sexuality in the mentally retarded. In J. L. Matson & F. Andrasik (Eds.), *Treatment issues and innovations in mental retardation* (pp. 581–643). New York: Plenum.

Murphy, W. D., Coleman, E. M., & Haynes, M. A. (1983). Treatment evaluation issues with the mentally retarded sex offender. In J. G. Greer & I. R. Stuart (Eds.), *The sexual aggressor: Current perspectives on treatment* (pp. 22–41). New York: Van Nostrand Reinhold.

Nezu, A. M., Nezu, C. M., Peacock, M. A., & Girdwood, C. P. (2004). Models of behavioral case formulation. In S. N. Haynes & E. Heiby (Eds.) & M. Hersen (Editor-in-Chief), *Behavioral assessment: Vol. 3. Comprehensive handbook of psychological assessment* (pp. 402–426). New York: Wiley.

Nezu, C. M., Nezu, A. M., & Arean, P. (1991). Assertiveness and problem-solving therapy for persons with mental retardation and dual diagnosis. *Research in Developmental Disabilities, 12*, 371–386.

Nezu, C. M., Nezu, A. M., & Dudek, J. A. (1998). A cognitive–behavioral model of assessment and treatment for intellectually disabled sexual offenders. *Cognitive and Behavioral Practice, 5*, 25–64.

Nezu, C. M., Nezu, A. M., & Gill-Weiss, M. J. (1992). *Psychopathology in persons with mental retardation: Clinical guidelines to assessment and treatment*. Champaign, IL: Research Press.

Nezu, C. M., Nezu, A. M., Good, W., & Saad, R. (1997). *Social problem solving task for persons with intellectual disabilities—Adapted for Sexual Offenders (PST-Sex Offenders; unpublished test and manual)*. Philadelphia, PA: Allegheny University of the Health Sciences.

Nichols, H. R., & Molinder, I. (1996). *Multiphasic Sex Inventory II*. Tacoma, WA: Nichols and Molinder Assessments.

O'Connor, W. (1996). A problem-solving intervention for sex offenders with an intellectual disability. *Journal of Intellectual and Developmental Disability, 21*, 219–236.

O'Connor, W. (1997). Towards an environmental perspective on intervention for problem sexual behaviour in people with an intellectual disability. *Journal of Applied Research in Intellectual Disabilities, 10*, 159–175.

Pitceathly, A. S., & Chapman, J. W. (1985). Sexuality, marriage and parenthood of mentally retarded people. *International Journal for the Advancement of Counseling, 8*, 173–181.

Prentky, R. A., & Knight, R. A. (1991). Identifying critical dimensions for discriminating among rapists. *Journal of Consulting and Clinical Psychology, 59*, 643–661.

Prentky, R. A., Knight, R. A., & Lee, A. F. S. (1997). Risk factors associated with recidivism among extrafamilial child molesters. *Journal of Consulting and Clinical Psychology, 65*, 141–149.

Prout, H. T., & Nowak-Drabick, K. M. (2003). Psychotherapy with persons who have mental retardation: An evaluation of effectiveness. *American Journal of Mental Retardation, 108*, 82–93.

Reiss, S. (1988). *The Reiss Screen for Maladaptive Behavior test manual*. Orland Park, IL: International Diagnostic Systems.

Reiss, S. (1993). Assessment of psychopathology in persons with mental retardation. In J. L. Matson & R. P. Barrett (Eds.), *Psychopathology in the mentally retarded* (2nd ed., pp. 17–40). Orlando, FL: Grune & Stratton.

Reiss, S., & Havercamp, S. (2001). *The Reiss profile of fundamental goals and motivation sensitivities for persons with mental retardation.* Worthington, OH: IDS.

Rice, M. E., Chaplin, T. C., Harris, G. T., & Couts, J. (1994). Empathy for the victim and sexual arousal among rapists and nonrapists. *Journal of Interpersonal Violence, 9,* 435–449.

Rush, A. J., & Frances, A. (2000). Expert consensus guideline series: Treatment of psychiatric and behavioral problems in mental retardation. *American Journal on Mental Retardation, 105,* 159–228.

Schilling, R. F., & Schinke S. P. (1989). Mentally retarded sex offenders: Fact, fiction, and treatment. *Journal of Social Work and Human Sexuality, 7*(2), 33–48.

Schoen, J., & Hoover, J. H. (1990). Mentally retarded sex offenders. *Journal of Offender Rehabilitation, 16,* 81–90.

Seghorn, T. K., Prentky, R. A., & Boucher, R. J. (1987). Childhood sexual abuse in the lives of sexually aggressive offenders. *Journal of the American Academy of Child and Adolescent Psychiatry, 26,* 262–267.

Stermac, L., & Sheridan, P. (1993). The developmentally disabled adolescent sex offender. In W. L. Marshall & H. E. Barbaree (Eds.), *The juvenile sex offender* (pp. 235–242). New York: Guildford Press.

Sulzer-Azaroff, B., & Mayer, G. R. (1991). *Behaviour analysis for lasting change.* Fort Worth, TX: Holt, Rinehart & Winston.

Szollos, A. A., & McCabe, M. P. (1995). The sexuality of people with mild intellectual disability: Perceptions of clients and caregivers. *Australia and New Zealand Journal of Developmental Disabilities, 20,* 205–222.

Tierny, D. W., & McCabe, M. P. (2002). Motivation for behavior change among sex offenders: A review of the literature. *Clinical Psychology Review, 22,* 113–129.

Timms, S., & Goreczny, A. (2002). Adolescent sex offenders with mental retardation: Literature review and assessment considerations. *Aggression and Violent Behavior, 7,* 1–19.

Tymchuk, A. (1984). *Social Behavior Inventory.* Portland, OR: Ednick Communications.

Van Dyke, D. C., McBrien, D. M., & Mattheis, P. J. (1996). Psychosexual behaviour, sexuality and management issues in individuals with Down's syndrome. In J. Rondal, J. Perera, L. Nadel, & A. Comblain (Eds.), *Down's syndrome. Psychological, psychobiological, and socio-educational perspectives* (pp. 191–206). San Diego, CA: Singular.

Ward, T., Hudson, S. M., & Marshall, W. L. (1995). Cognitive distortions and affective deficits in sexual offenders: A cognitive deconstructionist interpretation. *Sexual Abuse: Journal of Research and Treatment, 7,* 67–83.

Williams, S. (1991). Sex education. *Australia and New Zealand Journal of Developmental Disabilities, 17,* 217–219.

Wish, J. R., McCombs, K. F., & Edmonson, B. (1980). *The Socio-Sexual Knowledge and Attitude Test: Instruction manual.* Wood Dale, IL: Stoelting.

Wong, S. E., Gaydos, G. R., & Fuqua, R. W. (1982). Operant control of pedophilia: Reducing approaches to children. *Behavior Modification, 6,* 73–84.

Woodill, G. (1992). Controlling the sexuality of developmentally disabled persons: Historical perspectives. *Journal on Developmental Disabilities, 1*(1), 1–14.

Xenitidis, K. I., Henry, J., Russell, A. J., Ward, A., & Murphy, D. G. M. (1999). An inpatient treatment model for adults with mild intellectual disability and challenging behaviour. *Journal of Intellectual Disability Research, 43,* 128–134.

Zuker-Weiss, R. (1994). Sex, mental retardation and ethics. *International Journal of Adolescent Medicine and Health, 7,* 193–197.

33

Pharmacotherapy

MICHAEL G. AMAN and YASER RAMADAN

Ever since the discovery of antipsychotic drugs in the 1950s, pharmacotherapy has been common in people with mental retardation. Surveys differ greatly in reported prevalences, but most of the recent drug surveys within institutions have reported psychotropic drug rates between 30 and 40% (Rinck, 1998). Studies of adults living in community settings often report rates between 25 and 35% (Rinck, 1998). Prevalence of psychotropic medicines among individuals with autism (across the life span) is currently around 45% (Aman, Lam, & Collier-Crespin, 2003; Langworthy-Lam, Aman, & Van Bourgondien, 2002). It is clear that drug therapy is common among people with mental retardation and developmental disabilities, and hence workers interested in this field cannot afford to be uninformed about pharmacotherapy.

In the interests of brevity, we shall be summarizing the evidence from an authoritative text (Reiss & Aman, 1998; The International Consensus Handbook) and from the recent Expert Consensus guideline Series: Treatment of psychiatric and behavioral problems in mental retardation (Rush & Frances, 2000). The latter was derived from a scientific survey of approximately 100 prominent researchers and clinicians in the field. Other evidence presented here comes directly from the scientific literature.

Historically, the use of medicines in this field has been driven by two considerations. Some patients have been treated because of behavioral excesses, such as prominent aggression. Others have been treated because they present with a Diagnostic and Statistical Manual of Mental Disorders (DSM) (American Psychiatric Association, 2000) or International Classification of Diseases (ICD) (World Health Organization, 1992) psychiatric diagnosis, such as manic disorder. Most clinicians accept the use of pharmacotherapy for treating clear-cut psychiatric disorders, especially more severe ones like schizophrenia, major depressive disorder, and manic

---

MICHAEL G. AMAN and YASER RAMADAN • The Nisonger Center, The Ohio State University, Columbus, Ohio 43210.

disorder. However, many workers (especially those espousing the use of behavior therapy) may oppose the use of medicine to manage non-DSM behavioral excesses. Nevertheless, the medication experts responding to the Expert Consensus questionnaire did endorse the use of medication for managing certain behavioral excesses, such as self-injurious behavior, interpersonal aggression, and hyperactivity.

Our personal position is that pharmacotherapy is justified for managing certain behavioral excesses, provided that hard data show clear benefit from use of medicine and that a proper cost-benefit analysis is conducted before and during treatment. These are the same standards that should be applied for the use of *any* therapy. It is a fact that it can be exceptionally difficult (if not impossible) to establish many diagnoses (e.g., schizophrenia, major depressive disorder) in people with severe or profound retardation. Nevertheless, these individuals should not be denied access to potentially therapeutic agents just because we have not learned to identify possible underlying conditions. It is also possible that there is no underlying DSM condition but that, for reasons that are not understood, the behavior problem is responsive to drug treatment. In keeping with this view, we shall discuss the use of psychotropic medicines in well-established DSM and ICD conditions. Following this, we shall discuss use of pharmacotherapy of other conditions—not otherwise specified (NOS) (i.e., behavioral excesses).

DSM OR ICD MENTAL DISORDERS

Diagnosing psychiatric disorders in individuals with intellectual disability is a challenging task for clinicians and requires a developmental approach. This is ordinarily based on the patient's intellectual or developmental age, rather than chronological age. The greatest obstacle in diagnosing psychiatric disorders in people with severe or profound intellectual disability is a diminished ability to communicate adequately with the individual; therefore collateral information from the primary caregiver, school, and counselor is usually very helpful for evaluation and assessment.

The most frequently made diagnoses following a psychiatric consultation of individuals with intellectual disability are (a) impulse control disorder, (b) anxiety disorder, and (c) mood disorders. Others include (d) schizophrenia, (e) ADHD, and (f) conduct disorder or oppositional defiant disorder. For this reason, we structure our review of the available research around these conditions. To assist readers with the discussions that follow, we have summarized the most common psychotropic drugs in the Appendix that follows this chapter. We also offer a brief note about recent pharmaceutical developments. In the 1990s, the selective serotonin reuptake inhibitors (SSRIs) and the atypical antipsychotics were ushered in. In general, the SSRIs are safer than the older heterocyclic antidepressants (e.g., amitriptyline, doxepin, nortriptyline, etc.), which can cause ECG changes, drowsiness, and (uncommonly) epileptic seizures. The newer atypical antipsychotics are generally safer than the classical antipsychotics and are less likely to cause extrapyramidal side effects (dystonias, Parkinsonism, akathisia) or tardive dyskinesia (a neurological movement condition that

may follow long-term exposure to antipsychotics). However, some atypical antipsychotics may be more likely to cause weight gain than classical
antipsychotics. Both the SSRIs and the atypical antipsychotics appear to
have certain therapeutic advantages as well over their predecessors.

Mood Disorders

Mood in individuals with intellectual disability (mental retardation)
may be normal, elevated, or depressed; usually a sense of control is lost,
and the client may experience great distress. The coexistence of mood
disorders and mental retardation was not fully recognized until the early
1970s. Today, a consensus has been reached that individuals with intellectual disability are vulnerable to mood disorders, with an overall prevalence
rate as high as in the general population (Reiss, 1994, p. 82).

Poindexter et al. (1998) conducted a helpful review of the available
evidence on mood stabilizers in people with mental retardation. Lithium
(Lithane, Lithobid) has been assessed in a few small-scale studies, some
involving participants with manic depression and some with aggression
but without manic disorder. Modest benefits were seen in both manic and
in aggressive behavior. In general, these were poorly controlled studies;
some were based on retrospective chart reviews. There have been relatively few studies of other agents for managing manic symptoms in people
with mental retardation. One poorly controlled study did show a favorable response to valproic acid (Depakene) in 18 adults, especially among
those with a history of epilepsy (see Poindexter et al., 1998). Only case reports are available for clonazepine (Klonopin) and, on balance, these were
somewhat positive. One study comparing lithium only with lithium-plus-
carbamazepine (Tegretol) reported better outcomes with the latter.

The Expert Consensus guideline recommendations for treating mood
disorders in individuals with mental retardation are the same as for in the
general population. For treating bipolar disorder, depressive episode without psychotic features, the Expert Consensus guidelines recommended
treatment with lithium or valproic acid plus one of the following antidepressants (SSRI, bupropion [Wellbutrin], or venlafaxine [Effexor]). For bipolar disorder with psychotic features, the Expert Guidelines recommended
lithium or divalproex plus an antidepressant (SSRI, bupropion, or venlafaxine), plus a newer atypical antipsychotic.

Sovner et al. (1998) conducted a very good review of the research on
antidepressant medicines in people with mental retardation. They summarized nine reports of adults with either major depression or atypical
depression who were treated with a monoamine oxidase inhibitor ($n = 27$),
tricyclic antidepressant ($n = 7$), amoxapine (Asendin) ($n = 2$), or SSRI ($n =$
10; total $N = 46$). Two or three of these studies were properly controlled.
All but one indicated improvement, but the sole negative report was
one of the controlled investigations. Another of the controlled investigations was a single-subject study. Hence, most of the positive reports
for adults were case reports or case series. Sovner et al. (1998) also
summarized three reports involving children with mental retardation.
These addressed the effectiveness of tricyclic antidepressants ($n = 14$),

tryptophan-plus-nicotinamide ($n = 2$), or fluoxetine (Prozac) ($n = 4$; total $N = 20$). All three reports indicated some improvement. We could not determine if two of the studies (written in Dutch) were controlled; the third was not. Thus the empirical support for efficacy of all of the antidepressants in patients with mental retardation is weak, although the uncontrolled literature is largely positive. The problem with this is that workers may not be inclined to report their failures, so that there is often a bias in the type of reports that are published. For major depressive disorders, the Expert Consensus guidelines recommended starting treatment with an SSRI, but also to consider using venlafaxine.

Recently it has been reported that SSRIs are often (although certainly not always) helpful in the treatment of ritualistic, stereotyped, or compulsive behaviors in individuals with mental retardation (Aman, Arnold, & Armstrong, 1999; Branford, Bhaumik, & Naik, 1998 ; see in section "self-injury"). However several researchers working with children have had limited success managing ritualistic and other perseverative behaviors with SSRIs (L. E. Arnold, March 2003; C. McDougle, March 2003; L. Scahill, March 2003; all personal communications). It is possible that SSRIs are helpful for managing perseverative behavior in adults but that, for reasons yet to be determined, their role in children is more limited.

Schizophrenia

There is very little research on the use of antipsychotic drugs to manage schizophrenia in people with mental retardation. The reason is fairly obvious, namely the significant difficulty compiling samples (with both mental retardation and schizophrenia) large enough for meaningful statistical analyses.

Menolascino, Ruedrich, Golden, and Wilson (1985) carried out a comparison of thioridazine (Mellaril) and thiothixene (Navane) in 31 patients with mental retardation and schizophrenia and 30 with normal range IQ and schizophrenia. There was no placebo control. Both the subjects with mental retardation and those with normal range IQ (≥ 90) showed significant improvement with medication. However, no data were actually presented to show improvement. Those with mental retardation responded significantly more quickly to thiothixene, whereas those with normal range IQ responded faster (but not significantly so) with thioridazine. The clients with mental retardation required lower doses than the normal range IQ sample, although it was not clear if this difference was significant.

Craft and Schiff (1980) also reported an uncontrolled study of fluphenazine decanoate (Prolixin) in residents having both psychotic and nonpsychotic conditions; global improvements were reported. Sajatovic, Ramirez, Kenny, and Meltzer (1994) reported an open study of five adults with borderline IQ who met research diagnostic criteria for schizophrenia. Clozapine (Clozaril) in doses of 225–400 mg/day produced statistically significant improvement on several clinical rating scales.

Of course, the usefulness of antipsychotics for managing schizophrenia is well established in the general population, with about 75–80% of such patients showing a positive response (Baumeister, Sevin, & King,

1998). In the Expert Consensus survey, the experts most frequently chose (a) newer atypical antipsychotics (e.g., risperidone [Risperdal], olanzapine [Zyprexa]); (b) clozapine (in the case of numerous failed trials with other antipsychotics); and (c) long-acting depot antipsychotics (for patients who are noncompliant with oral medication—Rush & Frances, 2000). At this stage, it is safe to say that management of schizophrenia in individuals with mental retardation needs to be guided by researchers' and clinicians' experience in the general population.

Other Psychotic Disorders

There are other psychotic syndromes that do not meet the diagnostic criteria for schizophrenia, the major ones being schizophreniform disorder, schizoaffective disorder, delusional disorder, and brief psychotic disorder. To the best of our knowledge, none of these disorders has been the subject of proper controlled drug studies (Reiss & Aman, 1998).

The treatment for this group of psychotic disorders usually entails a comprehensive treatment plan, which involves bio-psycho-social aspects of the disorder. The use of antipsychotics is usually a major part of treatment. Clinically, antipsychotic drugs appear to be effective for treating many symptoms, including hyperactivity, aggression, tantrums, agitation, insomnia, and self-injury. Again, however, we are not aware of research data on antipsychotic management of other psychotic disorders in this population (Reiss & Aman, 1998). Despite the controversy that has surrounded the use of antipsychotic drugs in people with mental retardation over the years, they are widely prescribed for people with mental retardation and other psychotic disorders. The most highly recommended antipsychotics in the Consensus Survey for psychotic syndrome were risperidone and olanzapine (Rush & Frances, 2000).

Anxiety Disorders

Anxiety disorders are probably the most commonly undiagnosed psychiatric disorders in the general population. Obviously in individuals with mental retardation, the diagnosis will be more difficult due to lack of communication and altered expression of the common signs and symptoms of anxiety. The clinician's experience in observing signs or symptoms of anxiety is the cornerstone of diagnosis of anxiety in this population.

The DSM-IV lists 11 subtypes of anxiety disorder. Phobia is the most common type of anxiety disorder seen in people with mental retardation, whereas panic disorder is relatively uncommon and has only recently been reported for people with mental retardation (Szymanski et al., 1998). Posttraumatic stress disorder is indicated by a persistent tendency to reexperience a traumatic event in several ways. McNally and Shin (1995) found a negative correlation between the severity of PTSD symptoms over time and the IQ of combat soldiers. Reports of PTSD in people with ID have frequently focused on victims of physical and sexual abuse.

The actual research on anxiolytics in this field is extraordinarily limited. Werry (1998) reviewed the work on benzodiazepines (such as diazepam

[Valium]) and found that most of the published work has been done with children. Symptoms reflecting high-anxious behaviors were more responsive than symptoms of acting out, which often became *worse* with benzodiazepines. Furthermore, there are some data suggesting that individuals with conspicuous stereotypy and self-injury may respond paradoxically (i.e., with excitability and combativeness) to anxiolytics; lower IQ has also been a predictor of a paradoxical response. There are no research data on the effects of antihistamines on anxiety or sleep disorders in patients with mental retardation, and the very limited evidence for buspirone (BuSpar) is equivocal (Werry, 1998).

Faced with this lack of experimental evidence, clinicians are probably most likely to provide treatment based on symptoms present, symptom severity, and the clinician's own experience with various treatment modalities. The Expert Consensus guideline recommendations (Rush & Frances, 2000) for anxiety disorders in individuals with mental retardation consist of two categories of therapy, namely behavior therapy and medication therapy. Behavior therapy includes client and family education, applied behavior analysis, and managing the environment with cognitive and classical behavioral therapies. The preferred pharmacotherapy for anxiety disorders is to start with an SSRI or other agents such as venlafaxine, buspirone, and (in some cases) benzodiazepines.

ADHD

Attention-Deficit/Hyperactivity Disorder (ADHD) is one of the more common conditions among children with mental retardation (Benson & Aman, 1999). The mainstay of treatment for ADHD in typically-developing children is psychostimulant medication (such as methylphenidate [Ritalin], dextroamphetamine [Dexedrine], and amphetamine salts [Adderall]). Reviews of research in young people with mental retardation clearly show that these children also benefit with these medicines, although the response rate is lower (Aman, 1996; Arnold, Gadow, Pearson, & Varley, 1998). Aman (1996) calculated that 54% of participants in these studies were responders, as compared with approximately 75% in the general population.

Whereas stimulants may be the most thoroughly studied drug group for any specific DSM condition (i.e., ADHD) in mental retardation, many important questions remain unanswered. For example, Arnold et al. (1998) pointed out that the course of ADHD, duration of treatment effect, long-term side effects, and any development of tolerance all remain unstudied. Furthermore, there are now several relatively new and longer-acting preparations on the market such as Adderall and long-acting methylphenidate (Concerta, Metadate, Methypatch). We are not aware of any data on the efficacy of these newer agents in mental retardation.

Finally, a new agent, atomoxetine (Strattera), was recently approved by the FDA for the treatment of typically-developing children with ADHD. Arnold et al. (in press) conducted a crossover, placebo-controlled study with 16 children with autism spectrum disorders; six of the children (38%) also had mental retardation. Statistically significant improvement was observed on the Hyperactivity subscale of the Aberrant Behavior Checklist and on DSM-IV ADHD hyperactive/impulsive symptoms. No changes were seen on cognitive measures, including on a test of vigilance (attention span). We are not aware of any studies that have assessed atomoxetine for management of ADHD in children chosen exclusively for ADHD and mental retardation.

In the Expert Consensus guidelines, the following medicines were endorsed, in this order, for ADHD: (a) psychostimulants (first line treatment), (b) alpha-2-agonists (clonidine [Catapres] or guanfacine [Tenex]—second line), (c) bupropion (Wellbutrin), and (d) tricyclic antidepressants. We are not aware of any controlled studies among children with mental retardation that support (or contest use of) drug groups (b) through (d), above. Given that ADHD is perhaps the best studied disorder within mental retardation, this gives some idea of the challenges before us and the gaps in knowledge that currently exist.

Conduct Disorder (CD) and Oppositional Defiant Disorder (ODD)

CD and ODD are the main conditions comprising disruptive behavior disorders in children. CD with aggression has been found to have a higher prevalence in people with mental retardation than in the general population, with one survey giving a rate of 12.6% (Benson & Aman, 1999). CD, in particular, has a poor prognosis, with a high percentage of such individuals eventually engaging in substance abuse, criminal offenses, or eventually developing antisocial personality disorder.

There is a small literature on the effects of psychostimulants (e.g., methylphenidate, dextroamphetamine) on aggression in children of average IQ (Aman & Lindsay, 2002). For the most part, the literature suggests modest to moderate effects in reducing aggression. Presumably, the mechanism of effect is via reduction of impulsive acting out in such individuals. We are not aware of any literature on stimulant effects in aggressive children with mental retardation, although we assume that the effect would be similar and perhaps more modest.

Historically antipsychotic medicines have sometimes been used to manage aggression in children. Of the older (classical) antipsychotics, haloperidol (Haldol) is the best studied in this respect (Aman & Lindsay, in press). However, the tendency of the traditional antipsychotics to cause extrapyramidal effects or tardive dyskinesia probably makes them a suboptimal choice.

Recently, two controlled reports were published of the use of risperidone in children with either CD or ODD, prominent hostility, or aggression, and borderline IQ or mental retardation (Aman et al., 2002; Snyder et al., 2002). Both studies showed reductions in ratings of conduct problems by about 47% as compared with about 18% for placebo. These children were followed for nearly one year, and their behavior was found to remain stable, usually with mild to moderate side effects (Aman & Lindsay,

2003). We are not aware of similar controlled research with other atypical antipsychotics, although one report of clozapine indicated less aggression (Aman & Madrid, 1999).

Mood stabilizers (lithium carbonate, carbamazepine, sodium valproate, and others) have been assessed with clients having aggressive behavior and mental retardation and in aggressive individuals from the general population (Aman & Lindsay, 2003; Poindexter et al, 1998). These agents appear to reduce aggressive behavior to variable degrees, with the best results occurring with valproate (Depakote). However, most of this work is done with typically developing children.

In the Expert Consensus survey, practitioners were asked for their recommendations when a specific DSM-IV diagnosis could not be made and where the target symptom was physical aggression to people or property. The experts chose (a) newer atypical antipsychotics and (b) anticonvulsant/mood stabilizers as the first-line choices. They also chose (c) SSRIs and (d) beta blockers as second-line treatments. Whereas there are case series and uncontrolled reports of these latter agents (c and d), there is little or no controlled research on their value for this purpose in mental retardation (Fraser, Ruedrich, Kerr, & Levitas, 1998; Sovner et al., 1998).

Other Behaviors Not Otherwise Specified

Personality Disorder

Some investigators have identified several extreme personality characteristics that may occur in individuals with mental retardation (Zigler & Burack, 1989). They include over-dependency, low ideal self-image, limited aspirations, and an outer-directed style of problem solving. During the early developmental years, a combination of parental restrictiveness and overprotection, peer pressure and rejection, and low self-esteem and low confidence can lead to major problems with one's self-identity. The diagnosis and treatment of personality disorders in individuals with mental retardation is still controversial, but it seems that these individuals may have a higher rate of severe personality disorders than other groups.

The treatment of personality disorder in individuals with mental retardation is not different from the general population. It consists of psychotherapy or behavior therapy and pharmacotherapy. The latter depends on the IQ of the individual with mental retardation. In dealing with agitation, pharmacotherapy with an anti-anxiety agent such as diazepam (Valium) is usually sufficient, although sometimes it is necessary to use an antipsychotic; recently the atypical antipsychotics have become standard treatments when stronger agents are needed. We are not aware of any drug research involving personality disorders in this field (Reiss & Aman, 1998).

Aggression

This category was addressed above when CD and ODD were discussed. Suffice it to say that aggression (without a co-existing DSM disorder) has been a frequent target of treatment since the first psychotropic agents were synthesized. Much of this work was with the classical antipsychotics, which are now superseded by the atypical antipsychotics. In their review of antidepressants, Sovner et al. (1998) identified seven case reports and case series ($n = 9$ participants) showing improvement when treated with a variety of drugs. One patient had organic personality disorder and another had intermittent explosive disorder, but the remainder did not have DSM diagnoses normally considered to cause aggression. The antidepressants used included trazodone (Desyrel), fluoxetine (Prozac), and fluvoxamine (Luvox).

As noted above, the Expert Consensus guidelines identified atypical antipsychotics, antipsychotics in combination with mood stabilizers, SS-RIs, and beta blockers as the most likely to be helpful for aggressive behavior in the absence of a DSM diagnosis (Rush & Frances, 2000). This statement is based on expert *opinion* and awaits confirmation in rigorous controlled studies.

Pica

Eating inedible substances is fairly common in people with severe or profound mental retardation. In the Expert Consensus survey, the respondents most commonly recommended the following: (a) no medication ("first-line"), (b) SSRI, and (c) mineral or nutritional supplement (e.g., zinc, iron) (Rush & Frances, 2000). We do not know the rationale for using SSRIs and we are not aware of any research on this. The use of vitamin or mineral supplements makes sense if the pica reflects some sort of compensatory need and if it can be shown by laboratory tests that the individual has a vitamin or mineral deficiency.

Self-Injury

Self-injury of a repetitive nature is somewhat common in people with developmental disabilities, and its prevalence seems to increase with functional impairment. Approximately 10–15% of institutional residents display self-injury as compared with 1–2.5% in the community (Aman, 1993).

Virtually every type of psychotropic agent has been tried in the past in the hopes of reducing self-injury. In one review, the evidence seemed strongest for certain classical antipsychotics, lithium carbonate, and the opiate blocker naltrexone (Trexan—Aman, 1993). Among the atypical antipsychotics, risperidone, clozapine, and olanzapine have all been shown to reduce self-injury, although the methodology in most of the reports was found to be wanting (Aman & Madrid, 1999).

In the 1980s and 1990s there was considerable interest in the notion that self-injury might reflect a dysfunction in the patient's opiate system, and this generated a number of studies of naltrexone, a relatively pure opiate blocker (Sandman et al., 1998). Our reading of this literature is that naltrexone has not lived up to its initial promise, although a few patients do appear to get benefit from it. There has also been speculation that self-injury may reflect an underlying form of obsessive compulsive disorder or that it may be a symptom of underlying major depression, both of which could implicate serotonergic antidepressants as therapeutic agents. A review of SSRI reports identified 12 that were positive in outcome, one that was mixed, and two that were negative (Aman et al., 1999). The same review identified two positive studies with clomipramine (Anafranil) and one negative one. Thus, overall, the literature suggests some benefit with SSRIs, atypical antipsychotics, lithium carbonate, and natrexone, although sample sizes were often small and research methodology frequently weak. Some clinicians try to tailor treatment to patient characteristics by prescribing (a) antidepressants when there is a bout of depression, OCD, or evidence of affective disorder in family members; (b) antipsychotics when behavior presents as bizarre or there is a family history of psychosis; and (c) naltrexone when the self-harm is very repetitive with no apparent reinforcement to maintain it.

In the Expert Consensus survey, the respondents chose the following therapies in this order when asked how they would treat self-injury in the absence of a DSM diagnosis: (a) newer atypical antipsychotic, (b) anticonvulsant in combination with a mood stabilizer (a and b: "first-line" treatments), (c) serotonergic antidepressant, and (d) naltrexone ("second line" treatments). Conventional antipsychotics, beta blockers, and buspirone (an anxiolytic) were also mentioned.

Symptoms Accompanied by a General Medical Condition

The most common general medical condition associated with mental retardation is seizure disorder, which can present as generalized or partial seizures. The most common generalized seizures in adults are tonic-clonic seizures ("grand mal" convulsions). Partial seizures are either complex or simple partial seizures; seizures are associated with alterations of consciousness or somatosensory, autonomic, or mixed symptoms. Clinicians often treat combined mood disorder with seizures with divalproex sodium (Depakote) or carbamazepine (Tegretol), both of which are approved by the U.S. Food and Drug Administration for this purpose. It is widely accepted that higher doses of these two antiepileptic mood stabilizers are needed to treat combined mood and seizure disorders. Lithium, a mood stabilizer without antiepileptic properties, would not ordinarily be used to manage combined mood and seizure disorders.

DISCUSSION

State of the Field

There has been a proliferation of new psychotropic agents in the recent past. Examples include the atypical antipsychotics (with the recent addition of aripiprazole [Abilify] and ziprasidone [Geodon]), SSRIs (with citalopram [Celexa] and escitalopram [Lexapro] recently introduced to the U.S. market), several new anticonvulsants (e.g., lamotrigine, topiramate, gabapentin; many of which have found a place as mood stabilizers), and certain over-the-counter agents (e.g., St. John's Wort, melatonin). Suffice it to say that good research has not been able to keep pace with this rate of development. There are several major challenges that confront researchers in this field including the following. First, the numbers of individuals with mental retardation and a psychiatric problem are far smaller than in the general population, making recruitment for research very difficult. Second, this is an "orphan population," sufficiently small that many pharmaceutical companies may lack incentive for grooming new psychoactive agents. Third, it can be exceptionally difficult to make psychiatric diagnoses with confidence in this population, especially with people having severe or profound retardation, which further compounds difficulties in defining research samples. Fourth, by the very nature of mental retardation, many participants may find it difficult to cooperate with test procedures (e.g., perform cognitive tests) or provide valuable subjective feedback regarding sensation or emotion.

Consequently, it is exceptionally difficult to conduct research in this field. It is still true today, as it was 35 years ago (Sprague & Werry, 1971), that investigators often rush to assess the latest sexy drug. Scientific journals often publish such reports, even when the research methods are inferior. The reality is that we do not have much evidence for the efficacy of most agents based on research with patients having mental retardation. Much of the literature that is available is either poorly controlled or uncontrolled. Consequently, we do not have much hard evidence for the efficacy of most agents based on research with patients having mental retardation. Hence, many (perhaps most) practitioners try to work by inference or analogy from what is known in the general population. Having said that, we do have certain directions from past experience. For instance, clinicians are becoming more sophisticated in making dual diagnoses of developmental and mental disorders. In addition, many prescribers seem to appreciate important challenges posed by clients having mental retardation. For example, most experts appreciate that it is often necessary to start with lower doses (presumably because of central nervous system [CNS] dysfunction) and to titrate dosage more slowly when medicating patients with mental retardation (Rush & Frances, 2000).

Directions for the Future

In the short term, we cannot possibly assess all novel agents for all psychiatric conditions and target symptoms in this field. At the very least, then, we should strive for some sound investigations with at least a *prototype* of each medication class and for each major indication for these agents. For example, it would be rational to attempt to assess good candidates from among the atypical antipsychotics (currently numbering at least 7) and from the SSRIs (numbering 5 at time of this writing). The National Association for the Dually Diagnosed (NADD) and the American Psychiatric Association are working together to develop modified symptom criteria in people with mental retardation that are equivalent to symptoms among psychiatric patients in the general population (R. Fletcher, personal communication, February 2003). It is hoped that the guidelines will help future investigators to achieve better reliability when choosing study participants.

New imaging techniques are becoming more sophisticated and (perhaps) less invasive. Examples are functional MRI, SPECT and PET scan, which can locate areas of brain with metabolic hyperactivity. Both CT and MRI have been used successfully in identifying specific congenital disorders. It is likely that these tools will help us both to identify more appropriate participants and to understand the central nervous system effects that make a given drug therapeutic. We also have much greater sophistication than in the past in identifying metabolically (and genetically) determined etiological subgroups and behavioral phenotypes among people with mental retardation. If we conduct our research carefully, with documentation of such subgroups and attention to rational matches between conditions and pharmacological agents, we may be able to achieve breakthroughs in pharmacotherapy.

APPENDIX

Common Psychotropic Medicines Grouped by Class

Drug groups and examples	Brand names
Antipsychotics	
(Classical antipsychotics)	
chlorpromazine	Largactil, Thorazine
flupenthixol	Depixol
fluphenazine	Prolixin, Modecate
thioridazine	Mellaril
haloperidol	Haldol
loxapine	Loxitane
molindone	Moban
prochlorperazine	Compazine
(Atypical antipsychotics)	
aripiprazole	Abilify
clozapine	Clozaril
olanzapine	Zypreza
quetiapine	Seroquel
risperidone	Risperdal
sertindole	Serlect
ziprasidone	Geodon
Antidepressants	
(Heterocyclics)	
amitriptyline	Elavil
clomipramine	Anafranil
desipramine	Norpramin
doxepin	Sinequan
imipramine	Tofranil
nortriptyline	Aventyl, others

(Continued)

Drug groups and examples	Brand names
(Atypical antidepressants)	
amoxapine	Asendin
bupropion	Wellbutrin
maprotiline	Ludiomil
nefazadone	Serzone
trazodone	Desyrel
Selective serotonin reuptake inhibitors (SSRIs)	
citalopram	Celexa
escitalopram	Lexapro
fluoxetine	Prozac
fluvoxamine	Luvox
paroxetine	Paxil
sertraline	Zoloft
(Monoamine oxidase inhibitors)	
moclobemide[a]	Aurorix
phenelzine	Nardil
tranylcypromine	Parnate
Mood stabilizers	
carbamazepine[b]	Tegretol
clonazepam[b]	Klonopin, Rivotril
gabapentin[b]	Neurontin
lamotrigine[b]	Lamictal
lithium carbonate	Eskalith, others
valproic acid[b]	Depakote, Depakene
Psychostimulants	
amphetamine salts	Adderall
D-amphetamine	Dexedrine
methylphenidate	Ritalin, Metadate, Concerta, Methypatch
D-methylphenidate	Focalin
Norepinephrine reuptake inhibitor	
atomoxetine	Strattera
Alpha 2 adrenergic agonists	
clonidine	Catapres
guanfacine	Tenex
Anxiolytics/sedatives	
(Benzodiazepines and benzodiazepine analogue)	
alprazolam	Xanax
diazepam	Valium
flurazepam	Dalmane
lorazepam	Ativan
nitrazepam	Mogadon
temazepam	Restoril
zopiclone	Ambien
(Atypical anxiolytic)	
buspirone	BuSpar
(Antihistamines)	
diphenhydramine	Benedryl
hydroxyzine	Atarax
promethazine	Phenergan

[a] Not available in the United States.
[b] Main indication is as antiepileptic agent.

REFERENCES

Aman, M. G. (1993). Efficacy of psychotropic drugs for reducing self injurious behavior in the developmental disabilities. *Annals of Clinical Psychiatry, 5,* 171–188.

Aman, M. G. (1996). Stimulant drugs in the developmental disabilities revisited. *Journal of Developmental and Physical Disabilities, 8,* 347–365.

Aman, M. G., Arnold L. E., & Armstrong, S. C. (1999). Review of serotonergic agents and perseverative behavior in patients with developmental disabilities. *Mental Retardation and Developmental Disabilities Research Reviews, 5,* 279–289.

Aman, M. G., De Smedt, G., Derivan, A., Lyons, B., Findling, R. L., & The Risperidone Disruptive Behavior Study Group. (2002). Risperidone treatment of children with disruptive behavior disorders and subaverage IQ: A double-blind, placebo-controlled study. *American Journal of Psychiatry, 159,* 1337–1346.

Aman, M. G., Lam, K. L., & Collier-Crespin, A. (2003). Prevalence and patterns of psychoactive medicines among individuals with autism in the Autism Society of Ohio. *Journal of Autism and Developmental Disorders, 33,* 527–534.

Aman, M. G., & Lindsay, R. L. (2002, October). Psychotropic medicines and aggressive behavior. Part I: Psychostimulants. *Child and Adolescent Psychopharmacology News, 7*(5), 1–6.

Aman, M. G., & Lindsay, R. L. (2003, March). Psychotropic medicines and aggressive behavior. Part II: Antipsychotics and mood stabilizers. *Child and Adolescent Psychopharmacology News, 8*(2), 6–9, 12.

Aman, M. G., & Madrid, A. (1999). Atypical antipsychotics in persons with developmental disabilities. *Mental Retardation and Developmental Disabilities Research Reviews, 5,* 253–263.

American Psychiatric Association. (2000). *Diagnostic and statistical manual of mental disorders, 4th edition, text revision (DSM-IV-TR).* Washington, DC: American Psychiatric Press.

Arnold, L. E., Aman, M. G., Cook, A., Witwer, A., Hall, K., Thompson, S., & Ramadan, Y. (in press). *Atomoxetine for hyperactivity in autism spectrum disorders: Placebo-controlled crossover trial. Journal of the American Academy of Child and Adolescent Psychiatry.* Columbus: Ohio State University: Manuscript submitted for publication.

Arnold, L. E., Gadow, K. D., Pearson, D. A., & Varley, C. K. (1998). Stimulants. In S. Reiss & M. G. Aman (Eds.), *Psychotropic and developmental disabilities: The international consensus handbook.* Columbus, OH: The Ohio State University Nisonger Center.

Baumeister, A. A., Sevin, J. A., & King, B. H. (1998). Neuroleptic medications. In S. Reiss & M. G. Aman (Eds.), *Psychotropic medication and developmental disabilities: The international consensus handbook,* (pp. 133–150). Columbus, OH: The Ohio State University Nisonger Center.

Benson, B. B., & Aman, M. G. (1999). Disruptive behavior disorders in children with mental retardation. In H. C. Quay & A. E. Hogan (Eds.), *Handbook of disruptive behavior disorders* (pp. 559–578). New York: Plenum Press.

Branford, D., Bhaumik, S., & Naik, B. (1998). Selective serotonin re-uptake inhibitors for the treatment of perseverative and maladaptive behaviours of people with intellectual disability. *Journal of Intellectual Disability Research, 42,* 301–306.

Craft, M. J., & Schiff, A. A. (1980). Psychiatric disturbance in mentally handicapped patients. *British Journal of Psychiatry, 137,* 250–255.

Fraser, W. I., Ruedrich, S., Kerr, M., & Levitas, A. (1998). Beta-adrenergic blockers. In S. Reiss & M. G. Aman (Eds). *Psychotropic medications and developmental disabilities: The international consensus handbook* (pp. 271–289.) Columbus, OH: The Ohio State University Nisonger Center.

Langworthy-Lam, K. L., Aman, M. G., & Van Bourgondien, M. E. (2002). Prevalence and patterns of use of psychoactive medicines in individuals with autism in the Autism Society of North Carolina. *Journal of Child and Adolescent Psychopharmacology, 12,* 311–321.

McNally, R. J., & Shin, L. M. (1995). Association of intelligence with severity of posttraumatic stress disorder in Vietnam combat veterans (1995). *American Journal of Psychiatry, 152,* 936–938.

Menolascino, F. J., Ruedrich, S. L., Golden, C J., & Wilson, J. E. (1985). Diagnosis and phar-macotherapy of schizophrenia in the retarded. *Psychopharmacology Bulletin, 21,* 316–322.

Poindexter, A. R., Cain, N., Clarke, D. J., Cook, E. H., Corbett, J. A., & Levitas, A. (1998). Mood stabilizers. In S. Reiss & M. G. Aman (Eds.), *Psychotropic and developmental disabilities: The international consensus handbook* (pp. 215–228). Columbus, OH: The Ohio State University Nisonger Center.

Reiss, S (1994). *Handbook of challenging behavior: Mental health aspects of mental retardation.* Worthington, OH: IDS Publishing Corporation.

Reiss, S., & Aman, M. G. (1998). *Psychotropic medications and developmental disabilities: The international consensus handbook.* Columbus, OH: The Ohio State University Nisonger Center.

Rinck, C. (1998). Epidemiology and psychoactive medication. In S. Reiss & M. G. Aman (Eds.), *Psychotropic and developmental disabilities: The international consensus handbook* (pp. 31–44). Columbus, OH: The Ohio State University Nisonger Center.

Rush, A. J ., & Frances, A. (Eds.) (2000). Special Issue: the expert consensus guideline se-ries. Treatment of psychiatric and behavioral problems in mental retardation, *American Journal on Mental Retardation, 105,* 159–228.

Sandman, C. A., Thompson, T., Barrett, R. P., Verhoeven, W. M. A., McCubbin, J. A., Schroeder, S. R., et al. (1998). Opiate blockers. In S. Reiss & M. G. Aman (Eds.), *Psy-chotropic and developmental disabilities: The international consensus handbook.* Colum-bus, OH: The Ohio State University Nisonger Center.

Sajatovic, M., Ramirez, L. F., Kenny, J. T., & Meltzer, H. Y. (1994). The use of clozapine in borderline-intellectual-functioning and mentally retarded schizophrenic patients. *Com-prehensive Psychiatry, 35,* 29–33.

Snyder, R., Turgay, A., Aman, M. G., Binder, C., Fisman, S., Carroll, A., et al. (2002). Effects of risperidone on conduct and disruptive behavior disorders in children with subaverage IQs. *Journal of the American Academy of Child and Adolescent Psychiatry, 41,* 1026–1036.

Sovner, R., Pary, R., Dosen, A. Gedye, A., Barrera, F., Cantwell, D., et al. (1998). Antidepres-sant drugs. In S. Reiss & M. G. Aman (Eds.), *Psychopharmacology and developmental disabilities: The international consensus handbook* (pp. 179–200). Columbus, OH: The Ohio State University Nisonger Center.

Sprague, R. L. & Werry, J. S. (1971). Methodology of psychopharmacological studies with the retarded. In N. R. Ellis (Ed.), *International review of research in mental retardation* (Vol. 5, pp. 147–210). New York: Academic Press.

Szymanski, L. S., King, B., Goldberg, B., Reid, A., Tonge, B., & Cain, N. (1998). Diagnosis of mental disorders in people with mental retardation. *Psychopharmacology and devel-opmental disabilities: The international consensus handbook* (pp. 3–17). Columbus, OH: The Ohio State University Nisonger Center.

Werry, J. S. (1998). Anxiolytics and sedatives. In S. Reiss & M. G. Aman (Eds.), *Psychophar-macology and developmental disabilities: The international consensus handbook* (pp. 201–214). Columbus, OH: The Ohio State University Nisonger Center.

World Health Organization. (1992). *International statistical classification of diseases and re-lated health problems* (10th ed.) (ICD-10). Geneva, SW: Author.

Zigler, E. & Burack, J. A. (1989). Personality development and the dually diagnosed person. *Research in Developmental Disabilities, 10,* 225–240.

V

Ethical Issues

34

Ethical Issues in Clinical Services and Research

ROBERT L. SPRAGUE

PREFACE

In what may be the last chapter written of my professional career, I may cause considerable discussion and debate because the topic of this chapter is a many-faceted and complex issue rife with controversy and strong opinion held by people with opposing viewpoints. Two aspects of this review are obvious: first, I can only cover some (Sprague, 1994) of the many aspects of ethical issues surrounding individual with developmental disabilities, and second, even the relatively few issues that are covered may bring about strong dissent from the readers because the spread of opinions about these issues is so vast. But now, having little to fear about promotion and salary reviews that do not exist for me any more in retirement, I will plunge ahead into the controversial fray.

THE BREADTH OF ETHICAL ISSUES IN
DEVELOPMENTAL DISABILITIES

When one examines the area of ethics of developmental disability, very wide ranges of issues appear in the literature. Perhaps this can best be explained by referring to the bibliographic searches that were conducted as an aid in the preparation for this paper. Using the keywords "ethics" and "mental retardation," National Library of Medicine (NLM) lists 337 references plus another 13 using the keywords "ethics" and "developmental disabilities" giving a total of 350 references. ERIC, a bibliographic database primarily dealing with education, lists only a total of 20 references using all

ROBERT L. SPRAGUE • University of Illinois, Champaign, Illinois 61821.

the three keywords described above. PsychINFO, another bibliographic service, provided about 30 more references. However, when one examines the titles, keywords, and abstracts of these references, a very large set of issues is mentioned. To give the reader some understanding of the range of issues covered in the literature, some, but not all of these issues are: (1) abortion, (2) abuse and neglect, (3) accountability for providers of care, (4) advanced directives for end of life issues, (5) use of aversive stimulation for treatment, (6) behavior modification programs, (7) curriculum and training for both professional and paraprofessional in the field, (8) use of databases and privacy issues, (9) concerns about death and dying, (11) severe diseases, such as diabetes, kidney failure, and obesity, and associated treatment problems, (12) ethical codes, (13) eugenics, (14) genetics, (15) hospice care, (16) informed consent for treatment and research, (17) many issues involving institutional care, (18) solving disagreements among professional service providers, (19) psychopharmacology, (20) use of restraints, (21) sexuality, (22) sterilization, (23) transplantation of organs, and (24) appropriate treatments. This should be a long enough list of issues for anybody, and, certainly, more issues than may be reasonably handled in one chapter. However, I will make an attempt to pare down these numerous issues to a more reasonable number and hopefully more relevant to the readers of this book.

Several caveats should be mentioned at the start. Some issues are not covered, for example, legal competency, involvement with the police and their actions, court decisions, and other issues may only be briefly covered, for example, sterilization. There have been several reviews of legal actions and decision that should be studied if the reader is interested in this area (Ferleger & Boyd, 1979; Landau, 1996; Mason & Menolascino, 1976; Plotkin & Gill, 1979; Singh, Guernsey, & Ellis, 1992; Sprague, 1982a, 1982b; Sprague & Galliher, 1988). Even though sometimes relevant, usually foreign journals typically are not cited. There is a bias toward citing more recent references, those appearing in the decade of the 1990s, although this is certainly not an absolute rule. Finally, because there are numerous sides to each of these many issues, sometimes strongly and emotionally held by some proponents, the author does not try to present his answers to debates. Rather he attempts to present the issues and some of the relevant literature pertinent to each controversy.

HEALTH SERVICES

Community Care in Comparison with Institutional Care

The issue of whether people with mental retardation can be more appropriately cared for in an institution or in the community is debate that has been raging for a number of years, and it is likely to continue. Often the debate is taken to the courts. Although there are ethical aspects to this controversy, seldom have ethical issues been addressed as a single issue in writings about this issue. But even if the question of provision of quality service in the institution or in the community is not taken to court, the debate rages on in the literature (Eyman, 1998, Kalachnik, 1999; Rothman & Rothman, 1984). Sometimes the argument is exemplified by the use of quite colorful language: "The Mansfield Training School is closed: the swamp has been finally drained" (MacNamara, 1994). It has been argued that considerable ethical responsibility rightly bears on institutions to provide adequate care (Repp, 1978; Repp & Deitz, 1978).

Death and Dying Issues

A very difficult and controversial issue arises when a person with severe disability has a life-threatening illness or is judged terminally ill. At least two questions arise: first, who is the proper person from whom consent for major medical treatment should be requested, and second, how heroic should the medical treatment be, considering the severity of the impairment of the individual (Norris, 1979; Singer, 1983). In general, it is very difficult to give overall principles in this situation because each individual case varies so widely from one to another, often involving questions of the availability and closeness of the family to the patient, the seriousness of the illness, and the painfulness and likelihood of success of the medical treatment.

Examinations

There are many routine physical examinations that are either uncomfortable, painful, or potentially embarrassing that may be difficult to explain verbally to the person with an intellectual disability (ID) who has very limited verbal communication skills. Clearly many such examinations are beneficial to the health and welfare of the patient. A number of such situations can easily be mentioned: drawing of blood for diagnostic work, dental examinations and treatment, gynecological examinations (Brown, Rosen, & Elkins, 1992), X-ray examinations, and more advanced radiological assessments such as PET scan requiring confinement in a small tunnel. If the examination is essential to the health and welfare of the patient, it is quite common to sedate the person until the examination is complete, although this procedure is sometimes debatable.

Gene Therapy

Although there is now little practical value in gene therapy for people with ID, there is great, perhaps (Pollack, 2003), promise for the future of this therapeutic technique, possibly even reversing some of the disease conditions that result in severe cognitive impairment. The promise for the future of this new treatment is so great that it has been argued that ethical considerations of its use be examined today in preparation for future advances that might be extremely valuable to this population (Fletcher, 1995).

Informed Consent

Informed consent is deemed necessary for most medical procedures, but the problem obviously is how to obtain proper informed consent when the person may be so cognitively impaired that ordinary communication, especially the typically written medical consent form, is highly inappropriate. In this situation, many providers of service use substituted judgment of another cognitively competent person (a topic discussed in the section below). Many articles in the literature refer to the intriguing but extremely complex issues that arise in the practical application of ordinary educational, medical, and psychological services to this population of people with developmental disabilities.

Moon (Moon & Graber, 1985) presents the case of a person with mild ID whose kidneys failed in end-stage renal disease. Treatments for this disease usually involve two heroic procedures that involve considerable pain and great inconvenience (surgery for transplantation of kidneys or renal dialysis) that "Danny" apparently partially understood, and, consequently, he adamantly refused the dialysis option. Advocates on his behalf appeared and disagreed among themselves—that did not help the situation. After several years of discussion, it was finally agreed that considering his firm decision, his independence even in this life-and-death situation should be respected. However, and ironically, he died before the final decision was made. The obvious point of this case is that decisions, even very difficult ones, should not be made in such a cumbersome manner and instead made with all deliberate speed.

Cardiac surgery is a difficult decision for even the best-integrated and well-educated family. The ethical problems around such surgery for ward of the state who is adjudged cognitively incompetent becomes much more difficult (as described by Goldhaber, Reardon, Goulart, & Rubin, 1985). In this day of HMOs and a strong push for cost control, the difficulty is real when deciding between two cases that may be competing for the same services, one case a person with ID who is free of symptoms at the time but who will certainly develop symptoms in future, or another respectable symptomatic man with a family in the community. Clearly, there are no easy answers for these very tough ethical, legal, and economic problems. Similar ethical problems exist with treatment of children within the constraints of limited resources, clinical or financial (Shevell, 1998). Probably the best that can be done now is for individual ethics committees and physicians to make their own decisions based upon their understanding of all the unique factors involved in such complicated cases. General, rigid rules issued by some governmental unit certainly would not work in such complex situations although an agreed upon set of principles, not yet reached by consensus, would certainly be of assistance in making such decisions.

Electro-Convulsive Therapy

Another controversial treatment is the use of electro-convulsive therapy (ECT) with patients with ID and concurrent severe psychiatric disorders (van Waarde, Stolker, & van der Mast, 2001). Of course, one of the first issues is the reliability of the psychiatric diagnoses in such situations (Jacobson, 1982; Rojahn, Borthwick-Duffy, & Jacobson, 1993). Even if the diagnosis is reliable, many other ethical questions remain. However, some studies in this area indicate support for the use of ECT with such patients who cannot give their consent (van Waarde et al., 2001).

Treatment for Dementia

Perhaps even more difficult diagnostic task involves the issue of proper treatment for individuals with ID who also have senile dementia. One author has addressed the issue of coercive or forced treatment in such cases (Tannsjo, 1999). In some instances, nurses may need to engage in deception of the person with ID in order to provide the treatment thought to be necessary for the person with ID; two authors (Teasdale & Kent, 1995) have written about the situations in which deception may be properly used.

This brief discussion by no means exhausts the literature, and certainly not the manifold number of problems, interwoven with issues of informed consent. Some authors argue that parameters of self-determination should be decided by courts (Strudler, 1988), and other authors deal with a range of related issues (O'Sullivan & Borcherding, 2002; Relman, 1979; Sprague, 1972, 1977, 1978, 1982b). As could be expected often the writers take opposing views in this complicated area; Relman argues for considerable deference to physician's judgment, but Buchanan (1979) calls Relman's position medical paternalism (Kay, 1995).

Substituted Judgment

Quite often in cases of severe cognitive impairment the judgment of another person (family member, advocate, or court-appointed person) is sought when medical treatment is essential for continued health or even life itself. Should substituted judgment be used for people with ID? Support for such substituted judgment is made in cases such as end-stage renal disease cited above; in some cases the judgment was made not to start dialysis (Kujdych, Lowe, Sparks, Dottes, & Crook, 2000). Generally, most of the limited literature on substituted judgment in important medical matters seems to support substituted judgment although there are clearly some limitations to its application (Kluge, 1987; Martyn, 1994).

NEONATAL CONCERNS

Ethical issues may begin long before the individual with ID is even born. With the ability to diagnosis prenatal medical conditions, ethical issues may arise when a prenatal diagnosis is given. However, the presentation of a prenatal diagnosis to the expectant mother is not always given in some situations such as that of a very young adolescent mother (St Amant, Elkins, Brown, & Pastorek, 1993). Of course, the question then becomes if not the expectant mother, then who *should* be given the diagnosis? Even if there are no questions about presenting the prenatal diagnosis, there are many questions surrounding how the diagnosis should be presented and, particularly, what kinds of discussions to hold with the expectant mother and, possibly, father regarding the seriousness of the diagnosis, prognosis, and, if any, available treatments. Most of the issues are covered in the literature in a general way (Hauerwas, 1975; Hayes, Hayes, Moore, & Ghezzi, 1994; Hemphill & Freeman, 1977; Reich, 1987). It is generally recognized that recent advances in neonatal care have greatly increased the likelihood of survival of infants with serious medical conditions (Hauerwas, 1975), but this increased probability of survival comes at a large increase in cost at the neonatal intensive care unit and possible later medical costs throughout childhood and, perhaps, the life of the individual (Reynolds, 1978). Is there a limit to providing high technology neonatal care considering predictable massive future medical costs? Few such issues have been settled yet by a reaching of consensus and, in fact, these issues may be becoming more complex as medical procedures improve, extending the survival of infants with very serious central nervous system complications (Katzen, 1971; Reich, 1987) who even today are unlikely to survive. Quite often the wishes or beliefs of the parents may come into conflict with the moral beliefs of the nurses caring for the mothers and infants, and it has been pointed out that such conflicts require continuing discussion and attention within neonatal settings (Mims & Crisham, 1996).

PSYCHOPHARMACOLOGICAL TREATMENT

Many treatment modalities provoke ample ethical problems, and the issue of psychopharmacological medications to control behavior and treat psychiatric conditions has elicited many of the most contentious ethical issues and legal battles. There is a very large literature on this subject that can only be briefly covered in this section of one chapter. If the reader is interested in the general problem of psychopharmacology with mentally retarded people, there are several review articles on this topic (Aman & Singh, 1988, 1991; Crabbe & Handen, 1994; Freeman, 1966; Gadow & Poling, 1988; Lewis, Aman, Gadow, Schroeder, & Thompson, 1996; Poling, 1994; Schroeder, 1985; Sprague, 1995; Sprague & Baxley, 1978; Sprague & Werry, 1971; Werry & Aman, 1999). For at least 15 years, the ethical controversies regarding the use of psychotropic medications with people who have developmental disabilities have been so intense that many parents, advocates, and others have taken their issues to court, and a substantial literature has been generated reviewing the decisions and implications of these court orders (Patterson & Robinson, 1982; Plotkin & Gill, 1979; Singh et al., 1992; Sprague, 1978, 1982a, 1982b; Sprague & Galliher, 1988) that in turn impact on clinical medical practice. A review of this literature leaves no doubt that the many issues involved in the use of psychotropic medication are considered important enough by society, as determined by the courts, that standards and limits on the use of these medications for this impaired population of citizens are often set and enforced in both institutional and community settings.

There are some aspects of psychotropic medication usage that have attracted more attention and comment than other areas; one such issue is tardive dyskinesia (the development of abnormal movement symptoms due to the continued usage of this medication) that has prompted several authors to write on the topic (Gualtieri, Keppel, & Schroeder, 1986; Kalachnik & Sprague, 1994; Sprague & Kalachnik, 1991; Wigal et al., 1996; Wszola, Newell, & Sprague, 2001).

It also seems likely that more attention in the future will be paid to the effects of these medications on the learning and rehabilitation plans on cognitively impaired people than has been devoted to this topic in the past.

SEXUALITY

Sexuality and sexual activity of people limited by developmental disabilities is a major concern of many sectors of the general public. In the past, these concerns were expressed in sterilization laws that have been, for the most part, abandoned in the United States although there is still concern about the usefulness of such laws in other counties. But coverage of such laws and their overturn is not the main concern of this chapter. In 1978 rules of the U.S. Department of Health, Education, Welfare were promulgated regarding the use of federal funds for sterilization of women on welfare that also had implications for women with ID (Petchesky, 1979). A number of controls were applied to be certain that sterilization was voluntary, but there was concern about whether consent was adequately voluntary and informed on the part of people with ID.

There is general concern about the ability of parents with cognitive disabilities to care properly for their offspring, including questions of whether sexual predators may take advantage of children or parents, adequacy of information about sexually transmitted diseases, and related reproductive health matters. There is some literature that addresses adequacy of the sexual knowledge of the individual (Hall, Morris, & Barker, 1973), emphasis on normalization of sexuality even with the difficulties noted (Held, 1993), advisability of prenatal screening for all mothers (St Amant et al., 1993), differences between the attitudes of some caregivers and interpretation of normalization practices by staff and professionals (Zuker-Weiss, 1994), concern about the adequacy of training in this area for caregivers (Halstead, 2002), and issues regarding the attitudes of nurses toward liberalized standards (Aylott, 1999). Of course, the main concern expressed in the literature is for the care and welfare of pregnant woman with ID (Higgs, 1983; O'Hara, 1989).

EUTHANASIA

This topic appeared in the literature after the publicity about the Quinlan and Saikewicz cases in the late 1970s (Annas, 1978, 1979). The issue is whether the life of a person suffering from incurable and severely painful disease(s) should be ended. Much of the debate involved prenatal diagnosis of severe malformations (Bayley, 1980; Friedmann, 1971). One writer has held out the promise of gene therapy to correct several problems of prenatal life thus avoiding such difficult ethical questions about possible euthanasia (Ye, Mitchell, Newman, & Batshaw, 2001).

APPLIED BEHAVIOR MODIFICATION

Use of Aversive Stimulation

Should aversive stimulation in behavioral intervention programs be used with people with ID? The issue has elicited considerable debate with two camps forming, one against any use and another camp pointing out appropriate use in very difficult cases, such as self-injurious behavior (SIB). There are more cases of reported success using aversive stimulation in severe behavioral problems than can be reported here, thus only a few will be mentioned. In cases of SIB and other severe behavior problems, it has been useful (Corbett, 1975; Harris & Ersner-Hershfield, 1978; Meinhold, 1996; Smolev, 1971). Yet some government sponsored reports have seriously questioned the philosophy of using aversive stimulation (Abusing the Unprotected: A Study of the Misuse of Aversive Behavior Modification Techniques and Weaknesses in the Regulatory Structure (BBB19993), 1987). In another situation, apparently the report of a major National Institute of Child Health and Human Development report on this general topic publication was delayed due to ethical debates on the issue (Holden, 1990; National Institutes of Health, 1991). As has been pointed out several times in this chapter, obtaining appropriate consent for the use of aversive stimulation is a major problem (Cook, Altman, & Haavik, 1978; Murphy, 1993). The ethical debate in this area continues (Elder, 1996; Gerhardt, Holmes, Alessandri, & Goodman, 1991; Stolz, 1977). Various organizations with major interests in this area have proposed guidelines for the use of aversive stimulation that have been discussed by other authors (Hayes et al., 1994; Sajwaj, 1977; Schroeder & Schroeder, 1989; Stolz, 1977).

Differential Reinforcement of Inappropriate Behavior

Within the scope of behavior modification, there are a number of technical issues that have received some comment in the literature. DRI (I for Incompatible) schedules of reinforcement represent one of those more technical areas: relevant literature includes a case of ritualistic behavior treated in this fashion (Iqbal, 2002) and a commentary on the ethics of using this procedure to treat social isolation (Reinders, 2002a, 2002b).

Punishment, Restraints, and Seclusion

The use of punishment has brought a range of comments about its appropriateness (Butterfield, 1990; Mulick, 1990). Some research on the usefulness of punishment has been reported (Lerman, Iwata, Shore, & DeLeon, 1997). Restraint has been suggested as appropriate control in dental examinations and treatment (Connick, Palat, & Pugliese, 2000). On the other hand, methods to phase out seclusion in nursing practice have also been reported (McDonnell, 1996).

EDUCATION AND TRAINING

Some authors have been concerned about the adequacy of training in medical schools for physicians providing health care to people with developmental disabilities (Lesser, 1986), but other authors have conducted surveys regarding the training and perceptions of more numerous paraprofessional caregivers (Oliver, Yutrzenka, & Redinius, 2002). A topic related to training relates to information about and perceptions of caregivers regarding people with ID who make personal decisions to use harmful substances, such as tobacco (Burtner, Wakham, McNeal, & Garvey, 1995).

TRANSPLANTATION

In a highly specialized area of transplantation, some literature is available about the additional ethical problems involved with special populations of people with cognitive impairments beyond the usual multitude of ethical problems surrounding transplantation in general (Johnston & Orr, 1999; Orr, Johnston, Ashwal, & Bailey, 2000; Spike, 1997).

EXPERIMENTATION AND RESEARCH

One of the most basic issues that is highly relevant to this chapter is whether any research should be done with this population, considering that their cognitive impairment makes it difficult to impossible to obtain appropriate informed consent from the involved person, and allowing them to become a subject in a research study. Although some authors have taken a stand against conducting such research (Edwards, 2000), most writers have supported research with some limitations: appropriate consent of a surrogate (Freedman, 2001), a cost to people with ID if important research is not done (i.e., a palliative or curative intervention for a related health condition cannot be studied; Haywood, 1977). A famous editor of the *New England Journal of Medicine* has weighed in on research for children with and without ID (Ingelfinger, 1973), controversial researcher at Willowbrook has set forth arguments that support his hepatitis studies (Krugman, 1986), and others have argued in favor of general acceptance of important research (Weisstub & Arboleda-Florez, 1997; Weisstub, Arboleda-Florez, & Tomossy, 1996). Even though many authors support research in general, there are numerous other problems that have been mentioned: often difficult dilemmas arise (Baudouin, 1990), participation may conflict with emphasis on protecting the rights of the person with mental impairment (Clayton, 1972), and individual rights may come into conflict with the state government aims and rights (Davis & Mahon, 1984). One researcher has made a plea for others to follow international principles such as the *Declaration of Helsinki* and the *International Ethics Guidelines for Biomedical Research Involving Human Subjects*, prepared by the Council for International Organizations of Medical Sciences (CIOMS—Harris, 1999). As has been mentioned several times in this chapter, consent of a surrogate is often the key to conducting needed research; however, institutional boards should be very careful about consent obtained from guardians and others (Dresser, 1996); others argue that consent may be obtained from the individual if an adequate attempt is made (Melton & Stanley, 1996), and yet others point out that the researcher bears an added burden of responsibility to guard the rights of the subject because it is difficult to obtain consent (Rosenfeld, 2002).

In an article from a somewhat different area of investigation although with highly relevant comments, Weiss (2001) cogently discusses the interplay of the three basic principles involved in deciding whether research projects meet ethical standards: (1) *justice*, which involves who bears the burdens of the research and who reaps its benefits, (2) *beneficence*, which requires research maximize the potential benefits to the subjects and minimize the risk to them, and (3) *respect for persons*, which requires subjects enter into research voluntarily and with adequate information. Weiss points out that there are some areas of research endeavor in which it is not possible to fulfill the intent of all three principles but yet the research has great benefit. If all three principles cannot be met, the other two principles should be followed. For example, in Weiss' area of environmental neurotoxin research, seldom can the third principle of informed consent be obtained, because the study may involve group data from a whole population. Nevertheless, the research is vital. This seems to summarize nicely the situation for many researchers in the field of ID unless appropriate substituted consent may be obtained.

SUMMARY

Perhaps the most important point that may be gleaned from this review of ethical issues in clinical service and research for the population of people with intellectual disabilities is that the topic and its literature encompass almost every aspect of dealing with the problem of impaired cognitive ability. Closure has seldom been obtained in this large array of issues although in the United States consensus seems to have been reached in a very few areas; for example, sterilization is no longer generally accepted as a method of treating sexual problems. All of this to say is that the general consensus on ethical issues has a very long way to go to reach acceptance by large portions of the general population, or very often, even consensus among key participants in developmental services, including the people with disabilities, their family members, and paraprofessionals and professionals who serve them. If any young researcher can tolerate intense controversy yet operate in an important, developing area, ethics of this special population may be a field of scholarship and research that offers advancement and rewards.

REFERENCES

Abusing the Unprotected: A Study of the Misuse of Aversive Behavior Modification Techniques and Weaknesses in the Regulatory Structure (BBB19993). (1987). Albany, NY: New York State Commission on Quality of Care for the Mentally Disabled.

Aman, M. G., & Singh, N. N. (Eds.). (1988). *Psychopharmacology of the developmental disabilities*. New York: Springer-Verlag.

Aman, M. G., & Singh, N. N. (1991). Pharmacological intervention. In J. L. Matson & J. A. Mulick (Eds.), *Handbook of mental retardation* (pp. 347–372). New York: Pergamon Press, Inc.

Annas, G. J. (1978). The incompetent's right to die: The case of Joseph Saikewicz. *Hastings Center Report, 8,* 21–23.

Annas, G. J. (1979). Reconciling Quinlan and Saikewicz: Decision making for the terminally ill incompetent. *American Journal of Law and Medicine, 4,* 367–396.

Aylott, J. (1999). Is the sexuality of people with a learning disability being denied? *British Journal of Nursing, 8,* 438–442.

Baudouin, J. L. (1990). Biomedical experimentation on the mentally handicapped: Ethical and legal dilemmas. *Medicine and Law, 9,* 1052–1061.

Bayley, C. (1980). Terminating treatment: Asking the right questions. *Hospital Progress, 61,* 50–53.

Brown, D., Rosen, D., & Elkins, T. E. (1992). Sedating women with mental retardation for routine gynecologic examination: An ethical analysis. *Journal of Clinical Ethics, 3,* 68–75.

Buchanan, A. (1979). Medical paternalism or legal imperialism: Not the only alternatives for handling Saikewicz-type cases. *American Journal of Law & Medicine, 5,* 97–117.

Burtner, A. P., Wakham, M. D., McNeal, D. R., & Garvey, T. P. (1995). Tobacco and the institutionalized mentally retarded: Usage choices and ethical considerations. *Special Care in Dentistry, 15,* 56–60.

Butterfield, E. C. (1990). The compassion of distinguishing punishing behavioral treatment from aversive treatment [Comment]. *American Journal of Mental Retardation, 95,* 137–141.

Clayton, T. (1972). Human rights, retardation, and research. *Hospital and Community Psychiatry, 23,* 81–84.

Connick, C., Palat, M., & Pugliese, S. (2000). The appropriate use of physical restraint: Considerations. *Journal of Dentistry for Children, 67,* 256–262.

Cook, J. W., Altman, K., & Haavik, S. (1978). Consent for aversive treatment: A model form. *Mental Retardation, 16,* 47–49.

Corbett, J. (1975). Aversion for the treatment of self-injurious behavior. *Journal of Mental Deficiency Research, 19,* 79–95.

Crabbe, H. F., & Handen, B. L. (1994). Pharmacotherapy in mental retardation. In N. Bouras (Ed.), *Mental health in mental retardation: Recent advances and practices* (pp. 187–204). New York: Cambridge University Press.Davis, A. J., & Mahon, K. A. (1984). Research with the mentally retarded and mentally ill: Rights and duties versus compelling state interest. *Journal of Advanced Nursing, 9,* 15–21.

Dresser, R. (1996). Mentally disabled research subjects. The enduring policy issues. *JAMA, 276,* 67–72.

Edwards, S. D. (2000). An argument against research on people with intellectual disabilities. *Medicine, Health Care, and Philosophy, 3,* 69–73.

Elder, J. H. (1996). Behavioral treatment of children with autism, mental retardation, and related disabilities: Ethics and efficacy. *Journal of Child and Adolescent Psychiatric Nursing, 9*, 28–36.

Eyman, R. K. (1998, Spring). Predictors of mortality, politics, and deinstitutionalization. *Psychology in Mental Retardation and Developmental Disabilities*, 4–10.

Ferleger, D., & Boyd, P. (1979). Anti-institutionalization: The promise of the Pennhurst case. *Stanford Law Review, 31*, 717–751.

Fletcher, J. C. (1995). Gene therapy in mental retardation: Ethical considerations. *Mental Retardation and Developmental Disabilities Research Reviews, 1*, 7–13.

Freeman, R. (1966). Drug effects on learning in children—A selective review of the past thirty years. *Journal of Special Education, 1*, 17–43.

Freedman, R. I. (2001). Ethical challenges in the conduct of research involving persons with mental retardation. *Mental Retardation, 39*, 130–141.

Friedmann, T. (1971). Prenatal diagnosis of genetic disease. *Scientific American, 225*, 34–42.

Gadow, K. D., & Poling, A. D. (1988). *Pharmacotherapy and mental retardation*. Boston, MA: College-Hill.

Gerhardt, P., Holmes, D. L., Alessandri, M., & Goodman, M. (1991). Social policy on the use of aversive interventions: Empirical, ethical, and legal considerations. *Journal of Autism and Developmental Disorders, 21*, 265–277.

Goldhaber, S. Z., Reardon, F. E., Goulart, D. T., & Rubin, I. L. (1985). Cardiac surgery for adults with mental retardation. Dilemmas in management. *American Journal of Medicine, 79*, 403–406.

Gualtieri, C. T., Keppel, J. M., & Schroeder, S. R. (1986). Tardive dyskinesia: Facts, issues and new recommendations. *Psychiatric Aspects of Mental Retardation Reviews, 5*, 6.

Hall, J. E., Morris, H. L., & Barker, H. R. (1973). Sexual knowledge and attitudes of mentally retarded adolescents. *American Journal of Mental Deficiency, 77*, 706–709.

Halstead, S. (2002). Service-user and professional issues. *Journal of Intellectual Disability Research, 46*(Suppl.), 31–46.

Harris, J. (1999). The principles of medical ethics and medical research. *Cadernos de Saude Publica, 15*(Suppl. 1), 7–13.

Harris, S. L., & Ersner-Hershfield, R. (1978). Behavioral suppression of seriously disruptive behavior in psychotic and retarded patients: A review of punishment and its alternatives. *Psychological Bulletin, 85*, 1352–1375.

Hauerwas, S. (1975). The demands and limits of care—Ethical reflections on the moral dilemma of neonatal intensive care. *American Journal of the Medical Sciences, 269*, 223–236.

Hayes, L. J., Hayes, G. J., Moore, S. C., & Ghezzi, P. M. (Eds.). (1994). *Ethical issues in developmental disabilities*. Reno, NV: University of Nevada.

Haywood, H. C. (1977). The ethics of doing research. . . and of not doing it. *American Journal of Mental Deficiency, 81*, 311–317.

Held, K. R. (1993). Ethical aspects of sexuality of persons with mental retardation. In M. Nagler (Ed.), *Perspectives on disability text and readings on disability* (2nd ed., pp. 255–259). Waterloo, Ontario: University of Waterloo.

Hemphill, M., & Freeman, J. M. (1977). Ethical aspects of care of the newborn with serious neurological disease. *Clinics in Perinatology, 4*, 201–209.

Higgs, R. (1983). Making up her mind: Consent, pregnancy and mental handicap. *Journal of Medical Ethics, 9*, 219–226.

Holden, C. (1990). What's holding up "aversives" report. *Science, 249*, 980–981.

Ingelfinger, F. J. (1973). Ethics of experiments on children. *New England Journal of Medicine, 288*, 791–792.

Iqbal, Z. (2002). Ethical issues involved in the implementation of a differential reinforcement of inappropriate behavior program for the treatment of social isolation and ritualistic behavior in an individual with intellectual disabilities. *Journal of Intellectual Disability Research, 46*, 82–93.

Jacobson, J. W. (1982). Problem behavior and psychiatric impairment within a developmentally disabled population 1: Behavior frequency. *Applied Research in Mental Retardation, 3*, 121–139.

Johnston, J. K., & Orr, R. D. (1999). Ethical challenges in infant heart transplantation: A clinical case presentation. *Journal of Transplant Coordination, 9,* 263–265.

Kalachnik, J. E. (1999). Psychotropic medication monitoring: "You tell me it's the institution well you know you better free your mind instead." In N. A. Wieseler & H. R. Hanson (Eds.), *Challenging behavior of persons with mental disorders and severe developmental disabilities* (pp. 151–203). Washington, DC: AAMR Books.

Kalachnik, J. E., & Sprague, R. L. (1994). How well do physicians, pharmacists, and psychologists assess tardive dyskinesia movement? *The Annals of Pharmacotherapy, 28,* 185–190.

Katzen, M. (1971). The decision to treat myelomeningocele on the first day of life. *South African Medical Journal, 45,* 345–349.

Kay, B. (1995). Grasping the research nettle in learning disabilities nursing. *British Journal of Nursing, 4,* 96–98.

Kluge, E. H. (1987). After "Eve": Whither proxy decision-making? *Canadian Medical Association Journal, 137,* 715–720.

Krugman, S. (1986). The Willowbrook hepatitis studies revisited: Ethical aspects. *Reviews of Infectious Diseases, 8,* 157–162.

Kujdych, N., Lowe, D. A., Sparks, J., Dottes, A., & Crook, E. D. (2000). Dignity or denial? Decisions regarding initiation of dialysis and medical therapy in the institutionalized severely mentally retarded. *American Journal of the Medical Sciences, 320,* 374–378.

Landau, R. J. (1996). Professional advocacy and legal issues. In J. W. Jacobson & J. A. Mulick (Eds.), *Manual of diagnosis and professional practice in mental retardation* (pp. 413–422). Washington, DC: American Psychological Association.

Lerman, D. C., Iwata, B. A., Shore, B. A., & DeLeon, I. G. (1997). Effects of intermittent punishment on self-injurious behavior: An evaluation of schedule thinning. *Journal of Applied Behavior Analysis, 30,* 187–201.

Lesser, E. K. (1986). An overview of the medical school curriculum in mental retardation and strategies for change. *Annals of the New York Academy of Sciences, 477,* 339–345.

Lewis, M. H., Aman, M. G., Gadow, K. D., Schroeder, S. R., & Thompson, T. (1996). Psychopharmacology. In J. W. Jacobson & J. A. Mulick (Eds.), *Manual of diagnosis and professional practice in mental retardation* (pp. 323–340). Washington, DC: American Psychological Association.

MacNamara, R. D. (1994). The Mansfield Training School is closed: The swamp has been finally drained. *Mental Retardation, 32,* 239–242.

Martyn, S. R. (1994). Substituted judgment, best interests, and the need for best respect. *Cambridge Quarterly of Healthcare Ethics, 3,* 195–208.

Mason, G., & Menolascino, F. (1976). The right to treatment for mentally retarded citizens: An evolving legal and scientific interface. *Creighton Law Review, 10,* 124–166.

McDonnell, A. (1996). Phasing out seclusion through staff training and support. *Nursing Times, 92,* 43–44.

Meinhold, P. (1996, Fall). An advocate's story: Do we accept or challenge community views of behavioral treatments? *Psychology in Mental Retardation and Developmental Disabilities,* 12–17.

Melton, G. B., & Stanley, B. H. (1996). Research involving special populations. In B. H. Stanley & J. E. Sieber (Eds.), *Research ethics: A psychological approach* (pp. 177–202). Lincoln, NE: University of Nebraska Press.

Mims, J., & Crisham, P. (1996). Health care management of children with cognitive and physical disabilities: To treat or not to treat. *Journal of Neuroscience Nursing, 28,* 238–244.

Moon, J. B., & Graber, G. C. (1985). When Danny said no! Refusal of treatment by a patient of questionable competence. *Journal of Medical Humanities and Bioethics, 6,* 12–27.

Mulick, J. A. (1990). The ideology and science of punishment in mental retardation. *American Journal of Mental Retardation, 95,* 142–156.

Murphy, G. (1993). The use of aversive stimuli in treatment: The issue of consent. *Journal of Intellectual Disability Research, 37,* 211–219.

National Institutes of Health. (1991). *Treatment of destructive behavior in persons with developmental disabilities (DHHS Publication No. 91-2410).* Washington, DC: National Institutes of Health.

Norris, J. A. (1979). More on appropriate decision making for the terminally ill incompetent patient. *American Journal of Law and Medicine, 5*, 1–6.

O'Hara, J. (1989). Pregnancy in a severely mentally handicapped adult. *Journal of Medical Ethics, 15*, 197–199.

Oliver, M. N., Yutrzenka, B. A., & Redinius, P. L. (2002). Residential paraprofessionals' perceptions of and responses to work-related ethical dilemmas. *Mental Retardation, 40*, 235–242.

Orr, R. D., Johnston, J. K., Ashwal, S., & Bailey, L. L. (2000). Should children with severe cognitive impairment receive solid organ transplants? *Journal of Clinical Ethics, 11*, 219–229.

O'Sullivan, J. L., & Borcherding, B. G. (2002). Informed consent for medication in persons with mental retardation and mental illness. *Health Matrix, 12*, 63–92.

Patterson, P., & Robinson, R. (Eds.). (1982). *Drugs in litigation: Damage awards involving prescription and nonprescription drugs*. Indianapolis, IN: The Allen Smith Company.

Petchesky, R. P. (1979). Reproduction, ethics, and public policy: The federal sterilization regulations. *Hastings Center Report, 9*, 29–41.

Plotkin, R., & Gill, K. (1979). Invisible manacles: Drugging mentally retarded people. *Stanford Law Review, 31*, 637–678.

Poling, A. (1994). Pharmacological treatment of behavioral problems in people with mental retardation: Some ethical considerations. In L. J. Hayes, G. J. Hayes, S. C. Moore & P. M. Ghezzi (Eds.), *Ethical issues in developmental disabilities* (pp. 149–177). Reno, NV: University of Nevada.

Pollack, A. (2003, January 15). Gene therapy trials halted. *New York Times*.

Reich, W. T. (1987). Caring for life in the first of it: Moral paradigms for perinatal and neonatal ethics. *Seminars in Perinatology, 11*, 279–287.

Reinders, H. S. (2002a). The ethics of behavior modification: A comment on ethical issues in the implementation of a DRI program for the treatment of social isolation and ritualistic behavior in a learning disabled individual. *Journal of Intellectual Disability Research, 46*, 187–190.

Reinders, J. S. I. (2002b). The good life for citizens with intellectual disability. *Journal of Intellectual Disability Research, 46*, 1–5.

Relman, A. S. (1979). A response to Allen Buchanan's views on decision making for terminally ill incompetents. *American Journal of Law and Medicine, 5*, 119–123.

Repp, A. C. (1978). On the ethical responsibilities of institutions providing services for mentally retarded people. *Mental Retardation, 16*, 153–156.

Repp, A. C., & Deitz, D. E. (1978). Ethical issues in reducing responding of institutionalized mentally retarded persons. *Mental Retardation, 16*, 45–46.

Reynolds, E. O. (1978). Neonatal intensive care and the prevention of major handicap. *Ciba Foundation Symposium, 59*, 77–106.

Rojahn, J., Borthwick-Duffy, S. A., & Jacobson, J. W. (1993). The association between psychiatric diagnosis and severe behavior problems in mental retardation. *Annals of Clinical Psychiatry, 5*, 163–170.

Rosenfeld, B. (2002). Competence to consent to research: Where psychology, ethics, and the law intersect. *Ethics and Behavior, 12*, 284–287.

Rothman, D., & Rothman, S. (1984). *The Willowbrook wars*. New York: Harper and Row.

Sajwaj, T. (1977). Issues and implications of establishing guidelines for the use of behavioral techniques. *Journal of Applied Behavior Analysis, 10*, 531–540.

Schroeder, S. R. (1985). Issues and future research directions of pharmacotherapy in mental retardation. *Psychopharmacology Bulletin, 21*, 323–326.

Schroeder, S. R., & Schroeder, C. S. (1989). The role of the AAMR in the aversives controversy. *Mental Retardation, 27*, 3–5.

Shevell, M. I. (1998). Clinical ethics and developmental delay. *Seminars in Pediatric Neurology, 5*, 70–75.

Singer, P. (1983). Non-intervention in children with major disabilities. *Australian Paediatric Journal, 19*, 215–216.

Singh, N. N., Guernsey, T. F., & Ellis, C. R. (1992). Drug therapy for persons with developmental disabilities: Legislation and litigation. *Clinical Psychology Review, 12*, 665–679.

Smolev, S. R. (1971). Use of operant techniques for the modification of self-injurious behavior. *American Journal of Mental Deficiency, 76*, 295–305.

Spike, J. (1997). What's love got to do with it? The altruistic giving of organs. *Journal of Clinical Ethics, 8*, 165–170.

Sprague, R. L. (1972). Psychopharmacology and learning disabilities. *Journal of Operational Psychiatry, 3*, 56–67.

Sprague, R. L. (1977). Overview of psychopharmacology for the retarded in the United States. In P. Mittler (Ed.), *Research to practice in mental retardation—Biomedical aspects* (Vol. 3, pp. 199–203). Baltimore, MD: University Park Press.

Sprague, R. L. (1978). Psychopharmacology of the mentally retarded: Present and future. *Psychopharmacology Bulletin, 14*, 63–65.

Sprague, R. L. (1982a). Litigation legislation, and regulations. In S. E. Breuning & A. D. Poling (Eds.), *Drugs and mental retardation* (pp. 377–414). Springfield, IL: Charles C. Thomas.

Sprague, R. L. (1982b). *The rights of mentally retarded people.* Paper presented at Symposium at the meeting of the International Conference on Psychology and Law, Swansea, Wales.

Sprague, R. L. (1994). Ethics of treatment evaluation: Balancing efficacy against other considerations. In T. Thompson & D. B. Gray (Eds.), *Destructive behavior in developmental disabilities* (pp. 293–311). Thousand Oaks, CA: Sage Publications.

Sprague, R. L. (1995). *Basic concepts of psychopharmacology for people with developmental disabilities.* Algonquin, IL: Creative Core, Inc.

Sprague, R. L., & Baxley, G. (1978). Drugs for behavior management, with comment on some legal aspects. In J. Wortis (Ed.) *Mental retardation* (Vol. 10, pp. 92–129). New York: Brunner/Mazel.

Sprague, R. L., & Galliher, L. (1988). Litigation about psychotropic medication. In K. D. Gadow & A. D. Poling (Eds.), *Pharmacotherapy and mental retardation* (pp. 297–312). Boston, MA: College-Hill.

Sprague, R. L., & Kalachnik, J. E. (1991). Reliability, validity, and a total score cutoff for the dyskinesia identification system: Condensed User Scale (DISCUS) with mentally ill and mentally retarded populations. *Psychopharmacology Bulletin, 27*, 51–58.

Sprague, R. L., & Werry, J. (1971). Methodology of psychopharmacological studies with the retarded, *International Review of research in mental retardation* (Vol. 5, pp. 147–219). New York: Academic Press.

St Amant, M., Elkins, T. E., Brown, D., & Pastorek, J. G. (1993). Should all pregnant patients be offered prenatal diagnosis regardless of age? *Obstetrics and Gynecology, 82*, 315–316.

Stolz, S. B. (1977). Why no guidelines for behavior modification? *Journal of Applied Behavior Analysis, 10*, 541–547.

Strudler, A. (1988). Self-determination, incompetence, and medical jurisprudence. *Journal of Medicine and Philosophy, 13*, 349–365.

Tannsjo, T. (1999). Informal coercion in the physical care of patients suffering from senile dementia or mental retardation. *Nursing Ethics: An International Journal for Health Care Professionals, 6*, 327–336.

Teasdale, K., & Kent, G. (1995). The use of deception in nursing. *Journal of Medical Ethics, 21*, 77–81.

van Waarde, J. A., Stolker, J. J., & van der Mast, R. C. (2001). ECT in mental retardation: A review. *Journal of ECT, 17*, 236–243.

Weiss, B. (2001). Ethics assessment as an adjunct to risk assessment in the evaluation of developmental neurotoxicants. *Environmental Health Perspectives, 109*(Suppl. 6), 905–908.

Weisstub, D. N., & Arboleda-Florez, J. (1997). Ethical research with the developmentally disabled. *Canadian Journal of Psychiatry. Revue Canadienne de Psychiatrie, 42*, 492–496.

Weisstub, D. N., Arboleda-Florez, J., & Tomossy, G. F. (1996). Establishing the boundaries of ethically permissible research with special populations. *Health Law in Canada, 17*, 45–63.

Werry, J. S., & Aman, M. G. (Eds.). (1999). *Practitioner's guide to psychoactive drugs for children and adolescents* (2nd ed.). New York: Plenum Medical Book Company.

Wigal, T., Wigal, S. B., Fulbright, K. K., Ackerland, V., Dean, D. B., Swanson, J. M., et al. (1996). Standardized videotape procedure for evaluating withdrawal-emergent tardive dyskinesia in a public residential facility. *Journal of Developmental and Psychical Diseases, 8*, 375–389.

Wszola, B. A., Newell, K. M., & Sprague, R. L. (2001). Risk factors for tardive dyskinesia in a large population of youths and adults. *Experimental and Clinical Psychopharmacology, 9*, 285–296.

Ye, X., Mitchell, M., Newman, K., & Batshaw, M. L. (2001). Prospects for prenatal gene therapy in disorders causing mental retardation. *Mental Retardation and Developmental Disabilities Research Reviews, 7*, 65–72.

Zuker-Weiss, R. (1994). Sex, mental retardation and ethics. *International Journal of Adolescent Medicine and Health, 7*, 193–197.

35

Ethics and Values in Behavioral Perspective

LINDA J. HAYES and JONATHAN TARBOX

Ethical situations are complex circumstances in which actors take one or another course of action upon having engaged in evaluative responses with respect to the anticipated consequences of those actions (Hayes, Adams, & Rydeen, 1994). So analyzed, ethical conduct comprised two phases, a first phase in which the anticipated consequences of alternative courses of action are compared with reference to standards of right and wrong, and a second phase in which the course of action leading to the consequences deemed right by that comparison is taken. From this perspective, the responses to future (i.e., absent) circumstances implicated in the first phase of such situations are not held to arise from within the responding organism, but are rather assumed to be coordinated with substitute stimulus functions having their sources in currently participating verbal events; whereas the action taken in the second phase is interpreted as an end point in an historical continuity of action, also implying the absence of agency in such events.

This interpretation of ethical situations and ethical conduct is at odds with that prevailing in the culture at large. The conventional interpretation of ethical conduct implicates the participation of a metaphysical entity in such events, namely the soul or mind, along with its faculties of conscience and will (Kantor, 1991.) More explicitly, the conventional position holds that the first phase of ethical conduct, in which the consequences of alternative courses of action are considered, is guided by the soul's faculty of conscience; whereas the action taken in the second phase is interpreted an ahistorical choice arising from within the actor and being put into motion by the power of the will. By this account, the assumptions underlying the

LINDA J. HAYES • Psychology Department, University of Nevada, Reno, Reno, Nevada 89557.   JONATHAN TARBOX • Center for Autism and Related Disorders, Tarzana, California 91356 prevailing view of ethical situations and ethical conduct must be regarded as antithetical to the postulates of behavior science. Indeed, the prevailing view of ethical events reflects an understanding of human beings and human behavior that is diametrically opposed to that held by behavior analysts.

This circumstance should come as no surprise to behavior analysts. After all, behaviorism is a rogue philosophy, its views typically at odds with more conventional understandings, particularly as they pertain to the human condition. In fact, its break with tradition on such matters is one of the most distinguishing features of behaviorism as a philosophical system. At the center of this debate, ontologically considered, is the nature of all things—whether it be constituted of one "stuff" or two—along with the implications of these alternatives for the place of humankind in the universe.

Still, no matter how well aligned with the premises of a particular technical philosophy one's beliefs may be, no one is completely immune to influence from cultural sources, including behavior analysts. As such, behavior analysts may occasionally find themselves in the uneasy circumstance of holding conflicting beliefs about decidedly nontrivial issues; and given how deeply ingrained in conventional thinking is the assumption that values fall outside the boundaries of scientific consideration, this circumstance is especially likely to present itself when issues of value come into play. The outcome of this circumstance is that psychological events in which valuing acts figure prominently are especially likely to be misinterpreted by behavior scientists. Such is the case of ethical conduct.

ETHICS AND BEHAVIOR SCIENCE

Ethics are prescriptions for the instantiation of societal values. They characterize the fundamental affordances of a society to its members as members' rights. In the United States, for example, these affordances are specified in the *Bill of Rights*. In various domains of human activity below the level of the society at large, ethical prescriptions address threats to human welfare uniquely present in those domains. For example, in the domain of scientific research, clients are afforded the right of informed consent; whereas in the domain of habilitative services, clients are afforded the right of effective treatment.

At the societal level, as well as at the level of these more specific domains, rights tend to be articulated as descriptions of experiences reflecting particular societal values. Missing in ethical prescriptions is the means by which the prescribed outcomes are to be achieved. This is to say, rules for effective action on the parts of the guarantors of societal rights remain unspecified in such statements. As such, the values of a society are not revealed in the occurrence or nonoccurrence of particular actions on the parts of those responsible for their instantiation. Instead, they are revealed in the experiences of its members. The actual experiences of a society's members may or may not be aptly characterized by the descriptions of experiences articulated in statements of member's rights. However, to whatever extent they are characterized by these descriptions, that is the extent to which whatever actions have been taken by those responsible for bringing them about are held to have been successful and, in having been so, may also be held to be justifiable.

Operationally, peoples' experiences may be understood as the contingencies operating with respect to their behavior: They amount to what people do under various conditions and what happens as a result. From this perspective, the rights afforded by a society to its members may be understood as descriptions of contingencies prescribed for operation with respect to members' behavior, otherwise known as rules.

When the contingencies described in prescriptive rules match those in actual operation, the values of the society are upheld and their nature is revealed. This outcome is more likely to be achieved if prescriptions of this sort are articulated as complete rules than if some of their features are missing however; and, as discussed above, it is typical of such rules to leave unspecified the means by which the contingencies they prescribe may be brought about. Rules of this sort, in specifying no path to follow, are not followed in the ordinary sense in which rules serve as guides to effective action (Skinner, 1969). Instead, they constitute attempts to illustrate the values of a society by depicting what ought to happen when its members act in particular ways under particular conditions.

The notion that societal values are reflected in the actions of societal members under particular sets of conditions, along with the consequences of those actions, presents a sizeable opportunity for the field of behavior analysis. Behavior analytic strategies are unrivaled in their capacity to induce acts of particular sorts under particular conditions; and, importantly, this capacity extends to acts of arranging the conditions under which the actions of others may be induced. To take advantage of this opportunity, though, it must be deemed possible to find evidence of values in these sources, and an unconventional approach to the concept of values is entailed in the adoption of this premise.

The latter presents a significant challenge given that psychological events in which valuing acts figure prominently are especially prone to misinterpretation as a result of influence from cultural sources, as previously mentioned. To put it plainly, behavior scientists must be especially careful to resist corruption from conventional thinking on the subject of ethics if we are to take advantage of the opportunity the effectuality of our discipline affords in this context.

If the strength of behavior analysis is at least partially attributable to its opposition to traditional views, failing to stand our ground on the subject of ethics does not bode well for our future. More pointedly, in as much as the "future" may be understood as a verbal construction derived from elaborate descriptions of present circumstance (Hayes, 1997), the future has already arrived and we are already in trouble on this issue. Evidence of behavior analysts' alignment with conventional views on matters of ethics and values is already available. The most obvious indication of this alignment is seen in the participation of behavior analysts in deliberate efforts to afford rights of "self-determination" and "freedom of choice" to persons with profound cognitive disabilities. If the source of our discipline's strength and utility may be traced to its departure from conventional views, supporting practices compromised by their conformity to premises that are antithetical to those of behaviorism is decidedly not in our interest.

Our aim in this chapter, therefore, is to characterize ethical situations and ethical conduct from a behavioral perspective. Our purpose in doing so is to reaffirm our convictions as behaviorists and to foster whatever reconfigurations of our practices as are needed to bring them into greater accord with those convictions. In what follows, behavioral perspectives on the nature and participation of various aspects of ethical conduct are contrasted with more conventional interpretations of these phenomena for the purpose of isolating and clarifying the underlying premises of the former. As B. F. Skinner is the founder and foremost authority on the behavior analytic perspective in psychology, as well as the most prolific writer on the subject of ethics and value from this perspective, his views on these issues are taken as representative of those of behavior analysts at large. Accordingly, Skinner's (1953, 1957, 1969, 1971, 1974) contributions to these issues are examined in considerable detail, as well as subjected to critical evaluation. Out of these considerations, and in keeping with features of J. R. Kantor's (1958, 1981, 1991) analyses of these issues, we propose what we regard as a more coherent naturalistic interpretation of a more comprehensive set of ethical phenomena than has heretofore been available for consideration by the behavior analytic community. Finally, we discuss the implications of our interpretation of these phenomena for applications of the science of behavior to problems of human adjustment.

THE FIRST PHASE OF ETHICAL SITUATIONS: ETHICAL VALUATION

As previously mentioned, we view ethical situations as being divisible into two phases on the basis of the types of activity taking place in each. In the first of these phases, persons engage in valuative acts with respect to alternative courses of action, whereas in the second phase, the alternative deemed relatively more valuable is pursued. We begin, then, by considering the events of the first of these phases.

More precisely, during the first phase of an ethical situation, persons interact with the anticipated consequences of different courses of action, through which the relative values of those consequences, in meeting societal standards of right and wrong, are determined. As this is a complex set of events, with a number of significant implications for service delivery, further clarification as to the factors participating in such events is warranted. To be addressed in this context are the nature and provenance of ethical standards, the means by which knowledge of right and wrong is acquired, and the implications of these analyses for the concept of personal responsibility. Further, as this phase involves knowing and valuing acts, and both are occurring with respect to future (and thereby absent) conditions, these two types of activity are analyzed under conditions in which relevant stimuli are absent. Traditional views on these issues are provided to clarify the behavior analytic perspective through contrast. We begin with the issue of standards.

The Nature and Provenance of Ethical Standards

Ethical standards, as discussed herein, are roughly synonymous with the highest values of a particular group. More precisely, ethical standards are the criteria upon which events and/or conditions are able to be placed into dichotomous categories of right and wrong or good and bad. For example, if a group considers happiness to be more valuable than any other condition, then whatever maximizes happiness is held to be good or right, whatever diminishes it, bad or wrong. The nature and provenance of ethical standards are matters about which philosophers disagree. In the following sections we consider these disagreements. Two traditional perspectives are compared to behavior analytic views on these issues.

Traditional Perspectives

Broadly speaking, traditional ethicists are divided into two main groups with respect to the nature and provenance of ethical standards (Kantor, 1991.) One prominent group of ethical philosophers promotes the view that right and wrong are stable, absolute categories. In other words, what falls into each of these categories is not subject to interpretation in keeping with circumstantial variations. What is right is always right; what is wrong is always wrong.

The other group takes a relativistic view of these standards. The relativistic position (e.g., Cooper, 1978) holds that there are no stable criteria by which the rightfulness or wrongfulness of conduct may be judged, nor is there a rational basis for determining the rightfulness of different moral judgments. Instead, what falls into these categories amounts to whatever meets the needs of a particular group at a particular time. Accordingly, what is right for one group at one time is not necessarily right for another group at the same time or for the same group at a different time.

Different views as to the nature of ethical standards also imply different premises as to their provenance. As previously mentioned, ethical absolutists presume that right and wrong are stable categories. This argument demands that the source of these categories be of an otherworldly sort. To put it another way, given that the most fundamental characteristic of all natural things is change, that which is held to be unchanging in principle must be regarded as issuing from a supernatural source. By this logic, ethical absolutists hold that what is right or wrong is determined by an all-knowing deity. Moreover, in as much as no situation escapes the purview of an all-knowing deity, ethical standards are not merely absolute from this perspective. They are also universal, which is to say, they apply to all things, in all circumstances, for all time.

By contrast, having taken the position that what falls into the categories of right and wrong is whatever meets the needs of a particular group at a particular time, as argued by ethical relativists, there is no alternative but to suggest that ethical standards have their sources in the cultural circumstances of particular groups at particular times. From a relativistic perspective, ethical standards are culturally determined, and because cultural circumstances are ever changing and multitudinous, they are incapable of giving rise to stable or universal standards of right and wrong.

The Behavioral Position

Obviously, the position of ethical absolutists with respect to standards of right and wrong, as discussed above, is not a position to which behavior scientists may subscribe, at least not in their roles as scientists. Otherworldly entities of the sort implicated in this position have no existence from a scientific standpoint. Hence, an understanding of ethical situations and ethical conduct, articulated in terms of the roles played by such entities, must be excluded from scientific consideration.

By contrast, the obligation of a scientist in attempting to understand circumstances of these sorts is rather to identify the natural factors comprising them, along with their organization and interrelations. Among the factors involved are particular persons with particular histories interacting with particular materials in particular contexts (Kantor, 1953)—none of which has the character of "all things" for "all time." As Kantor (1991, p. 163) puts it, "There is lacking in most if not all philosophical systems the humility of appreciating that universal systems are really the constructions of particular persons with specific capacities and with a large or small fund of unique experiences throughout a particular behavior history."

The alternative proposed by ethical relativists falls short of behavior analytic sensibilities as well. At least this may be said of behaviorists following Skinner's lead in such matters. As it applies to the *nature* of ethical standards, Skinner does not subscribe to a position of ethical relativism. Although not a theist, as discussed above, Skinner asserts an absolute criterion against which conduct may be evaluated as right and wrong. That criterion is "survival" (Skinner, 1971). From Skinner's standpoint, whatever assures survival is held to be right or good, whereas whatever threatens it is regarded as wrong or bad.

It is important to recognize that adopting absolute standards of right and wrong does not imply standardization with respect to the actions productive of outcomes having these values. The survival of a species is a case in point. The survival of a species may be assured by one set of actions at a given point in its evolution whereas, at another point, actions of a different sort may have this effect. For example, Skinner (1974) explains that a heightened susceptibility to reinforcement by sugar, through which behaviors producing contact with this substance would be maintained at strength, was critical to the survival of the human species at a time when sugar, even in small quantities, was not readily available. As much greater quantities and concentrations of sugar became available, a heightened susceptibility to reinforcement by sugar would engender obesity in the population, therein posing a threat to its survival. In short, what achieves the good of survival for the species varies as circumstances vary.

Knowing Right from Wrong

Traditional and behavioral views also differ as to the means by which persons are assumed to have knowledge of ethical standards, and these differences point to different conclusions as to the matter of personal responsibility for ethical behavior. These issues are discussed below.

The Traditional Position

In accordance with their more general assumptions concerning the nature of ethical situations, ethical philosophers have proposed different means by which an individual comes to know right from wrong. Further elaboration of the theistically oriented, absolutist position suggests that a person's knowledge of right and wrong arises out of his or her special relation to the source of these standards. In essence, the presence of such knowledge defines the human condition. Accordingly, responsibility for the rightfulness or wrongfulness of persons' actions is theirs to bear, as are the consequences of such. Rightful conduct is thereby deserving of praise and reward, wrongful conduct of blame and punishment or, in the extreme, of eternal life and eternal damnation, respectively.

Relativists, by contrast, argue that knowledge of right and wrong is acquired over the course of a person's experiences as a member of a culture. The culture as a source of such knowledge is not typically taken to mean that the culture is also the source of control over behavior, however. Rather, it is generally assumed that knowledge of right and wrong, having been absorbed from this source, prevails thereafter as a personal possession. As such, it is available for consultation prior to the occurrence of actions having an ethical connotation. This is to say engaging in rightful or wrongful action is assumed to be knowingly done. A person is thereby responsible for his or her actions in this regard and, as such, is also deserving of the consequences for those actions as meted out by the society.

The Behavioral Position

From a behavior analytic perspective, knowledge is not a thing. It thereby cannot be instilled as a thing by a deity, nor can it be possessed as a thing by an organism, as argued by traditional ethical philosophers. Instead, knowing is behaving. Skinner explains, "We do not act by putting knowledge to use, our knowledge *is* action, or at least rules for action" (Skinner, 1974, p. 139, emphasis his). More technically, from Skinner's perspective, *knowing* is behaving, and knowledge is a way of referring to a behavioral repertoire. Specifically, knowledge is behavior that is not occurring at the present time but that has occurred previously and thereby has some potential of occurring again (Skinner, 1974). In his words, "(I)t is potential behavior which is called knowledge" (Skinner, 1957, p. 363).

Knowing right from wrong exemplifies the most complex category of knowing discussed by Skinner: It is a case of "contemplative knowing about." Skinner's concept of "knowing about," as distinguished from the simpler case of "knowing how," entails multiple forms of overt action with respect to a given set of circumstances (Skinner, 1957, 1974). In his words, "We know *about* electricity if we can work successfully, verbally and otherwise, with electrical things" (Skinner, 1974, p. 138, emphasis added).

Skinner's characterization of "contemplative knowing" is less clear. Acts of contemplative knowing, or "knowing short of action" (Skinner, 1974, p. 140), are interpreted as private events, and although private events are admissible subjects of inquiry from the perspective of Radical Behaviorism, Skinner is not inclined to speculate as to the characteristics of such events beyond denying their possession of nonnatural properties and dismissing their causal status with respect to public response events (Parrott, 1983b). Accordingly, Skinner's (1957, 1974) description of contemplative knowing lacks detail as to the nature of such events at the time of their occurrence (Parrott, 1983a). From his perspective, contemplative knowing is manifested as subsequent overt behavior occurring when circumstances appropriate for its occurrence are encountered (Skinner, 1974.) As he puts it, "The term 'know' refers to a hypothetical intermediate condition which is detected only at a later date" (Skinner, 1957, p. 363).

Whatever might be the utility of dismissing contemplative knowing as a hypothetical event under other analytical circumstances, it has little to recommend it in the present context. As previously mentioned, the second phase of an ethical situation is one in which one or another course of action, the consequences of which have been imagined in the first phase, is taken. Although it might be tempting to view such action as the missing overt behavior implicated in Skinner's analysis of contemplative knowing, to do so would suggest that "knowing what is right" is the same event as "engaging in rightful behavior" minus an appropriate opportunity for the latter. It seems obvious that a person can engage in wrongful behavior despite knowing what is right, though. Similarly, a person can engage in rightful behavior without knowing that it is right. Hence, it seems more fruitful to conceptualize the events of knowing right from wrong as distinct from the events of acting rightfully or wrongfully. The former are characteristic of the first phase of an ethical situation, the latter, of the second phase.

Toward this end, we would suggest that contemplative knowing, as a form of contemporaneous activity, may be viewed as a configuration of verbal and perceptual behaviors occurring with respect to immediately present sources of stimulation (Parrott, 1983a, 1986). Contemplative knowing of right and wrong, as applied to the anticipated consequences of alternative courses of action, may then be viewed as a more complex case of such activity, the complication arising from the absence of pertinent stimulus objects (i.e., the consequences of behaviors yet to occur) in the immediate environment.

Behaving with respect to absent stimulus objects, we would argue, is possible of occurrence if the stimulus functions of those objects operate from other, immediately present, object sources (Kantor, 1958; Parrott, 1983b). For example, if seeing an apple is simulated by an apple, and the verbal stimulus "apple" is also present in such circumstances, then seeing an apple may be stimulated by the stimulus "apple" when no actual apple is present. A great deal has been written about events of these sorts and the details of these interpretations are beyond the scope of the present argument. Our point in raising the issue here is to distinguish *knowing* what is right from *doing* what is right so as to provide a means of differentiating ethical from nonethical behavior under undifferentiated circumstances.

Although Skinner (1974) does not address the perceptual components of knowing acts in any detail (although, see Skinner, 1957, p. 22), he would agree as to the role of verbal activity in such circumstances. In his view, to behave rightfully (i.e., in such a way that one's survival is assured), is one thing; to "know" that one is behaving rightfully is quite another. Self-knowing or self-awareness, as involved here, is viewed as acting verbally with respect to one's own behavior in Skinner's system (1957, 1974). Hence, although it may be possible for a person to engage in rightful conduct without knowing that he/she does so, it is not possible for a person to know that he/she does so in the absence of a verbal repertoire.

Accordingly, in order for persons to participate in the first phase of an ethical situation, in which the consequences of alternative courses of action are considered in light of cultural standards of right and wrong, they must be equipped with verbal repertoires. Moreover, these repertoires must be sufficiently elaborate as to include the capacity to describe contingency relations, or rules, and to act under their control. This is the case because the alternatives present in ethical situations always include acts producing personal goods pitted against acts producing goods for others (or the culture), and acts of the latter sort cannot be sustained in the absence of a capacity for rule governance.

As to the issue of personal responsibility for ethical conduct, from a behavior analytic perspective knowing that one is engaging in rightful conduct (as well as doing so without this knowledge) is held to constitute a learned act, established by way of direct contact with contingencies or by exposure to contingency-specifying rules. What a person knows (and does) in an ethical situation is thereby entirely attributable to their experiences in and with such situations. Hence, the responsibility for ethical conduct lies not with the individual *per se* as a matter of inner virtue, but rather with the contingencies and rules to which an individual has been exposed as a member of a particular cultural group. Hence, from a behavioral perspective, praise for ethical conduct and blame for a lack of it are not heaped upon the individual but rather upon the conditions responsible for such conduct.

As previously asserted, ethical situations comprised two phases, the first entailing behavior with respect to the anticipated consequences of alternative courses of action in terms of their conformity to cultural standards of right and wrong. We have discussed the nature of such acts, the means by which they are acquired, and how they are enacted in such situations. We have also discussed the nature and provenance of the standards involved as well as the implications of these analyses for the concept of personal responsibility for ethical behavior.

THE SECOND PHASE OF ETHICAL SITUATIONS: ETHICAL CONDUCT

We turn now to the second phase of an ethical situation, in which one or the other of the alternative courses of action considered in the first phase is taken. We may regard the action in this phase as ethical conduct proper. Again, we examine both traditional and behavior analytic interpretations of these events.

Choosing Rightful or Wrongful Courses of Action

One of the most fundamental differences between the traditional and behavioral perspectives is revealed in their views on the issue of choice. So important for the organization of cultural practices is the traditional perspective on this issue that even those operating as behaviorists may fail to appreciate the logic and significance of the behavioral perspective on this issue. These differences are discussed below.

The Traditional Position

In traditional perspective, the circumstances under which an ethical act occurs, if it does, are those in which a person *could* have acted in an unethical manner. This is to say, the action taken in such circumstances is not viewed as an inevitable outcome of the person's behavioral history. Rather, the alternative courses of action in such circumstances are assumed to constitute real alternatives for the actor. As such, the action ultimately taken under such circumstances is regarded as secondary to the act of deciding which action among the available alternatives to take.

Further, as the act of deciding which action to take, like the action ultimately taken in an ethical situation, is conceptualized ahistorically, it must be assumed to arise from an independent and incorruptible part of the person, namely the mind or soul. The responsibility for ethical conduct is thereby borne by this internal entity, and its capacity to assume this responsibility is attributed to the various faculties and powers it is assumed to possess, among which are the faculty of conscience (i.e., knowledge of right and wrong), and the power of the will. Accordingly, the act of choosing among the alternative courses of action present in an ethical situation is held to be an act of conscience, instigated by the power of the will, and for which the individual bears personal responsibility.

The Behavioral Position

From a behavioral perspective, a person is not regarded as a duality of his or her behavior and a mysterious entity responsible for that behavior.

Rather, at a psychological level of analysis, a person is nothing more than his or her behavior, the responsibility for which lies with the environment. Further, the current behavior of a person is held to be continuous with his or her historical actions (Hayes, 1992.) As such, although an ethical situation may present alternative courses of action from the standpoint of an observer this does not imply that these alternatives exist for the person involved in an ethical situation. From a behavioral perspective, an ethical situation does not represent a circumstance in which a person *could* behave in one way or the other. Rather, the action taken is the action a person's history and current circumstances have prepared him or her to take. To put it another way, the only action that could be taken under such circumstances is the action that is taken.

This being the case, the "choice" made under such conditions is simply the action a person takes, not something upon which a person takes action. As Skinner puts it, "To exercise a choice is simply to act, and the choice a person is capable of making is the act itself" (1974, p. 113).

SURVIVAL AS AN ABSOLUTE STANDARD OF VALUE

Skinner's contributions to issues of value are much more extensive than what we have thus far addressed and our depiction of ethics from a behavioral perspective would be incomplete without further discussion of his contributions. As previously mentioned, Skinner (1971) adopts survival as the absolute standard of goodness for his system. He further articulates the meaning and significance of this standard in three distinct domains of inquiry, including: the phylogenies of species, the behaviors of organisms, and the practices of cultures.

Technically, however, the standard of survival is applicable only in the context of biological evolution. In this context, whatever genetic structure survives the selective action of the environment is held to be good by default. Something analogous to survival is needed for use in the psychological domain, and by abstracting the property of sustainability inherent in the concept of survival Skinner (1971) makes the case for the value of "reinforcement." More precisely, what is taken to be the standard of goodness or rightness in the domain of individual behavior is what functions as a reinforcer for that behavior (Skinner, 1971). Just as a particular genotype is sustained in the mix of animal life on the planet if its representatives survive, a particular operant is sustained in an individual's behavioral repertoire if its instances are reinforced. In Skinner's words, "To make a value judgment by calling something good or bad is to classify it in terms of its reinforcing effects" (1971, p. 105).

Having derived reinforcement as the value appropriate for the domain of individual behavior, Skinner (1971) goes on to suggest that this value is manifested in different degrees and that these differences are best depicted as a hierarchy. Included in this hierarchy, from least to most valuable, are behaving for the good of oneself, behaving for the good of others, and behaving for the good of the culture. In the following section, Skinner's views on these issues are examined.

Behaving for the Good of Oneself

Skinner (1971) argues that things are good or bad because of the contingencies of survival under which the species evolved. This is to say, the reinforcing values of things have their sources in universal, biological conditions as opposed to idiosyncratic, psychological circumstances. As Skinner puts it, "The effect of a reinforcer which cannot be attributed to its survival value in the course of evolution (the effect of heroin, for example) is presumably anomalous.... Conditioned reinforcers may seem to suggest other kinds of susceptibilities, but they are effective because of circumstances in a person's earlier history" (1971, p. 110).

This analysis suggests that given the capacity to engage in particular behaviors, and the absence of constraints on such engagements, organisms will *always* act to produce those things that are inherently good and/or to avoid those that are inherently bad. "Behaving for the good of oneself" in this sense constitutes what Skinner (1971) refers to as a first level of value.

Behaving for the Good of Others

As Skinner (1971) points out, the social life conditions of human beings are such that good and bad things often come at the hands of other people, and recognizing this circumstance give rise to the construction of a second level of value, namely that of "behaving for the good of others." In making the case for this conception, Skinner (1971) invokes the concept of intentionality. Reinforcement of a person's behavior by another person is said to be intentional if its delivery is maintained by the behavior of the person reinforced in this manner. Skinner (1971, p. 108) explains, "When other people intentionally arrange and maintain contingencies of reinforcement, the person affected by the contingencies may be said to be behaving 'for the good of others'."

Behaving for the good of others is not held by Skinner to have its sources in the behaving person. In his view, human beings are not held to be virtuous by nature, as often assumed by ethical philosophers operating on theistic foundations. Rather, the contingencies account for this behavior: People act for the good of others because this behavior is strongly reinforced by those others.

Behaving for the good of others means that one is not behaving for the good of oneself though, implying a conflict of values. This conflict calls for an explanation as to how people can be induced to behave for the good of others at personal cost, as well as raises an issue of fairness as to the distribution of reinforcement. Although Skinner's (1971) explanation is somewhat obtuse, he appears to suggest, simply, that under conditions in which more than one set of contingencies is operating, a person's behavior may be expected to come under the control of whichever is the more powerful set.

Determining the relative power of contingencies operating for the good of oneself versus the good of others cannot be accomplished merely by comparing the magnitude of the immediate consequences for the behaviors embodied in these two types of contingencies, though, as this comparison will always tip the balance in favor of those producing personal good. To understand how a person can be induced to behave for the good of others despite personal loss requires an appreciation of the more remote gains such contingencies are capable of delivering to those under their control. Skinner (1971) claims that when these remote gains are taken into account, contingencies operating for the good of others may emerge as the more powerful set, therein overriding the control exerted by contingencies operating for the good of oneself.

With regard to the issue of fairness as to the distribution of reinforcement, Skinner (1971) makes a point of saying that fairness is never guaranteed in value conflicts. Still, it would appear that in his view an individual is to be counted among the "others" for whom the more remote gains produced by behaving for the good of others are achieved. As such, he would argue that these more remote gains more than make up for the loss of personal reinforcers in the immediate situation. In short, people can be induced to behave for the good of others, rather than for the good of themselves, because the good achieved by doing the former is greater than that achieved by the latter. Further, it is clear from his discussion of these issues that behaving for the good of others is not merely a second level of value. It is also a *higher* value. As Skinner (1971, p. 122) puts it, "To be for oneself is to be almost nothing."

Behavior is not subject to direct control by remote consequences, though. Hence, to bring behavior under the control of remote consequences, more immediate consequences must be incorporated into contingencies operating for the good of others. For the most part, these more immediate consequences consist of verbal stimuli. That is, remote consequences of current behavior are brought to bear on this behavior by means of verbal specifications as to the relevant, longer term contingencies in operation. More technically, behavior with respect to the stimulus functions of remote, and thereby absent, consequences is possible of occurrence if those functions inhere in other immediately present stimuli, and verbal stimuli are particularly well suited to harbor substitutional functions of this sort (Parrott, 1984).

Behaving for the Good of the Culture

Skinner (1971) goes on to suggest that an even greater good than that achieved by behaving for the good of others is possible of attainment. The third and highest level of value in his system is demonstrated when people are induced to "behave for the good of the culture." The good achieved in this case is, again, that which is afforded when behavior is brought under the control of its remote consequences. In the case of behaving for the good of the culture even more remote consequences are engaged by way of verbal stimuli. As Skinner describes it, "The group supplies supporting contingencies when it describes its practices in codes or rules which tell the individual how to behave and when it enforces those rules with supplementary contingencies" (1971, p. 173). The main effect of this action on the part of the group "is to bring the individual under the control of the remoter consequences of his behavior." From Skinner's (1974) standpoint, a culture is essentially a complex network of such contingencies.

CRITICAL ANALYSIS OF SURVIVAL AS AN ABSOLUTE STANDARD OF VALUE

Over the course of biological evolution, factors emerge as random mutations and, generally speaking, are either sustained or eliminated by virtue of their relative contributions to survival. Nonetheless, the presence of a particular factor is not necessarily an indication of its survival value. This is the case because factors once relevant to survival may have become irrelevant over the course of changing environmental conditions yet continue to prevail as a result of having been carried along by their interrelations with survival-relevant factors. The same may be said of behaviors in the development of an individual's repertoire over his or her lifetime, as well as of cultural practices over the course of cultural evolution. Further, because the circumstances in each of these domains are continuously changing, it is also possible for them to configure in such a way that factors once merely irrelevant to survival become lethal.

Knowing Long-Term Consequences

This last possibility becomes an issue of some significance when the aim of an enterprise is not merely to describe the factors involved, but also to modify them for particular purposes, namely, to *enhance* their survival value. Aims of this sort imply knowledge as to the roles played by the various factors. When factors are assumed to be capable of elimination or modification by deliberate design, as exemplified in efforts to bring current actions under the control of remote consequences, their selection as targets for manipulation implies that the survival value of those selected is known. Otherwise, there is no rational basis for their selection and no reason thereby to assume that enhancing or eliminating those factors will have a positive impact on survival. In short, although bringing behavior under the control of its long-term consequences as a matter of deliberate design *may* promote survival this outcome depends on those long-term consequences being *known* to designers in advance.

This requirement is readily fulfilled in circumstances pertaining to Skinner's second level of value. As previously discussed, behaving for the good of others is induced by way of specification as to the more remote consequences of such behavior. Although the contingencies specified for this purpose may not have been contacted directly by the one whose behavior is being induced, they are very likely to have been contacted by other members of the group. In other words, the remote consequences of particular "actions in the interests of others" are known to the group. This being the case, actions known to promote survival may be selected for deliberate strengthening; whereas those known to threaten survival may be deliberately weakened.

The same cannot be said of acting for the good of the culture however. Because the life span of a culture is much longer than that of its members, the remote consequences of behaving in the interest of its survival are highly unlikely to have been directly experienced by any of its members and are, in this sense, unknown. In the absence of knowledge as to the consequences of prescribed practices, the survival value of those practices in future circumstances cannot be foretold, even on logical grounds. Added to this, and for the same reason, practices of unknown origin are always present in cultural circumstances and the fact of their presence is no more proof of their survival value in this domain than in any other. This is to say, it is not just in matters of prediction that assessing the survival value of cultural practices is problematic: Without knowledge as to the historical circumstances giving rise to *existing* practices, their survival value under *current* circumstances is also impossible to determine. Hence, although it may be assumed that some practices promote the survival of the culture better than others, it is not possible to say with any certainty which practices are valuable in this sense and which are not.

Speculating About Long-Term Consequences

Skinner (1971, 1974) makes some guesses in this regard. For example, he suggests that the extent to which a culture supports its own future may be observed in its treatment of leisure. He argues that although leisure affords opportunity for artistic, literary, and scientific productivity, such is unlikely in the absence of explicit design. In his view, therefore, a culture that controls what its members do when they have nothing to do is more likely to survive than one that does not attempt to capture this potential. Implicit in this argument is the premise that productivity of these sorts is a "good" that ought to be promoted by deliberate design.

Another guess in this regard is the suggestion that practices producing variety will be seen to have survival value (Skinner, 1971). Skinner's logic in this case is that regimented uniformity may work against the further evolution of the culture. Hence, he argues that cultural practices should not be left to emerge by accident but instead should be fostered by deliberate design. As he puts it, "The only hope is *planned* diversification, in which the importance of variety is recognized" (Skinner, 1971, p. 162, emphasis his).

As a final example of Skinner's speculations about long-term consequences, he argues that practices of experimentation have survival value and ought to be promoted. He likens the design of a culture to the design of an experiment, "Designing a culture is like designing an experiment; contingencies are arranged and effects are noted" (Skinner, 1971, p. 153). The value inherent in this suggestion is workability.

Critical Commentary on Skinner's Speculations

As plausible as these and other guesses might seem, they are still guesses. Moreover, they are guesses about future goods from the standpoint of current circumstances; and future circumstances may be very different. For instance, leisure may come to occupy a much greater proportion of the human experience than is currently the case due to the impact of technological advancements on the conditions of labor. Because a great deal of energy and resources are required to sustain productive behavior, it seems plausible that designing contingencies to strengthen such behavior under circumstances in which leisure is a dominant life condition might actually be detrimental to the survival of a culture.

Skinner's second strategy for enhancing survival value, namely planned diversification of cultural practices, would seem to hold greater promise, both because selection operates on variation and because no commitment to particular practices is entailed. Diversification happens in the absence of design, though, and the mosaic of practices prevailing in the absence of design reflects the historical and existing conditions of selection. It is not clear what Skinner envisioned as *planned* diversification in this context, though. For example, it is possible that pursuing a strategy of planned diversification amounts to nothing more sinister than the promotion of *tolerance* for diversity in cultural practices. A society in which diversity was tolerated would seem to constitute an ideal condition for the selection of valuable practices.

Alternatively, his vision of planned diversification may have been one in which new practices are deliberately induced. The survival value of this plan is not as obvious, especially if pursuing it necessitated the suppression of practices emerging "by accident." The success of this plan for sustaining the survival of a culture depends on the practices selected for induction, and the wisdom of their selection is neither known nor possible to predict. Moreover, any manipulation of the conditions upon which selection operates, of which the deliberate induction of new practices is an example, is likely to have the effect of reducing the absolute number of practices prevailing in a cultural circumstance as a simple matter of displacement. Even if the absolute number of practices were not directly diminished by this manipulation, it would necessarily change the distribution and prevalence of the various practices, wherein some might be rendered too weak to be sustained. In short, the risk inherent in attempting to increase diversity by deliberate design is that the opposite effect might be obtained.

Skinner's idea that experimentation with respect to cultural practices ought to be promoted is problematic in another sense. In the absence of deliberate design, cultural practices tend to emerge slowly, but once established, appear to sustain enormous momentum (Kantor, 1981). Hence, should a guess about the survival value of outcomes produced by deliberate design prove to be in error, the culture in which such an experiment were conducted might not survive long enough for the effects of a new experiment to be realized.

In short, there is no guarantee that practices designed to induce productivity during leisure, variability for its own sake, experimentation, or any other outcome, will assure the survival of a culture. In short, the deliberate design of cultural practices is no more likely to assure the culture's survival than it is to put its survival at risk. Our point here is not to suggest that deliberate design of cultural practices ought to be avoided in favor of their "accidental" development, but rather to raise awareness of our inability to make accurate predictions in this regard.

In summary, we are not convinced that survival constitutes a workable criterion upon which to judge the rightfulness or wrongfulness of cultural practices in that it cannot be applied to such events in a predictive sense. Survival is an outcome concept. As such, it cannot serve as a criterion by which to ascertain the advisability of practices designed to produce it, and efforts to design a better culture are thereby not able to be guided by it (Hayes, Adams, et al., 1994).

Direction in Evolution

Perhaps it is this realization that prompts Skinner (1971) to posit a strategy for the identification of survival value apart from the outcome of survival. In this regard, he suggests that the value of a particular factor—be it a genetic mutation, an individual behavior, or a cultural practice—may be determined by examining the extent to which it fulfills the purpose of evolution. The direction of change in biological as well as cultural evolution, he suggests, is to make organisms more sensitive to the consequences of their behavior.

Although Skinner's attempt to discover survival value by shifting the focus of inquiry from the outcome of survival to the process of achieving greater sensitivity to consequences is a laudable one, it does not solve the problem. In the first place, what distinguishes an event as a consequence is not something about the event but rather something about the way events are verbally constructed by scientists for purposes of analysis. That is to say, *events* do not come in categories of "antecedents" and "consequences." These are just the names given to events when scientists assume that they are arranged on a linear plane. The same events are described differently when other premises are adopted. To reiterate, "consequences" are verbal constructions, not events. Hence, to argue that organisms are becoming more sensitive to the consequences of their actions is to argue that they are becoming more sensitive to verbal constructions. The problem here is one of confusing events with their descriptions (Hayes, Adams, & Dixon, 1997).

A more plausible argument than sensitivity to consequences as the direction in which evolution is proceeding might be to suggest that organisms are becoming increasingly sensitive to their *environments*. However, in order for increasing sensitivity to the environment to constitute a valid measure of value, it is necessary to assume that at one time there were organisms that were substantially less sensitive to their environments. This is an unworkable premise. There have never been organisms that were even slightly insensitive to their environments. More-over, in the absence of this sensitivity, there would be no process of evo-lution about which to presume a purpose. As a process, evolution *is* this sensitivity.

More pointedly, from a scientific perspective, there is neither purpose nor direction in evolution. There is only change. In this light, it is only a measure of change that could conceivably constitute a workable *process* alternative to Skinner's outcome concept of survival.

SUMMARY OF ETHICAL SITUATIONS AND ETHICAL CONDUCT IN BEHAVIORAL PERSPECTIVE

Understanding ethical conduct as an historical continuity of action over which the individual has no ultimate control, as herein articulated, departs radically from the theistically inspired, traditional notion that eth-ical behavior occurs as spontaneous acts of choosing exercised by the free will. This departure reflects a difference between the two positions at the level of fundamental premises. Differences at this level cannot be resolved by compromise. This is to say, it is illogical to suggest that behavior is some-times environmentally determined and sometimes freely willed: If control by the will is *ever* present, it is *always* present. Having it both ways is not merely illogical. It has significant practical implications as well. Specif-ically, it is only if control by the will is categorically denied that behavior can be subjected to scientific study.

Our perspective on ethical situations and ethical conduct also differs in some respects from the behavior analytic position on these issues, as developed by Skinner (1953, 1971, 1974). One of these differences per-tains to the concept of knowing. As previously discussed, Skinner argues that contemplative knowing is essentially nothing until it eventuates in overt behavior indicative of its having occurred at a previous time. This interpretation precludes analytic consideration of contemplative knowing *per se*, presumably because nothing of value would be gained by such an analysis.

We have objected to this presumption, arguing that what is to be gained by an analysis of contemplative knowing as a contemporaneous event in its own right is a means of distinguishing ethical behavior from other classes of action. Ethical behavior is not properly isolated as a distinct class of action so long as instances of ethical behavior are defined simply as acting in a manner deemed right by the culture in that this definition permits acts having rightfulness as a matter of accident or coincidence to be included in the ethical class.

We argue instead that ethical situations are complicated by the par-ticipation of additional factors, namely by acts of considering the likely consequences of alternative courses of action in terms of their conformity to standards of right and wrong. Ethical behavior is "conscious" in this sense. Accordingly, acting in a manner deemed right by the culture exem-plifies ethical behavior only in so far as it has been conditioned by prior acts of contemplative knowing. For rightful action to meet the specifications for inclusion in the ethical class, its controlling conditions must include the products of prior knowing actions. Ethical behavior is "deliberate" in this sense.

A second difference concerns the utility of adopting survival as an absolute standard of goodness. As previously discussed, an absolute standard of goodness is needed if intentional control over behavior or cultural practices, such as to strengthen some such events at the expense of others, is to be justified. Particular events are selected for strengthening on the grounds that they embody relatively greater goodness than events not selected. We have argued that survival as an absolute standard of goodness is not well suited for such purposes in that it characterizes the end point of some set of events, rather than some characteristic of events known to come to a particular end. As such, there is no guarantee that the repertoires and cultures modified by deliberate design will have survival value, suggesting caution as to the certainty of claims to this effect.

We have also taken issue with Skinner's suggestion that direction in evolution may be observed in organisms' increasing sensitivity to the consequences of their actions. We have denied both purpose and direction in evolution categorically, and have further pointed out that Skinner's contention in this regard reflects a confusion of events with their descriptions (Hayes, Adams, & Dixon, 1998). Our disagreements with Skinner on these issues are possible of resolution through further discussion and compromise. The same does not apply to our disagreement with traditional views as to the nature of man. Disagreements of the latter sort can be "resolved" only by eliminating one of the contenders, and it would be foolhardy to imagine this to be the fate of the traditional position. Virtually all of our culture's institutions, including those of the political, military, economic, legal, and educational spheres are organized in accordance with the presumption that man is the agent of his own action. This understanding is also the source of our culture's values. As such, our aim in contrasting traditional and behavioral views on the subject of ethics was not intended as a call to arms against traditional misunderstandings of humankind. There is no getting rid of autonomous man. Instead, our aim was to reaffirm our philosophical convictions such that we might take proper advantage of certain weaknesses in the means by which traditional values are invoked in the application of behavior science to problems of human adjustment, to which we now turn.

ETHICAL APPLICATIONS OF BEHAVIOR SCIENCE IN BEHAVIORAL PERSPECTIVE

We may begin by reiterating our contention that deliberate applications of scientific understandings to matters of societal concern are always predicated on values of one sort or another. This is the case because the primary aim of applied work is to achieve control over particular behaviors such that their character or occurrence might be modified in some way, and it is not sensible to pursue this aim in the absence of a criterion against which the goodness of a thing may be judged. In other words, it is not sensible to modify a thing for applied purposes if doing so does not make it better. Accordingly, controlling behavior may be regarded as therapeutic only in so far as doing so produces outcomes deemed "better" than the status quo in light of some standard of value. Skinner's articulation of survival as an absolute standard of goodness shows awareness of this obligation.

Although we have denied the utility of this standard at the level of cultural design, we have not disputed its potential in matters of lesser scope and temporal distance. Moreover, a standard of some sort is needed to guide as well as justify that deliberate practices of behavior control, and survival (or its derivative of sustainability) are no less workable for this purpose than "happiness" or "freedom" or "good will" as have been proposed by others with the same need. We may proceed then to consider what adopting the standard of survival/sustainability implies for applications of the science of behavior to problems of human adjustment—applications that would be deemed *ethical* in behavioral perspective, as herein discussed. For purposes of illustration, we consider applications pertaining only to persons lacking verbal repertoires, as these circumstances bring a number of significant issues to bear.

Behaving for the Good of Others

"Behaving for the good of others" might seem to capture the professional activities of human service providers particularly well: These are persons who provide goods and services to those who are unable to provide these things for themselves. Behaving for the good of others has nothing to do with altruism, though. Indeed, there is no place in a behavior analytic understanding for "altruism," as conventionally conceived. Recall that behaving for the good of others is exemplified when a person's action is such as to sustain another person's intentional control over that action. In Skinner's (1971, p. 108) words, "When other people intentionally arrange and maintain contingencies of reinforcement, the person affected by the contingencies may be said to be behaving 'for the good of others'." As such, it would be the *consumer* of services—not the provider of the same—who might be said to exemplify action in keeping with Skinner's second level of value.

This suggestion would also miss the point though, at least for consumers lacking verbal repertoires. Behaving for the good of others, as herein defined, implies a relinquishing of immediate personal gain for a more remote shared gain on the promise that the good achieved by doing the latter will be greater than that achieved by the former. The "promise" here is a contingency specification or rule, and persons without verbal repertoires are not capable of behaving under the control of rules. Hence, it is not the nonverbal or minimally verbal consumers of services who are behaving for the good of others in such circumstances.

Instead, to examine "behaving for the good of others" on the parts of service providers, we must examine circumstances in which their behavior is under the control of contingencies that have been intentionally arranged by others. We may begin by identifying the "others" exerting intentional control over providers' behavior. We take these others to constitute collectivities of various sorts, among which are the culture as a whole, and numerous subdivisions of this collectivity reflecting specific disciplinary interests, such as the Behavior Analyst Certification Board, The Association for Behavior Analysis, The American Psychological Association, and so on. These more specific subdivisions are the relevant "others" for our purposes.

Behaving for the Good of Others as Ethical Conduct

Understood in the context of behavior analytic therapy, ethical situations are those in which therapists compare the anticipated consequences of alternative courses of therapeutic action, namely changes in clients' repertoires, as to their embodiment of the value of survival or sustainability, and subsequently take the course of action leading to the changes deemed most sustainable by that comparison. This is a complex set of circumstances involving three sets of interacting contingencies operating with respect to the actions of three classes of participants, including psychological collectivities, therapists, and clients.

The contingencies operating on the actions of psychological collectivities are established and maintained by the culture at large. The practices of the culture—of which "valuing" is a type—constitute a context in which psychological collectivities formulate rules to govern therapeutic actions such as to produce changes in the repertoires of disabled persons deemed valuable from the perspective of the culture at large. Rule-following on the parts of therapists responsible to these collectivities has three important outcomes. First, it reinforces *rule-giving* by the psychological collectivity, whereby the conditions under which behaving in the interest of others on the parts of therapists are preserved. The reinforcement of rule-giving completes the account of contingencies operating for the psychological collectivities. Second, rule-following by therapists produces valuable changes in clients' repertoires, which is to say, rule-following is reinforced by these changes and is thereby strengthened as an operant class (Parrott, 1987). This outcome completes the account of contingencies operating for therapists. Third, the actions taken by therapists under the control of the rules given by the psychological collectivities are such as to establish and maintain conditions under which clients' behavior is directly controlled, therein completing the account of contingencies operating at this level. In the following section, we examine the contingencies operating with respect to rule-giving and rule-following in greater detail, along with the opportunities they afford for the expansion of behavior analytic services to disabled persons.

CONTINGENCIES SUSTAINING RULE-GIVING BY PSYCHOLOGICAL COLLECTIVITIES

Disciplinary collectivities assure ethical conduct on the parts of therapists by means of aversive control: Failing to adhere to the rules of ethical conduct articulated by these collectivities results in disciplinary actions of various sorts. These may include a revocation of professional credentials, loss of membership in professional associations, or legal actions, depending on the nature and severity of the offense.

One of the difficulties therapists encounter in attempting to abide by ethical conduct rules has to do with the fact that these rules tend to be incomplete specifications of the relevant contingencies. More often than not, disciplinary collectivities articulate only the "goods" that clients should have as outcomes of therapeutic practices. For example, it is said that consumers should have meaningful and productive lives, that they should participate fully in their communities, and that they should live independently. Rarely is any mention made of the circumstances under which these rules apply (e.g., for consumers of moderate disability) or, more importantly, of the practices most likely to produce the outcomes specified. Hence, from the standpoint of those managing the contingencies operating with respect to therapists' behavior, the ends to be achieved by therapy would appear to be more important, or at least more important to prescribe, than the means by which they are to be achieved.

This emphasis on desired outcomes, as opposed to the practices that might be expected to produce them, affords a significant opportunity for behavior analysts. Specifically, if particular outcomes are *possible* to deliver, which is to say, if the human and environmental conditions are suited to the application of particular rules, then, from past evidence, we may assume that therapists operating from a behavior analytic perspective will be able to bring them about in a shorter period of time than will those operating from other perspectives be capable of doing. Further, if these are the outcomes deemed valuable from the standpoint of the professional collectivities involved, then producing them in a timely manner will strengthen the contingency management practices of these collectivities. In other words, behaving for the good of others, as herein defined, is more likely to be demonstrated by behavior analysts than by therapists of other persuasions.

The worth of our approach in this regard is not unconditional, however. It depends on whether the *speed* with which outcomes are achieved constitutes a standard of value for the professional collectivities involved. If speed of change is not explicitly valued by these collectivities, it would behoove behavior analysts to promote the adoption of this value. All things being equal, to bring about desired outcomes rapidly as opposed to slowly would not seem to be a difficult value to champion.

The worth of a behavior analytic approach in the eyes of relevant professional collectivities is circumscribed by another factor as well. Specifically, the means by which particular outcomes are achieved must not be such as to diminish valued outcomes of other sorts. Unfortunately for behavior analysts, some of these other outcomes are characterized as personal possessions. It is said, for example, that services should provide consumers with such goods as "self-determination." Outcomes of this sort pose a problem for behavior analysts as "self-determination" is not an end for which others controlling one's behavior can be a means, the implication being that if goods of this sort are possible to deliver, some means other than behavior analysis would be required to deliver them. Moreover, because goods of this sort are *concepts* rather than observable things or events, their actual receipt is a matter of interpretation. The same is true of the relationship between these outcomes and the practices assumed to be responsible for their production. In other words, because some of the goods clients ought to receive as a result of therapeutic practices are intangible, and their receipt is thereby uncertain, the practices by which they are delivered cannot be subjected to the sort of scrutiny that might lead to their improvement or elimination. Nonetheless, these are highly valued outcomes that can and must be delivered by some means other than behavior analysis.

This conclusion poses a problem that would not be solved by disputing the premise of autonomy on which it is based, at least not if "behaving for the good of others" on the parts of behavior analytic service providers is to be sustained. To solve the problem in this way amounts to forfeiting others' good in favor of one's own. Not being able to deliver the good of agreement on underlying premises does not mean abandoning the aim of behaving for the good of others, however. It just means that we must find another good to strengthen the collectivity's management of the contingencies under which we participate in service delivery.

To the extent that the professional collectivity is behaving for the good of an even larger collectivity, that is to say, the culture, one such good might pertain to resource allocation. All things being equal, to bring about desired outcomes—even intangible ones—at lesser as opposed to greater cost is hardly a controversial proposal, and to formulating the worth of behavior analytic services in these terms might thereby be a particularly useful means of generating support from the "others" managing the contingencies operating on our behavior. In this regard, over the long run, the cost of refusing to develop the limited behavioral repertoires of persons with severe disabilities on the grounds that such would undermine their freedom to do nothing is enormous compared to the more immediate cost of effectively developing those repertoires.

A culture's resources tend to be allocated across its various sectors in proportion to their ability to exert effective counter-control (Skinner, 1971), and when resources become scarce, allocations to those sectors least able to exert counter-control are disproportionately reduced. The human service sector is always at risk in this regard. This circumstance provides an opportunity for behavior analysts however, in that the more limited the resources are, the more likely are allocations to be made on the basis of cost-effectiveness. Analyses of this sort cannot be made unless the costs of achieving particular outcomes of particular magnitude can be calculated.

Intangible outcomes are not readily quantified and, under conditions of limited resources, this mismatch is much more likely to be solved by making the outcomes susceptible to quantification than by abandoning the aim of quantifying them. Articulating the worth of behavior analytic services in these terms will assist the professional collectivity in making its case for a more reasonable proportion of the culture's resources, and in so doing, will sustain its management of the contingencies controlling our behavior.

In summary, the emphasis on outcomes in ethical conduct rules, as opposed to the conditions under which the rules might apply and the practices by which the specified outcomes might be achieved, poses greater problems for applied behavior analysts than for other therapists of other persuasions. Hence, it is incumbent upon behavior analysts to encourage more complete specifications of contingencies in these rules. For example, the good of "making informed choices and decisions about one's life" does not apply rationally to all human circumstances and the circumstances to which it does apply, namely, to circumstances in which clients have verbal repertoires, need to be specified when such outcomes are prescribed as therapeutic goals. Similarly, some therapeutic practices have been shown to be more effective than others in producing particular outcomes, and these "best practices" or practice guidelines should also be specified in the rules governing the ethical behavior of therapists.

Contingencies Maintaining Rule-Following on the Parts of Therapists

As previously discussed, behaving for the good of others typically means forfeiting immediate personal goods for more remote shared goods. In as much as behavior is not subject to direct control by remote consequences, for contingencies of this sort to be effective they must be supplemented by immediate verbal substitutes for those consequences. To put it another way, behaving for the good of others must be understood as rule-following.

It is assumed that clients' repertoires will undergo valuable changes if therapists follow the rules of ethical conduct set out by psychological collectivities. If this outcome of rule-following is also valuable to therapists, achieving it will strengthen rule-following as an operant (see Parrott, 1987, for further discussion of rule-following as an operant class). Even if this outcome is not valuable to therapists, rule-following may be maintained by negative reinforcement so long as the consequences of not following rules are sufficiently aversive to allow this to occur.

Between these extremes, the strength of rule-following on the parts of therapists is subject to a number of conditions. One such condition has to do with how closely rules match the contingencies upon which they are based. This condition suggests that rule-following will be more probable if the consequences specified in rules are contacted when rule-following occurs than when this is not the case. (The same is true of aversive consequences for not following rules.) It further suggests that rule-following will be more likely if this contact occurs when the actions specified in the rule occur in the presence of the settings specified in the rule than when these settings are not present. In as much as unspecified events cannot be contacted by definition, these conditions suggest that the more completely and accurately ethical conduct rules describe the contingencies from which they were derived, the more likely it is that therapists will follow them.

As previously discussed, following rules set forth by psychological collectivities sustain rule-giving by these collectivities that provide opportunities for therapists to behave for the good of others. However, incomplete rules control behavior in incomplete ways, which is to say, incomplete rules fulfill their intended purposes less effectively than more complete rules and the immediate purpose of giving rules is having others follow them. To the extent that rule-giving by professional collectivities is reinforced by rule-following on the parts of therapists, the overemphasis on outcomes in these rules is subject to change. This circumstance bodes well for behavior analysts, as any move to increase rule-following by articulating more complete rules favors the behavior analytic approach to therapy.

Behaving for the Good of Others as Ethical Conduct Reflecting Survival Value

As behavior analysts following Skinner's lead, survival or its psychological derivative of sustainability, is held to constitute an absolute standard of goodness. In a psychological context, the continuation of particular operants in an organism's repertoire is assured if particular instances of those operants are reinforced. Hence, what remains to be considered is whether this standard is reflected in the actions of those participating in the therapeutic enterprise. We must ask whether the actions of psychological collectivities are explicitly designed to sustain rule-following by therapists, whether the actions of therapists are explicitly designed to sustain changes in clients' repertoires, and whether the actions of each might have greater survival value.

The Survival Value of Actions of Psychological Collectivities

The first of these questions has already been addressed. Ethical conduct rules emphasize desirable outcomes of therapeutic activity, to the neglect of the means by which these ends might be achieved. The rule-giving actions of psychological collectivities would exhibit greater survival value if such actions were products of more elaborate analytical activities as to the contingencies by which the outcomes specified in these rules might be achieved. This would permit specification of the therapeutic actions likely to produce these outcomes, and the human and environmental setting conditions predictive of success in this regard to be included in these rules. The addition of these elements in ethical conduct rules would increase the probability of rule-following by therapists and, in so doing, would increase the likelihood that the outcomes currently specified in these rules would be achieved.

The Survival Value of Actions of Therapists

We turn now to the survival value of therapists' actions as exhibited in sustained changes in clients' repertoires. We have not addressed this issue in any detail in this chapter as it has been the subject of many thoughtful discussions elsewhere (e.g., see Hayes, Hayes, Moore, & Ghezzi, 1994). Briefly, however, ethical behaving for the good of others with survival as a value on the part of therapists involves their comparing the anticipated outcomes of alternative courses of therapeutic action as to their embodiment of this value, and subsequently taking the course of action leading to the outcomes held to be most valuable by that comparison. In as much as the future is not known, anticipating the consequences of actions yet to occur amounts to reviewing the consequences known to have been produced by previous, similar, actions. In other words, behaving ethically is not an accidental matter. To behave ethically, one must act in whatever manner one knows will produce outcomes with the greatest survival value.

In this regard, a number of variables have been shown to impact the extent to which repertoire changes are sustained beyond the period of their initial development. We are speaking here of therapeutic practices known to be valuable with respect to transferring the control over behavior from deliberately imposed contingencies, involving arbitrary setting conditions and consequences, to the circumstances in which such behavior would ordinarily occur and its occurrence would produce nonarbitrary consequences. For example, the behavior of saying "hi" might be established under the stimulus control of therapist action in the form of "say hi," with occurrences of echoic responses being reinforced by small bits of preferred food. Therapeutic practices that are such as to bring this behavior under the stimulus control of another person's arrival and be reinforced by this other person's returned greeting, would exhibit survival value, as herein defined.

What behavior to establish is no less an ethical matter than how one goes about establishing it. More pointedly, establishing behaviors in a client that have no likelihood of occurring under ordinary circumstances and thereby no likelihood of being maintained by nonarbitrary consequences due to the limitations of that client's repertoire more broadly considered, must be regarded as unethical practice. For example, if a client's repertoire is so severely limited that the likelihood of her having a bank account is virtually zero, it would be unethical to establish the behavior of signing her name on a deposit slip.

Finally, in as much as clients would not require therapeutic services if their repertoires were normally developed the speed with which their repertoires are able to be expanded becomes an ethical consideration as well. Thus, those intervention strategies that have been shown to be most efficient might be deemed most ethical. Further, research that reveals the relative efficiency of various treatment approaches would likewise have ethical implications. In summary, the behaviors we elect to establish, the means by which they are established such as to be sustained in our absence, and the speed with which we do so, all have ethical implications.

EPILOGUE

We have examined the position of behavior analysts on the subject of ethics with the purposes of revealing the influence of conventional thinking upon it, suppressing the propagation of ineffectual practices derived from corrupt sources, providing the basis for a coherent, comprehensive, and thoroughly naturalistic alternative to the interpretation of these important events, and illustrating the implications of the latter in the context of ethical service provision. Our aim in examining these issues has been to reiterate, clarify, and refine the philosophical underpinnings of the science of behavior, in keeping with which its investigations have been fruitful, its practices have been effective, and its future may be secured.

REFERENCES

Cooper, D. E. (1978). Moral relativism. In P. A. Franch, T. E. Uehling Jr., H. K. Wettstein (Eds.), *Studies in ethical theory*. Morris: University of Minnesota Press.

Hayes, L. J. (1992). The psychological present. *The Behavior Analyst, 15*, 139–146.

Hayes, L. J. (1997). Scientific knowing in psychological perspective. In L. J. Hayes & P. N. Ghezzi (Eds.), *Investigations in behavioral epistemology* (pp. 123–141). Reno, NV: Context Press.

Hayes, L. J., Adams, M. A., & Dixon, M. (1997). Causal constructs and conceptual confusions. *Psychological Record, 47*, 97–112.

Hayes, L. J., Adams, M., & Rydeen, K. (1994). Ethics, choice and value. In L. J. Hayes, G. J. Hayes, S. C. Moore, & P. M. Ghezzi (Eds.), *Ethical issues in developmental disabilities* (pp. 11–39). Reno, NV: Context Press.

Hayes, L. J., Hayes, G. J., Moore, S. C., & Ghezzi, P. M. (Eds.). (1994). *Ethical issues in developmental disabilities*. Reno, NV: Context Press.

Kantor, J. R. (1953). *The logic of modern science*. Chicago: Principia.

Kantor, J. R. (1958). *Interbehavioral psychology*. Chicago: Principia.

Kantor, J. R. (1981). *Cultural psychology*. Chicago: Principia.

Kantor, J. R. (1991). *Interbehavioral philosophy*. Chicago: Principia.

Parrott, L. J. (1983a). Perspectives on knowing and knowledge. *Psychological Record, 33*, 171–184.

Parrott, L. J. (1983b). Systematic foundations for the concept of private events: A critique. In N. M. Smith, P. T. Mountjoy, & D. Ruben (Eds.), *Reassessment in psychology: The interbehavioral alternative*. New York: University of America Press.

Parrott, L. J. (1984). Listening and understanding. *The Behavior Analyst, 7*, 29–40.

Parrott, L. J. (1986). Ethical situations in interbehavioral perspective. *The Interbehaviorist, 14*, 35–41.

Parrott, L. J. (1987). Rule governed behavior: An implicit analysis of reference. In S. Modgil & C. Modgil (Eds.), *B. F. Skinner: Consensus and controversy*. Barcombe, UK: Falmer.

Skinner, B. F. (1953). *Science and human behavior*. New York: Free Press.

Skinner, B. F. (1957). *Verbal behavior*. New York: Appleton-Century-Crofts.

Skinner, B. F. (1969). *Contingencies of reinforcement*. New York: Appleton-Century-Crofts.

Skinner, B. F. (1971). *Beyond freedom and dignity*. New York: Knopf.

Skinner, B. F. (1974). *About behaviorism*. New York: Vintage.

Index

Printed in the United States of America.